Medications and Mathematics for the Nurse

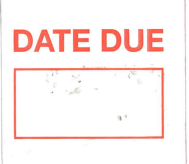

Medications and Mathematics for the Nurse

9TH EDITION

Jane Rice

DELMAR

THOMSON LEARNING™

Australia   Canada   Mexico   Singapore   Spain   United Kingdom   United States

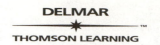

Medications and Mathematics for the Nurse

Jane Rice

Business Unit Director:
William Brottmiller

Executive Marketing Manager:
Dawn F. Gerrain

Project Editor:
David R. Buddle

Executive Editor:
Cathy L. Esperti

Developmental Editor:
Marjorie A. Bruce

Production Coordinator:
Anne Sherman

Acquisitions Editor:
Matthew Kane

Editorial Assistant:
Shelley Esposito

Art/Design Coordinator:
Jay Purcell

For permission to use material from this text or product, contact us by
Tel   (800) 730-2214
Fax   (800) 730-2215
www.thomsonrights.com

Library of Congress Cataloging-in-Publication Data
Rice, Jane.
    Medications and mathematics for the nurse /
Jane Rice—9th ed.
        p.   cm.
    Includes index.
    ISBN 0-7668-3080-2
    1. Pharmacology.   2. Drugs—Administration.
3. Pharmaceutical arithmetic.   4. Nursing.   I. Title.
RM125.R53   2001
615.5′8—dc21   2001042160

NOTICE TO THE READER

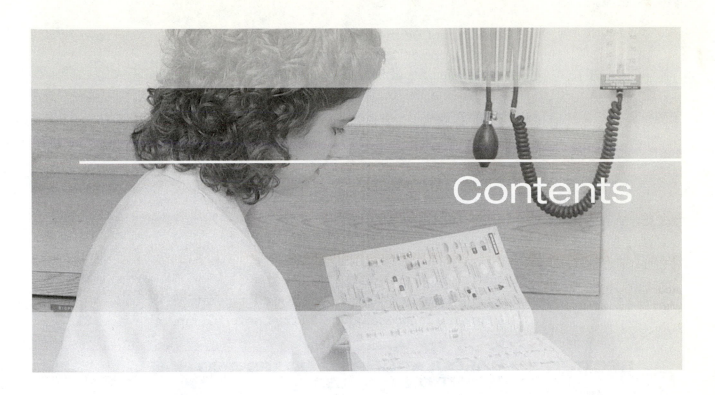

Contents

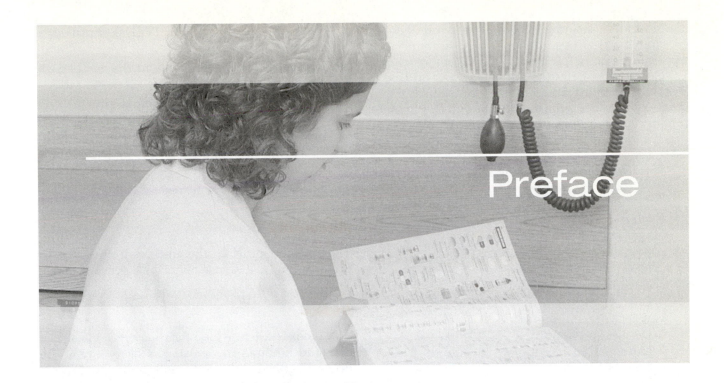

Preface

Medications and Mathematics for the Nurse, 9th edition is designed for the nurse. Although directed at the nurse, this text can be used by any health professional who needs essential information about mathematics and pharmacology.

The text reflects current and commonly used practices, procedures, medications, and drug preparations. The content is explained in a clear and easy to understand language. At all times, safety is emphasized—for the health professional administering the medications and for the client receiving the medications.

The text is divided into five sections. **Section 1—Basic Mathematics** explains how to work each mathematical process correctly, using a step-by-step format. Practice problems follow the mathematical presentation for immediate reinforcement. Self-Assessments at the end of each chapter allow the learner to assess his/her understanding of each chapter's content.

Section 2—Calculations of Doses and Solutions builds the mathematical skills necessary for the safe preparation and administration of medications to the adult and pediatric client. Each mathematical process is presented in a clear, concise, step-by-step format with numerous solved problems as examples. Practice problems are based upon actual clinical situations with the use of current drugs and dosages. Self-Assessments at the end of each chapter allow the learner to assess his/her understanding of each chapter's content.

Section 3—Administration of Medications provides a detailed explanation of topics essential to a thorough understanding of drug sources, legislation relating to drugs, drug references, forms of drugs, drug classifications and actions, the medication order, and basic principles for the administration of nonparenteral and parenteral medications.

Features of Section 3 include:

- Stresses the "six rights" of proper drug administration
- Stresses proper documentation: the "sixth right"
- Drugs cited are current and commonly used
- Numerous photographs, drawings, tables and examples of drugs and equipment are provided
- Multiple choice and matching questions are provided for each chapter
- Basic principles for the administration of medications are based upon the nursing process
- Emphasis is placed on legal implications and safety
- Drug administration procedures are presented in a step-by-step format.
- Self-Assessments at the end of each chapter allow the learner to assess his/her understanding of each chapter's content.

Section 4—Drugs and Related Substances presents essential information on antibiotics, anthelmintics, antiprotozoal agents, antiseptics, disinfectants, antifungal agents, antiviral agents, immunizing agents, antineoplastics, vitamins and minerals, psychotropic agents, and substance abuse.

Section 5—Effects of Medications on Body Systems provides the learner with an explanation of the effects of specific medications on the circulatory, respiratory, gastrointestinal, urinary, endocrine musculoskeletal, nervous, and reproductive systems.

Features of Sections 4 and 5 include:

- Tables summarizing currently used drugs
- Each major drug classification includes:
    —Description
    —Action
    —Uses
    —Adverse Reactions
    —Contraindications
    —Safety Precautions
    —Dosage and Route
    —Nursing Considerations
    —Clients' Instruction
    —Special Considerations
- Multiple choice and matching questions based on the nursing process, with numerous clinical situations described.

New to the Ninth Edition

- Added guidelines on preventing needlestick injuries and use of safety syringe-needle units
- New and expanded content on MedWatch, controlled substances, food- and water-borne infectious diseases, drug-resistant microorganisms, lipid-lowering drugs, drug therapy for Alzheimer's disease, hormone replacement therapy following menopause, and erectile dysfunction
- Added content on newer drug classifications: SSRIs (selective serotonin reuptake inhibitors), Cox-2 inhibitors, gastric-acid pump (or proton pump) inhibitors, leukotriene receptor antago-

nists, thiazolidinediones (TZDs), antitumor necrosis factor drugs

- Expanded Self-Assessments at the end of each chapter
- Procedures added for nonparenteral and parental routes of drug administration
- Web Activities section in selected chapters provides website addresses for pharmacology-related information
- New glossary of key terms

Appendix

The appendix provides the answers to the practice problems and self-assessments for Sections 1 and 2.

Index

Two indexes are provided for ready reference. The drug index allows the learner to locate any of the drugs described in the text, and a general index covers all other topics.

Supplement

An Instructor's Manual accompanies the text and contains the following information:

1. Suggestions for using *Medications and Mathematics for the Nurse*, 9th edition, in the classroom.
2. Suggested answers for the Spot Checks that appear in Chapters 18–31.
3. Answers to Practice Problems and Self-Assessments for Sections 1 and 2.
4. Comprehensive examinations and answer keys for Sections 1–5.
5. Post tests and answer keys for Chapters 11–31 (Sections 3–5).
6. Performance checklists.

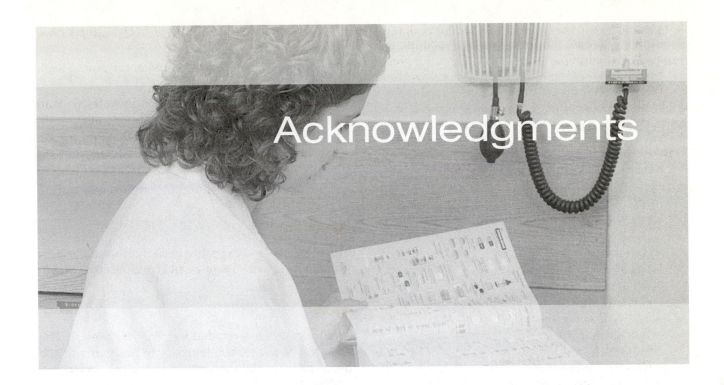

Acknowledgments

I wish to express my deepest appreciation to those individuals who assisted me in this revision of *Medications and Mathematics for the Nurse*. Thank you for your time, knowledge, encouragement, expertise, and your valuable input.

—The staff at Delmar Publishers: Matthew Kane, Marjorie A. Bruce, David Buddle, Anne Sherman, Jay Purcell, and Shelley Esposito.

—Husband and partner: Larry Rice

Reviewers

The author and staff at Delmar Publishers would like to thank the following individuals for their many suggestions for improvement in the manuscript. Their constructive evaluation contributed to an outstanding ninth edition of the text.

Judy Baker
Louisiana Technical College
Jena, LA

Susan Beggs, RN, MSN
Austin Community College
Austin, TX

Gyl Ann Burkhardt
Warners, NY

Tracylain Evans, APRN, MS, MPH, CCRN, CEN, ACNP
Norwalk Community-Technical College
Norwalk, CT

Betty R. Coffman
Coosa Valley Technical Institute
Rome, GA

Betty Kehl Richardson, PhD, RN, CS
Austin Community College
Austin, TX

Cindy Smith, RN, ADN
Foothills Technical Institute
Searcy, AR

Frances F. Swasey, RN, MN
College of Eastern Utah
Price, UTx

I would like to thank those companies and agencies that responded to my request for photographs and permission to use their materials.

Aventis Pharmaceuticals
Becton, Dickinson and Company
C.B. Fleet Company, Inc.

MedWatch, U.S. Food and Drug Administration
Merck & Company, Inc.
Pharmacia Corporation
SmithKline Beecham
TAP Pharmaceutical Products Inc.
United States Pharmacopeia

Section 1

BASIC MATHEMATICS

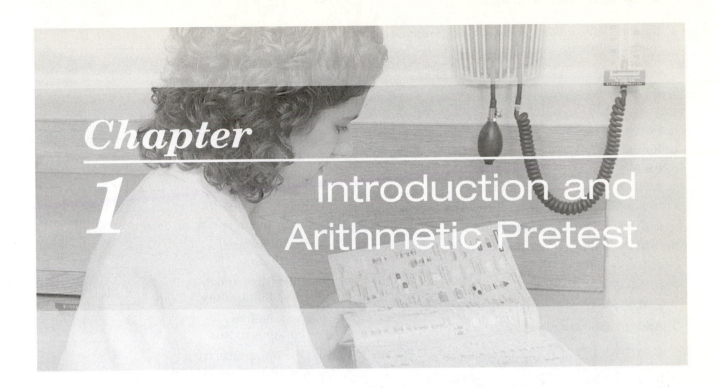

Chapter 1

Introduction and Arithmetic Pretest

Objectives

Upon completion of this chapter, you should be able to

- Explain why the knowledge of basic mathematics is so important to the safe preparation and administration of medications

- Determine areas in which improvement in basic arithmetic is needed

INTRODUCTION

The preparation and administration of medications is one of the most important and critical tasks that you can perform. Today, drugs are more potent and more likely to cause physiological changes in the body; therefore, anyone who administers medications must do so with extreme care.

Incorrectly calculated or measured dosages are the leading cause of error in the administration of medications. A drug error is a violation of a client's rights. It is important that you develop a working knowledge of mathematics, so that you will be able to calculate or measure accurately a medication that is to be administered to a client. As you progress through this textbook, you will acquire the knowledge and skill needed to administer medications safely, accurately, and efficiently.

In order to pinpoint individual weaknesses in arithmetic, the following pretest is recommended. Those areas that need improvement may be strengthened through study of the remaining chapters in this section.

ARITHMETIC PRETEST

1. Express the following as Roman numerals:

   a. 15 _____   e. 20 _____

   b. 19 _____   f. 1 _____

   c. 5 _____   g. 8 _____

   d. 4 _____   h. 7 _____

2. Express as Arabic numerals.

   a. X _____   e. III _____

   b. VI _____   f. XXIV _____

   c. IX _____   g. XIV _____

   d. XXVI _____ h. XIII _____

3. Express the following in words:

   a. 1,005,221 _____

   b. 125,936 _____

   c. 48,224 _____

   d. 2,001.5 _____

   e. 1,200,000 _____

4. Express the following as whole numbers or mixed numbers:

   a. $\frac{24}{12}$ = _____   d. $\frac{16}{3}$ = _____

   b. $\frac{9}{4}$ = _____   e. $\frac{500}{25}$ = _____

   c. $\frac{100}{25}$ = _____   f. $\frac{67}{15}$ = _____

5. Round the following numbers to the next largest number:

   a. 498 to the nearest hundred _____

   b. 2,597,500 to the nearest thousand _____

   c. 1,997,855 to the nearest million _____

6. Add the following decimals:

   a. 0.05 + 0.010 + 0.156 = _____

   b. 1.005 + 20.1 + 400.5 = _____

   c. 0.004 + 42.015 + 1,004.05 = _____

7. Add the following fractions:

   a. $\frac{1}{5} + \frac{1}{2} + \frac{1}{4}$ = _____

   b. $\frac{1}{6} + \frac{3}{8} + \frac{3}{4}$ = _____

   c. $2\frac{3}{4} + 4\frac{1}{8} + 5\frac{1}{2}$ = _____

8. Subtract the following fractions and mixed numbers:

   a. $\frac{2}{3} - \frac{1}{2}$ = _____

   b. $\frac{4}{5} - \frac{1}{3}$ = _____

   c. $4\frac{1}{2} - 2\frac{1}{3}$ = _____

   d. $10\frac{1}{4} - 6\frac{3}{8}$ = _____

9. Subtract the following:

   a. 2(5 + 3) − 4(2 + 1) = _____

   b. 4(3 − 2) − 3(4 − 3) = _____

   c. 4(3 − 1) − 2(2 − 2) = _____

   d. 5(5 + 5) − 3(5 + 3) = _____

10. Subtract the following decimals:

   a. 12.05 − 10.50 = _____

   b. 9.00 − 5.50 = _____

   c. 125.50 − 100.60 = _____

   d. 95.05 − 5.25 = _____

11. Multiply the following:

   a. 525 × 0.51 = _____

   b. 550.10 × 0.05 = _____

   c. 594.99 × 0.99 = _____

   d. 841.08 × 0.08 = _____

12. Divide the following:

   a. $\frac{3}{5} \div \frac{3}{10}$ = _____

   b. $\frac{4}{8} \div \frac{1}{16}$ = _____

   c. 14.25 ÷ 3.5 = _____

   d. 150.25 ÷ 0.25 = _____

13. Which is larger?

   a. $\frac{5}{6}$ or $\frac{5}{8}$ _____

   b. $\frac{3}{4}$ or $\frac{1}{3}$ _____

   c. 0.75 or 0.749 _____

   d. 0.25 or 0.255 _____

14. Express the following as decimals:

   a. Forty-five and
      five tenths _____

   b. Thirty-five and
      three hundredths _____

   c. Two and five
      ten thousandths _____

   d. One hundred sixty
      and three thousandths _____

15. Express the following fractions as decimals:

   a. $\frac{7}{10}$ = _____   c. $2\frac{1}{2}$ = _____

   b. $5\frac{1}{4}$ = _____   d. $\frac{1}{4}$ = _____

16. Express the following as percentages:

   a. $\frac{1}{2}$ _____   d. 0.05 _____

   b. 0.007 _____   e. $\frac{1}{4}$ _____

   c. $\frac{3}{4}$ _____   f. 0.50 _____

17. What is

   a. 5% of 75? _____

   b. 0.5% of 500? _____

   c. 6% of 400? _____

   d. 0.7% of 750? _____

   e. 10% of 500? _____

   f. 25% of 500? _____

18. Express the following as Arabic numerals:

   a. Four thousand two
      hundred and eighty _____

   b. Six hundred thousand _____

   c. Six million _____

   d. Forty thousand two
      hundred and eight _____

   e. Two hundred thousand
      and twenty _____

   f. Five hundred three
      and five tenths _____

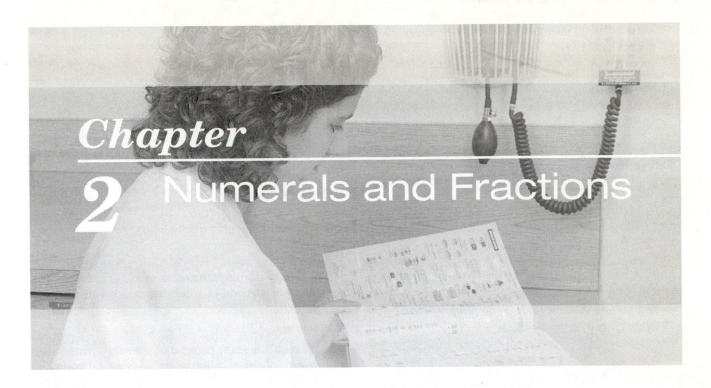

Chapter 2 Numerals and Fractions

Chapter Outline

- Determine the relative values of fractions
- Express improper fractions as mixed numbers
- Add, subtract, multiply, and divide fractions
- Use the process of cancellation whenever possible
- Work the practice problems correctly
- Complete the Self-Assessment

Key Terms

denominator

dividend

divisor

fraction

lowest common denominator (LCD)

minuend

numerator

subtrahend

Objectives

Upon completion of this chapter, you should be able to

- Define the key terms
- Express Arabic numerals as Roman numerals
- Express Roman numerals as Arabic numerals
- Express a fraction as a simple, compound, complex, proper, or improper fraction
- Express fractions as equivalents

INTRODUCTION

Medications are generally ordered and measured by amounts expressed in Arabic numbers: the familiar system of whole numbers, fractions, and decimals. However, some medication orders will be expressed in Roman numerals. The Roman system of counting dates back to ancient Rome. In this system, alphabetic letters are used to designate numeric amounts such as I, V, and X.

A numeral is a symbol or letter used alone or in combination with others to express a number. In this

TABLE 2-1 ARABIC AND ROMAN NUMERALS

Arabic Numerals	Roman Numerals	Arabic Numerals	Roman Numerals	Arabic Numerals	Roman Numerals
1	I	8	VIII	60	LX
2	II	9	IX	70	LXX
3	III	10	X	80	LXXX
4	IV	20	XX	90	XC
5	V	30	XXX	100	C
6	VI	40	XL	500	D
7	VII	50	L	1000	M

chapter, Arabic and Roman numerals are described for you as a basic mathematical review, as well as fractions. It is well to remember that fractions are the result of breaking whole numbers into parts.

ARABIC AND ROMAN NUMERALS

Arabic numerals are those we use in everyday calculations. They include the figures 0 through 9 or a combination of these figures.

Roman numerals are letters used to represent numeric values. They are a part of the apothecaries' system of measurement. Roman numerals may be used on prescriptions or medication orders. Table 2-1 shows some Arabic numbers and their Roman numeral equivalents.

Reading and Writing Roman Numerals

The following steps will guide you as you learn to read and write Roman numerals:

1. When using two Roman numerals of the same value that are repeated in sequence, you add their values. A Roman numeral may not be repeated more than three times.

   Example: XXX = 30

2. When a Roman numeral of a larger value is followed by one of a lesser value, you add the values.

   Example: XI = (10 + 1) = 11

3. When a Roman numeral of a lesser value is followed by one of a larger value, you subtract the values.

   Example: IV = (5 − 1) = 4

4. When a Roman numeral is placed between two numerals of a larger value, you subtract the lesser value from the following numeral.

   Example: XIV = (10 + 5 − 1) = 14

5. Roman numerals over 100 are seldom used in medicine. The basic Roman numerals you are likely to encounter and their Arabic equivalents are included in Table 2-2.

● PRACTICE PROBLEM

1. Express the following as Arabic or Roman numerals:

   a. 3 _____
   b. 5 _____
   c. 8 _____
   d. 10 _____
   e. 100 _____
   f. 7 _____
   g. 50 _____
   h. 60 _____

TABLE 2-2 BASIC ROMAN NUMERALS WITH ARABIC EQUIVALENTS

Roman Numerals	Arabic Numerals	Roman Numerals	Arabic Numerals
I	1	C	100
V	5	D	500
X	10	M	1000
L	50		

i. XXIV _____   m. IX _____

j. IV _____   n. VIII _____

k. XVI _____   o. XX _____

l. XIX _____

FRACTIONS

The word **fraction** literally means the result of breaking; dividing. It is used to indicate a small part that is broken off, a small amount, degree, or fragment. In mathematics, a fraction is a quantity that is less than a whole. It may be written in either of the following ways and still have the same value: 0.2 (decimal fraction) or $\frac{2}{10}$ (common fraction).

A common fraction is a part of a whole number. It is obtained by dividing a number into a **numerator** (the number above the line in a fraction; also known as the dividend) separated from the **denominator** (the number below the line in a fraction; also known as the divisor) by a horizontal line ($\frac{2}{10}$) or by a diagonal line ($^2/_{10}$). In the fraction $\frac{2}{10}$, the 2 is the numerator, and the 10 is the denominator. The line separating the numerator from the denominator expresses the process of division: the numerator is divided by the denominator.

Example: denominator $10)\overline{\begin{smallmatrix}0.2\\2.0\\2.0\end{smallmatrix}}$ numerator

Types of Common Fractions

Simple fractions are fractions that contain only one numerator and one denominator, such as $\frac{1}{3}, \frac{1}{4}$, and $\frac{2}{10}$.

Compound fractions are those in which an arithmetical process is necessary in either the numerator or denominator, as in $\frac{2\times4}{12} = \frac{8}{12}$ or $\frac{10}{6-4} = \frac{10}{2} = 5$.

Complex fractions may have simple fractions in either the numerator or the denominator, or both, as in

$\dfrac{1\frac{1}{2}\text{ numerator}}{6}$ $\dfrac{6}{1\frac{1}{2}\text{ denominator}}$ $\dfrac{1\frac{1}{2}}{6\frac{1}{2}}$ both.

Proper fractions have a numerator that is smaller than the denominator, as in $\frac{6}{8}$ or $\frac{4}{5}$.

Improper fractions have a numerator that is larger than the denominator, as in $\frac{16}{4}$ or $\frac{15}{3}$.

A mixed number contains a whole number and a fraction, as in $3\frac{1}{3}$ or $2\frac{1}{2}$.

Equivalent fractions are those that have the same value, as in $\frac{4}{8} = \frac{1}{2}$ or $\frac{5}{10} = \frac{1}{2}$.

Expressing Fractions as Equivalents

To express fractions as equivalents you must find the largest whole number that will divide evenly into both the numerator and the denominator. This is called reducing the fraction to lowest terms. It is easier and safer to work with smaller numbers than larger numbers.

Example: To reduce $\frac{27}{81}$ to lowest terms, divide the numerator and the denominator by 27.
$$\frac{27}{81} = \frac{1}{3}$$

● PRACTICE PROBLEM

2. Reduce the following fractions to lowest terms:

   a. $\frac{75}{100}$ = _____   d. $\frac{33}{66}$ = _____

   b. $\frac{34}{102}$ = _____   e. $\frac{60}{1200}$ = _____

   c. $\frac{14}{56}$ = _____   f. $\frac{21}{105}$ = _____

Expressing Improper Fractions as Mixed Numbers

To express improper fractions as mixed numbers, follow these steps:

1. Divide the numerator by the denominator.
2. Place the remainder as a fraction and reduce to lowest terms.

Example: $\dfrac{4}{3} = 3)\overline{\begin{smallmatrix}1\frac{1}{3}\\4\\3\end{smallmatrix}}$
                           1 (remainder)

● PRACTICE PROBLEM

3. Express the following improper fractions as mixed numbers and reduce to lowest terms:

   a. $\frac{16}{12}$ = _____   d. $\frac{8}{5}$ = _____

   b. $\frac{24}{18}$ = _____   e. $\frac{10}{9}$ = _____

   c. $\frac{9}{6}$ = _____   f. $\frac{15}{13}$ = _____

Expressing Mixed Numbers as Improper Fractions

To express mixed numbers as improper fractions, follow these steps:

1. Multiply the whole number by the denominator.
2. Add the numerator to the product of step 1.

3. Place the sum over the denominator.

Example: $2\frac{1}{2} = \frac{(2 \times 2) + 1}{2} = \frac{5}{2} = 2\frac{1}{2}$

● PRACTICE PROBLEM

4. Express the following mixed numbers as improper fractions. Check your work by changing the fractions back into mixed numbers.

a. $3\frac{1}{3} =$ _____   d. $6\frac{7}{10} =$ _____

b. $4\frac{1}{4} =$ _____   e. $7\frac{1}{7} =$ _____

c. $5\frac{2}{3} =$ _____   f. $9\frac{1}{9} =$ _____

RELATIVE VALUES OF FRACTIONS

To determine the relative values of a series of fractions, you need to determine which fraction is the largest. Which is the largest, $\frac{1}{4}$, $\frac{1}{15}$, or $\frac{1}{3}$? To assist you in determining which fraction is the largest, follow these steps:

1. Make each fraction a whole number. The fraction that takes fewer parts to make a whole number is the largest.

Example: $\frac{1}{3} + \frac{2}{3} = \frac{3}{3} = 1$

$\frac{1}{4} + \frac{3}{4} = \frac{4}{4} = 1$

$\frac{1}{15} + \frac{14}{15} = \frac{15}{15} = 1$

$\frac{1}{3}$ is the largest fraction in this series, because it takes 2 additional parts to make a whole.

$\frac{1}{4}$ is the next largest fraction, because it takes 3 additional parts to make a whole.

$\frac{1}{15}$ is the smallest fraction in this series, because it takes 14 additional parts to make a whole.

2. When the fractions have the same denominators, the fraction with the largest numerator is the largest, because it takes fewer parts to make a whole. Which is the largest, $\frac{2}{8}$, $\frac{4}{8}$, or $\frac{7}{8}$?

Example: $\frac{7}{8} + \frac{1}{8} = \frac{8}{8} = 1$

$\frac{4}{8} + \frac{4}{8} = \frac{8}{8} = 1$

$\frac{2}{8} + \frac{6}{8} = \frac{8}{8} = 1$

$\frac{7}{8}$ is the largest fraction in this series, because it takes 1 additional part to make a whole.

$\frac{4}{8}$ is the next largest fraction, because it takes 4 additional parts to make a whole.

$\frac{2}{8}$ is the smallest fraction, because it takes 6 additional parts to make a whole.

● PRACTICE PROBLEM

5. To determine the relative values of fractions, analyze each series of fractions that follows, noting the largest value on the first line and the smallest value on the second line:

	Largest Value	Smallest Value
a. $\frac{1}{3}$, $\frac{1}{8}$	_____	_____
b. $\frac{1}{30}$, $\frac{1}{4}$, $\frac{1}{150}$	_____	_____
c. $\frac{1}{5}$, $\frac{3}{20}$, $\frac{1}{100}$	_____	_____
d. $\frac{2}{5}$, $\frac{4}{5}$, $\frac{3}{5}$	_____	_____
e. $\frac{2}{40}$, $\frac{8}{40}$, $\frac{10}{40}$	_____	_____
f. $\frac{1}{150}$, $\frac{1}{125}$, $\frac{1}{100}$	_____	_____
g. $\frac{1}{4}$, $\frac{3}{8}$, $\frac{3}{4}$	_____	_____
h. $\frac{1}{3}$, $\frac{1}{2}$, $\frac{1}{5}$	_____	_____
i. $\frac{25}{100}$, $\frac{75}{100}$, $\frac{50}{100}$	_____	_____
j. $\frac{3}{10}$, $\frac{5}{10}$, $\frac{8}{10}$	_____	_____

ADDITION OF FRACTIONS

To add fractions, the denominators must be the same. Once the denominators are the same, you do not perform any mathematical calculation on the denominators.

Adding Common Fractions

When adding common fractions, the denominators must be the same. The following fractions can be added because their denominators are the same.

$$\frac{1}{4} + \frac{3}{4} = \frac{4}{4} = 1$$

To add fractions that have unlike denominators, follow these steps:

1. Express the fractions as equivalent fractions by finding the **lowest common denominator (LCD)** (the least number into which the denominators of two or more fractions will go evenly).

2. Add the numerators and place the sum over the lowest common denominator.

Example: $\frac{1}{4} + \frac{1}{2} = ?$

$$4 \text{ (LCD)}$$

$$\frac{1}{4} = \frac{1}{4}$$

$$\frac{1}{2} = \frac{2}{4}$$

$$\frac{1}{4} + \frac{2}{4} = \frac{3}{4}$$

Adding Mixed Numbers

When adding fractions and whole numbers, the denominators must be the same. When the denominators are the same, add the fractions, and then add the results to the whole numbers.

Example: $7\frac{1}{8}$

$$+6\frac{2}{8}$$

$$13\frac{3}{8}$$

To add fractions and whole numbers that have unlike denominators, follow these steps:

1. Express the fractions as equivalent fractions by finding the lowest common denominator (LCD).

2. Add the fractions and then add the whole numbers.

Example: $1\frac{1}{4} + 2\frac{5}{8} + 3\frac{1}{2} = ?$

Step 1.   8 (LCD)

$$\frac{1}{4} = \frac{2}{8}$$

$$\frac{5}{8} = \frac{5}{8}$$

$$\frac{1}{2} = \frac{4}{8}$$

Step 2. $1\frac{2}{8}$

$$+2\frac{5}{8}$$

$$+3\frac{4}{8}$$

$$6\frac{11}{8}$$

3. When addition of the fractions results in a numerator that is larger than the denominator, divide the numerator by the denominator and then add the results to the whole number.

Example: $6\frac{11}{8}$

$$\begin{array}{r} 1\frac{3}{8} \\ 8\overline{)11} \\ \underline{8} \\ 3 \text{ (remainder)} \end{array}$$

Step 3. 6

$$+1\frac{3}{8}$$

$$7\frac{3}{8}$$

● PRACTICE PROBLEM

6. Add the following fractions and reduce to lowest terms:

a. $\frac{1}{6}$ _____   g. $9\frac{1}{3}$ _____

   $+\frac{3}{4}$ $+33\frac{2}{3}$

b. $\frac{4}{7}$ _____   h. $18\frac{14}{12}$ _____

   $+\frac{1}{3}$ $+9\frac{20}{12}$

c. $\frac{6}{16}$ _____   i. $13\frac{2}{5}$ _____

   $\frac{7}{8}$ $16\frac{4}{10}$

   $+\frac{1}{4}$ $+7\frac{5}{30}$

d. $\frac{2}{5}$ _____   j. $24\frac{3}{9}$ _____

   $\frac{6}{10}$ $8\frac{16}{18}$

   $+\frac{8}{20}$ $+3\frac{40}{36}$

e. $22\frac{3}{4}$ _____   k. $\frac{1}{5}$ _____

   $+76\frac{1}{4}$ $\frac{14}{25}$

                                $+\frac{11}{50}$

f. $49\frac{1}{7}$ _____   l. $\frac{1}{4}$ _____

   $+106\frac{5}{7}$ $+\frac{3}{4}$

SUBTRACTION OF FRACTIONS

To subtract fractions, the denominators must be the same. Once the denominators are the same, you do not perform any mathematical calculation on the denominators.

Subtracting Common Fractions

When subtracting common fractions, the denominators must be the same. The following fractions can be subtracted because their denominators are the same.

$$\frac{3}{4} - \frac{1}{4} = \frac{2}{4} = \frac{1}{2}$$

To subtract fractions that have unlike denominators, follow these steps:

1. Express the fractions as equivalent fractions by finding the lowest common denominator (LCD).
2. Subtract the numerators and place your answer over the lowest common denominator.

Example: $\frac{1}{2} - \frac{1}{4} = ?$

4 (LCD)

$$\frac{1}{2} = \frac{2}{4}$$

$$\frac{1}{4} = \frac{1}{4}$$

$$\frac{2}{4} - \frac{1}{4} = \frac{1}{4}$$

Subtracting Mixed Numbers

When subtracting fractions and whole numbers, the denominators must be the same. When the denominators are the same, subtract the fractions, and then subtract the whole numbers.

Example:
$$7\frac{9}{10}$$
$$-\,2\frac{6}{10}$$
$$\overline{5\frac{3}{10}}$$

To subtract fractions and whole numbers that have unlike denominators, follow these steps:

1. Express the fractions as equivalent fractions by finding the lowest common denominator (LCD).
2. Subtract the fractions and then subtract the whole numbers.
3. When subtracting fractions in which the **subtrahend** (the number that is to be subtracted) is larger than the **minuend** (the number from which another is to be subtracted):
   a. Borrow one whole unit from the whole number.

b. Add the borrowed unit (1) to the fraction of the minuend.

c. Subtract the fractions then subtract the whole numbers.

Example:
$$10\frac{1}{5} \qquad 10\frac{1}{5}$$
$$-\,8\frac{3}{5} \qquad -\frac{5}{5} \quad (1)\ \text{borrow} \qquad \frac{5}{5} + \frac{1}{5} = \frac{6}{5}$$
$$\overline{\qquad\qquad 9\frac{6}{5}}$$

$$10\frac{1}{5} \ \text{becomes} \qquad 9\frac{6}{5}$$
$$-\,8\frac{3}{5} \ \text{now subtract}$$
$$\overline{\qquad\qquad 1\frac{3}{5}}$$

4. Check the accuracy of your work by adding the answer and the subtrahend together. The sum will equal the minuend.

$$8\frac{3}{5} \quad (\textbf{subtrahend})$$
$$+1\frac{3}{5} \quad (\textbf{answer})$$
$$\overline{9\frac{6}{5}} = 9\frac{6}{5} \ (\textbf{minuend})$$

● PRACTICE PROBLEM

7. Subtract the following fractions and reduce to lowest terms:

a. $\frac{7}{8}$ _____
   $-\frac{2}{16}$

g. $17\frac{9}{10}$ _____
   $-\,9\frac{12}{10}$

b. $\frac{4}{15}$ _____
   $-\frac{1}{45}$

h. $106\frac{7}{8}$ _____
   $-\,23\frac{3}{8}$

c. $\frac{16}{32}$ _____
   $-\frac{9}{32}$

i. $91\frac{45}{25}$ _____
   $-\,42\frac{7}{25}$

d. $66\frac{2}{3}$ _____
   $-\,33\frac{1}{3}$

j. $\frac{25}{75}$ _____
   $-\frac{16}{150}$

e. $21\frac{3}{9}$ _____
   $-\,5\frac{5}{9}$

k. $\frac{11}{12}$ _____
   $-\frac{5}{6}$

f. $14\frac{3}{15}$ _____
   $-\,5\frac{6}{30}$

l. $16\frac{5}{6}$ _____
   $-14\frac{3}{8}$

THE PROCESS OF CANCELLATION

When multiplying or dividing fractions, it is easier and more accurate to work with smaller numbers. To arrive at a smaller number, the process of cancellation is used.

Steps to Cancel

1. Divide the numerator and the denominator by the largest number contained in each.
2. After canceling, continue with the mathematical process of the problem.

   Example: *Multiplication*

   $$16 \times \frac{3}{8} = \frac{16}{1} \times \frac{3}{8}$$
   $$= 16 \div 8 = 2$$
   $$= 8 \div 8 = 1$$
   $$= \frac{\overset{2}{\cancel{16}}}{1} \times \frac{3}{\underset{1}{\cancel{8}}} \qquad \frac{2 \times 3}{1 \times 1} = \frac{6}{1}$$
   $$= 6$$

MULTIPLICATION OF FRACTIONS

To multiply fractions, you multiply the numerators and the denominators.

Multiplying Common Fractions

To multiply common fractions, multiply the numerator by the numerator and the denominator by the denominator. Reduce to lowest terms when possible.

   Example: $\frac{3}{7} \times \frac{4}{5} = \frac{(3 \times 4)}{(7 \times 5)} = \frac{12}{35}$

   Reduce to lowest terms:

   $$\frac{1}{6} \times \frac{3}{4} = \frac{(3 \times 1)}{(6 \times 4)} = \frac{3}{24} = \frac{(3 \div 3)}{(24 \div 3)} = \frac{1}{8}$$

Multiplying a Fraction and a Whole Number

To multiply a fraction and a whole number, follow these steps:

1. Change the whole number to a fraction by placing the whole number over one (1).
2. Then multiply the numerator by the numerator and the denominator by the denominator.
3. Reduce to lowest terms when possible.

   Example: $16 \times \frac{3}{8} =$

   $$\frac{16}{1} \times \frac{3}{8} = \frac{(16 \times 3)}{(1 \times 8)} = \frac{48}{8} = 48 \div 8 = 6$$

Multiplying Mixed Numbers

To multiply mixed numbers, follow these steps:

1. Change the mixed numbers to improper fractions.
2. Then multiply the numerator by the numerator and the denominator by the denominator.
3. Reduce to lowest terms when possible.

   Example: $2\frac{7}{8} \times \frac{3}{5}$

   $$8 \times 2 = 16 + 7 = \frac{23}{8} \times \frac{3}{5} = \frac{(23 \times 3)}{(8 \times 5)} =$$
   $$\frac{69}{40} = 69 \div 40 = 1\frac{29}{40}$$

● PRACTICE PROBLEM

8. Multiply the following fractions and reduce to lowest terms:

   a. $\frac{23}{9} \times \frac{7}{16} =$ _____

   b. $\frac{2}{5} \times \frac{1}{3} =$ _____

   c. $\frac{14}{8} \times \frac{2}{4} =$ _____

   d. $6\frac{10}{12} \times \frac{15}{3} =$ _____

   e. $91\frac{2}{3} \times \frac{4}{6} =$ _____

   f. $\frac{18}{24} \times 5\frac{1}{10} =$ _____

   g. $42 \times \frac{1}{2} =$ _____

   h. $56 \times \frac{9}{20} =$ _____

   i. $365 \times \frac{12}{30} =$ _____

   j. $18 \times \frac{2}{3} =$ _____

   k. $\frac{2}{3} \times \frac{3}{4} =$ _____

   l. $\frac{4}{5} \times \frac{1}{8} =$ _____

   m. $\frac{4}{9} \times \frac{3}{8} =$ _____

   n. $\frac{5}{7} \times 5\frac{1}{4} =$ _____

   o. $\frac{5}{12} \times 4\frac{3}{4} =$ _____

DIVISION OF FRACTIONS

To divide fractions, you invert the divisor (second fraction) and then follow the rules for multiplying fractions.

Dividing Common Fractions

To divide common fractions, invert the divisor (inverting a fraction means turning it upside down). It is most important that you invert the **divisor** (the number that is divided into another number or the number by which another can be divided; also known as the denominator) and not the **dividend** (the number that is divided; also known as the numerator). When $\frac{3}{4}$ is inverted, it becomes $\frac{4}{3}$.

To divide common fractions, follow these steps:

1. Invert the *divisor*.
2. Then multiply the numerator by the numerator and the denominator by the denominator.
3. Reduce to lowest terms when possible.

Example: $\frac{1}{6} \div \frac{3}{4}$ (divisor)

$$\frac{1}{6} \times \frac{4}{3} = \frac{(4 \times 1)}{(6 \times 3)} = \frac{4}{18} = \frac{2}{9}$$

Dividing a Fraction and a Whole Number

To divide a fraction and a whole number, follow these steps:

1. Change the whole number to a fraction by placing the whole number over one (1).
2. Invert the *divisor*.
3. Then multiply the numerator by the numerator and the denominator by the denominator.
4. Reduce to lowest terms when possible.

Example: $16 \div \frac{3}{8} = \frac{16}{1} \div \frac{3}{8}$

$$= \frac{16}{1} \times \frac{8}{3} = \frac{(16 \times 8)}{(1 \times 3)} = \frac{128}{3}$$

$$= 128 \div 3 = 42\frac{2}{3}$$

Dividing Mixed Numbers

To divide mixed numbers, follow these steps:

1. Change the mixed number to an improper fraction.
2. Invert the *divisor*.
3. Then multiply the numerator by the numerator and the denominator by the denominator.
4. Reduce to lowest terms when possible.

Example: $2\frac{7}{8} \div \frac{3}{5}$

$$2 \times 8 = 16 + 7 = \frac{23}{8}$$

$$\frac{23}{8} \div \frac{3}{5}$$

$$\frac{23}{8} \times \frac{5}{3} = \frac{(23 \times 5)}{(8 \times 3)} = \frac{115}{24} = 115 \div 24 = 4\frac{19}{24}$$

● PRACTICE PROBLEM

9. Divide the following fractions and reduce to lowest terms:

a. $\frac{23}{9} \div \frac{7}{16} =$ _____

b. $\frac{2}{5} \div \frac{1}{3} =$ _____

c. $\frac{14}{8} \div \frac{2}{4} =$ _____

d. $6\frac{10}{12} \div \frac{15}{3} =$ _____

e. $91\frac{2}{3} \div \frac{4}{6} =$ _____

f. $\frac{18}{24} \div 5\frac{1}{10} =$ _____

g. $42 \div \frac{1}{2} =$ _____

h. $56 \div \frac{9}{20} =$ _____

i. $\frac{7}{8} \div \frac{3}{4} =$ _____

j. $\frac{2}{3} \div \frac{1}{3} =$ _____

k. $\frac{1}{5} \div \frac{1}{10} =$ _____

l. $\frac{1}{150} \div \frac{1}{100} =$ _____

m. $\frac{2}{5} \div \frac{10}{15} =$ _____

n. $3 \div \frac{5}{3} =$ _____

o. $\frac{2}{3} \div 5\frac{1}{2} =$ _____

p. $\frac{3}{4} \div \frac{8}{9} =$ _____

● SELF-ASSESSMENT

This exercise is designed to assess your understanding of numerals and fractions. Follow the directions for each question.

1. Express the following as Arabic or Roman numerals:

   a. 15 _____   d. IV _____

   b. 25 _____   e. XIX _____

   c. 50 _____   f. XVI _____

2. Express the following mixed numbers as improper fractions:

   a. $5\frac{1}{2}$ _____   d. $6\frac{7}{8}$ _____

   b. $3\frac{1}{3}$ _____   e. $4\frac{2}{3}$ _____

   c. $8\frac{1}{6}$ _____   f. $2\frac{1}{2}$ _____

3. Express the following improper fractions as mixed numbers:

a. $\frac{9}{6}$ _____ d. $\frac{15}{2}$ _____

b. $\frac{7}{5}$ _____ e. $\frac{8}{6}$ _____

c. $\frac{6}{4}$ _____ f. $\frac{3}{2}$ _____

4. Reduce the following fractions to lowest terms:

a. $\frac{48}{96}$ _____ d. $\frac{60}{100}$ _____

b. $\frac{75}{100}$ _____ e. $\frac{14}{56}$ _____

c. $\frac{33}{66}$ _____ f. $\frac{3}{15}$ _____

5. Add the following fractions:

a. $\frac{1}{8} + \frac{3}{4}$ _____

b. $22\frac{14}{12} + 2\frac{1}{6}$ _____

c. $\frac{1}{7} + \frac{3}{21}$ _____

d. $9\frac{1}{3} + 31\frac{2}{3}$ _____

e. $\frac{1}{3} + \frac{1}{9}$ _____

f. $102\frac{5}{6} + 98\frac{1}{3}$ _____

6. Subtract the following fractions:

a. $\frac{3}{4} - \frac{1}{8}$ _____

b. $21\frac{3}{9} - 5\frac{5}{9}$ _____

c. $\frac{11}{12} - \frac{5}{6}$ _____

d. $31\frac{2}{3} - 9\frac{1}{3}$ _____

e. $\frac{25}{75} - \frac{16}{150}$ _____

f. $14\frac{3}{5} - 5\frac{6}{10}$ _____

7. Multiply the following fractions:

a. $\frac{4}{9} \times \frac{1}{8}$ _____

b. $365 \times \frac{12}{30}$ _____

c. $45 \times \frac{1}{5}$ _____

d. $6\frac{11}{12} \times \frac{7}{3}$ _____

8. Divide the following fractions:

a. $\frac{1}{150} \div \frac{1}{100}$ _____

b. $\frac{3}{4} \div \frac{8}{9}$ _____

c. $\frac{2}{3} \div 5\frac{1}{2}$ _____

d. $56 \div \frac{9}{20}$ _____

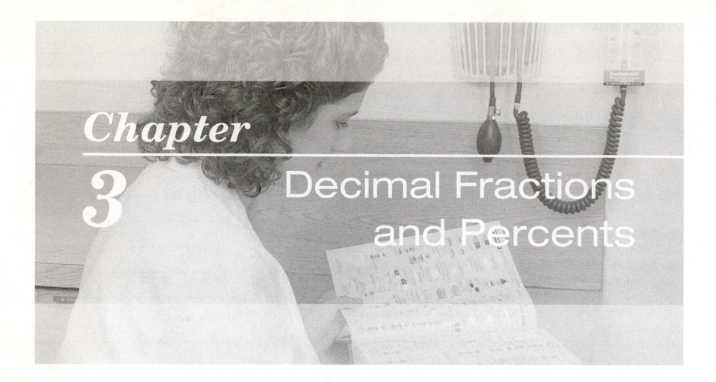

Chapter 3
Decimal Fractions and Percents

Chapter Outline

- Express a common fraction as a decimal fraction
- Express a decimal fraction as a common fraction
- Add, subtract, multiply, and divide decimals
- Express common fractions and decimal fractions as percents, and percents as common fractions and decimal fractions
- Work the practice problems correctly
- Complete the Self-Assessment

Key Terms

common fraction	percent
decimal	place value
decimal fraction	power of 10

Objectives

Upon completion of this chapter, you should be able to

- Define the key terms
- Read and write decimals correctly
- Define and use the powers of 10

INTRODUCTION

There is evidence that the decimal system dates back to the third century B.C. in India. The system was formalized during the Middle Ages and is now referred to as the Hindu-Arabic system. This number structure and place values were brought to Europe during the early thirteenth century by Fibonacci, an Italian mathematician. The decimal system is a number system based upon the number 10 or multiples of 10.

Percent means per hundred. It literally means to divide by 100 to find the value of the number. If a solution contains 10% of a concentrate, you would divide 10 by 100 and get 0.1. Medications and/or solutions may be ordered and measured in decimals and percent.

UNDERSTANDING DECIMAL FRACTIONS

A **decimal** is a mathematical form that represents a straight line of units described as a fraction. The decimal point is in the center of the line. All the numbers to the left of the decimal point are *whole* numbers. All the numbers to the right of the decimal point are *decimals* or **decimal fractions**. The position of the number to the left or the right of the decimal point is its **place value**. The value of each place left of the decimal point is ten times that of the place to its right. The value of each place right of the decimal point is one tenth the value of the place to its left. See Figure 3-1.

READING AND WRITING DECIMAL FRACTIONS

The following steps will guide you as you learn to read and write decimal fractions:

1. Note the place value of the decimal point.
2. Read the number to the right of the decimal point.
3. Use the name that applies to the decimal place of the last number.
4. Read using *th* or *ths* on the end of the denominator.

TABLE 3-1 READING DECIMALS

0.1	Read as one tenth.
0.01	Read as one hundredth.
0.001	Read as one thousandth.
0.0001	Read as one ten-thousandth.
0.00001	Read as one hundred-thousandth.
0.000001	Read as one millionth.

5. To read a whole number and a decimal fraction, the decimal point is read as *and* or *point*.
6. It is good practice to place a zero (0) before the decimal point. This is a safety measure that insures the reading of the number as a decimal and not as a whole number.
7. Study Table 3-1 and the examples given.

Examples

1. Note that the number is directly to the right of the decimal point (0.1). Read as one tenth.
2. Note that the number is two places to the right of the decimal point (0.01). Read as one hundredth.
3. Note that the number is three places to the right of the decimal point (0.001). Read as one thousandth.
4. Note that the number is four places to the right of the decimal point (0.0001). Read as one ten-thousandth.
5. Note that the number is five places to the right of the decimal point (0.00001). Read as one hundred-thousandth.
6. Note that the number is six places to the right of the decimal point (0.000001). Read as one millionth.
7. The number 10.1 is a whole number and a decimal fraction. Read as ten and one tenth or ten point one.

Powers of 10

The **power of 10** is the process of multiplying 10's together. The number of 10's multiplied determines the power. Remember that a decimal fraction is a fraction with an unwritten denominator of 10 or any power of 10. Study Table 3-2 for an understanding of the powers of 10.

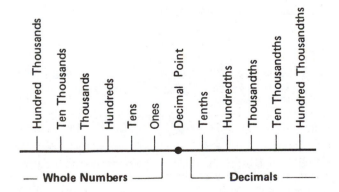

FIGURE 3-1

TABLE 3-2   POWERS OF 10

Power	Number	Name or Value
1st	10	ten
2nd	100	hundred
3rd	1,000	thousand
4th	10,000	ten thousand
5th	100,000	hundred thousand
6th	1,000,000	million
7th	10,000,000	ten million
8th	100,000,000	hundred million
9th	1,000,000,000	billion
10th	10,000,000,000	ten billion

● PRACTICE PROBLEMS

Complete the following statements that involve the use of decimals:

1. A _____ is a mathematical form that represents a straight line of units described as a fraction.

2. State the usage of a decimal.

3. All the numbers to the left of the decimal point are _____ numbers.

4. All the numbers to the right of the decimal point are _____ or _____.

5. The position of the number to the left or right of the decimal point is its _____ _____.

6. The value of each place left of the decimal point is _____ times that of the place to its right.

7. The value of each place right of the decimal point is _____ of the value of the place to its left.

8. A _____ _____ is a fraction with an unwritten denominator of 10 or a power of ten.

9. It is important to place a 0 before the decimal point because _____.

10. The _____ _____ _____ is the process of multiplying 10's together.

11. Write out the following fractions:

   a. $\frac{1}{10,000}$ _____

   b. $\frac{2}{10}$ _____

   c. $\frac{6}{100}$ _____

   d. $\frac{10}{100,000}$ _____

   e. $\frac{25}{1000}$ _____

12. Write out the following decimal fractions:

   a. 0.25 _____

   b. 0.7 _____

   c. 0.150 _____

   d. 0.4200 _____

   e. 0.00006 _____

13. Write out the following whole numbers and decimal fractions:

   a. 2.5 _____
   _____

   b. 9.25 _____
   _____

   c. 125.040 _____
   _____

   d. 15.0150 _____
   _____

   e. 4.00005 _____
   _____

EXPRESSING A COMMON FRACTION AS A DECIMAL FRACTION

A **common fraction** is part of a whole number. It is the result of the process of dividing a number into a numerator separated from the denominator by either a horizontal or diagonal line ($\frac{1}{2}$ or ½).

A **decimal fraction** is a fraction with an unwritten denominator of 10 or a power of 10 ($0.5 = \frac{5}{10}$).

To express a common fraction as a decimal fraction, follow these steps:

1. Divide the denominator of the fraction into the numerator.

$$\text{denominator} \quad 2\overline{)1} \quad \text{numerator}$$

2. Place a decimal point after the numerator.

$$2\overline{)1.} \quad \text{numerator}$$

3. Place a decimal point in the quotient (answer) directly over the decimal point of the numerator.

$$\overset{.}{2\overline{)1.}} \quad \begin{matrix}\text{quotient}\\\text{numerator}\end{matrix}$$

4. Place a 0 after the decimal point of the numerator.

$$\overset{.}{2\overline{)1.0}} \quad \text{numerator}$$

5. Now divide.

$$2\overline{)1.0}^{\,.5}\ \ \text{numerator}$$
$$\underline{1\,0}$$

6. Place a 0 before the decimal point of the quotient.

$$2\overline{)1.0}^{\,0.5}\ \ \text{quotient}$$
$$\underline{1\,0}$$

The common fraction $\frac{1}{2}$ is equal to the decimal fraction 0.5 ($\frac{5}{10}$). The number is 0.5 read as five tenths and can be reduced to

$$\frac{\overset{1}{\cancel{5}}}{\underset{2}{\cancel{10}}} = \frac{1}{2}$$

7. To check the accuracy of your work, multiply the quotient by the denominator (divisor). This will give you the same number as the numerator (dividend).

$$\begin{array}{r} 0.5 \quad \text{quotient} \\ \times\ 2 \quad \text{denominator (divisor)} \\ \hline 1.0 \quad \text{numerator (dividend)} \end{array}$$

EXPRESSING A DECIMAL FRACTION AS A COMMON FRACTION

To express a decimal fraction as a common fraction, follow these steps:

1. Read the decimal fraction.
2. The numerator is the number you get when you move the decimal point to the right past the last number.
3. The denominator is the number of spaces you moved the decimal point.
4. Remember that each space is represented by a factor of 10.
5. Reduce to lowest terms.

Example: 0.25   Read as twenty-five hundredths

0.25   Move the decimal point to the right of the last number; 0.25 becomes 25.

You moved two spaces to the right, which is hundredths.

$$0.25 = \frac{25}{100}\ \ \frac{\text{numerator}}{\text{denominator}}$$

Reduce to lowest terms.

$$\frac{\overset{1}{\cancel{25}}}{\underset{4}{\cancel{100}}} = \frac{1}{4}$$

● PRACTICE PROBLEMS

1. Express the following common fractions as decimal fractions:

a. $\frac{2}{3}$ = _____   d. $\frac{1}{5}$ = _____

b. $\frac{1}{4}$ = _____   e. $\frac{7}{8}$ = _____

c. $\frac{3}{4}$ = _____

2. Express the following decimal fractions as common fractions:

a. 0.4 _____   d. 0.0006 _____

b. 0.05 _____   e. 0.000002 _____

c. 0.010 _____

ADDITION OF DECIMALS

To add decimals, follow these steps:

1. Arrange the numbers in a column.
2. Line up the decimal points.
3. Make sure you form a straight line with the decimal points one under the other.
4. Add the numbers as in addition of whole numbers.
5. Now place the decimal point in your answer directly under the decimal points of the problem.

Examples:

$$\begin{array}{r} 0.5 \\ +0.50 \\ \hline 0.10 \end{array} \qquad \begin{array}{r} 0.75 \\ 0.125 \\ +0.1000 \\ \hline 0.9750 \end{array}$$

● PRACTICE PROBLEM

3. Add the following decimals:

a. 0.6 + 0.4 = _____

b. 0.1 + 0.6 + 0.3 = _____

c. 0.89 + 0.26 + 0.2 = _____

d. 0.25 + 0.001 + 0.100 = _____

e. 10.5 + 123.75 + 0.010 = _____

SUBTRACTION OF DECIMALS

To subtract decimals, follow these steps:

1. Arrange the numbers in a column.
2. Line up the decimal points.
3. Make sure you form a straight line with the decimal points one under the other.
4. Subtract the numbers as in subtraction of whole numbers.
5. Now place the decimal point in your answer directly under the decimal points of the problem.

Examples:

$$\begin{array}{r} 104.32 \\ -\ 76.21 \\ \hline 28.11 \end{array} \qquad \begin{array}{r} 0.098 \\ -0.010 \\ \hline 0.088 \end{array}$$

6. To subtract a smaller number from a larger number, place a zero (0) after the larger number. A zero (0) placed after the number will not alter or change the decimal place or the decimal value.

Examples:

$$\begin{array}{r} 0.1 \\ -0.03 \end{array} \qquad \begin{array}{r} 0.10 \\ -0.03 \\ \hline 0.07 \end{array}$$

7. Check the accuracy of your work by adding the answer and the lower numbers (subtrahend) together. The sum will equal the upper numbers (minuend).

Examples:

$$\begin{array}{ll} 0.098 & \text{minuend} \\ -0.010 & \text{subtrahend} \\ +0.088 & \text{answer} \\ \hline 0.098 & \text{minuend} \end{array} \qquad \begin{array}{ll} 0.10 & \text{minuend} \\ -0.03 & \text{subtrahend} \\ +0.07 & \text{answer} \\ \hline 0.10 & \text{minuend} \end{array}$$

● PRACTICE PROBLEM

4. Subtract the following decimals:

    a. $0.1 - 0.04 =$ _____
    b. $2.25 - 1.75 =$ _____
    c. $304.65 - 264.26 =$ _____
    d. $9.123 - 6.055 =$ _____
    e. $1.000 - 0.556 =$ _____
    f. $0.2 - 0.07 =$ _____
    g. $0.1 - 0.04 =$ _____
    h. $0.3 - 0.09 =$ _____
    i. $0.6 - 0.08 =$ _____
    j. $0.5 - 0.06 =$ _____

MULTIPLICATION OF DECIMALS

To multiply decimals, follow these steps:

1. Multiply decimals just as you multiply whole numbers.
2. Count the total number of decimal places in the problem.
3. Start on the right of your answer (product) and count off the number of decimal places you counted in the previous step.
4. Remember that you count off decimal places in the product from right to left.

Example:

$$\begin{array}{r} 2.14 \\ \times 0.76 \\ \hline 12\ 84 \\ 149\ 8 \\ 000 \\ \hline 1.6264 \end{array}$$

2.14 (2 decimal places)
× 0.76 (2 decimal places)

Product left → 1.6264 (count off 4 decimal places from right to left)
← right

Multiplying Decimals by Ten or Any Power of Ten

> **Rule:** When you multiply decimals by 10 or any multiple of 10, you move the decimal point to the right in the product as many places as there are 0's in the multiplier.

Example:

$$3.6 \times 10 = 36$$
(1)
$$3.6 \times 100 = 360$$
(2)
$$3.6 \times 1000 = 3,600$$
(3)
$$3.6 \times 10,000 = 36,000$$
(4)
$$3.6 \times 100,000 = 360,000$$
(5)

To multiply decimals by 10 or any power of 10, follow these steps:

1. When you multiply by 10, you move the decimal point one place to the right.

$$0.6 \times 10 =$$
$$0.6 \times 10 = 6$$

2. When you multiply by 100, you move the decimal point two places to the right.

$$0.6 \times 100 =$$
$$0.60. \times 100 = 60$$

3. When you multiply by 1000, you move the decimal point three places to the right.

$$0.6 \times 1000 =$$
$$0.600. \times 1000 = 600$$

4. When you multiply by 10,000, you move the decimal point four places to the right.

$$0.6 \times 10,000 =$$
$$0.6000. \times 10,000 = 6,000$$

5. When you multiply by 100,000, you move the decimal point five places to the right.

$$0.6 \times 100,000 =$$
$$0.60000. \times 100,000 = 60,000$$

● PRACTICE PROBLEM

5. Multiply the following decimals:
   a. $4.25 \times 3.10 =$ _____
   b. $3.75 \times 7.35 =$ _____
   c. $83.126 \times 8.12 =$ _____
   d. $66.66 \times 3.33 =$ _____
   e. $0.0044 \times 72.16 =$ _____
   f. $2.5 \times 100,000 =$ _____
   g. $10.4 \times 10,000 =$ _____
   h. $5.2 \times 1,000 =$ _____
   i. $1.1 \times 100 =$ _____
   j. $0.3 \times 10 =$ _____

DIVISION OF DECIMALS

The following methods of division of decimals are designed to guide you step by step through dividing decimals by whole numbers, dividing whole numbers by decimals, dividing decimals by decimals, and dividing decimals by 10 or any factor of 10. Master one step at a time and you will acquire a working understanding of division of decimals.

Dividing Decimals by Whole Numbers

To divide decimals by whole numbers, follow these steps:

1. Set up the division process as follows:

$$12.6 \div 2$$
$$2\overline{)12.6}$$

2. Place a decimal point on the answer line directly over the decimal point of the dividend.

$$\overset{\text{\Large .}}{2\overline{)12.6}} \quad \begin{array}{l}\text{answer line}\\\text{dividend}\end{array}$$

3. Now divide the dividend by the divisor.

$$\text{divisor} \quad 2\overline{\smash{)}12.6} \quad \begin{array}{l}6.3 \quad \text{quotient}\\ \;\; \text{dividend}\end{array}$$
$$\underline{12}$$
$$6$$
$$\underline{6}$$

4. $12.6 \div 2 = 6.3$

5. To check the accuracy of your work, multiply the quotient by the divisor. This will give you the same number as the dividend.

$$\begin{array}{r}6.3 \quad \text{quotient}\\ \times\; 2 \quad \text{divisor}\\ \hline 12.6 \quad \text{dividend}\end{array}$$

6. To divide a whole number (divisor) that will not go into the decimal (dividend), follow these steps:
   a. $0.016 \div 4 =$

$$4\overline{)0.016}$$

   b. Place a decimal point on the answer line directly over the decimal point of the dividend. To insure accuracy, place a 0 before the decimal point.

$$\overset{\text{\normalsize 0.}}{4\overline{)0.016}} \quad \begin{array}{l}\text{answer line}\\\text{dividend}\end{array}$$

   c. Since 4 will not go into 0, place a 0 on the answer line directly over the 0 of the dividend.

$$\overset{\text{\normalsize 0.0}}{4\overline{)0.016}} \quad \begin{array}{l}\text{answer line}\\\text{dividend}\end{array}$$

   d. Since 4 will not go into 1, place a 0 on the answer line directly over the 1 of the dividend.

$$\overset{\text{\normalsize 0.00}}{4\overline{)0.016}} \quad \begin{array}{l}\text{answer line}\\\text{dividend}\end{array}$$

e. Now 4 will go into 16, so divide.

$$4\overline{)0.016}$$
quotient 0.004, then 16

f. To check the accuracy of your work, multiply the quotient by the divisor. This will give you the same number as the dividend.

$$
\begin{array}{r}
0.004 \quad \text{quotient} \\
\times \quad\quad 4 \quad \text{divisor} \\
\hline
0.016 \quad \text{dividend}
\end{array}
$$

● PRACTICE PROBLEM

6. Divide the following decimals by whole numbers:

   a. $28.8 \div 4 =$ _____
   b. $36.12 \div 6 =$ _____
   c. $100.40 \div 20 =$ _____
   d. $56.14 \div 7 =$ _____
   e. $86.86 \div 43 =$ _____
   f. $0.018 \div 9 =$ _____
   g. $0.025 \div 5 =$ _____
   h. $0.035 \div 7 =$ _____
   i. $0.04 \div 10 =$ _____
   j. $10.33 \div 3 =$ _____

Dividing Whole Numbers by Decimals

To divide a whole number by a decimal, make the decimal (divisor) a whole number. There are two methods of making a decimal a whole number.

1. Move the decimal point to the right as many places as necessary to make a whole number.
2. Multiply the decimal by the place value of the decimal point.

Moving the Decimal Point to the Right

To move the decimal point to the right, follow these steps:

1. Place a decimal point at the end of the whole number of the dividend. $100 \div 0.1 =$

   $$0.1\overline{)100.}\quad \text{dividend}$$

2. Place a 0 after the marked-off decimal point.

   $$0.1\overline{)100.0}$$

3. Move the decimal point one place to the right in the divisor, and one place to the right in the dividend.

   divisor $0.1.$ $100.0.$ dividend

4. You have made the decimal (divisor) and the dividend whole numbers. Now divide.

   $$
   1\overline{)1000}
   $$
   1000

5. To check the accuracy of your work, change the whole number and the decimal to fractions and then divide.

   $$100 \div 0.1 = \frac{100}{1} \div \frac{1}{10} =$$
   $$\frac{100}{1} \times \frac{10}{1} = \frac{1000}{1} = 1000$$

Multiplying the Decimal by the Place Value of the Decimal Point

To multiply the decimal by the place value, follow these steps:

1. Multiply the decimal (divisor) and the dividend by the same value of the decimal point.

   $100 \div 0.1 =$

   0.1 (decimal, divisor) has a place value of 10

   $0.1 \times 10 = 1$

   $100 \times 10 = 1000$

2. The decimal (divisor) and the dividend are now whole numbers. Now divide.

   $$
   1\overline{)1000}
   $$
   1000

Moving the decimal point to the right as many places as necessary to make a whole number, and multiplying the decimal by the place value of the decimal point to make a whole number, are two processes that will give the same result.

0.1̣. = 1

0.1 × 10 = 1

Moving the decimal one place to the right is the same as multiplying by the place value of 10.

0.0̣1. = 1

0.01 × 100 = 1

Moving the decimal two places to the right is the same as multiplying by the place value of 100.

0.0̣01. = 1

0.001 × 1000 = 1

Moving the decimal three places to the right is the same as multiplying by the place value of 1000.

0.0̣001. = 1

0.0001 × 10,000 = 1

Moving the decimal four places to the right is the same as multiplying by the place value of 10,000.

0.0̣0001. = 1

0.00001 × 100,000 = 1

Moving the decimal five places to the right is the same as multiplying by the place value of 100,000.

● PRACTICE PROBLEM

7. Divide the following whole numbers by decimals:

a. 20 ÷ 0.2 = _____

b. 60 ÷ 0.03 = _____

c. 150 ÷ 0.75 = _____

d. 100 ÷ 0.10 = _____

e. 1000 ÷ 0.01 = _____

f. 72 ÷ 0.009 = _____

g. 500 ÷ 0.0005 = _____

h. 86 ÷ 0.43 = _____

i. 60 ÷ 0.012 = _____

j. 36 ÷ 0.4 = _____

Dividing Decimals by Decimals

To divide decimals by decimals, follow these steps:

1. Make the divisor a whole number by moving the decimal point to the right as many places as necessary or by multiplying the decimal by the place value of the decimal point.

0.0016 ÷ 0.02 =   divisor   0.02)̅0̅.̅0̅0̅1̅6̅

Moving the decimal 0.0̣2. or multiplying 0.02 by the place value of 100 = 2.

$$
\begin{array}{r}
0.02 \\
\times\ 100 \\
\hline
0\ 00 \\
00\ 0 \\
002 \\
\hline
002.00
\end{array}
$$

2. Now do the same thing to the dividend that you did to the divisor.

0.0016 ÷ 0.02 =   0.02)̅0̅.̅0̅0̅1̅6̅   dividend

Moving the decimal 0.0̣0.16 or multiplying by the place value of 100 = .16.

$$
\begin{array}{r}
0.0016 \\
\times\ \ \ \ 100 \\
\hline
0\ 0000 \\
00\ 000 \\
000\ 16 \\
\hline
000.1600
\end{array}
$$

3. Set up the problem as follows:

2)̅.̅1̅6̅

To insure accuracy, place a 0 before the decimal point of the dividend.

2)̅0̅.̅1̅6̅   dividend

Place a decimal point on the answer line directly over the new decimal place of the dividend.

  .̅   answer line
2)0.16   dividend

Place a 0 before the marked-off decimal point.

  0.
2)̅0̅.̅1̅6̅

4. Now you have 0.16 ÷ 2. Divide.

  0.   answer line
2)̅0̅.̅1̅6̅   dividend

5. But, 2 will not go into 1, so place a 0 on the answer line directly over the 1 of the dividend.

  0.0   answer line
2)̅0̅.̅1̅6̅   dividend

6. Now 2 will go into 16.

  0.08
2)̅0̅.̅1̅6̅
  1̅6̅

7. To check the accuracy of your work, multiply the quotient (answer) by the divisor. This will give you the same number as the dividend.

$$
\begin{array}{r}
0.08 \quad \text{quotient (answer)} \\
\times \quad 2 \quad \text{divisor} \\
\hline
0.16 \quad \text{dividend}
\end{array}
$$

● PRACTICE PROBLEM

8. Divide the following decimals:

   a. $0.0024 \div 0.03 = $ _____

   b. $0.054 \div 0.18 = $ _____

   c. $0.02 \div 0.2 = $ _____

   d. $0.86 \div 0.43 = $ _____

   e. $0.2 \div 0.002 = $ _____

   f. $7.5 \div 2.5 = $ _____

   g. $0.49 \div 0.007 = $ _____

   h. $0.81 \div 0.9 = $ _____

   i. $0.0138 \div 0.46 = $ _____

   j. $0.06 \div 0.6 = $ _____

Dividing Decimals by Ten or Any Power of Ten

Rule: When you divide by 10 or any multiple of 10, move the decimal point to the left in the dividend as many places as there are 0's in the divisor.

$$3.6 \div 10 = 0.36$$
$$(1)$$
$$3.6 \div 100 = 0.036$$
$$(2)$$
$$3.6 \div 1000 = 0.0036$$
$$(3)$$
$$3.6 \div 10,000 = 0.00036$$
$$(4)$$
$$3.6 \div 100,000 = 0.000036$$
$$(5)$$

To divide decimals by 10 or any power of 10, follow these steps:

1. When you divide by 10, move the decimal point one place to the left.

$$0.6 \div 10 =$$
$$.0.6 \div 10 = 0.06$$

2. When you divide by 100, move the decimal point two places to the left.

$$0.6 \div 100 =$$
$$.00.6 \div 100 = 0.006$$

3. When you divide by 1000, move the decimal point three places to the left.

$$0.6 \div 1000 =$$
$$.000.6 \div 1000 = 0.0006$$

4. When you divide by 10,000, move the decimal point four places to the left.

$$0.6 \div 10,000 =$$
$$.0000.6 \div 10,000 = 0.00006$$

5. When you divide by 100,000, move the decimal point five places to the left.

$$0.6 \div 100,000 =$$
$$.00000.6 \div 100,000 = 0.000006$$

● PRACTICE PROBLEM

9. Divide the following decimals by the powers of 10:

   a. $2.5 \div 100,000 = $ _____

   b. $10.4 \div 10,000 = $ _____

   c. $5.2 \div 1000 = $ _____

   d. $1.1 \div 100 = $ _____

   e. $0.3 \div 10 = $ _____

   f. $88.8 \div 10 = $ _____

   g. $0.150 \div 100 = $ _____

   h. $0.66 \div 100,000 = $ _____

   i. $0.7 \div 10,000 = $ _____

   j. $0.100 \div 1000 = $ _____

PERCENTAGE

Percent means per hundred. Its symbol, %, indicates that the preceding number is a percentage. The whole is expressed as 100 percent. Therefore, a certain percent indicates parts of 100. For example, 34% means $\frac{34}{100}$ or 0.34, or 340% means $\frac{340}{100}$ or 3.4 or $3\frac{2}{5}$. Since the strength of solutions is expressed in percentage, it is necessary for the nurse to be able to express percents as decimal fractions and common fractions. This is done by considering the percent sign as a denominator of 100, and then dividing the number by this 100.

- To express a percent as a fraction, remove the percent sign and write the percent as the numerator of a fraction. Write 100 as the denominator of the fraction and express the fraction in lowest terms.

  Example: $50\% = \dfrac{50}{100} = \dfrac{1}{2}$

- If the percent is a mixed number or a fraction, the numerator of the complex fraction is divided by the denominator (100). The process may be simplified by merely multiplying the percent by $\dfrac{1}{100}$.

  Examples: a. $5.5\% = 5\dfrac{1}{2}\% = \dfrac{5\frac{1}{2}}{100} = \dfrac{11}{2} \div 100$

  $$= \dfrac{11}{2} \times \dfrac{1}{100} = \dfrac{11}{200}$$

  b. $\dfrac{1}{4}\% = \dfrac{\frac{1}{4}}{100} = \dfrac{1}{4} \div 100$

  $$= \dfrac{1}{4} \times \dfrac{1}{100} = \dfrac{1}{400}$$

- To express a fraction as a percent, multiply by 100 and add the percent sign.

  Examples: a. $\dfrac{3}{4} = \dfrac{3}{\cancel{4}} \times \dfrac{\overset{25}{\cancel{100}}}{1} = 75\%$

  b. $\dfrac{29}{400} = \dfrac{29}{400} \times \dfrac{100}{1} = \dfrac{2900}{400} = \dfrac{29\cancel{00}}{4\cancel{00}}$

  $$= \dfrac{29}{4} = 7\dfrac{1}{4}\%$$

- To express a percent as a decimal, simply remove the percent sign and move the decimal point two places to the left. This is the same as dividing by 100. If the percent has a fraction, the fraction must be expressed in decimal form before the decimal point may be moved.

  Examples: $50\% = 0.5$ $5.5\% = 0.055$

  $\dfrac{1}{4}\% = 0.25\% = 0.0025$

- To express a decimal as a percent, move the decimal point two places to the right and add the percent sign. You are actually multiplying by 100.

  Examples: $0.3 = 30\%$ $0.35 = 35\%$

  $0.355 = 35.5\%$ $0.0355 = 3.55\%$

● PRACTICE PROBLEMS

10. Express the following common fractions as percents:

    a. $\dfrac{1}{4}$ = _____   d. $\dfrac{2}{3}$ = _____

    b. $\dfrac{1}{3}$ = _____   e. $\dfrac{3}{25}$ = _____

    c. $\dfrac{2}{5}$ = _____

11. Express the largest decimal in each of the following series as a percent:

    a. 0.001   1.25   1.09   _____
    b. 0.07   0.69   0.349   _____
    c. 0.08   0.8   0.185   _____
    d. 0.495   4.95   0.049   _____
    e. 0.125   0.005   0.025   _____

12. Change each of the following percents to a fraction and a decimal:

    a. 2%   _____ and _____
    b. $4\dfrac{3}{4}\%$ _____ and _____
    c. 40%   _____ and _____
    d. 19.3%   _____ and _____
    e. 64%   _____ and _____

DETERMINING QUANTITY IF A PERCENT IS GIVEN

- To find the percentage of a given number, express the percent as a decimal or fraction; multiply the whole number by the decimal or fraction.

  Example: How much is 5% of 48?

(Conversion to decimal)	*(Conversion to fraction)*
$5\% = 0.05$	$5\% = \dfrac{5}{100}$ or $\dfrac{1}{20}$
$48 \times 0.05 = 2.4$	
Note: $2.4 = 2\dfrac{2}{5}$	$48 \times \dfrac{1}{20} = \dfrac{48}{20} = 2\dfrac{8}{20} = 2\dfrac{2}{5}$

● PRACTICE PROBLEM

13. Solve each of the following problems and give the answer as a decimal and as a fraction:

Problem	*Decimal*	*Fraction*
a. How much is 20% of 36?	_____	_____
b. How much is 8% of 60?	_____	_____
c. How much is $\dfrac{1}{2}\%$ of 750?	_____	_____
d. How much is 350% of 15?	_____	_____
e. How much is 2% of 10?	_____	_____

● SELF-ASSESSMENT

This exercise is designed to assess your understanding of decimal fractions and percents. Complete the statements or follow the directions as provided.

1. All the numbers to the left of the decimal point are _____ numbers.

2. All the numbers to the right of the decimal point are _____ or _____ _____.

3. The value of each place left of the decimal point is _____ times that of the place to its right.

4. The value of each place right of the decimal point is _____ of the value of the place to its left.

5. Write out the following fractions, decimal fractions, whole numbers, and decimal fractions:

   a. $\frac{5}{10}$ _____   d. 0.00005 _____

   b. $\frac{10}{1000}$ _____   e. 2.25 _____

   c. 0.50 _____   f. 8.75 _____

6. Express the following as decimal fractions:

   a. $\frac{1}{3}$ _____   b. $\frac{1}{4}$ _____

7. Express the following as common fractions:

   a. 0.5 _____   b. 0.00005 _____

8. Add the following:

   a. 0.5 + 0.5 _____

   b. 0.98 + 0.76 _____

9. Subtract the following:

   a. 0.6 − 0.08 _____

   b. 9.123 − 6.055 _____

10. Multiply the following:

    a. 66.66 × 3.33 _____

    b. 1.1 × 100 _____

11. Divide the following:

    a. 0.018 ÷ 9 _____

    b. 0.04 ÷ 10 _____

    c. 86 ÷ 0.43 _____

    d. 60 ÷ 0.012 _____

    e. 0.06 ÷ 0.6 _____

    f. 0.49 ÷ 0.007 _____

12. Express the following as percents:

    a. $\frac{1}{3}$ _____   c. $\frac{2}{3}$ _____

    b. $\frac{1}{4}$ _____

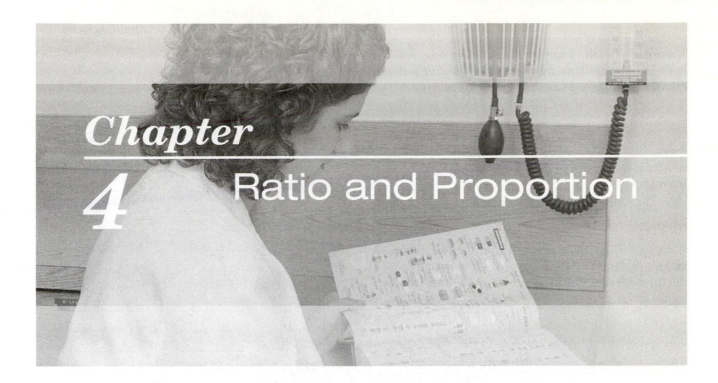

Chapter 4
Ratio and Proportion

Chapter Outline

Objectives
Key Terms
Introduction
Understanding Ratio
Understanding Proportion
Self-Assessment

- Work the practice problems correctly
- Complete the Self-Assessment

Key Terms

extremes	proportion
means	quotient
proof	ratio

Objectives

Upon completion of this chapter, you should be able to

- Define the key terms
- Express a ratio as a quotient, as a fraction, and as a decimal
- Name the four terms of a proportion
- State why the proportion is a useful mathematical tool
- Solve for x
- Solve for x when only a part of the term is unknown
- Solve for x when a fraction of the term is unknown
- Solve for x when decimals are used in the proportion
- Prove all of your answers

INTRODUCTION

Ratio and proportion are two mathematical concepts that are used to solve various types of problems. They may be used to determine an unknown number, quantity, substance, or degree between two similar components. Understanding ratio and proportion will enable you to accurately prepare and administer a variety of medications and treatments.

UNDERSTANDING RATIO

Ratio is a way of expressing the relationship of a number, quantity, substance, or degree between two similar components. For example, the relationship of one to five is written 1 : 5. Note that the numbers are side by side and separated by a colon.

In mathematics a ratio may be expressed as a quotient, a fraction, or a decimal.

Ratio Expressed as a Quotient

A **quotient** is the number found when one number is divided by another number. One is to five written as a quotient is $1 \div 5$.

Ratio Expressed as a Fraction

A fraction is the result of dividing or breaking a whole number into parts. One is to five written as a fraction is $\frac{1}{5}$.

Ratio Expressed as a Decimal

A decimal is a linear array of numbers based on 10 or any multiple of 10. To express one is to five as a decimal, divide the denominator (5) into the numerator (1).

$$\text{denominator} \quad 5\overline{)1.0}^{\,0.2} \quad \text{numerator}$$

The ratio 1 : 5 may be expressed as:		
A QUOTIENT	A FRACTION	A DECIMAL
$1 \div 5$	$\frac{1}{5}$	0.2

● PRACTICE PROBLEMS

Express the following numbers as ratios, quotients, fractions, or decimals and reduce to lowest terms when possible:

1. Express as a Ratio / Reduce to Lowest Terms

a. $\frac{1}{25}$ _____ _____

b. $\frac{2}{100}$ _____ _____

c. $\frac{10}{40}$ _____ _____

d. $\frac{25}{75}$ _____ _____

e. $\frac{8}{64}$ _____ _____

f. $\frac{1}{2}$ _____ _____

g. $\frac{1}{3}$ _____ _____

h. $\frac{1}{250}$ _____ _____

i. $\frac{6}{1000}$ _____ _____

j. $\frac{5}{2}$ _____ _____

2. Express as a Quotient / Reduce to Lowest Terms

a. 24 : 48 _____ _____

b. 12 : 6 _____ _____

c. 76 : 304 _____ _____

d. 5 : 25 _____ _____

e. 2 : 92 _____ _____

f. 18 : 108 _____ _____

g. 10 : 50 _____ _____

h. 17 : 51 _____ _____

i. 11 : 22 _____ _____

j. 55 : 165 _____ _____

3. Express as a Fraction / Reduce to Lowest Terms

a. 33 : 66 _____ _____

b. 4 : 10 _____ _____

c. 75 : 100 _____ _____

d. 22 : 88 _____ _____

e. 43 : 86 _____ _____

f. 2 : 13 _____ _____

g. 7 : 49 _____ _____

h. 4 : 100 _____ _____

i. 1 : 150 _____ _____

j. 12 : 36 _____ _____

4. Express as a Decimal / Reduce to Lowest Terms

a. 1 : 50 _____ _____

b. 8 : 100 _____ _____

c. 6 : 1000 _____ _____

d. 3 : 4 _____ _____

e. 1 : 500 _____ _____

f. 2 : 25 _____ _____

g. 5 : 4 _____ _____

h. 1 : 1000 _____ _____

i. 1 : 200 _____ _____

j. 1 : 2 _____ _____

UNDERSTANDING PROPORTION

Proportion is a way of expressing the comparative relationship between a part, share, or portion with regard to size, amount, or number. In mathematics, a proportion expresses the relationship between two ratios. In setting up a proportion, the ratios are separated by : : or an = sign. In this text, the equal sign (=) is used to separate ratios.

Example: $3:4 = 1:2$

Read: Three is to four equals one is to two.

The four terms of a proportion are given special names. The **means** are the inner numbers or the second and third terms of the proportion.

Example: $3:4 = 1:2$
      (4)   (1)
      means

The **extremes** are the outer numbers or the first and fourth terms of the proportion.

Example: $3:4 = 1:2$
      (3)   (2)
      extremes

In a *true* proportion, the product of the means equals the product of the extremes.

Example: *means*
      $8:16 = 1:2$
      extremes
      $16 \times 1 = 16$ (*means*)
      $8 \times 2 = 16$ (*extremes*)

Solving for x

The proportion is a very useful mathematical tool. When a part, share, or portion of the problem is unknown, x represents the unknown factor. You can determine the unknown by solving for x. The unknown factor x may appear any place in the proportion.

To solve for x in the problem $3:4 = x:12$, follow these steps:

1. Multiply the terms that contain the x and place the product to the left of the equal sign ($4x$).
2. Multiply the other terms and place the product to the right of the equal sign (36).
3. To find x, divide the product of x into the product of the other terms ($36 \div 4$).
4. Your answer will be equal to x (9).

Example: $3:4 = x:12$

      $4x = 36$
      $x = 36 \div 4 = 9$
      $x = 9$

After finding the unknown factor, check your mathematical skills by determining if you have a true proportion. This stage in resolving the accuracy of your work is called **proof** or *proving* your answer. To prove your answer,

1. Place the answer you found for x back into the formula where you once had x.
2. Multiply the *means* by the *means*, and the *extremes* by the *extremes*.
3. The results will equal each other.
   Example: Formula: $3:4 = x:12$
            Proof: $3:4 = 9:12$
                  $36 = 36$

● PRACTICE PROBLEM

5. Solve the following for x and prove your answers:

   a. $4:5 = x:10$ _____
   b. $25:x = 5:10$ _____
   c. $50:x = 25:1000$ _____
   d. $8:10 = x:30$ _____
   e. $4:8 = x:16$ _____
   f. $9:15 = x:5$ _____
   g. $500:x = 5:25$ _____
   h. $4:28 = x:84$ _____
   i. $9:x = 5:300$ _____
   j. $x:600 = 4:120$ _____

To solve for x when only a part of the term is unknown, as in $4:(x-2) = 6:3$, follow these steps:

1. Multiply the terms that contain the portion of x and place the product to the left of the equal sign.
2. Multiply the other terms and place the product to the right of the equal sign.
3. To find x when there is a negative (minus) or positive (plus) sign involved, change the sign as you transpose the number across the equal sign. A minus will become a plus, and a plus will become a minus.
4. To find x, divide the product of x into the product of the other terms.
5. Your answer will be equal to x.

   Example: $4:(x-2) = 6:3$
            $6(x-2) = 6x - 12$
            $6x - 12 = 4 \times 3 = 12$
            $6x - 12 = 12$
               $6x = 12 + 12 = 24$
               $6x = 24$
               $x = 24 \div 6$
               $x = 4$

6. Now prove your answer. Remember to multiply *means* by *means*, and *extremes* by *extremes*.

Proof:
$$4:(4-2) = 6:3$$
means $\quad (4-2) = 2 \times 6 = 12$
extremes $\quad 4 \times 3 = 12$
means $\quad 12 = extremes\ 12$
$$12 = 12$$

● **PRACTICE PROBLEM**

6. Solve the following for x and prove your answers:

a. $6:(x-10) = 1:6$ _____

b. $8:(x-4) = 2:6$ _____

c. $5:(x+4) = 4:40$ _____

d. $2:(x-2) = 4:24$ _____

e. $140:(x+10) = 1:100$ _____

f. $4:(x-6) = 2:6$ _____

g. $5:(x-32) = 5:9$ _____

h. $(x+40):25 = 150:30$ _____

i. $12:(x+3) = 6:9$ _____

j. $7:(x-14) = 2:28$ _____

To solve for x when a fraction of the term is unknown, as in $\frac{1}{2}x:1000 = 1:500$, follow these steps:

1. Multiply the fraction with the x by the appropriate term and place the product to the left of the equal sign.

2. Multiply the other terms and place the product to the right of the equal sign.

3. To find x, divide the product of x into the product of the other terms.

4. Your answer will be equal to x.

5. Prove your answer.

Example:
$$\frac{1}{2}x:1000 = 1:500$$
$$\frac{1}{2} \times \frac{500}{1} = 250$$
$$250x = 1000$$
$$x = 1000 \div 250 = 4$$
$$x = 4$$

Proof:
$$\frac{1}{2}\left(\times \frac{4}{1}\right) = 2$$
$$2:1000 = 1:500$$
$$1000 = 1000$$

● **PRACTICE PROBLEM**

7. Solve for x and prove your answers.

a. $\frac{1}{2}:x = 1:8$ _____

b. $\frac{1}{4}:x = 20:400$ _____

c. $\frac{1}{6}:\frac{5}{6} = 4:x$ _____

d. $\frac{1}{2}:1000 = x:500$ _____

e. $\frac{3}{4}:x = \frac{9}{10}:\frac{2}{3}$ _____

f. $\frac{1}{1000}:\frac{1}{100} = x:60$ _____

g. $\frac{1}{4}:500 = x:1000$ _____

h. $\frac{1}{1000}:\frac{1}{50} = x:60$ _____

i. $\frac{1}{10}x:2000 = 1:100$ _____

j. $\frac{1}{6}:1 = \frac{1}{8}:x$ _____

To solve for x when decimals are used in the formula, as in $0.6:0.4 = 9:x$, follow these steps:

1. Multiply the terms containing the x and place the product to the left of the equal sign. Remember the steps on multiplying decimals.

2. Multiply the other terms and place the product to the right of the equal sign.

3. To find x, divide the product of x into the product of the other terms. Remember your steps on how to divide decimals.

4. Your answer will be equal to x.

5. Prove your answer.

Example: $0.6:0.4 = 9:x$
$$0.6x = 3.6$$
$$x = 3.6 \div 0.6 \qquad 0.6\overline{)3.6} \quad \begin{array}{r}0.6\\ \hline\end{array}$$
$$x = 6 \qquad\qquad 3\,6$$

Proof: $0.6:0.4 = 9:x$
$$3.6 = 3.6$$

● **PRACTICE PROBLEM**

8. Solve for x and prove your answers.

a. $0.4:0.2 = 6:x$ _____

b. $0.2:4 = 25:x$ _____

c. $0.7:x = 70:500$ _____

d. $0.5:15 = x:60$ _____

e. $0.3:30 = 10:x$ _____

f. $0.7:70 = x:1000$ _____

g. $0.002:x = 0.4:100$ _____

h. $0.6:24 = 0.75:x$ _____

i. $0.2:8 = 25:x$ _____

j. $0.25:5 = x:100$ _____

● SELF-ASSESSMENT

This exercise is designed to assess your understanding of ratio and proportion. Follow the directions as provided.

1. Express the following numbers as a ratio, a quotient, a fraction, and a decimal:

	Ratio	Quotient	Fraction	Decimal
a. $\frac{1}{25}$	_____	_____	_____	_____
b. $12:6$	_____	_____	_____	_____
c. $33:66$	_____	_____	_____	_____
d. $1:50$	_____	_____	_____	_____
e. $\frac{25}{75}$	_____	_____	_____	_____

2. Solve for x in each of the following:

a. $\frac{1}{2}:x = 1:8$ $x =$ _____

b. $9:x = 5:300$ $x =$ _____

c. $\frac{1}{100}:\frac{1}{10} = x:6$ $x =$ _____

d. $\frac{1}{4}:500 = x:1000$ $x =$ _____

e. $36:12 = \frac{1}{100}:x$ $x =$ _____

f. $6:24 = 0.75:x$ $x =$ _____

g. $x:600 = 4:120$ $x =$ _____

h. $0.7:70 = x:1000$ $x =$ _____

i. $4:(x-6) = 2:6$ $x =$ _____

j. $6:12 = \frac{1}{4}:x$ $x =$ _____

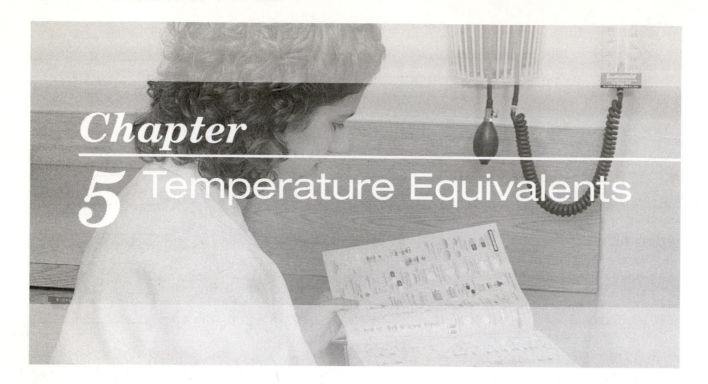

Chapter

5 Temperature Equivalents

Chapter Outline

Objectives

Upon completion of this chapter, you should be able to

● Define the key terms

● Change a temperature reading from Celsius to Fahrenheit

● Change a temperature reading from Fahrenheit to Celsius

● Work the practice problems correctly

● Complete the Self-Assessment

Key Terms

Celsius   Fahrenheit

INTRODUCTION

The normal human body temperature range is 97° to 99° Fahrenheit (F) and 36.1° to 37.2° Celsius (C). The average human body temperature is 98.6°F or 37° C.

A client's body temperature can be measured with a Fahrenheit, Celsius, or electronic thermometer. In the United States, both the Fahrenheit and Celsius scales are used; in some countries, the Celsius scale is preferred. See Figure 5-1.

The mercury thermometer was developed by Gabriel Fahrenheit. Using a mixture of salt and ice, Fahrenheit experimented with temperature. The coldest mixture he could make he called "zero." He noted that water froze at 32° and it boiled at 212°. The **Fahrenheit** temperature scale is based on Gabriel Fahrenheit's experiment with the freezing point of water at 32° and the boiling point at 212°.

Anders Celsius suggested a temperature scale based on the freezing point of water being 0° and its boiling point being 100°. The **Celsius** temperature scale is used in the metric system. This is a temperature scale with the freezing point of water at 0° and the boiling point at 100°.

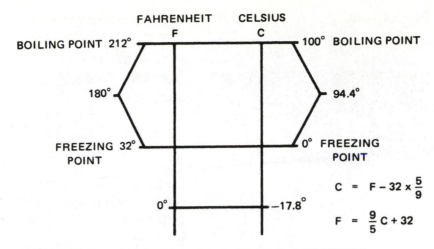

FIGURE 5-1   FAHRENHEIT AND CELSIUS TEMPERATURE EQUIVALENTS

MATHEMATICAL FORMULAS TO CONVERT TEMPERATURE

Five degrees on the Celsius scale corresponds to nine degrees on the Fahrenheit scale. Zero degrees on the Celsius scale corresponds to 32 degrees on the Fahrenheit scale. Several mathematical formulas are used to convert from one temperature scale to the other.

To convert a temperature from Fahrenheit to Celsius, subtract 32, multiply by 5, and divide by 9.

$$C = (F - 32) \times \frac{5}{9}$$

To convert a temperature from Celsius to Fahrenheit, multiply by 9, divide by 5, and add 32.

$$F = \frac{9 \times C}{5} + 32$$

● PRACTICE PROBLEM

1. Using the foregoing formulas, convert each of the following temperatures:

   a. 40°C = _____ F

   b. 35°C = _____ F

   c. 95°F = _____ C

   d. 99°F = _____ C

USING THE PROPORTIONAL METHOD TO CONVERT TEMPERATURE

Converting 37° Celsius to Fahrenheit

Formula: $C : (F - 32) = 5 : 9$

- Use the given formula for converting temperature.

- Substitute the known temperature in its proper place in the formula.

- Using the proportional method, solve for the unknown temperature.

   Problem: $37 : (F - 32) = 5 : 9$

Step 1.   Multiply the means by the means:

   $(F - 32) \times 5$
   $5\,F - 160$

Step 2. $5\,F - 160$ becomes the left side of the proportion: $5\,F - 160 =$

Step 3.   Multiply the extremes by the extremes:
   $37 \times 9 = 333$

Step 4.   333 becomes the right side of the proportion: $= 333$

Step 5.   Now, set up the proportion:
   $5\,F - 160 = 333$

Step 6. Solve for the unknown:

$$5\,F - 160 = 333$$
$$5\,F = 333 + 160$$
$$5\,F = 493$$
$$F = \frac{493}{5}$$
$$F = 98.6°$$

● You have converted 37° Celsius to 98.6° Fahrenheit.

Converting 98.6° Fahrenheit to Celsius

Formula: $C : (F - 32) = 5 : 9$

● Use the given formula for converting temperature.

● Substitute the known temperature in its proper place in the formula.

● Using the proportional method, solve for the unknown temperature.

Problem: $C : (98.6° - 32) = 5 : 9$

Step 1. Subtract: $98.6° - 32 = 66.6$

Step 2. Place 66.6 in the formula: $C : 66.6 = 5 : 9$

Step 3. Multiply the means by the means: $66.6 \times 5 = 333$

Step 4. $= 333$ becomes the right side of the proportion

Step 5. Multiply the extremes by the extremes: $C \times 9 = 9\,C$

Step 6. 9 C becomes the left side of the proportion: $9\,C =$

Step 7. Now, set up the proportion: $9\,C = 333$

Step 8. Solve for the unknown:

$$9\,C = 333$$
$$C = \frac{333}{9}$$
$$C = 37°$$

● You have converted 98.6° Fahrenheit to 37° Celsius.

● Prove your answer using the same process as proving any proportional answer.

$$C : (F - 32) = 5 : 9$$
$$37 : (98.6 - 32) = 5.9$$
$$333 = 333$$

● PRACTICE PROBLEM

2. Using the proportional method, convert each of the following temperatures:

   a. 102.2°F = _____ C

   b. 97.8°F = _____ C

   c. 99.6°F = _____ C

   d. 103°F = _____ C

   e. 104°F = _____ C

   f. 36°C = _____ F

   g. 37.2°C = _____ F

   h. 37.8°C = _____ F

   i. 38.3°C = _____ F

   j. 39°C = _____ F

● SELF-ASSESSMENT

This exercise is designed to assess your understanding of temperature equivalents. Write your answer in the space provided.

1. The normal human body temperature range is _____ to _____ Fahrenheit and _____ to _____ Celsius.

2. Boiling point on the Fahrenheit scale is _____ degrees.

3. Freezing point on the Celsius scale is _____ degrees.

4. Convert the following temperatures to Fahrenheit or Celsius:

   a. 99°F = _____ C

   b. 98.6°F = _____ C

   c. 101°F = _____ C

   d. 39°C = _____ F

   e. 36°C = _____ F

   f. 41°C = _____ F

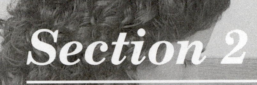

Section 2

CALCULATIONS OF DOSES AND SOLUTIONS

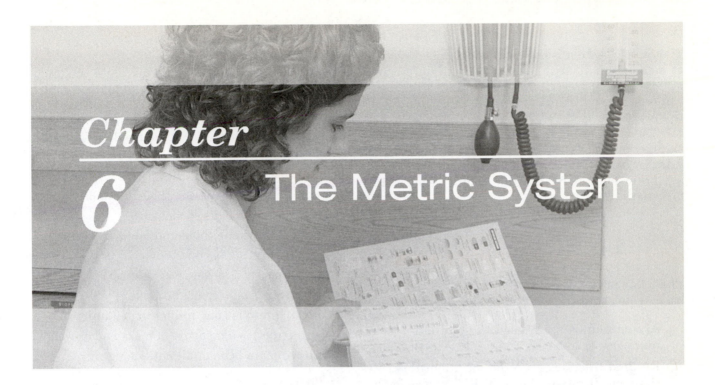

Chapter

6

The Metric System

Objectives

Upon completion of this chapter, you should be able to

- Define the key terms

- State why the metric system is used as the universal system of measurement

- List ten guidelines you will use as you work with the metric system

- Name the seven common prefixes used in the metric system

- Name the fundamental units of the metric system

- State why you place a zero before the decimal point

- Write the metric equivalents for length, volume, mass, and weight

- Write the abbreviations for the metric equivalents of length, volume, mass, and weight

- Name the metric equivalents that are most frequently used in the medical field

- Use the proportional method to convert from one metric unit to another

- Use moving the decimal method to convert from one metric unit to another

- Work the practice problems correctly

- Complete the Self-Assessment

Key Terms

conversion	meter
grain	microgram
gram	milliliter
kiloliter	millimeter
liter	minim

INTRODUCTION

The metric system is the most widely used system of measurement in the world. It is the preferred system used in prescribing and administering medications. It is a decimal system based on 10 or multiples of 10.

The language of the metric system is a simple, flexible, and accurate form of communication. The primary units of measurement of the metric system are gram for weight, liter for volume, and meter for length.

METRIC SYSTEM GUIDELINES

The following guidelines will help you as you learn basic facts about the metric system:

1. Arabic numbers are used to designate whole numbers: 1, 250, 500, 1000, and so forth.

2. Decimal fractions are used for quantities less than one: 0.1, 0.01, 0.001, 0.0001, and so forth.

3. To insure accuracy, place a zero before the decimal point: 0.1, 0.001, 0.0001, and so forth.

4. The Arabic number precedes the metric unit of measurement: 10 grams, 2 milliliters, 5 liters, and so forth.

5. The abbreviation for gram should be written as g.

6. The abbreviation for liter is capitalized L.

7. Prefixes are written in lowercase letters: milli, centi, deci, deka, and so forth.

8. Capitalize the measurement and symbol when it is named after a person: Celsius (C).

9. Periods are no longer used with most abbreviations or symbols.

10. Abbreviations for units are the same for singular and plural. An "s" is not added to indicate a plural.

THE LANGUAGE OF THE METRIC SYSTEM

In the metric system, 14 prefixes are used to denote the size of a metric unit. Each prefix is based upon a multiple or submultiple of 10. These prefixes are tera, giga, mega, kilo, hecto, deka, deci, centi, milli, micro, nano, pico, femto, and atto. You will not have to learn all 14 prefixes; however, you will need to know the 7 common metric prefixes that are used in the medical field.

The Seven Common Metric Prefixes

Study the following list of prefixes. Once you know these prefixes, you will have a solid foundation for determining metric equivalents. When you combine a metric prefix with a root of physical quantity, you will know the multiples or submultiples of the metric system.

Example:

milli (prefix) means one thousandth of a unit

meter (root) means to measure

millimeter is one thousandth of a meter

kilo (prefix) means one thousand units

liter (root) is a measure of volume

kiloliter is one thousand liters

micro (prefix) is one millionth of a unit

gram (root) is a measure of mass and/or weight

microgram is one millionth of a gram

Prefixes:

micro (mi′kro) = one millionth of a unit
written as 0.000001

milli (mil′i) = one thousandth of a unit
written as 0.001

centi (sen′ti) = one hundredth of a unit
written as 0.01

deci (des′i) = one tenth of a unit
written as 0.1

deka (dek′a) = ten units
written as 10

hecto (hek′to) = one hundred units
written as 100

kilo (kil′o) = one thousand units
written as 1000

FUNDAMENTAL UNITS

The following are the fundamental units of the metric system:

meter (m)—length

liter (L)—volume

gram (g)—weight

The **meter** is the fundamental unit of length in the metric system and originally formed the foundation for the entire system (Table 6-1). A meter is equal to 39.37 inches, which is slightly more than a yard, or 3.28 feet.

A **millimeter** is one thousandth of a meter. It is about the width of the head of a pin. It takes ap-

TABLE 6-1   FUNDAMENTAL UNIT OF LENGTH

Meter (m)	=	Length
1 millimeter (mm)	=	0.001 of a meter
1 centimeter (cm)	=	0.01 of a meter
1 decimeter (dm)	=	0.1 of a meter
1 meter (m)	=	1 meter
1 dekameter (dam)	=	10 meters
1 hectometer (hm)	=	100 meters
1 kilometer (km)	=	1000 meters

TABLE 6-3   FUNDAMENTAL UNIT OF WEIGHT

Gram (g)	=	Weight
1 microgram (mcg, μg)	=	0.000001 gram
1 milligram (mg)	=	0.001 of a gram
1 centigram (cg)	=	0.01 of a gram
1 decigram (dg)	=	0.1 of a gram
1 gram (g)	=	1 gram
1 dekagram (dag)	=	10 grams
1 hectogram (hg)	=	100 grams
1 kilogram (kg)	=	1000 grams

TABLE 6-2   FUNDAMENTAL UNIT OF VOLUME

Liter (L)	=	Volume
1 milliliter (ml)	=	0.001 of a liter
1 centiliter (cl)	=	0.01 of a liter
1 deciliter (dl)	=	0.1 of a liter
1 liter (L)	=	1 liter
1 dekaliter (dal)	=	10 liters
1 hectoliter (hl)	=	100 liters
1 kiloliter (kl)	=	1000 liters

TABLE 6-4   METRIC EQUIVALENTS

Length
2.5 centimeters (cm) = 1 inch (in.)

Volume
1000 milliliters (ml) or
1000 cubic centimeters (cc) = 1 liter (L)

Weight	
1000 micrograms (mcg)	= 1 milligram (mg)
1000 milligrams (mg)	= 1 gram (g)
1000 grams (g)	= 1 kilogram (kg)
1 kilogram	= 2.2 pounds (lb)

proximately $2\frac{1}{2}$ centimeters to make an inch; a decimeter is approximately 4 inches.

The **liter** is the metric unit of volume (Table 6-2). A liter is equal to 1.056 quarts, which is 0.26 of a gallon, or 2.1 pints.

A **milliliter** is equivalent to one cubic centimeter (cc), because the amount of space occupied by a milliliter is equal to one cubic centimeter. The weight of one milliliter of water equals approximately one gram. It takes approximately 15 milliliters to make one tablespoon.

A **minim** is a small amount of liquid measure. It takes 15 or 16 minims to make one milliliter or one cubic centimeter. A minim is equal to 1/60 of a fluidram, or 0.00376 of a cubic inch.

The **gram** is the metric unit of weight. (Table 6-3). It equals approximately the weight of one cubic centimeter, or one milliliter of water. A gram is equal to approximately 15 grains, or 0.035 of an ounce.

A **grain** is the smallest unit of weight used in the United States and Great Britain. It is equal to 0.0648 of a gram, which was originally the weight of a grain of wheat.

Metric equivalents most frequently used in the medical field are shown in Table 6-4.

● **PRACTICE PROBLEMS**

Write your answer in the space provided.

1. The fundamental units of the metric system are
   a. _____ length   c. _____ weight
   b. _____ volume

2. Write the name of the prefix for each of the following:
   a. _____ one thousand units
   b. _____ one tenth of a unit
   c. _____ one millionth of a unit
   d. _____ one hundred units
   e. _____ one thousandth of a unit
   f. _____ ten units
   g. _____ one hundredth of a unit

3. _____ _____ are used for quantities less than one.

4. To insure accuracy, place a _____ before the decimal point.

5. A meter is equal to _____ inches.

6. Write in the correct equivalent for each of the following:

   a. 1 mm = _____   e. 1 dam = _____

   b. 1 cm = _____   f. 1 hm = _____

   c. 1 dm = _____   g. 1 km = _____

   d. 1 m = _____

7. It takes approximately _____ centimeters to make an inch.

8. A liter is equal to _____ quarts.

9. It takes _____ or _____ minims to make one milliliter.

10. A gram equals approximately the weight of _____ _____ _____ or _____ _____ of water.

11. Write in the correct equivalent for each of the following:

    a. 1 ml = _____ L   e. 1 dal = _____ L

    b. 1 cl = _____ L   f. 1 hl = _____ L

    c. 1 dl = _____ L   g. 1 kl = _____ L

    d. 1 L = _____ L

12. A gram is equal to approximately _____ grains or _____ of an ounce.

13. Write in the correct equivalent for each of the following:

    a. mcg, μg = _____ g   e. 1 g = _____ g

    b. 1 mg = _____ g   f. 1 dag = _____ g

    c. 1 cg = _____ g   g. 1 hg = _____ g

    d. 1 dg = _____ g   h. 1 kg = _____ g

14. Name the metric equivalents that are most frequently used in the medical field. Start with the smallest and go to the largest.

    Volume

    a. _____   b. _____

    Weight

    a. _____   c. _____

    b. _____   d. _____

15. Write the correct abbreviation and unit of measurement for each of the following:

    a. one gram _____

    b. twenty-five hundredths of a liter _____

    c. two hundred milligrams _____

    d. two tenths of a milliliter _____

    e. twelve kilograms _____

16. Write in the abbreviation for the unit that makes the equivalent correct.

    a. 1000 ml = 1 _____

    b. 2000 mg = 2 _____

    c. 1000 mcg, μg = 1 _____

    d. 2 kg = 4.4 _____

    e. 0.5 g = 500 _____

CONVERSION

The process of changing into another form, state, substance, or product is known as **conversion**. In the metric system, changing from one unit to another involves multiplying or dividing by 10, 100, 1000, and so forth. This can be done by the proportional method or by moving the decimal in the correct direction.

Proportional Method for Converting Metric Equivalents

There are six basic steps in the proportional method, plus an additional step to prove your answer. The following example will serve as a model for future applications of the proportional method of converting metric equivalents. Study this example and then proceed to the practice problem.

Converting 1500 milligrams to grams.

1500 mg = _____ g

Step 1. Since the unknown factor in the given formula is the number of grams contained in 1500 milligrams, you will substitute the symbol x for grams in the equation.

Step 2. Setting up the proportion requires that you know your metric equivalents. For example, in this problem you have to know that 1000 milligrams (mg) = 1 gram (g).

Step 3. Since you know that 1000 mg is equal to 1 g, you can create one-half of the equation. Write the equivalent that you know and place it on the left of the equal sign.

1000 mg : 1 g =

Step 4. Now that you have the left side of the equation, set up the right side by using the designated metric value 1500 mg : x g. Always write the smallest equivalent as to the largest equivalent: mg : g. By being consistent, you will be less likely to make errors.

1000 mg : 1 g = 1500 mg : x g

Step 5. Note that you have an equal equation: mg : g = mg : g. The first values on either side of the equal sign are milligrams, and the second values on either side are grams.

Step 6. Now solve for the unknown (x) by multiplication and division. Remember, multiply the means by the means and the extremes by the extremes.

> **Note:** Once you have the proportion correctly set up, you may simply use the numbers as you multiply and divide.

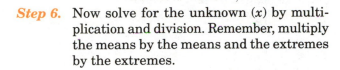

$$1000 : 1 = 1500 : x$$
$$1000x = 1500$$
$$x = 1500 \div 1000$$
$$x = 1.5$$

$$\begin{array}{r} 1.5 \\ 1000\overline{)1500.0} \\ \underline{1000} \\ 500\ 0 \\ \underline{500\ 0} \end{array}$$

Step 7. To make sure that you have a correct answer, prove your work: Place your answer 1.5 g into the formula where you once had x. Now multiply the means by the means and the extremes by the extremes.

$$1000 \text{ mg} : 1 \text{ g} = 1500 \text{ mg} : 1.5 \text{ g}$$
$$1500 = 1500$$

● PRACTICE PROBLEM

1. Using the proportional method, convert each of the following metric equivalents:

   a. 250 ml = _____ L
   b. 0.5 L = _____ ml
   c. 2 g = _____ mg
   d. 500 mg = _____ g
   e. 0.0300 g = _____ mg
   f. 0.05 mg = _____ g
   g. 1 mcg, μg = _____ mg
   h. 2 ml = _____ cc
   i. 1000 g = _____ kg
   j. 2 kg = _____ lb

Moving the Decimal Method for Converting Selected Metric Equivalents

Four basic steps are used to move the decimal in the correct direction. It is essential that you understand the following concepts. Study this example and then proceed to the practice problem.

Converting 2.5 grams to milligrams.

$$2.5 \text{ g} = \underline{\hspace{2cm}} \text{ mg}$$

Step 1. Establish the placement of the decimal in the unit that is to be converted to another unit.

convert 2.5 g to mg

Step 2. Determine if you are converting a larger unit to a smaller unit or a smaller unit to a larger unit.

convert g (larger) unit to mg (smaller) unit

Step 3. When converting from a larger unit to a smaller unit, you multiply by 1000, which is the same as moving the decimal point three places to the right.

Larger unit	$\dfrac{\times}{\text{multiply}}$	to smaller unit
milligram		microgram
gram		milligram
liter		milliliter
kilogram		gram

Convert: 2.5 g to _____ mg

Multiply

Moving the decimal point

$$\begin{array}{r} 2.5 \\ \times\ 1000 \\ \hline 2500.0 \end{array}$$

2.500.

1,2,3 places to the right

Step 4. When converting a smaller unit to a larger unit, you divide by 1000, which is the same as moving the decimal point three places to the left.

Smaller unit	$\dfrac{\div}{\text{divide}}$	to larger unit
microgram		milligram
milligram		gram
milliliter		liter
gram		kilogram

Convert: 2500 mg to _____ g

Divide

Moving the decimal point

$$\begin{array}{r} 2.5 \\ 1000\overline{)2500.0} \\ \underline{2000} \\ 500\ 0 \\ \underline{500\ 0} \end{array}$$

2500. 2.500.

3,2,1 places to the left

● PRACTICE PROBLEM

2. Using the moving the decimal method, convert each of the following metric equivalents:

   a. 60 mg = _____ g

   b. 0.005 L = _____ ml

   c. 200 ml = _____ L

   d. 1 g = _____ kg

   e. 0.0065 g = _____ mg

   f. 3.5 cc = _____ L

   g. 4 kg = _____ g

   h. 1 ml = _____ L

   i. 0.1 L = _____ ml

   j. 0.05 mg = _____ g

CALCULATING DOSAGE ACCORDING TO KILOGRAM OF BODY WEIGHT

It may be your responsibility to calculate the amount of dosage ordered by the physician according to the client's body weight. Today, many medications are ordered in this manner; therefore, it is essential that you learn how to calculate dosage according to this method. The following example will guide you step by step through the mathematical process of calculating dosage according to kilogram of body weight.

Remember there are 2.2 pounds in one kilogram.

Example: The physician ordered an anti-epileptic agent, Depakene (valproic acid) 15 mg/kg/day capsules for Clark McGee, who weighs 110 pounds. The medication is to be given in three divided doses.

Step 1. To express pounds in kilograms, divide the weight in pounds by 2.2.

Convert the client's weight to kilograms.

$110 \div 2.2 = 50$ kilograms

Step 2. Now, calculate the prescribed dosage by placing 50 in the appropriate place.

15 mg/50/day

$15 \times 50 = 750$ mg/day

Step 3. To determine the amount of each dose, divide 750 by 3 (divided doses).

$750 \div 3 = 250$ mg per dose

> Depakene is available in 250 mg capsules and 250 mg/5 ml syrup. The physician ordered the medication in capsules, so Clark will receive a 250 mg capsule every 8 hours.

Using the Proportional Method to Calculate Kilogram of Body Weight

Example: The physician ordered an anti-epileptic agent, Depakene (valproic acid) 15 mg/kg/day capsules for Clark McGee, who weighs 110 pounds. The medication is to be given in three divided doses.

Step 1. To convert 110 pounds to kilograms, set up the proportion as follows:

2.2 lb : 1 kg = 110 lb : x kg

Step 2. Now, solve for x.

$2.2 : 1 = 110 : x$

$2.2x = 110$

$x = 50$

Step 3. Now, calculate the prescribed dosage by placing 50 in the appropriate place.

15 mg/50 kg/day

$15 \times 50 = 750$ mg/day

Step 4. To determine the amount of each dose, divide 750 by 3 (divided doses).

$750 \div 3 = 250$ mg per dose

● PRACTICE PROBLEMS

3. Convert the following:

   a. 184 lb = _____ kilograms

   b. 210 lb = _____ kilograms

   c. 85 lb = _____ kilograms

   d. 54 lb = _____ kilograms

   ● To express kilograms as pounds, multiply the kilogram weight by 2.2

   Example: 25 kilograms × 2.2 = 55 lb

4. Convert the following:

   a. 30 kilograms = _____ lb

   b. 45 kilograms = _____ lb

   c. 65 kilograms = _____ lb

   d. 75 kilograms = _____ lb

5. The physician ordered Moxam (moxalactam disodium) 50 mg/kg every 6–8 hours, IM, for a pediatric client who weighs 88 pounds. Convert pounds to kilograms and then calculate the prescribed dosage.

6. The physician ordered Amoxil (amoxicillin) capsules 20 mg/kg/day in divided doses every 8 hours for a pediatric client who weighs 66 pounds. Convert pounds to kilograms and then calculate the prescribed dosage.

7. The physician ordered Garamycin (gentamicin sulfate) 3 mg/kg/day in three equal doses every 8 hours, IM, for a client who weighs 176 pounds. Convert pounds to kilograms and then calculate the prescribed dosage.

8. The physician ordered Lanoxin (digoxin) tablets 10 mg/kg as a rapid digitalization dose given as 50% of the dose initially and additional fractions given at 4–8 hr intervals for a client who weighs 154 pounds. Convert pounds to kilograms and then calculate the prescribed dosage.

9. The physician ordered Zovirax (acyclovir) capsules 5 mg/kg every 8 hours times 7 days for a client diagnosed with herpes zoster. The client weighs 132 pounds. Convert pounds to kilograms and then calculate the prescribed dosage.

10. The physician ordered Rocephin (ceftriaxone sodium) 50 mg/kg in two divided doses for a pediatric client who weighs 44 pounds. Convert pounds to kilograms and then calculate the prescribed dosage.

● **SELF-ASSESSMENT**

This exercise is designed to assess your understanding of the metric system. Write your answer in the space provided.

1. The fundamental units of the metric system are
   a. _____ length   c. _____ weight
   b. _____ volume

2. Write the prefix for each of the following:
   a. _____ one thousand units
   b. _____ one tenth of a unit
   c. _____ one millionth of a unit
   d. _____ one hundred units
   e. _____ one thousandth of a unit
   f. _____ ten units
   g. _____ one hundredth of a unit

3. It takes approximately _____ centimeters to make an inch.

4. A liter is equal to _____ quarts.

5. It takes _____ or _____ minims to make one milliliter.

6. Write in the abbreviation for the unit that makes the equivalent correct.
   a. 1000 ml = 1 _____
   b. 2000 mg = 2 _____
   c. 1000 mcg = 1 _____
   d. 2 kg = 4.4 _____
   e. 0.5 g = 500 _____

7. Convert each of the following metric equivalents:
   a. 1 mcg = _____ mg
   b. 4 g = _____ kg
   c. 5 kg = _____ g
   d. 0.2 L = _____ ml
   e. 1 ml = _____ L
   f. 3.5 mg = _____ g

8. Convert the following pounds to kilograms:
   a. 176 lb = _____ kg
   b. 100 lb = _____ kg
   c. 64 lb = _____ kg

9. The physician ordered Aquachloral (chloral hydrate) 25 mg/kg for a pediatric client who weighs 55 pounds. Convert pounds to kilograms and then calculate the prescribed dosage.

10. The physician ordered Chloromycetin (chloramphenicol sodium) 50 mg/kg/day in divided doses at 6-hour intervals. The client weighs 110 pounds. Convert pounds to kilograms and then calculate the prescribed dosage.

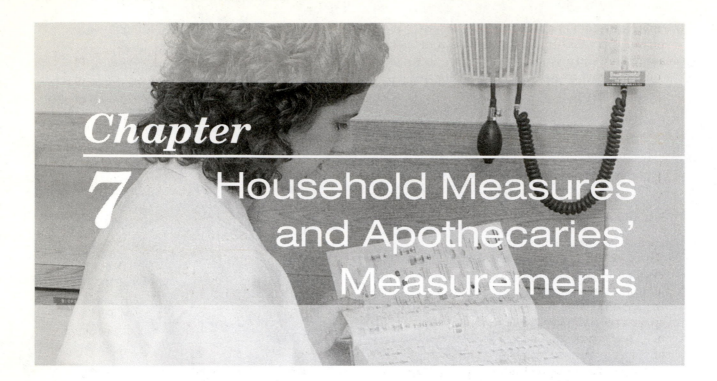

Chapter

7 Household Measures and Apothecaries' Measurements

Chapter Outline

- State the household approximate equivalents and the apothecaries' measurements that are given in this chapter
- Use the proportional method to convert household and apothecaries' measurements
- Work the practice problems correctly
- Complete the Self-Assessment

Key Terms

apothecaries'
    measurements
bore

household measures
viscosity

Objectives

Upon completion of this chapter, you should be able to

- Define the key terms
- Explain why a working knowledge of household measures and apothecaries' measurements is important
- List five factors that may vary or alter the size of a drop
- Write the abbreviations of the household measures and the apothecaries' measurements

INTRODUCTION

The apothecary system was the first system of medication measurement used by apothecaries (pharmacists) and physicians. It originated in Greece and made its way to Europe via Rome and France. The English used this system during the late 1600s and the colonists brought it to America. The household system of measurement is a modified system evolved from the apothecaries' system. Large liquid volumes were based on familiar trading measurements, such as pints, quarts, and gallons, which originated as apothecaries' measurements. Although the metric system is a more precise system of measurement, the apothecaries' system and household measurements are still being used on occasion in the ordering and measuring of medications.

HOUSEHOLD MEASURES

Household measures are more frequently used in the home than in the medical field. However, it may be your responsibility to instruct clients about preparing solutions for gargles, enemas, or douches, and your understanding of household equivalents will assist you in this matter.

Household measures are approximate measurements. Most household measuring devices lack standardization, and they are not accurate for measuring medications. For example, there are 3 or 4 teaspoons per tablespoon, depending upon the reference source and the size of each utensil. A teaspoon may vary in size from 4 to 5 milliliters or more. The American Standards Institute (ASI) has set the standards for an American teaspoon at 5 milliliters. In this text, the American standard is used.

When the physician orders a medication to be dispensed by drops, instruct the client and/or family to use the dropper that comes with the medicine. The size of a drop depends upon the following factors:

- The dropper size depends upon the diameter of the **bore** (the interior or diameter of a tube or needle; a hole); therefore, the size of the drop may vary due to the size of the hole.

- The angle at which the dropper is held may vary the size of the drop. For example, when you hold the dropper at a 90° angle, you will have a more uniform drop than if you hold the dropper at a 60° angle.

- The pressure used to squeeze the dropper may alter the number and size of the drop.

- The type or **viscosity** (the state of being thick and sticky) of the liquid being dispensed may alter the size of the drop.

- The temperature of the liquid being dispensed may alter the size of the drop.

HOUSEHOLD ABBREVIATIONS AND EQUIVALENTS

Household abbreviations (Table 7-1), household equivalents (Table 7-2), and common household measures (Table 7-3) should be learned before you proceed to the practice problems.

TABLE 7-1   HOUSEHOLD ABBREVIATIONS

drop (drops)	gtt	pint	pt
teaspoon	t or tsp	quart	qt
tablespoon	T or tbsp	gallon	gal
teacup	tcp	ounce	oz
cup	C		

TABLE 7-2   HOUSEHOLD EQUIVALENTS

60 gtt	=	1 t or tsp		
3 t or tsp	=	1 T		
180 gtt	=	1 T	=	$\frac{1}{2}$ oz
2 T	=	1 oz	=	6 t or tsp
360 gtt	=	2 T		
1 oz	=	30 cc or 30 ml		
6 oz	=	1 tcp		
8 oz	=	1 C or 1 glass		
2 C	=	1 pt	=	16 oz
2 pt	=	1 qt	=	32 oz
4 C	=	1 qt	=	32 oz
4 qt	=	1 gal	=	128 oz

TABLE 7-3   COMPARING HOUSEHOLD UNITS

Drop (gtt) = approximate liquid measure depending on kind of liquid measured and the size of the opening from which it is dropped	
60 drops	1 teaspoon (t or tsp)
1 dash	Less than $\frac{1}{8}$ teaspoon
3 teaspoons	1 tablespoon (T or tbsp)
2 tablespoons	1 ounce (oz)
4 ounces	1 juice glass
6 ounces	1 teacup
8 ounces	1 glass or cup
16 tablespoons or 8 ounces	1 measuring cup (c)
2 cups	1 pint (pt)
2 pints	1 quart (qt)
4 quarts	1 gallon (gal)

Comparing Household Units

Figure 7-1 illustrates the progression of the various units of volume in the household system of measurement.

● PRACTICE PROBLEMS

Write your answer in the space provided.

1. Write the abbreviation for each of the following:

   a. _____ drops   f. _____ cup

   b. _____ teaspoon   g. _____ pint

   c. _____ tablespoon   h. _____ quart

   d. _____ ounce   i. _____ gallon

   e. _____ teacup

2. Indicate the smallest to the largest household measurement by placing a number from one to nine in the appropriate space. One will be placed in the space by the smallest measurement, two will be placed by the measurement that is larger than one, and so on.

   a. tablespoon _____   f. teaspoon_____

   b. cup _____   g. teacup _____

   c. drop _____   h. pint _____

   d. ounce _____   i. gallon _____

   e. quart _____

3. Write in the correct abbreviation for each of the following:

   a. 180 _____ = 3 tsp

   b. 1 _____ = $\frac{1}{60}$ tsp

   c. 2 _____ = 1 oz

   d. 1 _____ = 6 tsp

   e. 6 _____ = 1 tcp

   f. 16 _____ = 2 C

   g. 4 _____ = 2 pt

   h. 2 _____ = $\frac{1}{2}$ gal

   i. 32 _____ = 1 qt

   j. 1 _____ = 16 oz

PROPORTIONAL METHOD FOR CONVERTING HOUSEHOLD MEASUREMENTS

Converting 2 tablespoons to teaspoons:

2 T = _____ tsp

Step 1. Setting up the proportion requires that you know your household measurements. For example, in this problem you have to know that 3 teaspoons equal 1 tablespoon.

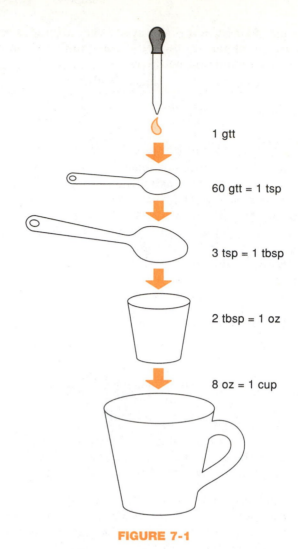

1 gtt

60 gtt = 1 tsp

3 tsp = 1 tbsp

2 tbsp = 1 oz

8 oz = 1 cup

FIGURE 7-1

Step 2. Since you know that 3 tsp = 1 T, you can create one-half of the equation. Write the equivalent that you know and place it on the left of the equal sign.

3 tsp : 1 T =

Step 3. Now that you have the left side of the equation, set up the right side by using the designated household measures: x tsp : 2 T. Always write the smallest equivalent as to the largest equivalent: tsp : T. By being consistent, you will be less likely to make errors.

3 tsp : 1 T = x tsp : 2 T

Step 4. Note that you have an equal equation tsp:T = tsp:T. The first values on both sides of the equal sign are teaspoons, and the second values on both sides are tablespoons.

Step 5. Now solve for the unknown (x) by multiplication and division. Remember, multiply the means by the means and the extremes by the extremes. Divide the number on the left of the equal sign into the number on the right.

$$3 \text{ tsp} : 1 \text{ T} = x \text{ tsp} : 2 \text{ T}$$
$$1x = 6 \text{ tsp}$$
$$x = 6$$

Step 6. To make sure that you have a correct answer, prove your work: Place your answer, 6 tsp, into the formula where you once had x. Now multiply the means by the means and the extremes by the extremes.

$$3 \text{ tsp} : 1 \text{ T} = 6 \text{ tsp} : 2 \text{ T}$$
$$6 = 6$$

Four-Step Conversion

Converting 3 tablespoons to drops:
3 T = _____ gtt

Step 1. Setting up the proportion requires that you know your household measurements. For example, in this problem you need to know that 60 drops equal 1 teaspoon, and 3 teaspoons equal 1 tablespoon.

Step 2. In the four-step conversion, you will first find out how many drops are in 3 teaspoons. Since you know that 60 gtt = 1 tsp, set up the proportion as follows:

$$60 \text{ gtt} : 1 \text{ tsp} = x \text{ gtt} : 3 \text{ tsp}$$
$$1x = 180 \text{ gtt}$$
$$x = 180 \text{ gtt}$$

Step 3. Since 3 teaspoons are equal to 1 tablespoon, 180 gtt are equal to 1 T. Now use this measurement to set up the second proportion.

$$180 \text{ gtt} : 1 \text{ T} = x \text{ gtt} : 3 \text{ T}$$
$$1x = 540 \text{ gtt}$$
$$x = 540 \text{ gtt}$$

You have determined that there are 540 gtt in 3 T.

Step 4. Prove your answer.

$$180 \text{ gtt} : 1 \text{ T} = 540 \text{ gtt} : 3 \text{ T}$$
$$540 = 540$$

● PRACTICE PROBLEM

1. Using the proportional method, convert each of the following household equivalents:

a. $2\frac{1}{2}$ tsp = _____ gtt

b. 10 oz = _____ pt

c. 12 T = _____ oz

d. $2\frac{1}{2}$ T = _____ tsp

e. 20 oz = _____ qt

f. 320 T = _____ oz

g. 1 oz = _____ gtt

h. $1\frac{1}{2}$ pt = _____ C

i. 4 tcp = _____ qt

j. $2\frac{1}{2}$ qt = _____ oz

APOTHECARIES' MEASUREMENTS

Apothecaries' measurements (a system of weights and measures based on 480 grains equals one ounce, and 12 ounces equal one pound) are rarely used today, but they must be included in a textbook as a reference for anyone who has a need to understand this system of measurement. You will note that some of the apothecaries' measurements are also used as household measures. However, in the apothecaries' system, 12 ounces is equal to one pound, whereas in the household system 16 ounces is equal to one pound.

Units of Weight and Liquid Volume

Tables 7-4 and 7-5 show the units of weight and liquid measurements of the apothecaries' system.

TABLE 7-4 APOTHECARIES' UNITS OF WEIGHT

60 grains (gr)	= 1 dram (dr) ʒ
8 drams (dr)	= 1 ounce (oz) ʒ
12 ounces (oz)	= 1 pound (lb)

TABLE 7-5 APOTHECARIES' UNITS OF LIQUID VOLUME

60 minims (♏)	= 1 fluidram (fldr)
8 fluidrams (fldr)	= 1 fluidounce (floz)
16 fluidounces (floz)	= 1 pint (pt)
2 pints (pt)	= 1 quart (qt)
4 quarts (qt)	= 1 gallon (gal)

PROPORTIONAL METHOD FOR CONVERTING APOTHECARIES' EQUIVALENTS

Converting 4 ounces to drams: 4 oz = _____ dr

Step 1. Setting up the proportion requires that you know the apothecaries' measurements. For example, in this problem you need to know that 8 drams is equal to 1 ounce.

Step 2. Since you know that 8 dr = 1 oz, you can create one-half of the equation. Write the equivalent that you know and place it on the left of the equal sign.

8 dr : 1 oz =

Step 3. Now that you have the left side of the equation, set up the right side by using the designated apothecaries' measures: x dr : 4 oz. Always write the smallest equivalent as to the largest equivalent.

8 dr : 1 oz = x dr : 4 oz

Step 4. Note that you have an equal equation:

dr : oz = dr : oz.

Step 5. Now solve for the unknown (x) by multiplication and division. Remember, multiply the means by the means and the extremes by the extremes. Divide the number on the left of the equal sign into the number on the right.

8 dr : 1 oz = x dr : 4 oz
$1x$ = 32 oz
x = 32 oz

Step 6. Prove your answer.

8 dr : 1 oz = 32 dr : 4 oz
32 = 32

● PRACTICE PROBLEM

2. Using the proportional method, convert each of the following apothecaries' equivalents:

a. 8 drams = _____ grains

b. $\frac{3}{4}$ dram = _____ grains

c. 3 ounces = _____ drams

d. 45 minims = _____ fluidrams

e. 3 pints = _____ quarts

f. 1 grain = _____ dram

g. 4 drams = _____ ounce(s)

h. $\frac{1}{2}$ pound = _____ ounces

i. $\frac{3}{4}$ pint = _____ quart

j. $\frac{1}{2}$ pint = _____ quart

TABLE 7-6 APPROXIMATE EQUIVALENTS AMONG METRIC, APOTHECARIES', AND HOUSEHOLD SYSTEMS

Metric	Apothecaries'	Household
Dry		
60 mg* =	1 gr	
1 g =	15 gr	
15 g =	4 dr	= 1 tbsp (3 tsp)
30 g =	1 oz (8 dr)	= 1 oz (2 tbsp)
	16 oz	= 1 lb (avoirdupois)
1 kg =		= 2.2 lb
Liquid		
1 ♏		= 1 gtt
1 ml =	15 ♏	= 15 gtt
4 ml =	1 dr	
5 ml* =	75 ♏	= 1 tsp
15 ml =	4 dr	= 1 tbsp (3 tsp)
30 ml =	1 oz (8 dr)	= 1 fl oz (2 tbsp)
500 ml† =	16 oz (1 pt)	= 16 oz (1 pt or 2 cups)
1000 ml† =	32 oz (1 qt)	= 32 oz (1 qt)
Length		
2.5 cm		= 1 in.
1 M		= 39.4 in.

*Approximate equivalents sometimes fall within a range, e.g., 60–65 mg = 1 gr, 4–5 ml = 1 dr, 15–16 ♏ = 1 ml. For purposes of calculations in this text, the numbers in Table 7-6 will be used.

†In common practice, these numbers are rounded up from 480 ml and 960 ml.

● SELF-ASSESSMENT

This exercise is designed to assess your understanding of household and apothecaries' measures. Write your answer in the space provided.

1. Write the abbreviation for each of the following:

a. _____ gallon f. _____ ounce

b. _____ quart g. _____ tablespoon

c. _____ pint h. _____ teaspoon

d. _____ cup i. _____ drops

e. _____ teacup

2. Write in the abbreviation for each of the following:

   a. 120 _____ = 2 tsp

   b. 1 _____ = $\frac{1}{60}$ tsp

   c. 1 _____ = 6 tsp

   d. 1 _____ = 8 oz

   e. 4 _____ = 2 oz

   f. 1 _____ = 3 tsp

   g. 6 _____ = 1 tcp

   h. 2 _____ = 1 pt

   i. 5 _____ = 10 C

3. Convert each of the following household equivalents:

   a. $2\frac{1}{2}$ T = _____ tsp

   b. 3 oz = _____ tsp

   c. 60 tsp = _____ T

   d. 540 gtt = _____ tsp

   e. 24 oz = _____ qt

4. Write in the abbreviation for each of the following:

   a. 60 _____ = 1 dram

   b. 8 _____ = 1 ounce

   c. 12 _____ = 1 pound

5. Convert each of the following apothecaries' equivalents:

   a. 4 drams = _____ ounce

   b. $\frac{3}{4}$ dram = _____ grains

   c. 1 grain = _____ dram

   d. 3 ounces = _____ drams

   e. 45 minims = _____ fluidrams

   f. $\frac{1}{2}$ pt = _____ quart

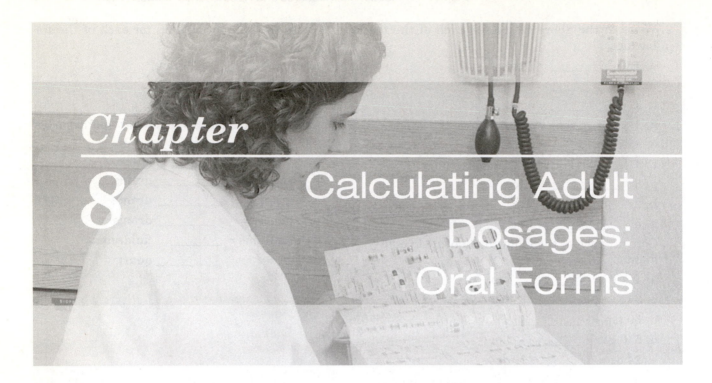

Chapter

8

Calculating Adult Dosages: Oral Forms

Chapter Outline

Objectives

Key Terms

Introduction

Calculating Oral Dosages Using the Proportional
   Method

Calculating Oral Dosages Using the Formula
   Method

Self-Assessment

Objectives

Upon completion of this chapter, you should be able
to

- Define the key terms

- Describe the oral route of drug administration

- Name two measures used to determine the
  amount of medication to be administered and
  give an example of each measure

- Define unit dose

- Calculate oral dosages using the proportional
  method

- Calculate oral dosages using a formula method

- Work the practice problems correctly

- Complete the Self-Assessment

Key Terms

multiple dose

oral route   unit dose

INTRODUCTION

The **oral route** of drug administration (by mouth,
po) is the route most commonly used. It provides
the safest, most convenient, and most economical
means of giving a medication. Drugs administered
by mouth may be in a solid or a liquid form. Solid
forms include tablets, capsules, caplets, powders,
and lozenges. Liquid preparations include solutions,
elixirs, and syrups.

Two measures are used to determine the
amount of medication to be administered: weight
and volume. The weight of a medication may be
expressed as any of the following: milliequivalents
(mEq), micrograms (mcg, μg), milligrams (mg),
grams (g), grains (gr), and units (U). The volume of
a medication may be expressed in milliliters (ml),
cubic centimeters (cc), minims (℥), drams (dr),
ounces (oz), and by a variety of household measures,
such as the teaspoon (tsp).

The amount of medication in the *average dose*
for an adult or a child is based upon the age and
weight of an *average client* in each category. The average client is between 10 and 60 years of age, and
weighs 150 pounds. In children, the dosage is de-

termined by BSA (body surface area) or kilogram of body weight

Medications prepared for oral administration may be dispensed in multiple dose form (solid and liquid) or in unit dose form (solid and liquid). The physician orders the medication using one of the various types of medication orders described in Chapter 13. On the order, the physician designates the name of the drug, the dosage, the frequency and route of administration, and the purpose for which it is prescribed. It then becomes the nurse's responsibility to follow the physician's order and administer the medication correctly.

Today, most oral medications are prepared and dispensed in unit dose form. A **unit dose** is a pre-measured amount of medication that is individually packaged on a per-dose basis. Occasionally, you may have to measure the dosage from a **multiple dose** (more than one dose per container) supply. This usually occurs when the medication strength ordered is not available in unit dose. To measure medications from a multiple dose supply, you must be familiar with the systems of measure and the formulas used for calculating dosages.

Many different methods can be used when calculating the dosage to be administered. Two of the most useful methods, the proportional method and the formula method, are described in this chapter. Study each method and practice computing dosages. This will prepare you in the event that you are required to calculate a dosage of medication.

CALCULATING ORAL DOSAGES USING THE PROPORTIONAL METHOD

Example: The physician orders 0.2 g of Equanil (meprobamate) tabs. The dose on hand is 400 mg tabs.

Step 1. Determine whether the medication ordered and the medication on hand are available in the same unit of measure.

Step 2. If the medication ordered and the medication on hand are not in the same unit of measure, convert so that both measures are expressed using the same unit of measure. (If you need to review this process, refer to Chapter 6.)

CONVERSION: To change 0.2 g to mg

$1000 \text{ mg} : 1 \text{ g} = x \text{ mg} : 0.2 \text{ g}$

$\qquad x = 200 \text{ mg}$

or

multiply $0.2 \times 1000 = 200$

Step 3. Now use the following proportion to calculate the dosage. Remember, you converted 0.2 g to 200 mg.

Known unit on hand	:	Known dosage form	=	Dose ordered	:	Unknown amount to be given
400 mg	:	1 tab	=	200 mg	:	x tab

$$400x = 200$$

$$x = \dfrac{\overset{1}{\cancel{200}}}{\underset{2}{\cancel{400}}} \quad \text{(Reduce fraction to lowest terms)}$$

$$x = \frac{1}{2} \text{ tab}$$

Step 4. Prove your answer. Remember to place your answer in the original formula in the x position.

$$400 \text{ mg} : 1 \text{ tab} = 200 \text{ mg} : \tfrac{1}{2} \text{ tab}$$

$$200 = 200$$

> Scored tablets have been bisected by a groove, making it easier for the user to break the tablet into halves or quarters, thereby varying the dosage.

● PRACTICE PROBLEM

1. Using the proportional method, calculate the following dosages:

   a. The physician ordered Sorbitrate (isosorbide dinitrate) chewable tabs, 2.5 mg. Available are Sorbitrate chewable tabs, 5 mg. How many tablets will you give?

   b. The physician ordered Xanax (alprazolam) tablets, 0.5 mg. Available are Xanax tablets, 0.25 mg. How many tablets will you give?

   c. The physician ordered Penicillin V Potassium (phenoxymethyl-penicillin potassium) tabs, 500 mg. On hand are Penicillin V Potassium tabs, 250 mg (400,000 U). How many tablets will you give?

   d. The physician ordered Omnipen (ampicillin) liquid oral suspension, 250 mg. Available is Omnipen liquid, 125 mg per 5 ml. How many milliliters will you give?

e. The physician ordered 0.5 g of Penicillin V Potassium (phenoxymethyl-penicillin potassium) tabs. Available are Penicillin V Potassium tabs, 250 mg (400,000 U). How many tablets will you give?

f. The physician ordered 0.250 mg of Lanoxin (digoxin) tabs. On hand are Lanoxin 0.125 mg tabs. How many tablets will you give?

g. The physician ordered 20 mg of Lasix (furosemide) tabs. On hand are Lasix 40 mg tabs. How many tablets will you give?

h. The physician ordered 150 mg of Tagamet (cimetidine) liquid. On hand is 300 mg/5 ml. How many milliliters will you give?

i. The physician ordered 500 mg of Ultracef (cefadroxil). On hand are 1 g tablets. The client will receive _____ tabs.

j. The physician ordered 1 g of Aquachloral (chloral hydrate). On hand are 500 mg capsules. How many capsules will you give?

CALCULATING ORAL DOSAGES USING THE FORMULA METHOD

Example: The physician orders 0.2 g of Equanil (meprobamate) tabs. The dose on hand is 400 mg tabs.

Step 1. Determine whether the medication ordered and the medication on hand are available in the same unit of measure.

Step 2. If the medication ordered and the medication on hand are not in the same unit of measure, convert so that both measures are expressed using the same unit of measure.

CONVERSION: To change 0.2 g to mg

$$1000 \text{ mg} : 1 \text{ g} = x \text{ mg} : 0.2 \text{ g}$$
$$x = 200 \text{ mg}$$

or

multiply $0.2 \times 1000 = 200$

Step 3. Now use the following formula to calculate the dosage:

$$\frac{\text{Dose ordered (desired)}}{\text{Dose on hand}} \times \text{Quantity (Q)} = \begin{array}{l}\text{Amount to give}\\ \text{(form of drug)}\end{array}$$

or

$$\frac{D}{H} \times Q = \text{Amount to give}$$

The physician ordered 0.2 g of Equanil tabs (0.2 g converts to 200 mg). The dose on hand is 400 mg tabs.

$$\frac{200 \text{ mg}}{400 \text{ mg}} \times 1 \text{ tab} = \frac{\overset{1}{\cancel{200}}}{\underset{2}{\cancel{400}}} \text{ or } \frac{1}{2} \text{ tab}$$

● PRACTICE PROBLEM

2. Using the formula method, calculate the following dosages:

a. The physician ordered Mycostatin (nystatin) oral tabs, 1,000,000 units. Available are Mycostatin oral tabs, 500,000 units. How many tablets will you give?

b. The physician ordered Penetrex (enoxacin) tabs, 200 mg. The dose on hand is Penetrex tabs, 400 mg. How many tablets will you give?

c. The physician ordered 3.75 mg of Coumadin (warfarin sodium) tabs. Available are Coumadin, 7.5 mg tabs. How many tablets will you give?

d. The physician ordered 600 mg of Equanil (meprobamate) tabs. The dose on hand is Equanil, 400 mg tabs. How many tablets will you give?

e. The physician ordered 62.5 mg of Diamox (acetazolamide) tabs. On hand are Diamox, 125 mg tabs. How many tablets will you give?

f. The physician ordered 200 mg of Thorazine (chlorpromazine hydrochloride), twice a day, po. On hand are 100 mg tablets. How many tablets will you give?

g. The physician ordered Amoxil (amoxicillin) 250 mg chewable tabs every 8 hours. On hand are 125 mg tabs. How many tablets will you give?

h. The physician ordered 0.25 mg of Lanoxin (digoxin). On hand are Lanoxin tabs, 0.125 mg. How many tablets will you give?

i. The physician ordered 1000 mg of Carafate (sucralfate). On hand are Carafate tabs, 1 g. How many tablets will you give?

j. The physician ordered 10 mg of Hydrocortone (hydrocortisone). On hand are 20 mg tablets. How many tablets will you give?

● SELF-ASSESSMENT

This exercise is designed to assess your understanding of calculating adult dosages. Answer the questions.

1. The physician ordered Lanoxin (digoxin) tabs, 0.125 mg. Available are Lanoxin tabs, 0.25 mg. How many tablets will you give?

2. The physician ordered Coumadin (warfarin sodium) tabs, 2.5 mg. Available are Coumadin tabs, 5 mg. How many tablets will you give?

3. The physician ordered Tylenol (acetaminophen) tabs, 650 mg. Available are acetaminophen tabs, 325 mg. How many tablets will you give?

4. The physician ordered Carafate (sucralfate) tabs, 500 mg. Available are Carafate tabs, 1 g. How many tablets will you give?

5. The physician ordered Duricef (cefadroxil monohydrate) tabs, 1500 mg. Available are Duricef tabs, 1 g. How many tablets will you give?

6. The physician ordered Diuril (chlorothiazide) tabs, 250 mg. Available are Diuril tabs, 0.25 g. How many tablets will you give?

7. The physician ordered Amoxil (amoxicillin) caps, 500 mg. Available are Amoxil caps, 250 mg. How many capsules will you give?

8. The physician ordered Lasix (furosemide) oral solution, 30 mg to be given as a single dose. Available is Lasix oral solution, 60 ml bottle that contains 10 mg/ml. How many milliliters will you give?

9. The physician ordered Decadron (dexamethasone) Elixir, 0.75 mg a day. Available is Decadron Elixir, 0.5 mg per 5 ml. How many milliliters will be given in a day?

10. The physician ordered Prelone (prednisolone) Syrup, 7.5 mg a day. Available is Prelone Syrup, 15 mg per 5 ml. How many milliliters will be given in a day?

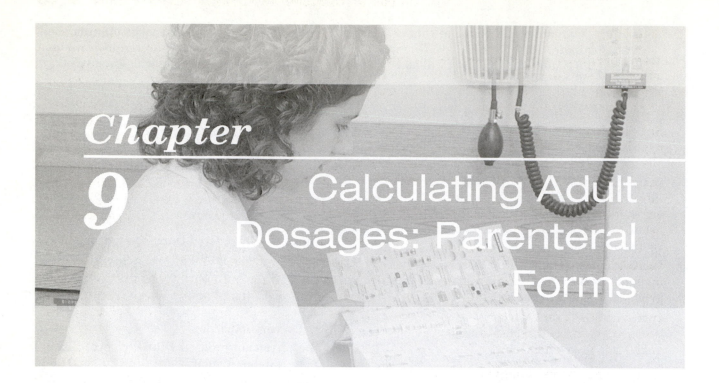

Chapter 9
Calculating Adult Dosages: Parenteral Forms

Chapter Outline

Objectives

Key Terms

Introduction

Calculating Parenteral Dosages Using the Proportional Method

Calculating Parenteral Dosages Using the Formula Method

Medications Measured in Units

Insulin

How to Calculate Unit Dosages

Calculating Intravenous Drip Rate

Self-Assessment

Objectives

Upon completion of this chapter, you should be able to:

- Define the key terms
- List the most frequently used parenteral routes
- State an advantage to using the parenteral route of drug administration
- Calculate parenteral dosages using the proportional method
- Calculate parenteral dosages using the formula method
- List six medications that are measured in units
- Define insulin
- List four categories of diabetes mellitus
- Explain why the exact dosage of insulin is so important
- List the precautions to be kept in mind when administering insulin
- Recognize rapid-acting, intermediate-acting, and slow-acting insulins
- Calculate unit dosages by the proportional or formula method
- Calculate an IV drip rate
- Work the practice problems correctly
- Complete the Self-Assessment

Key Terms

ampule

cartridge-needle unit

intradermal

intramuscular

intravenous

intravenous solution

parenteral

subcutaneous

vial

INTRODUCTION

The term **parenteral** is used to describe the injection of a liquid substance into the body via a route other than the alimentary canal. The most frequently used parenteral routes are

Subcutaneous (SC, SQ): Beneath the skin; hypodermic. A subcutaneous injection is usually given at a 45° angle.

Intramuscular (IM): Within the muscle. An intramuscular injection is given at a 90° angle, passing through the skin and subcutaneous tissue, and penetrating deep into muscle tissue.

Intradermal (ID): Within the epidermal layer of the skin. An intradermal injection is given at an angle between 10° and 15°.

Intravenous (IV): Within a vein. An intravenous injection is inserted (at less than a 15° angle) into the client's vein.

Medications that have been prepared for use by injection are available in multiple dose form (vials) and in unit dose form (ampules and cartridge-needle units). Injectable medications are also packaged for use with intravenous solution systems.

Vial: A small, sterile, prefilled glass bottle containing a hypodermic solution. See Figure 9-1.

Ampule: A small, sterile, prefilled container that usually holds a single dose of a hypodermic solution. See Figure 9-2.

Cartridge-needle unit: A disposable unit containing a premeasured amount of medication. This unit is designed for use in a nondisposable cartridge-holder syringe such as the Tubex® or Carpuject®.

Intravenous solutions: These medications are intended for intravenous use only and may be supplied in vials, ampules, and ready injectables (premeasured medicine packaged as a syringe-needle intravenous unit).

Because parenteral medications are intended for use by injection, they must be supplied as liquids. As such, the amount of medication is expressed in terms of volume (cubic centimeters, milliliters, or minims). The strength of the drug contained in the liquid is usually expressed in terms of its weight (milliequivalents, micrograms, milligrams, grams, grains, or units).

The parenteral route of drug administration offers an effective mode of delivering medication to a client when a rapid and direct result is desired. Since the effect of a parenteral medication is faster than by the oral route, the accuracy of dosage calculation is very important.

CALCULATING PARENTERAL DOSAGES USING THE PROPORTIONAL METHOD

Example: The physician orders Librium (chlordiazepoxide) 50 mg IM. The dose on hand is Librium 100 mg per 2 ml.

Step 1.   Determine if the medication ordered and the medication on hand are available in the same unit of measure.

Step 2.   If the medication ordered and the medication on hand are not in the same unit of measure, convert so that both measures are expressed using the same unit of measure.

Step 3.   Use the following proportion to calculate the dosage:

Known unit on hand	:	Known dosage form (volume)	=	Dose ordered	:	Unknown amount to give (volume)
100 mg	:	2 ml	=	50 mg	:	x ml

$$100x = 100$$
$$x = 1 \text{ ml}$$

Step 4.   Prove your answer. Remember that you place your answer in the position occupied by x in the original formula.

$$100 \text{ mg} : 2 \text{ ml} = 50 \text{ mg} : 1 \text{ ml}$$
$$100 = 100$$

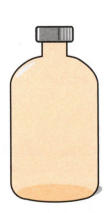

FIGURE 9-1   VIAL
(Courtesy of James Russell, Jr.)

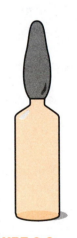

FIGURE 9-2   AMPULE *(Courtesy of James Russell, Jr.)*

● **PRACTICE PROBLEM**

1. Using the proportional method, calculate the following dosages:

   a. The physician ordered Demerol (meperidine hydrochloride), 75 mg IM. On hand is Demerol, 100 mg per 2 ml. How much Demerol will you administer?

   b. The physician ordered cyanocobalamin (vitamin B_{12}), 200 mcg IM or SQ. Available is cyanocobalamin, 1000 mcg per ml. What is the correct dosage to give to your client?

   c. The physician ordered Lasix (furosemide), 20 mg IM. On hand is Lasix, 10 mg per ml. What will you administer to your client?

   d. The physician ordered Bicillin L-A (penicillin G benzathine), 600,000 units for deep IM injection. On hand is Bicillin L-A, 1,200,000 units per 2 ml. What is the correct dosage?

   e. The physician ordered streptomycin, 250 mg IM. Available is streptomycin, 0.5 g per 2 ml. How many ml will you give?

CALCULATING PARENTERAL DOSAGES USING THE FORMULA METHOD

Example: The physician ordered Librium (chlordiazepoxide), 50 mg IM. The dose on hand is Librium, 100 mg per 2 ml.

Step 1. Determine if the medication ordered and the medication on hand are available in the same unit of measure.

Step 2. If the medication ordered and the medication on hand are not in the same unit of measure, convert so that both measures are expressed using the same unit of measure.

Step 3. Now, use the following formula to calculate the dosage:

$$\frac{\text{Dose ordered (desired)}}{\text{Dose on hand}} \times \text{Quantity (Q)} = \text{Amount to give}$$

$$\frac{D}{H} \times Q = \text{Amount to give}$$

$$\frac{50 \text{ mg}}{100 \text{ mg}} \times 2 \text{ ml} = \frac{50}{100} \times \frac{2}{1} = \frac{100}{100} = 1 \text{ ml}$$

● **PRACTICE PROBLEM**

2. Using the formula method, calculate the following dosages:

   a. The physician ordered Phenergan (promethazine hydrochloride), 75 mg IM. On hand is Phenergan, 50 mg per ml. How many milliliters will you give?

   b. The physician ordered Kantrex (kanamycin sulfate), 500 mg IM. Available is Kantrex, 0.5 g per ml. How many milliliters will you give?

   c. The physician ordered Dramamine (dimenhydrinate), 35 mg IM. On hand is Dramamine, 50 mg per ml. How many milliliters will you give?

   d. The physician ordered Dilantin (phenytoin sodium), 25 mg IM. On hand is Dilantin, 50 mg per ml. How many milliliters will you give?

   e. The physician ordered Garamycin (gentamicin sulfate), 60 mg IM. Available is Garamycin, 40 mg per ml. How many milliliters will you give?

   f. The physician ordered Nubain (nalbuphine hydrochloride), 10 mg IM. On hand is a 1 ml ampule that contains 20 mg/1 ml. What is the correct dosage?

g. The physician ordered Dilaudid (hydromorphone hydrochloride), 25 mg IM. On hand is a 5 ml ampule that contains 50 mg/5 ml. What is the correct dosage?

h. The physician ordered Compazine (prochlorperazine), 10 mg IM. On hand is a 10 ml vial that contains 5 mg/ml. What is the correct dosage?

i. The physician ordered Depo-Medrol (methylprednisolone acetate), 40 mg IM. On hand is a 5 ml vial that contains 80 mg/ml. What is the correct dosage?

j. The physician ordered Norflex (orphenadrine), 30 mg IM. On hand is a 60 mg/2 ml ampule. What is the correct dosage?

MEDICATIONS MEASURED IN UNITS

Such medications as insulin, heparin, some antibiotics, hormones, vitamins, and vaccines are measured in units (U). These medications are standardized in units based on their strengths. The strength varies from one medicine to another, depending upon the source, condition, and method in which they are obtained.

INSULIN

Insulin is a chemical substance (hormone) secreted by the beta cells of the islets of Langerhans. It is essential for the proper metabolism of carbohydrates, fats, and proteins. An inadequate secretion of insulin leads to a complex disorder known as diabetes mellitus. The National Diabetes Data Group of the National Institutes of Health organized the various forms of diabetes into the following categories:

- Type I: Insulin-dependent diabetes mellitus (IDDM)

- Type II: Noninsulin-dependent diabetes mellitus (NIDDM)

- Type III: Women who develop glucose intolerance in association with pregnancy. This is referred to as gestational diabetes.

- Type IV: Other types of diabetes associated with pancreatic disease, hormonal changes, adverse effects of drugs, or genetic or other anomalies

Individuals with Type I insulin-dependent diabetes mellitus (IDDM) must take insulin injections on a regular basis to maintain life. The dosage of insulin is expressed in units, U-100, and is individualized by the physician for each client. The amount of insulin that a person must take is based on blood glucose levels, diet, exercise, and the individual's needs.

Note: *It is extremely important that the exact dosage of insulin be taken by the client.* Too little or too much insulin can cause serious problems, ranging from a blood sugar level too low or too high, to coma, and even death. It may be your responsibility to administer insulin, and/or to teach clients or their families how to administer insulin themselves.

When administering insulin, the U-100 syringe (1 cc, LO-DOSE® $\frac{1}{2}$ cc, or very low dose $\frac{1}{3}$ cc) is preferred. U-100 means there are 100 units of insulin per milliliter or cubic centimeter. Insulin dosage should always be expressed in units rather than in milliliters or cubic centimeters. For example, if the physician orders 30 units of U-100 NPH insulin, you would use a U-100 syringe and draw up 30 units of U-100 NPH insulin.

Precautions to Keep in Mind When Administering Insulin

- Be sure to use the proper insulin, the one ordered by the physician.

- Do not substitute one insulin for another.

- Use the correct syringe U-100.

- Dosage of insulin is always measured in units and is individualized for each client.

- Check the label for the name and type of insulin, strength, and expiration date.

- Make sure the insulin has the proper appearance. (See Tables 9-1 and 9-2.)

Insulin that has been frozen should not be used. Unused insulin should be stored in a refrigerator at 2–8°C or 36–46°F. After opening, an insulin vial should be discarded after 3 months if kept at 2–8°C or after 1 month if kept at room temperature (25°C

TABLE 9-1 RAPID-ACTING INSULIN

Selected Insulin Preparations U-100				
Rapid-acting	Onset of Action	Peak	Duration	Appearance
Humalog	15 min	30–90 min	5 hr	Clear, colorless
Humulin R	15 min	1 hr	4–12 hr	Clear, colorless
Velosulin BR	$\frac{1}{2}$ hr	1–3 hr	8 hr	Clear
Novolin R	$\frac{1}{2}$ hr	$2\frac{1}{2}$–5 hr	8 hr	Clear

TABLE 9-2 INTERMEDIATE-ACTING AND SLOW-ACTING INSULIN

Selected Insulin Preparations U-100				
Intermediate-acting	Onset of Action	Peak	Duration	Appearance
NPH	$1\frac{1}{2}$ hr	4–12 hr	24 hr	Cloudy
Novolin L	$2\frac{1}{2}$ hr	7–15 hr	22 hr	Cloudy
Novolin N	$1\frac{1}{2}$ hr	4–12 hr	24 hr	Cloudy
Humulin N	1 hr	4 hr	24 hr	Cloudy
Slow-acting				
Humulin U	4 hr	10–20 hr	28 hr	Cloudy

or 77°F). In hot climates where refrigeration is not available, cooling jars or a cool wet cloth around the insulin will help to preserve the insulin activity. Direct sunlight or warming damages insulin.

- When insulin is not in use, store it in a cool place and avoid freezing.
- Avoid shaking an insulin bottle. Roll gently in palms of hand to mix. This method prevents bubbles in the medication.
- When calculating an insulin dosage, always have another nurse check your calculations.

HOW TO CALCULATE UNIT DOSAGES

When calculating medications that are ordered in units, you may use either the proportional or formula method.

Example: The physician ordered 4000 USP units of heparin to be administered deep subcutaneously. On hand is heparin, 5000 USP units per milliliter.

The Proportional Method

Step 1. Use the following proportion to calculate the dosage:

$$\frac{\text{Known unit on hand}}{5000\,U} : \frac{\text{Known dosage form (volume)}}{1\,ml} = \text{Dose ordered} : \frac{\text{Unknown amount to give (volume)}}{x\,ml}$$

$$\frac{\text{Known unit on hand}}{5000\,U} : \frac{\text{Known dosage form (volume)}}{1\,ml} = \frac{\text{Dose ordered}}{4000\,U} : \frac{\text{Unknown amount to give (volume)}}{x\,ml}$$

$$5000x = 4000$$

$$x = \frac{4000}{5000} = \frac{4}{5}\text{ ml or } 0.8\text{ ml}$$

You may use a tuberculin syringe to draw up 0.8 ml, or convert $\frac{4}{5}$ ml to minims. See step 2.

Step 2. If you choose to convert $\frac{4}{5}$ ml to minims, use the following example:

Converting Minims

There are 15 to 16 minims per milliliter. You will use 15 when the denominator of the fraction will go into 15 evenly. You will use 16 when the denominator of the fraction will go into 16 evenly.

To convert $\frac{4}{5}$ to minims, multiply

$$\frac{4}{5} \times \frac{15}{1} = \frac{4}{\cancel{5}} \times \frac{\cancel{15}}{1}^{3} = 12 \text{ minims}$$

You will administer 12 minims (4000 U) to the client.

The Formula Method

Example: The physician ordered 450,000 units of Bicillin L-A (penicillin G benzathine) for deep IM injection. Available is Bicillin L-A, 600,000 units per milliliter.

Step 1. Use the following formula to calculate the dosage:

$$\frac{\text{Dose ordered (desired)}}{\text{Dose on hand}} \times \text{Quantity (Q)} = \text{Amount to give}$$

$$\frac{450,000 \text{ U}}{600,000 \text{ U}} \times 1 \text{ ml} =$$

$$\frac{\cancel{450,000}^{3} \text{ U}}{\cancel{600,000}_{4} \text{ U}} \times 1 \text{ ml} = \frac{3}{4} \text{ ml}$$

Step 2. You may choose to convert to minims. If so, multiply $\frac{3}{4}$ by 16.

$$\frac{3}{\cancel{4}_{1}} \times \frac{\cancel{16}^{4}}{1} = 12 \text{ minims}$$

You will administer 12 minims (450,000 U) to the client.

● PRACTICE PROBLEM

3. Use the proportional or formula method to calculate the following:

   a. The physician ordered 20 units of Acthar (adrenocorticotropic hormone) IM. Available is Acthar, 40 units per milliliter. How many milliliters will you administer?

   b. The physician ordered 8000 USP units of heparin to be administered deep subcutaneously. On hand is heparin, 10,000 USP units per ml. How much heparin will you administer?

   c. The physician ordered Bicillin L-A (penicillin G benzathine), 600,000 units for deep IM injection. The dose on hand is Bicillin L-A, 1,200,000 units per 2 milliliters. How many milliliters will you administer?

   d. The physician ordered 32 units of U-100 NPH insulin. Shade in the correct dosage on the U-100 syringe pictured below.

   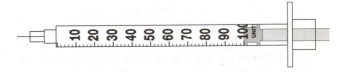

   e. The physician ordered 64 units of U-100 Humulin N insulin. Shade in the correct dosage on the U-100 syringe pictured below.

   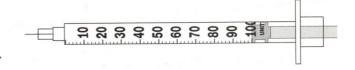

CALCULATING INTRAVENOUS DRIP RATE

The type, amount, and flow rate of an intravenous fluid is determined by the physician. The physician assesses the client's needs and physical condition. Intravenous fluids are used as replacements for fluids and electrolytes, and as a means to deliver routine or emergency medications. When the physician orders that a vein be kept open (KVO), a solution of 5% dextrose in water, D_5W, may be used. The drip rate may be 20 cc/hr (500 cc/24 hr) or 40 cc/hr (1000 cc/24 hr). It is very important to maintain the prescribed drip rate to prevent fluid and electrolyte imbalance.

Special preparation is required of those approved to start intravenous infusions and/or administer IV medications. A drug that is introduced directly into a client's bloodstream produces an immediate effect. Therefore, those administering medications by this method should be well versed in the ethical and legal implications accompanying such responsibility.

An intravenous solution is ordered by the physician in milliliters per hour. When an infusion control device or a dosage calculator is not available, the nurse must mathematically determine the flow rate in drops (gtt) per minute. Various formulas are used to calculate intravenous drip rate. In this chapter, the following formula is used:

$$\frac{(ml \div hr) \times calibrations\ (gtt/ml - drop\ factor)}{min}$$

Before you calculate the drip rate, you need to know several important factors.

- You need to know the total volume (amount) of solution that is to be infused.

- Next, you need to know the length of time (hours) that the fluid is to be infused.

- You need to know the calibrations (gtt/ml) of the infusion set that is to be used. The *drop factor* is identified on the package label. Be sure to read the label carefully. A *macro*drop may deliver 10 gtt/ml, 15 gtt/ml, or 20 gtt/ml, depending on the manufacturer. A *micro*drop delivers

60 gtt/ml, since this is standardized by all manufacturers. See Figure 9-3.

How to Calculate IV Drip Rate

Example: The physician ordered D$_5$W (5% dextrose in water) 1000 ml to be infused over 8 hours. The infusion set is calibrated to deliver 15 gtt/ml.

Step 1. Divide milliliters by hours (ml ÷ hr)

$$\frac{1000\ ml}{8\ hr} = 125\ ml/hr$$

Step 2. Multiply the answer you found by dividing milliliters by hours (125) by the calibrations (gtt/ml = 15).

125 ml × 15 gtt = 1875 gtt

Step 3. Divide the answer you found in step 2 by 60 min (1 hour).

$$\frac{1875\ gtt}{60\ min} = 31.25\ gtt/min$$

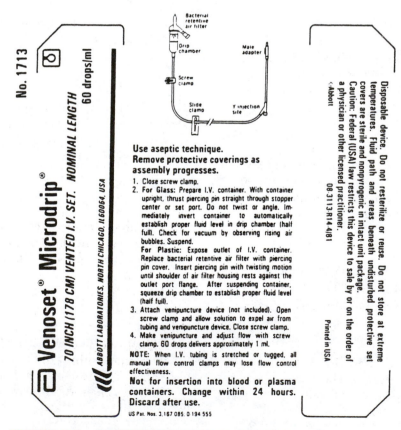

FIGURE 9-3 VENOSET MICRODRIP IV SET; 60 DROPS/ML *(Reprinted with permission from Abbott Laboratories, Hospital Products Division)*

TABLE 9-3   IV FLOW RATES/1 L IN GTT/MIN

Tubing Delivers	4 Hours	6 Hours	8 Hours	10 Hours	12 Hours
15 gtt/ml	62	42	31	25	21
10 gtt/ml	42	28	21	17	14
60 gtt/ml	250	167	125	100	83

Now let's review the total process.

$$\frac{(ml \div hr) \times calibrations\ (gtt/ml)}{min}$$

$$\frac{125 \times 15}{60} = \frac{1875}{60} = 31.25\ gtt/min\ (rate\ of\ flow)$$

- Round number to nearest whole number: 31 gtt/min. See Table 9-3.

● PRACTICE PROBLEM

4. Using the formula given in this chapter, calculate the following IV drip rates:

   a. The physician ordered D_5W 1000 ml to be infused over 8 hours. The infusion set delivers 20 gtt/ml (drop factor).

   b. The physician ordered D_5R/L (5 percent dextrose Ringers/Lactate) 1000 ml to be infused over 12 hours. The infusion set delivers 60 gtt/ml (drop factor).

   c. The physician ordered D_5NS (5 percent dextrose in normal saline) 1000 ml to be infused over 10 hours. The infusion set delivers 10 gtt/ml (drop factor).

   d. The physician ordered D_5W 2500 ml to be infused over 24 hours. The infusion set delivers 10 gtt/ml (drop factor).

   e. The physician ordered D_5NS 1200 ml to be infused over 16 hours. The infusion set delivers 15 gtt/ml (drop factor).

● SELF-ASSESSMENT

This exercise is designed to assess your understanding of calculating adult parenteral dosages. Answer the questions.

1. The physician ordered Demerol (meperidine hydrochloride), 50 mg IM. On hand is Demerol, 100 mg per 2 ml. How many milliliters will you give?

2. The physician ordered Robaxin (methocarbamol), 200 mg IM. On hand is Robaxin, 100 mg per ml. How many milliliters will you give?

3. The physician ordered Bicillin L-A (penicillin G benzathine), 800,000 units for deep IM injection. On hand is Bicillin L-A, 1,200,000 units per 2 ml. How many minims will you give?

4. The physician ordered Phenergan (promethazine hydrochloride), 100 mg IM. On hand is Phenergan, 50 mg per ml. How many milliliters will you give?

5. The physician ordered 30 units of Acthar (adrenocorticotropic hormone) IM. Available is Acthar, 40 units per milliliter. How many minims will you give?

6. The physician ordered D_5W 1000 ml to be infused over 8 hours. The infusion set delivers 20 gtt/ml (drop factor). Calculate the correct IV drip rate.

7. The physician ordered D_5NS (5 percent dextrose in normal saline) 1000 ml to be infused over 10 hours. The infusion set delivers 10 gtt/ml (drop factor). Calculate the correct IV drip rate.

8. The physician ordered Polycillin (ampicillin), 500 mg IM. On hand is Polycillin, 250 mg per ml. How many milliliters will you give?

9. The physician ordered Compazine (prochlorperazine), 10 mg IM. On hand is Compazine, 5 mg per ml. How many milliliters will you give?

10. The physician ordered Librium (chlordiazepoxide), 25 mg IM. On hand is Librium, 100 mg per 2 ml. How many milliliters will you give?

11. The physician ordered Depo-Medrol (methylprednisolone), 60 mg IM. On hand is Depo-Medrol, 80 mg per ml. How many milliliters will you give? Convert your answer to minims.

12. The physician ordered Dilor (dyphylline), 500 mg. On hand is Dilor, 500 mg per ml. How many milliliters will you give?

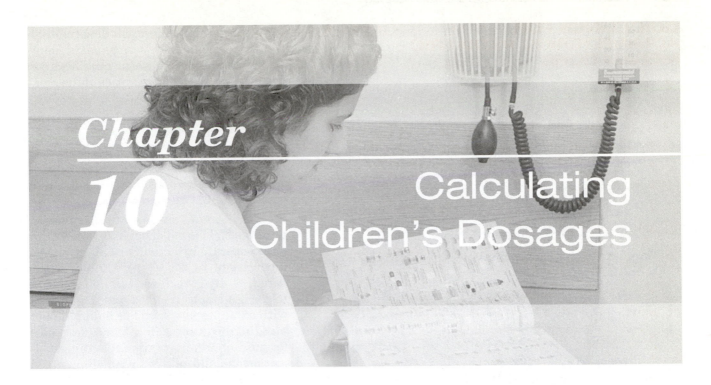

Chapter 10

Calculating Children's Dosages

Chapter Outline

Objectives

Key Terms

Introduction

Guidelines for Administering Pediatric Medications

Calculating Dosage per Kilogram of Body Weight

Body Surface Area (BSA)

Self-Assessment

Objectives

Upon completion of this chapter, you should be able to

- Define the key terms

- Give the guidelines for administering pediatric medications

- Calculate children's dosages according to kilogram of body weight and body surface area (BSA)

- Complete the practice problems correctly

- Complete the Self-Assessment

Key Terms

child

infancy

nomogram

puberty

INTRODUCTION

Each child is an individual, with differences in age, size, and weight. A **child** is any human between infancy and puberty. **Infancy** is the stage of life from the time of birth through the completion of one year. **Puberty** is the stage of life at which members of both sexes become functionally capable of reproduction. It is a period of rapid physical, mental, and emotional changes that occur from ages 13 to 15 in boys and ages 9 to 16 in girls. Since each child does not develop in the same way during a given time span, medication dosages for pediatric clients are determined by two methods.

The methods used to calculate children's dosages are according to kilogram of body weight and body surface area (BSA). The body weight method is generally the method of choice, since most medications are ordered in this way and it is easier to calculate. The body surface area (BSA) is an exact method, but one must use a formula and a nomogram to determine a correct dosage. Both of these methods are described in this chapter along with numerous practice problems.

GUIDELINES FOR ADMINISTERING PEDIATRIC MEDICATIONS

1. Follow the "Six Rights" of proper drug administration.
   - The Right Dose
   - The Right Drug
   - The Right Route
   - The Right Time
   - The Right Client
   - The Right Documentation

2. Carefully assess each pediatric client according to the following factors:
   - Age
   - Weight
   - Body size
   - Physical state
   - Disease process
   - Mental and emotional state
   - Level of understanding
   - Allergies

3. Gain parental cooperation.
   - Identify yourself. Call the parent and the child by name. Explain the procedure.
   - Whenever possible, allow the parent to assist you.
   - At times, it may be necessary to ask the parent to leave the room, as the parent's behavior may be upsetting to the child. When this is the case, explain to the parent and child that the procedure will only take a few minutes and you will ask another nurse to assist you.

4. Establish rapport with the child.
   - Use a positive and straightforward approach. Do not waste time. The longer it takes to accomplish a procedure, the more apprehensive the child will become.
   - Never lie to a child.
   - Explain the procedure at the level of the child's understanding.
   - Whenever possible, allow the child to assist you.
   - Show approval for positive behavior by the child. Clap, laugh, and reward with a "treat" if possible.

5. The route of administration will depend upon the child's age, weight, body size, physical, mental, and emotional state, disease process, level of understanding, specific properties of the medication, and the physician's order.
   - *Oral route:* Never force or give an oral medication to a crying child.
     - Liquid medications may be administered by dropper or an appropriate device such as an oral syringe or calibrated medication cup. See Figure 10-1.
     - Solid medications are generally not ordered until the child is old enough to understand and cooperate by actually swallowing the medication. In the event a tablet is ordered, always check with the pharmacist to see if it can be crushed and then mixed with an appropriate food or liquid (do not mix the medication in a baby's formula) for ease of administration. Certain medications should not be crushed or mixed with food.
   - *Parenteral route:* Two people will be needed when administering an injection to a child: one to assist in maintaining a proper body position and the other to give the injection. Administer subcutaneous, intramuscular, and/or intravenous medications with extreme care.
   - *Rectal route:* Consider the significance the child places on this part of his/her body. A toddler who is in the process of toilet training may resist this form of drug administration, while older children may feel as though this is an invasion of privacy and may react with embarrassment and resentment.

6. *Caution: When calculating children's dosages, be extremely careful. It is advisable to have someone check your mathematical solutions. Be sure to compare the normal dose range with the dosage you plan to administer. If there is any doubt, contact the physician and/or pharmacist.*

CALCULATING DOSAGE PER KILOGRAM OF BODY WEIGHT

As a nurse, it may be your responsibility to calculate the amount of dosage ordered by the physician according to the child's body weight. The physician will usually order the medication dosage per kilogram of body weight.

There are two methods of calculating dosage according to kilogram of body weight.

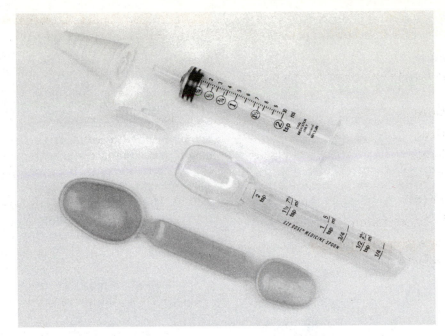

FIGURE 10-1   DEVICES FOR ADMINISTERING ORAL MEDICATIONS TO A CHILD

Method 1: Dividing Pounds by 2.2 and Multiplying Dose Ordered by kg of Body Weight

Step 1.   To convert pounds to kilograms, divide the pounds by 2.2 as 1 kg = 2.2 lb.

Step 2.   Multiply the dose ordered by kilogram of body weight.

Step 3.   If the dose is ordered in divided doses, divide the number of times into the answer you obtained in step 2.

Example: The physician orders Rocephin (ceftriaxone sodium), 100 mg/kg of body weight, in divided doses every 12 hours (not to exceed 4 g), for Alice Potts, who weighs 66 pounds. How many milligrams will Alice receive?

Step 1.   Convert pounds to kilograms.

$$\frac{66 \text{ lb}}{2.2} = x \text{ kg}$$

$$2.2\overline{)66.0}$$ → 30
$$\underline{66}$$
$$0$$
$$\underline{0}$$

66 lb = 30 kg

Step 2.   Multiply the dose ordered by kilogram of body weight.

100 mg/kg
100 × 30 = 3000 mg = 3 g

Step 3.   Determine the amount of each dose.

Divide 3000 by 2 to arrive at the divided dose = 1500 mg.

Alice will receive 1500 mg of Rocephin every 12 hours, as ordered by the physician.

Method 2: Using the Proportional Method to Calculate Kilogram of Body Weight

Example: The physician orders Rocephin (ceftriaxone sodium), 100 mg/kg of body weight, in divided doses every 12 hours (not to exceed 4 g), for Alice Potts, who weighs 66 pounds. How many milligrams will Alice receive?

Step 1.   To convert 66 pounds to kilograms, set up the proportion as follows:

2.2 lb : 1 kg = 66 lb : x kg

Step 2.   Now solve for x.

2.2 : 1 = 66 : x
2.2x = 66
x = 30

Step 3. Now calculate the prescribed dosage by placing 30 in the appropriate place:

100 mg/30 kg

$100 \times 30 = 3000$ mg $= 3$ g

Step 4. To determine the amount of each dose, divide 3000 by 2 (every 12 hours).

$3000 \div 2 = 1500$ mg

Alice Potts will receive 1500 mg of Rocephin every 12 hours, as ordered by the physician.

● PRACTICE PROBLEM

1. Calculate the following dosages according to kilogram of body weight:

   a. The physician orders Duricef (cefadroxil), 30 mg/kg of body weight, for John Knight, who weighs 44 pounds. The dose is to be divided and given every 12 hours. How many milligrams will you give?

   b. The physician orders codeine phosphate CII, 0.5 mg/kg of body weight, for pain. The client weighs 50 pounds. The medication may be given every 4–6 hours. How many milligrams will the client receive?

   c. The physician orders Cefadyl (cephapirin sodium), 20 mg/kg every 6 hours, for a child who weighs 46 pounds. How many milligrams will you give?

   d. The physician orders Claforan (cefotaxime), 60 mg/kg divided into four equal doses, for a child who weighs 42 pounds. What is the amount to be given in four equal doses?

   e. The physician orders Garamycin (gentamicin sulfate), 6 mg/kg/day, for a child who weighs 52 pounds. How many milligrams will be given daily?

BODY SURFACE AREA (BSA)

The body surface area (BSA) is considered to be one of the most accurate methods of calculating medication dosages for infants and children up to 12 years of age. This method requires the use of a **nomogram** (a device graph that shows the relationship among numerical values) that estimates the body surface area of the client according to height and weight. Refer to Figure 10-2.

The body surface area is determined by drawing a straight line from the client's height to the client's weight. The intersection of the line with the surface area column is the estimated BSA. This figure is then placed in the following formula:

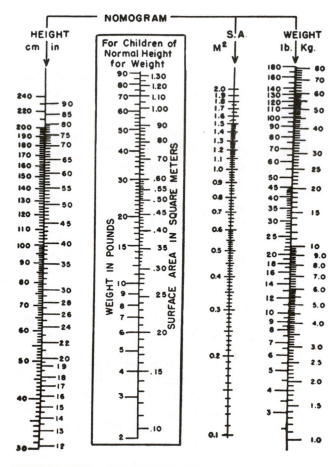

FIGURE 10-2. BODY SURFACE AREA (BSA) IS DETERMINED BY DRAWING A STRAIGHT LINE FROM THE CLIENT'S HEIGHT IN THE LEFT COLUMN TO HIS OR HER WEIGHT IN THE FAR RIGHT COLUMN. THE INTERSECTION OF THE LINE WITH THE SURFACE AREA (SA) COLUMN IS THE ESTIMATED BSA. FOR INFANTS AND CHILDREN OF NORMAL HEIGHT FOR WEIGHT, BSA MAY BE ESTIMATED FROM WEIGHT ALONE BY REFERRING TO THE ENCLOSED AREA. *(Reprinted from Behrman, R. E., and Vaughan, V. C., Nelson Textbook of Pediatrics, 12th ed. W. B. Saunders Company, Philadelphia, 1983. Used with permission from W. B. Saunders Company and R. E. Behrman, M.D., Case Western Reserve University, School of Medicine, Cleveland, Ohio.)*

$$\frac{\text{BSA of child (m}^2)}{1.7 \text{ (m}^2)} \times \text{adult dose} = \text{child's dose}$$

This formula is based on the average adult who weighs 140 lb and has a body surface area of 1.7 square meters (1.7 m²).

Example: Marion Green is a 4-year-old child who is 40 inches tall and weighs 38 lb (BSA 0.7). The physician has ordered Demerol (meperidine hydrochloride) for pain. The average adult dose of Demerol is 50 mg per ml. What dosage will be given to Marion according to the BSA method?

$$\frac{0.7 \text{ (m}^2)}{1.7 \text{ (m}^2)} \times \frac{50 \text{ mg}}{1} = \text{child's dose}$$

$$\frac{0.7 \text{ (m}^2)}{1.7 \text{ (m}^2)} \times \frac{50 \text{ mg}}{1} = \frac{35}{1.7}$$

$$= 20.5 \text{ mg}$$

$$= 21 \text{ mg}$$

Now use the formula

$$\frac{\text{Desired}}{\text{Have}} \times \text{Quantity}$$

to convert mg to ml.

$$\frac{21 \text{ mg}}{50 \text{ mg}} = x \text{ ml}$$

$$\frac{21}{50} = 0.42 \text{ ml (administered with a tuberculin syringe)}$$

● PRACTICE PROBLEM

2. Calculate the following dosages according to body surface area (BSA):

   a. If the adult dose of Microsulfon (sulfadiazine) is 250 mg IM three times a day, what is the dosage for a 3-year-old child, 36 inches tall, weighing 30 pounds (BSA 0.6)?

   b. If the adult dose of Amoxil (amoxicillin) is 250 mg every 8 hours, what is the dosage for a 2 $\frac{1}{2}$-year-old child, 28 inches tall, weighing 25 pounds (BSA 0.5)?

   c. If the adult dose of Amoxil (amoxicillin) is 250 mg, what is the dosage for a child with a BSA of 0.41?

   d. If the adult dose of a medication is 1000 units, what is the dosage for a child with a BSA of 0.56?

   e. If the adult dose of a medication is 500 units, what is the dosage for a child with a BSA of 0.5?

● SELF-ASSESSMENT

This exercise is designed to assess your understanding of calculating children's dosages. Answer the questions.

1. A 4-year-old child has a body surface area (BSA) of 0.7. The adult dose of medication is 50 mg per ml. What dosage will be given to the child?

2. The child weighs 66 pounds and the physician has ordered a medication to be given 30 mg/kg of body weight. What dosage will be given to the child?

3. The child weighs 44 pounds and the physician has ordered a medication to be given 30 mg/kg of body weight. What dosage will be given to the child?

4. If the adult dose of Microsulfon (sulfadiazine) is 250 mg IM, what is the dosage for a 3-year-old child, 36 inches tall, weighing 30 pounds (BSA 0.6)?

5. If the adult dose of E.E.S. (erythromycin ethyl-succinate) chewable tabs is 400 mg every 6 hours, what is the dosage for a child who is 35 inches tall and weighs 28 pounds (BSA 0.57)?

6. If the adult dose of Pen-Vee K (penicillin V potassium) is 250 mg every 6–8 hours, what is the dosage for a child who is 24 inches tall and weighs 35 pounds (BSA 0.56)?

7. The physician ordered Augmentin (amoxicillin and potassium clavulanate), 20 mg/kg/day, for a pediatric patient who weighs 72 pounds. The dose is to be divided and given every 8 hours for 10 days. What is the total dose? What is the amount to be given every 8 hours?

8. The physician ordered Cefadyl (cephapirin sodium), 40 mg/kg, for a pediatric patient who weighs 78 pounds. The dose is to be divided into four equal doses. What is the total dose? What is the amount to be given in four equal doses?

9. The physician ordered Garamycin (gentamicin sulfate), 2.0 mg/kg every 8 hours, for a child who weighs 86 pounds. What dosage will be given to the child?

10. The physician ordered Phenergan (promethazine hydrochloride), 1 mg/kg, as a preoperative medication for a pediatric client who weighs 44 pounds. What dosage will be given to the child?

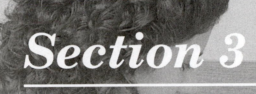

Section 3

ADMINISTRATION OF MEDICATIONS

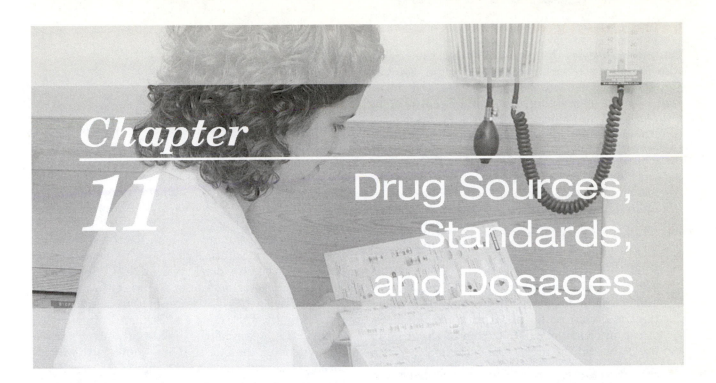

Chapter 11

Drug Sources, Standards, and Dosages

Chapter Outline

Objectives

Key Terms

Introduction

Drugs

Sources of Drugs

Drug Legislation

Drug References/Standards

Drug Dosage

Self-Assessment

Objectives

Upon completion of this chapter, you should be able to

- Define the key terms

- Define pharmacology

- Describe the five subdivisions of pharmacology

- State the five medical uses for drugs

- Give the three names assigned to a drug

- List the five main sources for drugs, giving examples from each source

- State the importance of the Federal Food, Drug and Cosmetic Act

- Explain the significance of the Controlled Substances Act of 1970

- Define the five controlled substances' schedules and give examples of drugs listed in each

- Explain storage and record keeping for controlled substances

- List two reasons for the standardization of drugs

- Define the terms used in describing various types of dosages

- Differentiate between and correctly use the following drug reference books:

  — *United States Pharmacopeia/National Formulary (USP/NF)*
  — *New Drugs*
  — *Physicians' Desk Reference (PDR)*

- Define dosage

- List the factors that affect drug dosage

- Define the terms used in describing dosage

- Complete the Self-Assessment

Key Terms

administer	dosage
controlled substance	drug
controlled substance analogue	pharmacology
	prescribe
dispense	

INTRODUCTION

Pharmacology is the study of drugs; the science that is concerned with the history, origin, sources, physical and chemical properties, uses, and the effects of drugs upon living organisms. Because of the complexity of the subject, pharmacology has evolved into the following subdivisions:

- *Pharmacodynamics.* The study of drugs and their actions on living organisms. It involves the biochemical and physiological effects of drugs upon living organisms as well as their actions.

- *Pharmacognosy.* The science of natural drugs and their physical, botanical, and chemical properties.

- *Pharmacokinetics.* The study of the metabolism and action of drugs within the body. It involves the time required for absorption to take place, duration of action, distribution of the drug in the body, and the method of excretion.

- *Pharmacotherapeutics.* The study of drugs and their relationships to the treatment of disease. It involves determining which drug is most or least appropriate for a specific disease and the required dosage to achieve beneficial results.

- *Toxicology.* The study of poisons; the science concerned with toxic substances. It involves the study of the chemistry and pharmacological actions of substances and establishing antidotes, treatment, prevention, and methods for controlling exposure to harmful substances.

DRUGS

A **drug** can be defined simply as a medicinal substance that may alter or modify the functions of a living organism. In general, there are five medical uses for drugs.

- *Therapeutic use.* Certain drugs such as antihistamines may be used in the treatment of an allergy to relieve the symptoms or to sustain the client until other measures are instituted.

- *Diagnostic use.* Certain drugs such as Ethiodol are used in conjunction with radiology to allow the physician to pinpoint the location of a disease process.

- *Curative use.* Certain drugs such as antibiotics kill or remove the causative agent of a disease.

- *Replacement use.* Certain drugs such as hormones and vitamins are used to replace substances normally found in the body.

- *Preventive or prophylactic use.* Certain drugs such as immunizing agents are used to ward off or lessen the severity of a disease.

Drug Names

Most drugs have the following three types of names: chemical, generic, and trade or brand name. The *chemical* name describes the drug's molecular structure and identifies its chemical structure. The *generic* name is the drug's *official* name and is assigned to the drug by the U.S. Adopted Names (USAN) Council.

A generic drug can be manufactured by more than one pharmaceutical company. When this is the case, each company markets the drug under its own unique *trade* or *brand* name. A trade or brand name is registered by the U.S. Patent Office as well as approved by the U.S. Food and Drug Administration (FDA). The ® symbol that follows the drug's trade name denotes the fact that this name is the registered trademark used by the manufacturer. Some trade (brand) names are followed by the letters TM, which also indicate that the name is registered and protected by laws that govern the use of trademarks.

Example: Chemical name: 4-amino-l-hydroxybutylidene

Generic name: alendronate sodium

Trade or brand name: Fosamax® (first letter capitalized). See Figure 11-1.

SOURCES OF DRUGS

Drugs prepared from roots, herbs, bark, and other forms of plant life are among the earliest known pharmaceuticals. Their origin can be traced back to primitive cultures where they were first used to evoke magical powers and drive out evil spirits. In South America, the Carib Indians coated the tips of their arrows with a poisonous substance obtained from trees, thereby improving their chances of success in hunting. The pharmacologically active ingredients of this substance (Curare) facilitate muscle relaxation, and, like many of the compounds discovered by primitive groups, are still used by drug manufacturers as components of modern-day medications.

Having discovered that certain plants were pharmacologically useful, early humans began a search for other potential sources of drugs that continues to this day. In addition to plants, drugs are

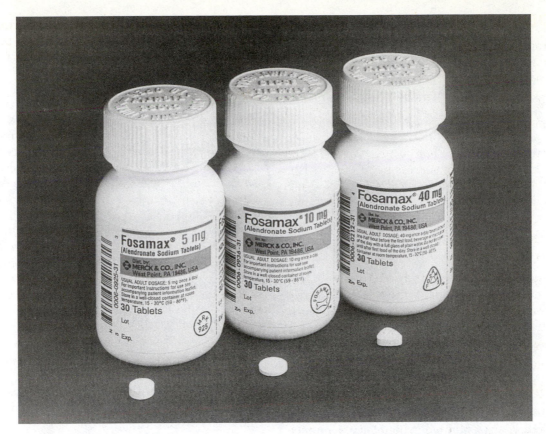

FIGURE 11-1   FOSAMAX® (ALENDRONATE SODIUM) 5 MG, 10 MG, AND 40 MG TABLETS *(Courtesy of Merck & Company, Inc.)*

now derived from animals and minerals, and are produced in laboratories utilizing chemical and biochemical processes.

Plants

As previously mentioned, the leaves, roots, stems, or fruit of certain plants may contain medicinal properties. The dried leaf of the purple foxglove plant is a source for digitalis, a cardiac glycoside used in the treatment of congestive heart failure.

The kelp plant is a rich source of iodine, a nonmetallic element. Iodine is not only used as a disinfectant, but is essential for the proper development and functioning of the thyroid gland. See Figure 11-2.

Another example of a drug derived from a plant source is Cenestin (synthetic conjugated estrogens), which is synthesized from soy and yam plants. This drug is prescribed for menopausal and postmenopausal women as estrogen replacement therapy.

Researchers have concluded that an extract from the saw palmetto plant (*Serenoa repens*) appears to be effective in easing the symptoms of be-

nign prostatic hyperplasia (BPH). Benign prostatic hyperplasia is a common age-related swelling of the prostate gland that is thought to affect up to 40 percent of men age 70 and older. This condition is characterized by frequent urges to urinate, and, if untreated, can lead to bladder infections and kidney damage.

Animals

There only a few drugs that are made from the fluids, tissues, organs, and/or glands of animals. Premarin (conjugated estrogens) is produced from the urine of a pregnant mare. This drug is prescribed for menopausal and postmenopausal women as estrogen replacement therapy.

Adrenaline and cortisone are two compounds that can be extracted from the adrenal glands of animals. See Figure 11-2. Adrenaline is a sympathomimetic drug used to relieve respiratory distress, relieve hypersensitivity reactions, and prolong the action of infiltration anesthetics. Cortisone is an anti-inflammatory agent used in the treatment of rheumatoid arthritis and certain skin conditions.

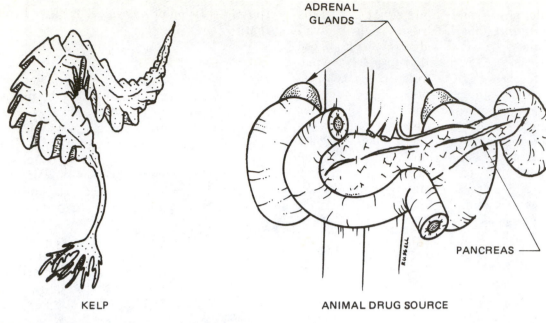

FIGURE 11-2 SOURCES OF DRUGS *(Courtesy of James Russell, Jr.)*

Minerals

Some naturally occurring mineral substances are used in medicine in a highly purified form. One such mineral is sulfur, a nonmetallic element that has been used for many years as a key ingredient in certain bacteriostatic drugs. Now prepared synthetically, sulfa drugs have widespread use in the treatment of urinary and intestinal tract infections.

Synthetic Drugs

By combining various chemicals, scientists can produce compounds that are identical to a natural drug, or they can create entirely new substances. These drugs are synthetic medications prepared in pharmaceutical laboratories.

For example, Chloromycetin may be produced naturally by organic means, or it may be created synthetically from ingredients that make up its chemical formula. Other drugs, such as sulfathiazole, cannot be produced by organic means, and are available only as a result of synthetic processes. Two advantages of synthetically prepared drugs are that they can be produced in great volume, and, consequently, are usually less expensive than organically derived medications.

Genetically Engineered Pharmaceuticals

Genetic engineering is a biotechnology that has revolutionized agriculture, industry, health, and med-

icine. Scientists are now capable of creating new strains of bacteria using a technique known as *gene splicing*. Through this process, hybrid forms of life have been created that benefit humankind by providing an alternate source of drugs, such as insulin (Humulin®) for the diabetic patient, and interferon for use in the treatment of cancer.

Genetic engineering has proved to be one of the most extraordinary sources of drugs ever known to humans. The application of recombinant DNA technology in pharmaceuticals grows every day. Recombinant technology can harness bacteria to make certain drugs or hormones. This technique has been used to make human insulin using *Escherichia coli (E. coli)*. Examples of other drugs that have been produced using biotechnology are Activase (alteplase, recombinant), a tissue-plasminogen activator that may be used for clients with heart attacks, acute ischemic strokes, and/or acute massive pulmonary embolism; Nutropin (somatropin-rDNA origin), a human growth hormone; Protropin (somatrem), a growth hormone; and Pulmozyme (dornase alfa, recombinant) for the management of cystic fibrosis.

DRUG LEGISLATION

Qualified medical practitioners who **prescribe** (to order or recommend the use of a drug, diet, or other form of therapy), **dispense** (to prepare and give out), or **administer** (to give) drugs must comply with federal and state laws governing the manufacture, sale, possession, administration, and dispensing and prescribing of drugs. All drugs available for legal use are controlled by the Federal Food, Drug and Cosmetic Act. This law protects the public by insuring the purity, strength, and composition of food, drugs, and cosmetics. It also prohibits the movement, in interstate commerce, of adulterated and misbranded food, drugs, devices, and cosmetics. Enforcement of the Federal Food, Drug and Cosmetic Act is the responsibility of the Food and Drug Administration (FDA), which is a part of the Department of Health and Human Services (HHS) of the U.S. government.

Controlled Substances Act of 1970

The Controlled Substances Act of 1970 controls the manufacture, importation, compounding, selling, dealing in, and giving away of drugs that have the potential for addiction and abuse. These drugs, known as **controlled substances**, include opium and cocaine and their derivatives, narcotics, stimulants, and depressants. The Drug Enforcement Administration (DEA) of the U.S. Justice Department enforces the act, which is also known as the Comprehensive Drug Abuse Prevention and Control Act. Under federal law, medical practitioners who prescribe, administer, or dispense controlled substances must register with the DEA, and physicians are required to renew their registration every 3 years.

Drug Schedules

Controlled substances are classified according to five drug schedules. Table 11-1 lists the five drug schedules and gives examples of the controlled substances in each classification.

Controlled substance analogues are a new class of substances created by the Anti-Drug Abuse Act of 1986. A **controlled substance analogue** is a substance with a chemical structure substantially similar to the chemical structure of a controlled substance in Schedule I or II.

Registration

Any person who handles or intends to handle controlled substances must obtain a registration issued by the Drug Enforcement Administration. A unique number is assigned to the importer, exporter, manufacturer, distributor, hospital, pharmacy, practitioner, and researcher. Exceptions include physicians who are interns, residents, from a foreign country, or on the staff of a Veterans Administration facility, who prescribe and dispense controlled substances using a special code under the registration of a hospital or other health care institution.

Record Keeping

Controlled substances may be dispensed by a practitioner by direct administration, by prescription, or by dispensing from office supplies. Records of Schedule II substances must be maintained separately from all other records. Schedule III, IV, and V records must be maintained separately or otherwise be readily retrievable from the ordinary professional and business records. This also includes computer-generated records. This data system is maintained on a daily basis and kept for a minimum of 2 years (3 years in some states). The Controlled Substances Act does not require the practitioner to maintain copies of prescriptions, but certain states require the use of multiple copy prescriptions for Schedule II and other specified controlled substances.

Security

Controlled substances must be kept separate from other drugs. They must be placed in a double-locked compartment such as a securely locked box placed in a locked safe or a substantially constructed cabinet. The number of employees with access to controlled substances must be kept to a minimum. The person responsible for the administration of controlled substances must keep the narcotic keys protected from possible misuse.

DRUG REFERENCES/ STANDARDS

The *United States Pharmacopeia/National Formulary* (USP/NF) is recognized by the U.S. government as the official list of standardized drugs. Published every 5 years by the United States Pharmacopeial Convention, this reference book includes only those drugs that have been tested and certified as having met established standards of quality, purity, and potency. Such testing may involve *assay*, whereby the ingredients of the drug are identified and measured, and/or *bioassay*, wherein the dosage necessary to produce a therapeutic effect is established utilizing animal studies. Each revision of the USP/NF includes new drugs and drops those older products that have been replaced by safer or more effective drugs.

Upon release by the FDA, the drug may be listed in *New Drugs* until it has been proved to be of sufficient value to be included in the *United States Pharmacopeia/National Formulary*. The

TABLE 11-1 DRUG SCHEDULES WITH EXAMPLES OF CONTROLLED SUBSTANCES

Schedule	Description with Examples
Schedule I (C-I)	Drugs that have a high potential for abuse and are not accepted for medical use within the United States (examples: heroin, LSD, marijuana, mescaline, nicocodeine, peyote, psilocybin, psilocyn)
Schedule II (C-II)	Drugs that have a high potential for abuse, but do have an accepted medical use within the United States (examples: Amytal, cocaine, codeine, Dexedrine, Dilaudid, Demerol, fentanyl citrate, morphine, opium, Percodan, Numorphan, Nembutal, Preludin, Ritalin [see Figure 11-3], Seconal)
Schedule III (C-III)	Drugs that have a low to moderate potential for physical dependency, yet have a high potential for psychological dependency. They do have an accepted medical use within the United States (examples: anabolic steroids, barbiturates, Doriden, Nalline, Noludar, paregoric, Tylenol with codeine).
Schedule IV (C-IV)	Drugs that have a low potential for abuse relative to Schedule III drugs. They do have an accepted medical use within the United States (examples: Ativan, barbital, chloral hydrate, Clonopin, Equanil, Librium, Placidyl, Serax, Valium, Xanax).
Schedule V (C-V)	Drugs that have the lowest abuse potential of controlled substances. They do have an accepted medical use within the United States (examples: Actifed with codeine, Donnagel, Lomotil, Robitussin A-C syrup).

Federal Food, Drug and Cosmetic Act specifies that a drug is official when it is listed in the USP/NF.

New Drugs, published annually by the Council on Pharmacy of the American Medical Association, lists all drugs having reached a certain frequency of use. Listing does not imply endorsement of any drug by the AMA. This publication provides health professionals with an up-to-date listing of drugs new to the market.

The *Physicians' Desk Reference* (PDR) is a useful drug information book for physicians and health professionals. Published annually by Medical Economics Company, Inc., in cooperation with pharmaceutical companies, it is an excellent drug reference book (see Figure 11-4). Supplements to the PDR are provided to purchasers of the book as they become available throughout the year, thereby keeping this reference current.

The *PDR Nurse's Drug Handbook* (or Delmar's Nurse's Drug Handbook for the 2003 version and beyond) is an authoritative source of information on prescription medications. Published annually by Delmar Thomson Learning, it is organized for quick, easy access by generic name. Dosage forms and routes are delineated and correlated, when appropriate, with the target disease state. Boldface italics highlight life-threatening side effects. For fast emergency reference, symptoms and treatment of overdose are summarized in each drug's "Overdose Management" section. Nursing considerations are presented in nursing process format, with assessment, intervention, teaching, and evaluation guidelines all clearly labeled. Specific criteria for evaluating the outcomes of drug therapy are easily found in the "Outcomes/Evaluate" section. Instant Internet updates are available at the handbook's Web site at www.delmar.com.

What's in the PDR?

Contents

Manufacturers' Index (white pages). Section 1: Alphabetical arrangement of all pharmaceutical manufacturers participating in the PDR. Includes addresses, phone numbers, and emergency contacts. Shows each manufacturer's products and the page number of those described in the PDR.

Brand and Generic Name Index (pink pages). Section 2: Gives the page number of each product by brand and generic name.

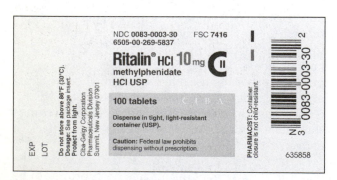

FIGURE 11-3 EXAMPLE OF A SCHEDULE II DRUG *(Courtesy of Akorn Manufacturing, Inc., Decatur, Illinois)*

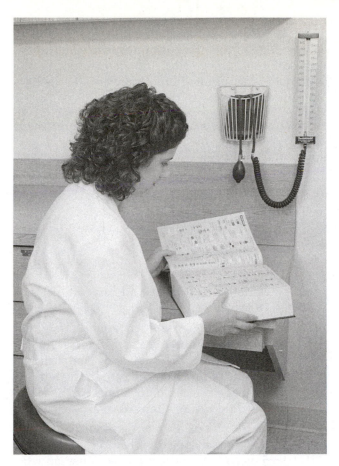

FIGURE 11-4 THE *PHYSICIANS' DESK REFERENCE* IS A USEFUL DRUG INFORMATION SOURCE.

Product Category Index (blue pages). Section 3: Lists all fully described products by prescribing category.

Product Identification Guide (gray pages). Section 4: Presents full-color, actual-size photos of tablets and capsules, plus pictures of a variety of other dosage forms and packages. Arranged alphabetically by manufacturer.

Product Information (white pages). Section 5: Provides prescribing information. This section includes an alphabetical arrangement by manufacturer of over 2500 products. The general format of this section is as follows:

Brand Name [phonetic spelling]

Generic Name

Description

Clinical Pharmacology

Indications and Usage

Contraindications

Warnings

Precautions

Adverse Reactions

Dosage and Administration

How Supplied

Diagnostic Product Information (green pages). Section 6: Gives usage guidelines for a variety of common diagnostic agents. Included in this section you will find

Certified Poison Control Centers

Discontinued Products

U.S. Food and Drug Administration Telephone Directory

Key to Controlled Substances Categories

Key to FDA Use-In-Pregnancy Ratings

Drug Information Centers

Note: All controlled substances listed in the PDR are indicated with the symbol C, with the Roman numeral II, III, IV, or V printed inside the C to designate the schedule in which the substance is classified.

Example: DURAMORPH® Ⓒ

morphine sulfate injection, USP

How to Use the PDR

Drugs contained in the *Physicians' Desk Reference* are listed according to

- Brand name and generic name (pink section)
- Classification or category (blue section)
- Alphabetical arrangement by manufacturers (white section)

The following guidelines will assist you as you learn to use the PDR:

1. If you know the brand name of the drug, turn to the pink section and locate the drug in the alphabetical listing. The manufacturer's name will be in parentheses, followed by a page number, or two page numbers. The first number is the product identification page number. The second number is the product information section (white).

Example: Look up Achromycin V capsules in the current PDR.

Achromycin® V

[a-kro-mi-cin]

tetracycline HCL

for ORAL USE

Note all the information provided about the drug.

Description. Gives the origin and chemical composition of the drug.

Clinical Pharmacology. Indicates the effect of the drug upon the body and the process by which the drug exerts this effect

Indications. States the various conditions, diseases, types of microorganisms, etc., that the drug is used for

Contraindications. This drug is contraindicated in persons who have shown hypersensitivity to any of the tetracyclines.

Warnings. Gives the potential dangers of the drug

Precautions. States the possible unfavorable effects that the drug may have upon a client

Adverse Reactions. Lists the side effects of the drug

Dosage and Administration. States the amount (usual daily dose for adults and children) and time sequence of administration

How Supplied. Lists the various forms of the drug and their dosages

2. If you know the classification of the drug, turn to the blue section and locate the category of the drug.

Example: Antibiotics, Systemic

Tetracyclines

Achromycin V capsules (Lederle)

3. On occasion you may not find the drug that you are looking for listed in the PDR. When this happens,

a. Refer to another drug reference book

b. Refer to the product information insert that comes in the drug package

c. Ask a pharmacist about the drug

An important source of information about a particular drug is the *product information insert* that most manufacturers provide with their product. This is a brief description of the drug, its clinical pharmacology, indications and usage, contraindications, warnings, precautions, drug interactions, adverse reactions, overdosage, dosage, and administration. The package insert can be a valuable source of information about new drugs that might not be listed elsewhere.

DRUG DOSAGE

The **dosage** is the amount of medicine that is prescribed for administration. It is determined by the physician or a qualified practitioner who considers the following factors in the decision:

● Weight, sex, and age of the client

Age. The usual adult dose is usually suitable for the 20–60 age group. Infants, young children, adolescents, and the aged require individualized dosage.

Pediatric clients are usually divided into three age groups:

Newborn—0 to 4 weeks

Infant—5 to 52 weeks

Child—1 to 16 years; adolescent—12 to 16 years

Pediatric clients require a smaller amount of a medication because of differences in gastrointestinal function, body composition, metabolism, and reduced renal function. The dosage is often determined by the size of the child rather than the age.

Geriatric clients are not necessarily divided into a specific age group because of the wide variance in the aging process. A person who is 60 years old or older may or may not be considered a geriatric client. Therefore, the physician will consider all factors, including the mental and physical state of the individual, to determine an appropriate dosage regimen. The geriatric client requires special considerations because of the following factors:

— Decreased gastrointestinal function that may cause poor absorption. Geriatric clients often suffer from constipation.

— Impaired or reduced metabolism

— Changes in body composition; limitations, deformities

— Alterations in circulation, liver and kidney function

— Changes in body functioning; systems, eyes, ears, and speech

— Sensitivity to drugs

— Number of medications the client is taking; drug interactions

— Psychosocial changes

Alertness

Confusion

Attitude

Forgetfulness

Misunderstanding of directions

Memory loss

— Disease process; multiple conditions

— Self-medication; over-the-counter (OTC) drugs

— Cost

— Living conditions; alone, with mate, skilled nursing facility or other care facility

— Poor water intake

- Pregnancy and lactation
- The physical and emotional condition of the client
- The disease process
- The presence of another disease process
- The causative microorganism and the severity of the infection
- The client's past medical history, allergies, idiosyncrasies, and so forth
- The safest method, route, time, and amount to effect the desired maximum result

Terms Used to Describe Dosages

- An *initial dose* is the first dose.
- An *average dose* is the amount of medication proven most effective with minimum toxic effect.
- A *maintenance dose* is the amount that will keep concentrations of the drug at a therapeutic level in the client's bloodstream.
- A *maximum dose* is the largest amount of a medication that can be given safely to a client.
- A *minimum dose* is the smallest dose that will be effective.
- A *therapeutic dose* is the amount needed to produce the desired effect.
- A *divided dose* is a fractional portion administered at short intervals.
- A *unit dose* is a premeasured amount of the medication, individually packaged on a per dose basis.
- A *cumulative dose* is the summation of the drug present in the body after repeated medication.
- A *lethal dose* is the amount of the medication that could kill a client.
- A *toxic dose* is the amount of a drug that causes signs and symptoms of drug toxicity.

● SELF-ASSESSMENT

Give answers to the following statements by the method indicated.

Source

p. 70   1. List the five general medical uses for drugs mentioned in this chapter:

_____ ,

_____ ,

_____ ,

_____ , and

_____ , or

_____ .

p. 70   2. Most drugs have three types of names: chemical, generic, and trade (or brand). Of these, the official name for the drug is the _____ name.

p. 71   3. In the chapter, _____ is given as an example of a drug the source of which is a living animal's urine. This drug is prescribed for _____ replacement therapy.

p. 72   4. True or False (circle one) The chapter lists two specific advantages that synthetic drugs have over other medicinal forms. These are the purity of the substance and their increased compatibility with other drugs.

p. 73   5. True or False (circle one) Although it is illegal under the Controlled Substances Act of 1970 to either manufacture, import, or sell a controlled substance, it is usually permissible to give away samples of such drugs.

p. 74   6. The primary factor that separates Schedule I (C-I) from Schedule II drugs is that C-II drugs have _____.

p. 73–74   7. Four publications mentioned in the chapter as recognized drug references are:

The _____ (USP/NF),

The _____ (PDR),

The _____ ,

and _____ .

p. 76   8. You read a label that lists the usual adult dose. According to this chapter, the usual adult dose is suitable for persons between _____ and _____ years.

p. 76   9. Pediatric dosages are often determined by the _____ of the child rather than the _____ of the child.

p. 77   10. Supply the missing word to complete the following statements:

- The _____ dose is the smallest dose that will be effective.

- The _____ dose is the amount that could kill a client.

- The _____ dose is a fractional portion given at short intervals.

- The _____ dose is the largest dose that can be safely administered.

- The _____ dose is the first dose administered.

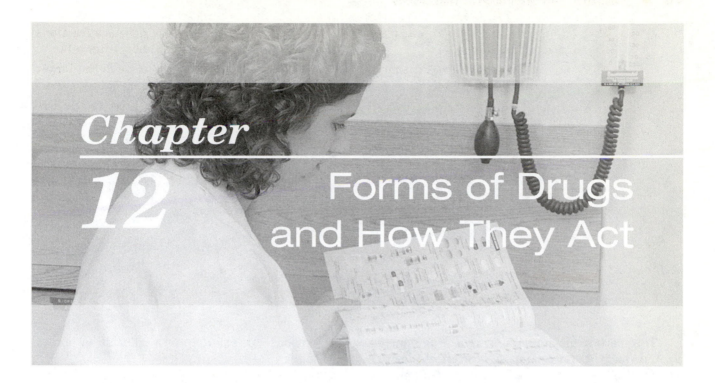

Chapter 12

Forms of Drugs and How They Act

Chapter Outline

- Define selected classifications of drugs and give examples of each
- List the three general ways that drugs may be grouped
- Define the actions of drugs according to the descriptive terms listed in this chapter
- Describe the factors that affect drug action
- Describe the undesirable actions of drugs
- Complete the Self-Assessment

Objectives

Upon completion of this chapter, you should be able to

- Define the key terms
- List the forms in which drugs are prepared, and give examples of these preparations
- List the routes used for drug administration
- Classify drugs according to preparation and therapeutic action

Key Terms

adverse reaction	side effect
depressant	solvent
interaction	stimulant

INTRODUCTION

Drugs are compounded in three basic types of preparations: liquids, solids, and semisolids. The ease with which a drug's ingredients can be dissolved largely determines the variety of forms manufactured. Some drug agents are soluble in water, others in alcohol, and yet others in a mixture of several **solvents** (that in which a substance is dissolved).

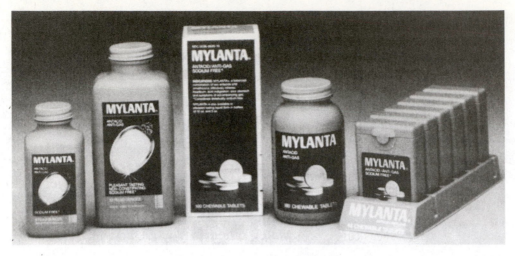

FIGURE 12-1   MYLANTA LIQUID AND TABLETS *(Courtesy of Stuart Pharmaceuticals)*

The method for administering a drug depends upon its form, its properties, and the effects desired. See Figure 12-1. When given orally, a drug may be in the form of a liquid, powder, tablet, capsule, or caplet. If it is to be injected, it must be in the form of a liquid. For topical use, the drug may be in the form of a liquid, a powder, or a semisolid. Oral and injectable medications are examples of preparations designed for internal use.

FORMS OF DRUGS

The forms of drugs described in this chapter are liquid preparations, solid and semisolid preparations, and other drug delivery systems.

Liquid Preparations

Liquid preparations are those containing a drug that has been dissolved or suspended. Depending upon the solvent used, the drug may be further classified as an aqueous (water) or alcohol preparation. When prescribed for internal use, liquid preparations other than emulsions are rapidly absorbed through the stomach or intestinal walls. The following are types of liquid preparations:

- *Emulsions.* Emulsions consist of fine droplets of an oil in water or water in oil. They separate into layers after standing for long periods of time and must be shaken vigorously before they are ready for use. An example of an emulsion is castor oil.

- *Solutions.* One or more drugs can be dissolved in an appropriate solvent to make a solution. The solution will appear to be clear and homo-geneous. An example of a solution is normal saline.

- *Mixtures and suspensions.* Drugs that have been mixed with a liquid, but not dissolved, are called mixtures or suspensions. These preparations must be shaken before being administered to the client. Milk of magnesia is an example of a mixture or suspension.

- *Syrups.* Drugs dissolved in a solution of sugar and water and then flavored are called syrups. An example is Benylin DM cough syrup.

- *Elixirs.* Drugs dissolved in a solution of alcohol and water that has been sweetened and flavored are elixirs. When prepared in this manner, the bitter or salty taste of the drug is disguised. For this reason, elixirs are frequently used for children's medications. An example of an elixir is Donnatal® (phenobarbital, hyoscyamine sulfate, atropine sulfate, and scopolamine hydrobromide). Donnatal is also available in tablets and capsules. See Figure 12-2.

- *Tinctures.* Tinctures are drugs dissolved in alcohol or alcohol and water. For the most part, they are made to represent a 10 percent solution of the drug agent. An example is tincture of digitalis. Another example, tincture of iodine, is an exception to the 10 percent rule. It may be found as a 7 percent or 2 percent tincture.

- *Spirits.* Alcoholic solutions of volatile (easily vaporized) drugs are called spirits. A spirit is also called an essence. Examples are spirits of peppermint and aromatic spirits of ammonia.

- *Fluidextracts.* Drugs that have been processed to a concentrated strength using alcohol as the solvent are called fluidextracts. Examples in-

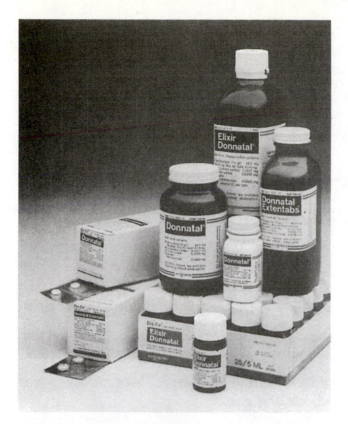

FIGURE 12-2   DONNATAL ELIXIR, TABLETS, EXTENTABS, AND CAPSULES *(Courtesy of A. H. Robins Company)*

clude fluidextract of ergot, fluidextract of ipecac, and cascara sagrada fluidextract.

- *Lotions.* Aqueous preparations of suspended ingredients used externally (without massage) to treat skin conditions are lotions. They may be a clear solution, suspension, or emulsion. Examples are Calamine lotion and Caladryl.

- *Liniments.* Liniments are drugs that are used externally, with massage, to produce a feeling of heat to the area. An example is methyl salicylate.

- *Sprays.* As the name implies, sprays are drugs prepared to such a consistency that they may be administered by an atomizer. They are used primarily to treat nose and throat conditions. Some drugs administered by this method function as astringents and produce a shrinking or contracting effect. Others function as antiseptics and inhibit the growth of bacteria. Oil is usually used as a solvent. An example of a spray is Neosynephrine.

- *Aerosols.* These preparations may contain medications, ointments, creams, lotions, powders, or liquids. They utilize a propellant, such as butane, and are packaged in pressurized units. An

example is Azmacort inhaler in a metered-dose aerosol unit. Azmacort is an anti-inflammatory steroid. (See Figure 15-20 in Chapter 15.

Solid and Semisolid Preparations

Tablets, capsules, caplets, troches or lozenges, suppositories, and ointments are examples of solid and semisolid preparations. These products offer great flexibility as a means of dispensing different dosages of drugs. See Figure 12-3. The following describes these products in detail:

- *Capsules* are small two-part containers (hard or soft shell) that are usually made of a gelatin substance that is designed to dissolve in the stomach or gastrointestinal tract. Some capsules contain drug-impregnated beads (sustained action) that are designed to release the medication at different rates.

- *Caplets* have the size and shape of a capsule, but the consistency of a tablet. They are coated, solid preparations for oral administration.

- *Tablets* are medication in the form of a powder compressed into a small, disklike shape. Tablets come in various sizes, shapes, colors, and compositions. The following are some of the descriptive names for certain tablets:

  — *Enteric-coated* tablets are designed to pass through the stomach without dissolving. Their special coating will dissolve in the small intestine.

  — *Buccal* tablets are formulated to be dissolved and absorbed when placed between the cheek and gum.

  — *Sublingual* tablets are designed to be placed under the tongue where they dissolve and are absorbed.

  — *Chewable* tablets are designed to be chewed. They contain a base of flavored and/or colored mannitol (a sugar alcohol). They are a preferred dosage form for antacids and for some vitamins. Chewable tablets are often used for children. A new form of chewable tablets is called quick dissolve. This unique form dissolves quickly in the mouth. An example is Quick Dissolve Maalox, which is used to quickly relieve heartburn and acid indigestion.

  — *Effervescent* tablets are made with granular effervescent salts and/or other materials that release gas. When placed in water, they dispense active ingredients into the solution. An example is Alka-Seltzer effervescent tablets.

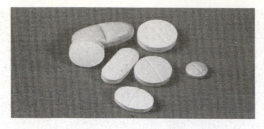

A. SCORED TABLETS

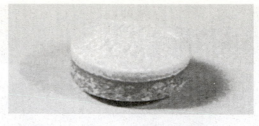

B. LAYERED TABLET

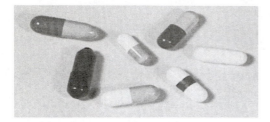

C. HARD GELATIN CAPSULES

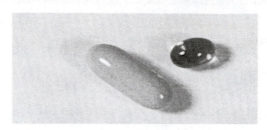

D. SOFT GELATIN CAPSULES

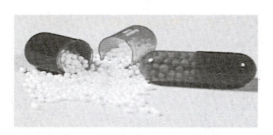

E. SUSTAINED ACTION CAPSULES

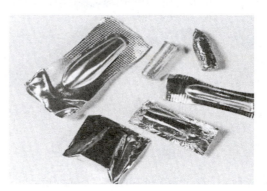

F. SUPPOSITORIES

FIGURE 12-3   EXAMPLES OF SOLID AND SEMISOLID PREPARATIONS

—*Vaginal* tablets are designed to be placed into the vagina via an applicator. They dissolve in the vagina and are absorbed into the vaginal mucosa. An example is Mycostatin antifungal vaginal tablets.

—*Layered* tablets contain two or more layers of ingredients, or the same ingredient that has been treated to provide a different absorption rate.

—*Scored* tablets are those whose surfaces have been grooved or scored to make it easy for the user to break them into halves or quarters in order to vary the dosage. See Figure 12-4.

● *Troches* or *lozenges* are hard, circular or oblong disks that consist of a medication in a candy-like base. They dissolve in the mouth and are commonly used to treat a sore throat. The effec-

tiveness of this medication is destroyed by drinking liquids too soon after use.

● *Suppositories* are semisolid preparations designed for insertion into the rectum, vagina, or urethra. A suppository consists of a drug agent or agents combined with a base of soap, glycerinated gelatin, or cocoa butter oil. These bases are selected because they are readily fusible (will melt) when subjected to body heat. Suppositories are usually shaped like a cylinder or cone and are classified as drugs for external use. Often supplied in a foil or other wrapper that must be removed before insertion, suppositories are usually lubricated with a water-soluble jelly.

● *Topical* preparations are designed for use on the skin. They exert either a local or systemic effect. Their mode of action depends upon the composition of the drug or drugs contained

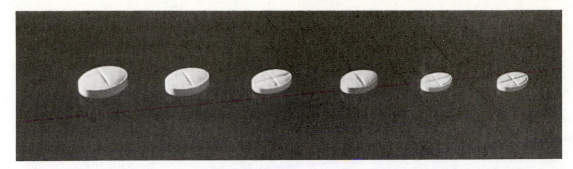

FIGURE 12-4   MEDROL GROOVED (SCORED) TABLETS (2, 4, 8, 16, 24, AND 32 MG) *(Courtesy of Pharmacia &*
Upjohn Company)

within the preparation. They may be compounded with an oily base (ointments) or a water base (lotions, creams). See Figure 12-5 for an example of a cream. Other topical preparations may be in the form of a liniment, oil, gel, foam, soap, or powder.

Other Drug Delivery Systems

Technological advances have introduced new ways by which drugs can be introduced into the client. In addition to the conventional preparations already covered, the following miniature therapeutic systems offer "special delivery" of medication to targeted areas.

Transdermal System

The transdermal system is a small adhesive patch that may be applied to intact skin near the treatment site. For example, Transderm Scop may be applied behind the ear to prevent motion sickness; Transderm-Nitro may be applied to the chest to prevent angina pectoris; Estraderm may be applied to the trunk to treat menopausal symptoms; and Nicoderm® may be applied to any area above the waist to relieve the body's craving for nicotine. A transdermal system generally consists of four layers (see Figure 12-6):

1. An impermeable backing that keeps the drug from leaking out of the system
2. A reservoir containing the drug
3. A membrane with tiny holes in it that controls the rate of drug release
4. An adhesive layer or gel that keeps the device in place

Ocular Therapeutic System

The ocular therapeutic system is another innovative drug delivery system in which a drug contained between two ultrathin plastic membranes is placed inside the lower eyelid. It appears to cause little or no discomfort and provides a controlled release of the medication for an extended period of time. Pilocarpine, a miotic that causes contraction of the pupil, is being used in this method for the treatment of glaucoma.

Implantable Devices

These devices come in several shapes and sizes and are positioned just beneath the skin, near blood vessels that lead directly to an area to be medicated. For example, an infusion pump that is about the size of a hockey puck can be implanted below the skin, near the waist, to provide continuous delivery of chemotherapy to clients with liver cancer. This

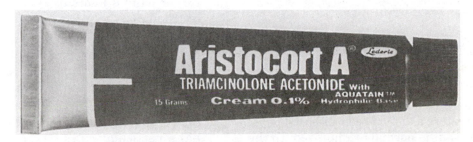

FIGURE 12-5   ARISTOCORT A® CREAM 0.1% *(Courtesy of Lederle Laboratories Division of*
American Cyanamid Company)

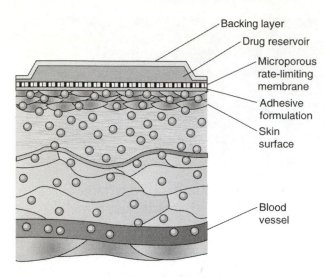

Backing layer
Drug reservoir
Microporous rate-limiting membrane
Adhesive formulation
Skin surface
Blood vessel

FIGURE 12-6 THE MULTILAYER UNIT COMPRISING TRANSDERM-NITRO® DELIVERS NITROGLYCERIN INTO THE BLOODSTREAM IN A CONSISTENT, CONTROLLED MANNER FOR 24 HOURS. THE VERY THIN UNIT CONTAINS A BACKING LAYER, A RESERVOIR OF NITROGLYCERIN, A UNIQUE RATE-LIMITING MEMBRANE, AND AN ADHESIVE LAYER THAT HAS A PRIMING DOSE OF NITROGLYCERIN. *(Courtesy of CIBA Pharmaceutical Company)*

device, which has a refillable drug reservoir, is connected by an outlet catheter to the client's blood vessel. In addition to providing a continuous supply of medication, these devices have the advantage of delivering higher doses with fewer side effects than can be realized through the systemic route.

CLASSIFICATION OF DRUGS/ THERAPEUTIC ACTION

There are many ways that drugs are classified. Two of these ways are by preparation and by therapeutic action. The therapeutic action of the drug involves the process of treating, relieving, or obtaining results through the action of the medication upon the body. Table 12-1 includes selected classifications, action, and examples.

PRINCIPAL ACTIONS OF DRUGS

Drugs may be used as a cure for disease. They may also be used to restore a disturbed or diseased physical state to one that is normal or improved. In the latter case, drugs assist the body to overcome its own difficulties by causing a change in cell activity

without altering basic cell functions. In general, drugs may be grouped as follows:

- Those that act directly upon one or more tissues of the body
- Those that act upon microorganisms invading the body (chemotherapy and antibiotics)
- Those that replace body chemicals and secretions (hormones)

Certain drugs are prescribed because of the selective actions that result when they are administered. The following descriptive terms have been applied to drugs because of the action that takes place:

- *Selective action* is a term applied to drugs that act upon certain tissues or on specific organs of the body. They are principally the stimulants and depressants.
  - **Stimulants** are drugs that increase cell activity. An example is caffeine, which acts to stimulate the cerebrum.
  - **Depressants** are drugs that decrease cell activity. An example is morphine, which acts to depress the respiratory center in the brain.
- *Agonist action* is that in which a drug has affinity for the cellular receptors (specific sites in certain cells) of another drug or natural substance and initiates/produces a drug response.
- *Antagonist action* is that in which a drug binds to a cellular receptor for a hormone, neurotransmitter, or another drug blocking the action of that substance without producing any drug effect itself.

> **Note:** A receptor is a receiver, a cell component that combines with a hormone, neurotransmitter, or drug to alter the function of the cell.

- *Local action* is the term applied to an external drug designed to act on the area to which it is administered. An example is methyl salicylate, a medication that is often applied to sore muscles or painful joints by rubbing it into the affected area.
- *Remote action* is the term applied to a drug affecting a part of the body that is distant from the site of administration. An example is an apomorphine injection into the arm to stimulate the vomiting center in the brain.
- *Specific action* is the term applied to a drug that has a particular effect on a certain pathogenic organism. An example is the action of primaquine on the malarial parasite.

TABLE 12-1   SELECTED DRUG CLASSIFICATION

Classification	Action	Examples
Analgesic	An agent that relieves pain without causing loss of consciousness	acetaminophen (Tylenol) aspirin ibuprofen (Advil, Motrin)
Anesthetic	An agent that produces a lack of feeling. May be local or general depending upon the type and how administered	lidocaine HCl (Xylocaine) procaine HCl (Novocain)
Antacid	An agent that neutralizes acid	Amphojel, Gelusil, Mylanta, Aludrox, Milk of Magnesia
Antianxiety	An agent that relieves anxiety and muscle tension	benzodiazepines: diazepam (Valium) and chlordiazepoxide HCl (Librium)
Antiarrhythmic	An agent that controls cardiac arrhythmias	lidocaine HCl (Xylocaine) propranolol HCl (Inderal)
Antibiotic	An agent that is destructive to or inhibits growth of microorganisms	penicillins (Pentids, Duracillin, Polycillin, Pipracil, Augmentin) cephalosporins (Keflin, Mandol, Rocephin)
Anticholinergic	An agent that blocks parasympathetic nerve impulses	atropine, scopolamine, trihexyphenidyl HCl (Artane)
Anticoagulant	An agent that prevents or delays blood clotting	heparin sodium, Dicumarol, warfarin sodium (Coumadin)
Anticonvulsant	An agent that prevents or relieves convulsions	carbamazepine (Tegretol) phenytoin (Dilantin) ethosuximide (Zarontin)
Antidepressant	An agent that prevents or relieves the symptoms of depression	monoamine oxidase (MAO) inhibitors: isocarboxazid (Marplan), phenelzine sulfate (Nardil), amitriptyline HCl (Elavil), imipramine HCl (Tofranil)
Antidiarrheal	An agent that prevents or relieves diarrhea	Lomotil, Pepto-Bismol, Kaopectate
Antidote	An agent that counteracts poisons and their effects	naloxone (Narcan)
Antiemetic	An agent that prevents or relieves nausea and vomiting	Tigan, Dramamine, Phenergan, Reglan, Marinol
Antifungal	An agent that destroys or inhibits the growth of fungi	Monistat, Nizoral, Lotrimin, Diflucan, Lamisil, Terazol
Antihistamine	An agent that acts to prevent the action of histamine	Dimetane, Benadryl, Allegra, Claritin, Zyrtec
Antihypertensive	An agent that prevents or controls high blood pressure	methyldopa (Aldomet) clonidine HCl (Catapres) metoprolol tartrate (Lopressor)
Anti-inflammatory	An agent that prevents inflammation	naproxen (Naprosyn), corticosteroids, aspirin, ibuprofen (Advil, Motrin)
Antilipemic	An agent that is used to lower abnormally high blood levels of fatty substances (lipids)	Nicobid, Mevacor, Lopid, Zocor, Lipitor

(continued)

TABLE 12-1 *(Continued)*

Classification	Action	Examples
Antimanic	An agent used for the treatment of the manic episode of manic-depressive disorder	lithium
Antineoplastic	An agent that prevents the replication of neoplastic cells	busulfan (Myleran), cyclophosphamide (Cytoxan)
Antiparkinsonian	An agent used for palliative relief of major symptoms of Parkinson's disease	Tasmar, Requip, Symmetrel, L-Dopa
Antipyretic	An agent that reduces fever	aspirin, acetaminophen (Tylenol)
Antitubercular	An agent used in the treatment of tuberculosis	Myambutol, INH, PZA, Mycobutin, Rifadin, Priftin, Streptomycin
Antitumor necrosis factor	An agent that seems to slow, if not halt altogether, the destruction of the joints by disrupting the activity of tumor necrosis factor (TNF)	Enbrel
Antitussive	An agent that prevents or relieves cough	codeine, dextromethorphan Benylin, Tessalen
Antiulcer	An agent used in the treatment of active duodenal ulcer and for pathological hypersecretory conditions	Tagamet, Pepcid, Axid, Zantac
Antiviral	An agent that combats a specific viral disease	Zovirax, Famivir, Retrovir, Denavir, Tamiflu, Relenza
Bronchodilator	An agent that dilates the bronchi	isoproterenol HCl (Isuprel), albuterol (Proventil)
Cardiac glycoside	An agent that exerts a positive inotropic effect on the heart	Digitalis preparations: Cedilanid-D, Crystodigin, Digitalin, Lanoxin
Contraceptive	Any device, method, or agent that prevents conception	Enovid-E 21, Ortho-Novum 10/11-21; 10/11-28 Triphasil-21
COX-2 inhibitor	An agent that inhibits cyclooxygenase (COX-2). An enzyme found in joints and other areas affected by inflammation	Celebrex, Vioxx, Mobic
Decongestant	An agent that reduces nasal congestion and/or swelling	oxymetazoline (Afrin), phenylephrine HCl (Neo-Synephrine), pseudoephedrine HCl (Sudafed)
Disease-modifying antirheumatic drugs (DMARDs)	An agent that may influence the course of the disease progression of rheumatoid arthritis	Ridaura, Rheumatrex, Cytoxan, Arava, Cuprimine
Diuretic	An agent that increases the excretion of urine	chlorothiazide (Diuril), furosemide (Lasix), mannitol (Osmitrol)
Emetic	An agent used to induce vomiting	Apomorphine HCl, Ipecac syrup
Expectorant	An agent that facilitates removal of secretion from broncho-pulmonary mucous membrane	guaifenesin (Robitussin)
Gastric acid pump inhibitor	An agent that suppresses gastric acid secretion by specific inhibition of the $H+/K+$ ATPase enzyme system. Used for gastroesophageal reflux disease (GERD)	Prilosec, Aciphex, Prevacid, Protonix

(continued)

TABLE 12-1   *(Continued)*

Classification	Action	Examples
Hemostatic	An agent that controls or stops bleeding	Humafac, Amicar, vitamin K
Hypnotic	An agent that produces sleep or hypnosis	secobarbital (Seconal), chloral hydrate, ethchlorvynol (Placidyl)
Hypoglycemic	An agent that lowers blood glucose level	insulin, chlorpropamide Diabinese, Glucophage, Actos, Precose
Immunologic	An agent administered to induce immunity and thereby prevent infectious disease	Diphtheria, Tetanus, and Pertussis (DTaP); Mumps, Rubeola, Rubella (MMR); Varivax, Havrix, Infanrix, Engerix-B, LYMErix
Laxative	An agent that loosens and promotes normal bowel elimination	Metamucil powder, Dulcolax
Leukotriene receptor antagonist (blocker)	An agent used for the treatment and management of asthma	Accolate, Zyflo, Singulair
Mucolytic	An agent that breaks chemical bonds in mucus, thereby lowering the viscosity	Mucomyst
Muscle relaxant	An agent that produces relaxation of skeletal muscle	Robaxin, Norflex, Paraflex, Skelaxin, Valium
Neuroleptic	An agent that modifies psychotic behavior	Thorazine, Mellaril, Stelazine, Haldol, Zyprexa, Clozaril, Risperdal
Sedative	An agent that produces a calming effect without causing sleep	amobarbital (Amytal), butabarbital sodium (Buticaps), phenobarbital
Selective serotonin reuptake inhibitors (SSRIs)	An agent that selectively inhibits serotonin reuptake and results in a potentiation of serotonergic neurotransmissions	Prozac, Luvox, Paxil, Zoloft
Serotonin nonselective reuptake inhibitors (SNRIs)	An agent that inhibits the reuptake of both serotonin and norepinephrine	Effexor
Thrombolytic	An agent that dissolves an existing thrombus when administered soon after its occurrence	Kabikinase, Streptase, Eminase, Activase, Abbokinase
Vasodilator	An agent that produces relaxation of blood vessels; lowers blood pressure	isosorbide dinitrate (Isordil), nitroglycerin
Vasopressor	An agent that produces contraction of muscles, capillaries, and arteries; elevates blood pressure	metaraminol (Aramine), norepinephrine (Levophed)

● *Systemic action* is the term applied to a drug that, when in the bloodstream as a result of injection or absorption, is carried throughout the body.

UNDESIRABLE ACTIONS OF DRUGS

Most drugs have the potential for causing an action other than their intended action. For example, certain antibiotics that are administered orally may disrupt the normal bacterial flora of the gastrointestinal tract and cause gastric discomfort. This type of reaction is known as a side effect. A **side effect** is an undesirable action of the drug and may limit the usefulness of the drug.

An **adverse reaction** is an unfavorable or harmful unintended action of a drug. Using a recent edition of the *Physicians' Desk Reference*, look up Demerol and note the adverse reactions. Lightheadedness, dizziness, sedation, nausea, and sweating are the most frequent adverse reactions to Demerol. To report an adverse reaction to a drug, you may call 1-800-FDA-1088.

A drug **interaction** may occur when one drug potentiates or diminishes the action of another drug. These actions may be desirable or undesirable. Drugs may also interact with various foods, alcohol, tobacco, and other substances. It is recommended that a pharmacist be consulted any time there is the possibility of a drug interaction.

FACTORS THAT AFFECT DRUG ACTION

The principal factors that affect drug action are absorption, distribution, biotransformation, and elimination. These factors depend upon the individual client, the form and chemical composition of the drug, and the method of administration.

● *Absorption* is the process whereby the drug passes into body fluids and tissues. The rate of absorption depends on the route of administration, the drug, differences in gastrointestinal function (pediatrics and geriatrics), and individual differences.

● *Distribution* is the process whereby the drug is transported from the blood to the intended site of action, site of biotransformation, site of storage, and site of elimination. The rate and extent of distribution depends upon the physical and chemical properties of the drug, the ability of the drug to bind to plasma proteins, and individual differences (such as cardiovascular function).

● *Biotransformation* is the chemical alteration that a substance (drug) undergoes in the body. Through this process enzymes may be activated to break down the drug and prepare it for elimination. Most biotransformation occurs in the liver.

● *Elimination* is the process whereby a substance is excreted from the body. Many drugs are eliminated via the kidneys, while others may be eliminated via the gastrointestinal tract, respiratory tract, the skin, mucous membranes, and mammary glands (breast-feeding).

LOSS OF DRUG POTENCY

The factors that determine the life of a drug include date of manufacture, the type of container in which it is packaged, the method of storage, and the drug's unique properties. Drugs, such as antibiotics, have an expiration date imprinted on their packages. Beyond this date, the product should not be used due to its gradual deterioration or change in potency.

Glass and/or plastic containers are often used to package medications because they allow the contents to be seen without exposure to air. Most unit dose medications are packaged within individual clear plastic envelopes that have a foil backing. Other medications require dark (opaque) containers to prevent deterioration due to exposure to light. Certain medications, such as reconstituted antibiotics, must be refrigerated to prevent deterioration. Other drugs require the presence of an absorbent material to remove moisture from the air within the container; otherwise, the moisture would be absorbed by the drug, affecting its potency.

● SELF-ASSESSMENT

Give answers to the following statements by the method indicated.

Source

p. 80   1. A liquid medicine has separated into distinct layers after sitting for a long time and must be shaken vigorously before use. Of the types mentioned in the chapter, this describes _____.

p. 81   2. A tablet has been designed to pass through the stomach without dissolving. Of the types mentioned, this describes _____.

p. 84   3. True or False (circle one) A drug that binds to a cellular receptor for a hormone, neurotransmitter, or another drug, thereby blocking the action of that substance without producing any drug effect itself is called an agonist.

p. 85   4. Aspirin, ibuprofen, and acetaminophen are agents that relieve pain without causing loss of consciousness. As such these drugs can be classified as _____.

p. 85   5. Aspirin, ibuprofen, and naproxen prevent inflammation; therefore, they can be classified as _____ agents.

p. 86   6. Ipecac syrup is used to induce vomiting; therefore, it can be classified as an _____ agent.

p. 87   7. Amicar and Humafac are agents that control or stop bleeding; therefore, they can be classified as _____ agents.

p. 87   8. True or False (circle one) Due to its effects on the client, nitroglycerin is an appropriate example of a vasodilator.

p. 88   9. In the spaces provided, list the four principal factors that affect drug actions. _____ , _____ , _____ and _____.

p. 87   10. Certain terms are used to describe an agent's unintended action. Write in the term that is best described by the following statements:

- _____ is descriptive of an undesirable action of a drug and may limit the drug's usefulness.

- _____ is descriptive of an unfavorable or harmful unintended action of a drug.

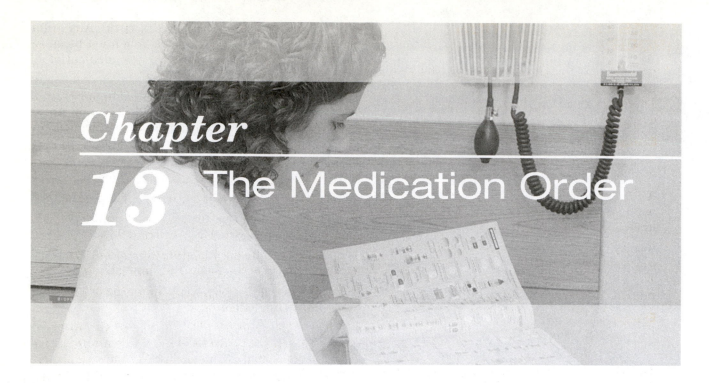

Chapter
13 The Medication Order

Chapter Outline

Objectives
Key Terms
Introduction
Types of Medication Orders
Medication Record Forms
The Medication Label
Time Schedule for Routine Medicines
Abbreviations
Self-Assessment

- Give the time schedule that may be used for routine medications
- Read and write the common medical abbreviations given in this chapter
- Complete the Self-Assessment

Key Terms

inscription   subscription
signature   superscription

Objectives

Upon completion of this chapter, you should be able to

- Define the key terms
- Describe the following types of medication orders: prn, routine, single, standing, stat, written, verbal, telephone, and prescription
- State the essential information that is included on a medication order
- List nine guidelines for understanding the medication order
- Understand medication labels (prescription and nonprescription)

INTRODUCTION

It is the physician's responsibility to diagnose the cause of an illness and to prescribe a medication. The drug prescribed is generally referred to as a *medication* or *medicine order*. Once prescribed, it is the responsibility of a legally approved health professional to carry out the medication order. Thus, it is essential that those whose duties include giving medications be familiar with the methods used to give such orders.

The medicine order is for a specific client. The order designates the drug to be used, the dosage, the form of the drug, the time or frequency for administration, and the method or route by which it is to be given.

TYPES OF MEDICATION ORDERS

- *prn order.* With this type of order, the medication is given "as necessary" or "when needed." The order includes the name of the drug, the dosage, frequency, route, and purpose.

  Example: Demerol (meperidine hydrochloride), 75 mg IM q̄ 4h prn, for severe pain

  A prn order for a narcotic is permissible, but must be rewritten every 3 to 5 days, depending upon the policy of the health care facility.

- *Routine order.* This is a prescribed, detailed course of action that is to be followed regularly. The order includes the medication, dosage, route, frequency, and purpose.

  Example: Tylenol, 1–2 tabs by mouth q̄ 4–6h, for a temperature above 100°F or 37.8°C

  This type of order is not permissible for narcotic drugs or barbiturates.

- *Single order.* This type is given one time only. The order includes the medication, dosage, route, time for administration, and purpose.

  Example: Demerol (meperidine hydrochloride), 100 mg IM, 1h before surgery

- *Standing order.* A type of protocol that is predetermined by a physician (or group of physicians) that sets forth specific instructions, guidelines, procedures, treatments, and/or medications for various client care situations

  Example: Dulcolax suppository ī q̄ am for constipation.

- *Stat order.* An order for immediate administration of a medication. The physician may write it as NOW rather than *stat* to guarantee that the medication is given at once. The physician gives the name of the drug, dosage, route, and time for administration (NOW).

  Example: Lasix (furosemide), 25 mg IM, NOW

- *Written order.* One that is inscribed by a physician (or other qualified practitioner) onto one of the following: the physician's order sheet, or a prescription for a client. Legally, this is the best type of medication order. Courts usually do not question the legality of a drug order that was written and signed by a physician; nor do they usually question an order written by another health professional and countersigned by a physician (as long as such order is

a safe drug, safe dose, and so forth). Any order that is illegible or questionable must be clarified by the physician before the medication is administered.

- *Verbal order (VO).* One expressed by speech and not written out. Student nurses should never take a verbal or telephone order. Licensed or certified health care providers should protect themselves by

  1. Writing down the order exactly as heard
  2. Repeating the order back to the physician
  3. Following the "Six Rights" of proper drug administration (See Chapter 14.)
  4. Carefully documenting all appropriate information about the administration
  5. Having the physician cosign the order within 24 hours

- *Telephone order (TO).* A type of verbal order that is transmitted via a telecommunication system. Telephone and verbal narcotic orders are approved, with reluctance, by the Narcotics Bureau. The bureau has made this major concession to hospitals for use in a true emergency situation. Whenever possible, it is a good idea to have another person listen on an extension phone when verbal orders are transmitted via the telephone. Many agencies have a policy to not accept any telephone orders for controlled substances.

- *Prescription.* A prescription is a separate written order that is not a part of the client's chart. Its purpose is to control the sale and use of drugs that can be used safely or effectively only under the supervision of a physician. A prescription is not needed for over-the-counter (OTC) drugs.

Parts of a Prescription

Refer to Figure 13-1. A prescription must include the following information:

1. The physician's name, address, telephone number, and registration number
2. The client's name, address, and the date on which the prescription is written
3. The **superscription** that includes the symbol ℞ ("take thou")
4. The **inscription** that states the names and quantities of ingredients to be included in the medication
5. The **subscription** that gives directions to the pharmacist for filling the prescription

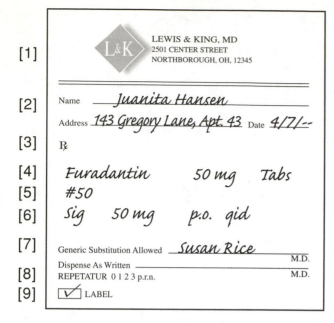

[1]	**LEWIS & KING, MD** 2501 CENTER STREET NORTHBOROUGH, OH, 12345
[2]	Name _Juanita Hansen_
	Address _143 Gregory Lane, Apt. 43_ Date _4/7/--_
[3]	℞
[4]	_Furadantin_ _50 mg_ _Tabs_
[5]	_#50_
[6]	_Sig_ _50 mg_ _p.o._ _qid_
[7]	Generic Substitution Allowed _Susan Rice_
	Dispense As Written ———————————————— M.D.
[8]	REPETATUR 0 1 2 3 p.r.n. M.D.
[9]	☑ LABEL

FIGURE 13-1   PARTS OF A PRESCRIPTION

Name of Drug: Trade/Brand   _____

Generic   _____

Clinical Pharmacology:

Indications:

Contraindications:

Warnings:

Precautions:

Adverse Reactions:

Dosage and Administration:

FIGURE 13-2   SAMPLE DRUG CARD

6. The **signature** (Sig) that gives the directions for the client

7. The physician's signature blanks. Where signed, indicates if a generic substitute is allowed or if the medication is to be dispensed as written

8. REPETATUR 0 1 2 3 prn. This is where the physician indicates whether the prescription can be refilled.

9. ☐ LABEL. Direction to the pharmacist to label the medication appropriately

> **Note:** Controlled substances such as opiates or Ritalin require a triplicate prescription whereby the physician retains a copy and the pharmacist retains two copies.

Guidelines for Understanding the Medication Order

1. It is the responsibility of the nurse to become knowledgeable about the medications that the physician prescribes.
   - Make a list of the drugs and use a drug reference book to learn about the medication.
   - Make a drug card for each drug. See Figure 13-2.
2. Write down each verbal order exactly as heard.
3. Repeat the order back to the physician.
4. Make sure you understand the medication order before administering any drug.

5. If there are any questions, ask before giving.

6. If you are ever in doubt, seek the assistance of the physician.

7. Be knowledgeable of new drugs on the market, especially any new drugs that the physician may order for specific disease processes.

8. When checking the medication administration record (MAR), if the ordered medicine is highlighted in a color, the order has been changed or discontinued.

MEDICATION RECORD FORMS

The medication record may consist of a physician's order sheet or a prescription, a medication sheet, a pharmacy patient profile, a medication administration form (Kardex, Medex), a controlled substance record book and audit form, the nurse's notes, and/or a computerized medication administration record.

Selected examples of typical medication record forms, with accompanying illustrations, have been included to acquaint you with these important documents.

The Physician's Order Sheet is a triplicate document containing a place for the date, time, medication order, and a client's drug sensitivity. The physician, using one order form per client, writes the medications to be administered, and signs the order. The original is maintained on the client's chart, a copy goes to the pharmacy, and a copy goes to the medication nurse. See Figure 13-3 for an example of a physician's order sheet.

ALBANY MEDICAL CENTER HOSPITAL
Physician's Order Sheet

INSTRUCTIONS:
1. Imprint patient's plate before placing in chart.
2. After each set of orders are written, remove first yellow copy and send to PHARMACY.
3. "X" out remaining unused lines after last copy is used.
4. Imprint new set and place in chart.

ALLERGIES:

Date Ordered	Time Ordered	Time Executed	Time Posted	USE BALL POINT PEN ONLY
				Present Weight lbs. kg. Present Height in. cm.
				"ALL ORDERS SHOULD BE PRECEDED BY THE NUMBER AND TITLE OF THE PROBLEM TO WHICH THEY REFER. NUMBER ONE (# 1) IS RESERVED FOR ROUTINE ADMISSION AND MAINTENANCE ORDERS."

FIGURE 13-3   EXAMPLE OF A PHYSICIAN'S ORDER SHEET. ALWAYS REMEMBER TO IMPRINT THE CLIENT'S IDENTIFICATION PLATE IN THE SPACE PROVIDED IN THE UPPER RIGHT-HAND CORNER. *(Courtesy of Albany Medical Center, Albany, New York)*

The physician's order is then transcribed onto a medical administration form. The transcribed order is initialed by the transcriber, who may be the charge nurse, the medication nurse, a ward secretary, or other person authorized by the employer to perform this task. The nurse giving the medication is ultimately responsible for the proper transcription of the medication order. If there is any reason for doubt, the order and transcription are checked for accuracy and completeness.

Medex is the name given to a medication record system used by some hospitals, nursing homes, and personal care facilities. The Medex may be a large, one-piece card of stiff paper. Its format divides it into several sections, each devoted to a specific type of medication order. The first section usually is used for recording prn medications. The inside section of the folded Medex card is for routine medications. This part of the form contains the greatest number of spaces for medication entries and has a section for signatures of those who administered the medicines. The third and final section is where changes are recorded. These may include tubing changes, op-site changes, filter changes, or setup changes.

A Medex card is prepared for each client. Along its lower edge are spaces for the room number, client's name, diagnosis, and physician's name. The format of this record allows the nurse to document the administration of various types of medications for a period of 8 days.

Kardex is a trade name for a large, one-piece record form printed on stiff paper. When folded, the Kardex becomes an $8\frac{1}{2} \times 11$ inch, three- or four-page client record. Typically a Kardex provides for client identification, diagnosis, the attending physician's name, the client's room number, and the admission data. The form may be divided into parts, with one part devoted to lab work and/or diagnostic tests, another part to the client care plan and is a section for medication orders. See Figure 13-4.

A *computerized medication administration record* (MAR) may be used by hospitals and other health care facilities that are furnished with the proper equipment. There are various medication administration computerized programs and record forms. The drug order is written by the physician on a *physician's order sheet*, then these data are transmitted to the pharmacy or entered into the computer, depending upon the system used for medication administration. Information from the medication administration record can also be used by the business office for the posting of charges. A hard copy of the MAR is posted in the client's chart. See Figure 13-5.

Client data and drug information that has been previously entered into the computer system, such as drug allergies, drug incompatibilities, usual dosage range, recommended administration time, recommended route of administration, and injection sites, can be assessed by the pharmacist and nurse. This provides a valuable means of assuring that the correct drug, dosage, time, and route of administration is provided for the correct client.

Hospitals that provide computers at each nurse's station allow the nurse to access the data and evaluate the drug order before administration. They also allow for direct documentation of the administration of the drug after it has been given to the client.

In long-term-care facilities where the client is a resident, drug orders are filled 30 days at a time and prepared in a bubble package. This method of drug preparation reduces the risk of error.

THE MEDICATION LABEL

The medication label can be a source of valuable information to the nurse and the client. Regardless of whether one is administering a prescription drug or taking a nonprescription drug product, an understanding of the information provided on the label is essential to the safe and effective use of any medicine. In addition to the name and address of the manufacturer, the following are the most important items of information that may be on a medication label. See Figure 13-6.

- The trade or brand name for the medication
- The generic name (or listing of active and inactive ingredients)
- The National Drug Code (NDC) numbers that can be used to identify the manufacturer, the product, and the size of the container
- The dosage strength in a given amount of the medication
- The usual dosage and frequency of administration
- The form in which the drug is supplied
- CAUTION. May also include warnings and cautionary statements
- The expiration date for the medication and the lot or batch code. This lot number must be documented on the client record when administering immunizations.
- The manufacturer's name
- The total number and /or volume of the drug contained

Other information that may be on a prescription label are the directions for storage and the

KARDEX FORM

ALLERGIES: ☐ NO   ☐ YES

SPECIAL
CONSIDERATIONS:

ADM DATE	AGE	REL	COND:		HO:	
DIAGNOSIS:						
OP DATE	OPERATION:					
MED HX:						
SURG HX:						
NOTES:						

D/C PLAN: ☐ HOME   ☐ OTHER: HELP AVAIL:

DATE	TREATMENTS

DATE ORD	DATE DONE	TEST/CONSULTS

DATE	DIET

DATE	ACTIVITY

DATE ORD	UP DATE	NURSING DIAGNOSES/PROBLEMS
		ACTIVITIES OF DAILY LIVING

11/86

(continued)

FIGURE 13-4   KARDEX

ALLERGIES: ☐ NO ☐ YES

STANDING MEDICATIONS

ORD DATE	INIT	REORD DATE	INIT	MEDICATION DOSAGE ROUTE FREQ	TIMES	DC DATE	INIT

PRN MEDICATIONS

ORD DATE	INIT	REORD DATE	INIT	MEDICATION DOSAGE ROUTE FREQ	TIMES	DC DATE	INIT

FIGURE 13-4 *(continued)*

PHARMACY MAR

START	STOP	MEDICATION	SCHEDULED TIMES	OK'D BY	0001 HRS. TO 1200 HRS.	1201 HRS. TO 2400 HRS.
08/31/xx 1800 SCH		PROCAN SR 500 MG TAB-SR 500 MG Q6H PO	0600 1200 1800 2400	JD	0600GP 1200 GP	1800 MS 2400 JD
09/03/xx 0900 SCH		DIGOXIN (LANOXIN) 0.125 MG TAB 1 TAB QOD PO ODD DAYS-SEPT	0900	JD	0900 GP	
09/03/xx 0900 SCH		FUROSEMIDE (LASIX) 40 MG TAB 1 TAB QD PO	0900	JD	0900 GP	
09/03/xx 0845 SCH		REGLAN 10 MG TAB 10 MG AC&HS PO GIVE ONE NOW!!	0730 1130 1630 2100	JD	0730 GP 1130 GP	1630 MS 2100 MS
09/04/xx 0900 SCH		K-LYTE 25 MEQ EFFERVESCENT TAB 1 EFF. TAB BID PO DISSOLVE AS DIR START 9-4	0900 1700	JD	0900 GP	1700 GP
09/03/xx 1507 PRN		NITROGLYCERIN 1/50 GR 0.4 MG TAB-SL 1 TABLET PRN* SL PRN CHEST PAIN		JD		
09/03/xx 1700 PRN		DARVOCET-N 100* 1 TAB Q4-6H PO PRN MILD–MODERATE PAIN		JD		
09/03/xx 2100 PRN		MEPERIDINE* (DEMEROL) INJ 50 MG Q4H IM PRN SEVERE PAIN W PHENERGAN		JD		2200 Ⓗ MS
09/03/xx 2100 PRN		PROMETHAZINE (PHENERGAN) INJ 50 MG Q4H IM PRN SEVERE PAIN W DEMEROL		JD		2200 Ⓗ MS

		NURSE'S SIGNATURE	INITIAL		
Gluteus A. Right B. Left	**Thigh** H. Right I. Left	7–3 G. Pickar, R.N.	GP	ALLERGIES: NKA	Patient: Patient, John D. Patient # 3-81512-3
Ventro Gluteal C. Right D. Left E. Abdomen	J. Right K. Left	3–11 M. Smith, R.N.	MS		Admitted: 08/31/xx Physician: J. Physician, MD
1 2 / 3 4		11–7 J. Doe, R.N.	JD	DIAGNOSIS: CHF	Room: PCU-14 PCU

730-13 (12/xx)

FIGURE 13-5   COMPUTERIZED MEDICATION ADMINISTRATION RECORD

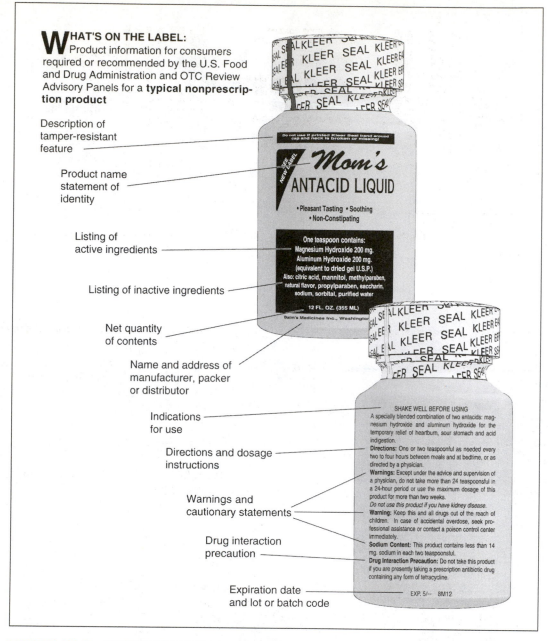

WHAT'S ON THE LABEL:
Product information for consumers required or recommended by the U.S. Food and Drug Administration and OTC Review Advisory Panels for a **typical nonprescription product**

Description of tamper-resistant feature

Product name statement of identity

Listing of active ingredients

Listing of inactive ingredients

Net quantity of contents

Name and address of manufacturer, packer or distributor

Indications for use

Directions and dosage instructions

Warnings and cautionary statements

Drug interaction precaution

Expiration date and lot or batch code

Do not use if printed Kleer Seal band around cap and neck is broken or missing!

Mom's ANTACID LIQUID

• Pleasant Tasting • Soothing
• Non-Constipating

One teaspoon contains:
Magnesium Hydroxide 200 mg.
Aluminum Hydroxide 200 mg.
(equivalent to dried gel U.S.P.)
Also: citric acid, mannitol, methylparaben, natural flavor, propylparaben, saccharin, sodium, sorbital, purified water

12 FL. OZ. (355 ML)

Balm's Medicines Inc., Washington

SHAKE WELL BEFORE USING
A specially blended combination of two antacids: magnesium hydroxide and aluminum hydroxide for the temporary relief of heartburn, sour stomach and acid indigestion.
Directions: One or two teaspoonful as needed every two to four hours between meals and at bedtime, or as directed by a physician.
Warnings: Except under the advice and supervision of a physician, do not take more than 24 teaspoonful in a 24-hour period or use the maximum dosage of this product for more than two weeks.
Do not use this product if you have kidney disease.
Warning: Keep this and all drugs out of the reach of children. In case of accidental overdose, seek professional assistance or contact a poison control center immediately.
Sodium Content: This product contains less than 14 mg. sodium in each two teaspoonful.
Drug Interaction Precaution: Do not take this product if you are presently taking a prescription antibiotic drug containing any form of tetracycline.

EXP. 5/-- 8M12

FIGURE 13-6 **WHAT'S ON THE LABEL?** *(Courtesy of The Proprietary Association)*

directions for mixing or reconstituting a powdered form of the drug. Prescription medications that are listed in the Federal Controlled Substances Act are so identified on the label by the symbols ℂ, ℂ, ℂ, ℂ, ℂ.

Understanding the Medication Label

Refer to Figure 13-7: Sample of a medication label: Ceclor. Note the following information as it relates to this label:

1. The trade or brand name for the medication: Ceclor

2. The generic name: cefaclor

3. The National Drug Code (NDC) numbers that can be used to identify the manufacturer, the product, and the size of the container: 0002-3062-02

4. The dosage strength in a given amount of the medication: 500 mg

5. The usual dosage and frequency of administration: usual adult dose—250 mg three times a

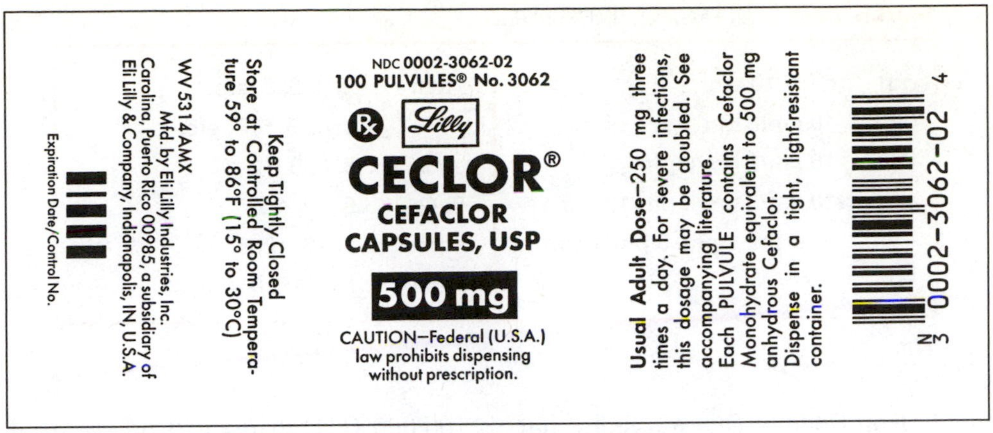

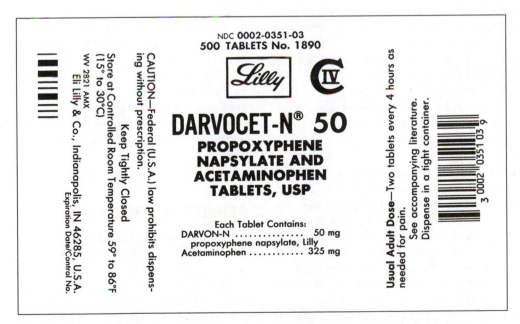

FIGURE 13-7   SAMPLE OF A MEDICATION LABEL: CECLOR® *(Courtesy of Eli Lilly & Company, Indianapolis, Indiana)*

day. For severe infections, this dosage may be doubled.

6. The form in which the drug is supplied: capsules, USP

7. CAUTION: Federal (USA) law prohibits dispensing without prescription.

8. The expiration date for the medication and the lot or batch code: Expiration date not given on the sample label. Lot or batch code No. 3062

9. The manufacturer's name: Lilly

10. The total number and/or volume of the drug contained: 100 pulvules

   Refer to Figure 13-8: Sample of a medication label: Darvocet-N 50 Ⓒ. Note the following information as it relates to this label:

1. The trade or brand name for the medication: Darvocet-N 50

2. The generic name: propoxyphene napsylate and acetaminophen

FIGURE 13-8   SAMPLE OF A MEDICATION LABEL: DARVOCET-N® 50 *(Courtesy of Eli Lilly & Company, Indianapolis, Indiana)*

TABLE 13-1 AN EXAMPLE TIME SCHEDULE

qd	daily 10 am	q2h	2, 4, 6, 8, etc.
bid	10 am/6 pm		or 1, 3, 5, 7, etc.
tid	10 am/2 pm/6 pm	q3h	3, 6, 9, 12
qid	10 am/2 pm/6 pm/10 pm	q4h	8, 12, 4, 8
	or 9 am, 1 pm, 5 pm, 9 pm	q6h	12, 6, 12, 6
		q8h	8, 4, 12, 8

3. The National Drug Code (NDC) numbers that can be used to identify the manufacturer, the product, and the size of the container: 0002-0351-03

4. The dosage strength in a given amount of the medication: Darvon-N® 50 mg propoxyphene napsylate and acetaminophen 325 mg

5. The usual dosage and frequency of administration: usual adult dose: two tablets every 4 hr prn

6. The form in which the drug is supplied: tablets, USP

7. CAUTION: Federal (USA) law prohibits dispensing without prescription.

8. The expiration date for the medication and the lot or batch code: Expiration date not given on the sample label. Lot or batch code No. 1890

9. The manufacturer's name: Lilly

10. The total number and/or volume of the drug contained: 500 tablets

Nonprescription medications, also known as over-the-counter (OTC) products, are intended for use without medical supervision. As such, the labeling of these products is very important to their safe and proper use by the consumer.

Consumers should always be cautious in taking OTC drugs when they are on prescribed medications. OTC drugs may aggravate the condition for which the prescribed medicine is indicated. The client is advised to read the warning on the label of the OTC drug and to call the physician if there are any questions. For example, a client with hypertension should not take many of the cold and/or allergy drugs that are on the market, and children and teenagers should not use aspirin products for chicken pox or flu symptoms before a physician is consulted because of Reye's syndrome, a rare but serious illness reported to be associated with aspirin.

In March 1999, the Food and Drug Administration's regulation to provide new, easy-to-understand labeling for over-the-counter (OTC), nonprescription drugs was approved. All of the more than 100,000 OTC drugs will be required to adopt the new labeling within the next 6 years. Titled "Drug Facts," the new labeling makes it easier for consumers to identify active ingredients, which are listed at the top, followed by uses, warnings, directions, and inactive ingredients. The rule also sets minimum font type sizes and other graphic features for the standardized format, including options for modifying the format for various package sizes and shapes.

TIME SCHEDULE FOR ROUTINE MEDICINES

Table 13-1 gives an example time schedule that may be helpful in the administration of routine medications. Bear in mind that schedule times vary. For example, every 6 hours may be 12–6, 12–6 or it could 2–8, 2–8, depending upon the time the medication was initiated. When possible, times are scheduled to allow a client to sleep with as few interruptions as necessary. Nursing units may also vary; for example, cardiac units often put tid drugs on an every-8-hour schedule.

Note that some medications may require administration with the client's meals, whereas other medications may require that they be given on an empty stomach. It is very important that you administer the medication as ordered and at the right time.

ABBREVIATIONS

Abbreviations are the shorthand of the medical field. They are a clear and concise means for writing orders. This medical shorthand is an international language used by professional and nonprofessional people who are concerned with client care. All of the abbreviations listed in Table 13-2 should be learned in order to properly fulfill your role in the administration of medications.

TABLE 13-2   ABBREVIATIONS AND THEIR MEANINGS

Abbreviation	Meaning	Abbreviation	Meaning
a̅a̅	of each	MO	mineral oil
ac	before meals	MOM	milk of magnesia
ad lib	as desired, as much as needed	MS	morphine sulfate
agit	shake, stir	MTD	maximum tolerated dose
alt dieb	alternating days	noct	at night
am	morning	N/S	normal saline
amp	ampule	O_2	oxygen
aq	water	OD	overdose
bid	two times a day, twice daily	OD	right eye
buc	bucally	OS	left eye
c̅	with	OU	both eyes
cap	capsule	OTC	over the counter (drugs)
CBI	continuous bladder irrigation	pc	after meals
cc	cubic centimeter	PL	placebo
chem	chemotherapy	pm	afternoon
DC	discontinue	PMI	patient medication instruction
DEA	Drug Enforcement Administration	pr	per rectum
dil	dilute	prn	as necessary, when needed
disp	dispense	pt	per tube
D/NS	dextrose in normal saline	pwd	powder
D/S	dextrose and saline	q	every
DW	distilled water	qd	every day
D/W	dextrose in water	qh	every hour
Eq	equivalent	q2h	every two hours
FDA	Food and Drug Administration	q3h	every three hours
fl	fluid	q4h	every four hours
fl oz	fluid ounce	qid	four times a day
FM	flowmeter	qam	every morning
garg	gargle	qpm	every night
(H)	hypodermic	qod	every other day
h, hr	hour	qs	quantity sufficient
hs	hour of sleep	R	rectal
H_2O	water	Rx	"take thou"
IM	intramuscular	S, Sig	give the following directions
inf	infusion	s̅	without
IU	international unit	SC, SQ	subcutaneous
IV	intravenous	subq	subcutaneous
L/min	liters per minute	s̅s̅	one-half
med	medicine	i̅s̅s̅	one and a half
mEq	milliequivalent	stat	immediately
ml, mL	milliliter	tid	three times a day
mn	midnight	tinct	tincture

(continued)

TABLE 13-2 *(Continued)*

Abbreviation	Meaning	Abbreviation	Meaning
TO	telephone order	dr	dram
tus	cough	oz	ounce
U	unit	lb	pound
vag	vagina	♏	minim
ves	bladder	gtt	drops
VO	verbal order	t, tsp	teaspoon
		T, tbs	tablespoon
Measurements		tab	tablet
cm	centimeter	C	cup, Celsius
mcg, μg	microgram	pt	pint
mg	milligram	qt	quart
g	gram	gal	gallon
kg	kilogram	F	Fahrenheit
cc	cubic centimeter	ʒ	dram
mL, ml	milliliter	℥	ounce
L	liter		
gr	grain		

● SELF-ASSESSMENT

Complete the following statements:

Source

p. 90   **1.** A medication order designates the drug to be used, the _____, the form of the drug, the time or frequency for administration, and the method or route by which it is to be given.

p. 91   **2.** When used in a medication order, the abbreviation *prn* stands for _____.

p. 92   **3.** It is the responsibility of the nurse to be knowledgeable of medications typically prescribed by physicians with whom he or she works. Write in one of the two methods suggested by this text to accomplish this purpose. _____.

p. 92   **4.** The physician's order sheet is a triplicate document. Indicate where each of the three pages are routed by completing the following:

     ● The original is maintained on _____.

     ● A copy goes to the _____.

     ● The remaining copy goes to the _____.

p. 94   **5.** Some medical centers utilize networked computers to store medication records. What is the source document mentioned in this text for a computerized medication administration record (MAR) of a drug order? _____.

p. 94   **6.** An understanding of the information provided on the label of a medication is essential to the _____ use of any medicine.

p. 101   **7.** In a medication time schedule, one may find such abbreviations as qd, qid, q3h. In these three examples, what word does q represent? _____.

p. 102   **8.** What word does the abbreviation tab represent? _____.

p. 101   **9.** The abbreviation OD can have two meanings. On the lines provided, give the two meanings given in this text: _____ and _____.

p. 101   **10.** The abbreviations for *give the following directions* are _____.

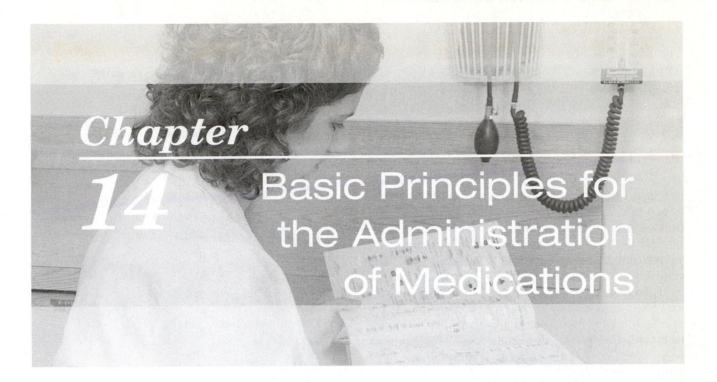

Chapter 14

Basic Principles for the Administration of Medications

Chapter Outline

Objectives
Key Terms
Introduction
The Nursing Process
Legal Implications
Standard Precautions
Safety Measures for Drug Administration
Safe Storage of Medications
Reactions to Medications
Medication Error
Self-Assessment

- List the basic medication guidelines
- List safety measures for drug administration
- Describe safe storage of medications
- Describe a general procedure for reporting an adverse drug reaction
- List signs of drug hypersensitivity according to body system affected
- List ten types of medication errors
- Explain the proper steps to take if a medication error occurs
- Complete the Self-Assessment

Objectives

Upon completion of this chapter, you should be able to

- Define the key terms
- Describe the five steps of the nursing process
- Give the legal implications of administering medications
- State the "Six Rights" of proper drug administration

Key Terms

assessment	evaluation
body substance isolation (BSI)	implementation
	meniscus
diagnosis	planning

INTRODUCTION

Basic principles for the administration of medications are based upon the nursing process. This process is the framework of nursing practice and involves the client, family, and community.

THE NURSING PROCESS

The five steps of the nursing process are assessment, diagnosis, planning, implementation, and evaluation. For this text, only the pharmacological aspects of the nursing process will be considered.

Step 1: Assessment

The systematic gathering, organizing, and interpretation of data to determine a client's nursing needs is called **assessment**. This process begins upon a client's admission to a hospital and continues until the client is discharged. Assessment on each client must be done every shift and prn if the condition of the client changes. When a client is discharged from a hospital setting and admitted to an extended care facility, or when home health care is given, the nursing process continues. In a physician's office or clinic, this same process is used, as each client is treated as an individual, with individual needs.

Medication History

It is essential that you know your client. Besides the person's name, occupation, diagnosis, age, and weight, you need to be familiar with the client's medication history. The following are some of the questions that may be asked to determine a client's medication history:

1. Do you have any allergies?
   a. To medicines (list)
   b. To food (list)
   c. To insects (list)
2. What medicines are you currently taking?
   a. Prescription
   b. Over-the-counter
   c. Home remedies
3. What condition(s) are you taking these medications for?

   Examples: headache, hypertension, chest pain.
4. Do they work for you?
5. How long have you been taking these medicines?
6. What other medicines have you taken in the past month, 6 months, year?
7. Have you experienced any problems when taking medications?

   Examples: Skin rash, nausea/vomiting, drowsiness, constipation, diarrhea,

dry mouth, blurred vision, ringing in the ear, loss of hair, tremors.
8. Do you have any difficulty taking medications?
   a. Can't swallow pills
   b. Forget to take medicine
   c. Forget which medicine you took
   d. Have to crush medicine
   e. Have to take with food
9. Do you ever give your medicine to others?
10. Do you ever take medicine that is not yours?
11. Do you follow the prescription order?
    a. Dosage
    b. Time
    c. Duration
12. Do you use tobacco, alcohol?
    a. How often?
    b. Amount?

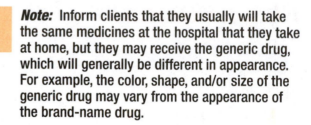

Note: Inform clients that they usually will take the same medicines at the hospital that they take at home, but they may receive the generic drug, which will generally be different in appearance. For example, the color, shape, and/or size of the generic drug may vary from the appearance of the brand-name drug.

Step 2: Diagnosis

The term **diagnosis** means "through knowledge." A nursing diagnosis is a clinical judgment about individual, family, or community responses to actual and potential health problems/life processes. Nursing diagnoses provide the basis for selection of nursing interventions to achieve outcomes for which the nurse is accountable.

Four steps are involved in the formulation of a nursing diagnosis.

1. A database is established by acquiring information about the client from all available sources. This database is continually updated.
2. Analysis of client's needs, problems, concerns, and human responses
3. Organization of data and clustering to make a diagnostic statement that summarizes the client information obtained
4. Evaluation of the sufficiency and accuracy of the database

Examples of appropriate diagnoses are as follows:

Elimination	Possible Cause
Bowel incontinence	Excessive use of laxatives
Constipation	Adverse reaction to Basaljel
Diarrhea	Adverse reaction to milk of magnesia

Step 3: Planning

Planning involves the development of nursing actions designed to enhance the client's responses to treatment or to prevent drug-related problems. The planning segment of the nursing process involves

1. Set goals.
2. Develop outcomes that the client will be able to do as a result of nursing actions.
3. Develop nursing interventions that describe how the nurse can assist the client to achieve outcomes.
4. Document the plan.

Examples of appropriate nursing interventions are as follows:

Nursing Interventions for Problems Related to Drug Therapy If Not Contraindicated	
Constipation	Encourage fluids.
	Encourage a diet rich in fiber.
	Encourage regular exercise.
	Encourage regular pattern of elimination.
Diarrhea	Monitor intake and output.
	Maintain hydration (clear fluids).
	Encourage nonirritating foods.
	Reduce stress.
	Encourage proper handwashing and body hygiene.
	Apply ointment to rectal area.

Step 4: Implementation

Implementation is the process of putting into effect, fulfillment, or carrying through with the plan of action. In the nursing process this step involves all aspects of actual caring for the client and requires full knowledge of the assessment and planning steps. Included in this step are client care areas such as hygiene, physical and mental comfort, assistance in daily living habits such as feeding and elimination, maintaining and controlling the client's physical environment, and teaching the client about factors that are important to his/her care and what actions to take to help facilitate recovery.

In drug therapy, implementation may involve psychological and physical care measures to help enhance the effectiveness of the medication(s), to reduce the need for certain medications, to consult with the physician or pharmacist regarding changes in the drug regimen, and client teaching.

Example: Client Teaching
Jane Rice
June 3, XXXX
Cephalexin 250 mg cap
20 capsules
Take one (1) cap 4 times daily until all used.

About Your Medicine

Cephalexin is an antibiotic that is used to treat bacterial infections. It does not work for colds, flu, or other viral infections.

Before Using This Medicine

Inform your doctor, nurse, and pharmacist if you:
- Are allergic to any medicine
- Are pregnant
- Are breast-feeding
- Are taking medication, especially probenecid (Benemid—used for gout)
- Have a history of stomach or intestinal disease

Proper Use of This Medicine

Cephalexin may be taken on a full or empty stomach. It may be taken with food or crushed and mixed with food. You must take the medicine 4 times daily (9 am, 1 pm, 5 pm, 9 pm) and take all of the medicine.

Precautions

If your symptoms do not improve within a few days, or if they become worse, inform your physician.

Safety Precaution: For patients with diabetes, this medicine may cause false test results with some urine sugar tests.

If diarrhea occurs, inform your physician. Do not take any diarrhea medicine without checking with your physician.

Do not give this medicine to other people.

Possible Side Effects—Report to Your Physician Immediately

Abdominal or stomach cramps, pain, and bloating (severe); convulsions (seizures); diarrhea (watery, severe, bloody); fever; increased thirst; joint pain; loss of appetite; nausea or vomiting; skin rash, itching, redness, or swelling; unusual tiredness or weakness; weight loss (unusual)

Step 5: Evaluation

Evaluation, the judgment of anything, is an integral part of each step of the nursing process. It ascertains the quality and effectiveness of the plan of care for the client and allows you to reflect upon the worth of the process. Remember that the nursing process is always changing and the care plan should reflect revision and addition/resolution of problems identified. Some questions you may ask are

1. Did the prescribed medication(s) alleviate the signs and symptoms of disease? How effective was the medication?
2. Were there any adverse reactions to the medication? If so, did you take appropriate action?
3. Did the client understand the prescribed medication regimen? Did the client understand the purpose, effects, precautions, and any bodily changes that could occur as a result of a medicine?
4. Did you consult with the physician or pharmacist to approve the client's drug regimen?
5. Did you follow the "Six Rights" of proper drug administration?

LEGAL IMPLICATIONS

Members of the health care profession who prepare and administer medications are ethically and legally responsible for their own actions. Under the law, these individuals are required to be licensed, registered, or otherwise authorized by a physician.

Each state has enacted laws governing the practice of medicine, nursing, and pharmacy. These laws vary from state to state; therefore, it is essential that one become familiar with the laws of the state in which one is employed before giving any medication. In some states, the only health professional authorized to give injections, other than a physician, is the registered nurse. On the other hand, legislation in some states gives physicians broad authority to delegate responsibility for giving medications. Other states have passed laws that specify which qualified and properly trained persons may perform certain medical acts.

Regardless of the differences in state authorization laws, the courts will not permit the careless actions of health care workers to go unpunished, especially when such actions result in harm to or the death of the client. Under the law, those administering medications are expected to be familiar with the drugs administered and the effects they might have on a client. In that there are thousands of drugs on the market, the task of keeping up with current information on each medication is overwhelming. Therefore, it is necessary to keep drug reference books handy and to refer to them every time there is any question about a drug. The following precautions should guide the administration of any medication:

P   Patients (clients) are individuals who depend upon the nurse for proper care.

R   Right Client, Right Dose, Right Drug, Right Route, Right Time, Right Documentation.

E   Explain to the clients the effects the drug should (or could) have on the body.

C   Check for contraindications before giving a medication.

A   Always check for drug allergies to the medication being given.

U   Understand the drug, its uses and actions.

T   Toxic effects; know the symptoms to look for.

I   Information on unfamiliar medications should be obtained before its administration.

O   Observe the client for signs of superinfection when administering antibiotics.

N   Never administer medications without the proper authorization

S   Side effects; be alert for signs of drug hypersensitivity.

The "Six Rights" of Proper Drug Administration

The "Six Rights" have been developed as a checklist of activities to be followed by those who give medications. This easy-to-remember list should always be followed to insure the proper administration of any drug. See Figure 14-1.

● *Right Drug* (Figure 14-1A): To be sure that the correct drug has been selected, compare the medication order with the label on the medica-

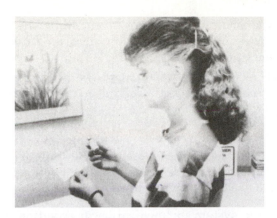

(A) *THE RIGHT DRUG.* THE NURSE COMPARES THE MEDICATION LABEL WITH THE PHYSICIAN'S ORDER.

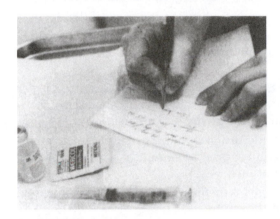

(B) *THE RIGHT DOSE.* THE NURSE CALCULATES THE CORRECT DOSE OF MEDICATION.

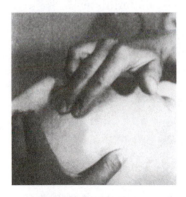

(C) *THE RIGHT ROUTE.* THE NURSE USES A PRACTICE MODEL TO LOCATE THE RIGHT ROUTE FOR AN IM INJECTION.

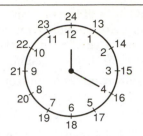

From midnight to noon, the 12-hour clock and the 24-hour clock are identical (numbers inside the circle). From noon to midnight, add 12 to each hour to arrive at the 24-hour clock (the numbers outside the circle).

12 M/N	2400	12:00 N	1200
1:00 am	0100	1:00 pm	1300
2:00 am	0200	2:00 pm	1400
3:00 am	0300	3:00 pm	1500
4:00 am	0400	4:00 pm	1600
5:00 am	0500	5:00 pm	1700
6:00 am	0600	6:00 pm	1800
7:00 am	0700	7:00 pm	1900
8:00 am	0800	8:00 pm	2000
9:00 am	0900	9:00 pm	2100
10:00 am	1000	10:00 pm	2200
11:00 am	1100	11:00 pm	2300

(D) *THE RIGHT TIME.* YOU ARE RESPONSIBLE FOR ADMINISTERING MEDICATION TO A CLIENT AT THE PROPER TIME. CHECK THE MEDICATION ORDER TO INSURE THAT A DRUG IS GIVEN AT THE PRESCRIBED INTERVAL. FOR A DRUG TO BE MAINTAINED AT THE PROPER BLOOD LEVEL, IT MUST BE ADMINISTERED ON TIME.

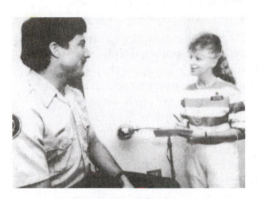

(E) *THE RIGHT CLIENT.* THE NURSE IDENTIFIES THE CLIENT.

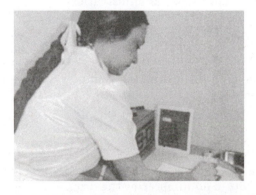

(F) *THE RIGHT DOCUMENTATION.* THE NURSE ENTERS DRUG ADMINISTRATION DATA INTO A CLIENT'S CHART.

FIGURE 14-1   THE "SIX RIGHTS" OF PROPER DRUG ADMINISTRATION

tion. A frequent check of the medication label is a good way to avoid a medication error. One should make a practice of reading the label on each of the following three occasions:

1. When the medication is taken from the storage area

2. Just before removing it from its container

3. Upon returning the medication container to storage or prior to discarding the empty container

● *Right Dose* (Figure 14-1B): It is essential that the client receive the right dose. If the dose ordered and the dose on hand are not the same, carefully determine the correct dose through mathematical calculation. When calculating dosage, it is advisable to have another qualified person verify the accuracy of your calculations before the medication is administered.

● *Right Route* (Figure 14-1C): Check the medication order to be sure that you have the right route of administration.

● *Right Time* (Figure 14-1D): You are responsible for medicating the client at the proper time. Check the medication order to insure that a drug is administered according to the time interval prescribed. For a drug to be maintained at the proper blood level, care must be taken to administer it at the right time.

● *Right Client* (Figure 14-1E): Before administering any medication, always be sure that you have the right client. A good safety practice is to correctly identify the client on each occasion when you administer a medication. In a hospital, always check the client's identification bracelet. In a physician's office or other health care facility, call the client by name or ask the client to state his or her name.

● *Right Documentation* (Figure 14-1F): A client's chart is a legal document. It is essential that the following data about drug administration be entered correctly:

— The client's name

— The date and time of administration

— The name of the medication and the amount (dosage) administered

— The route by which the medication was administered

— Any adverse reactions experienced by the client

— Any complications in administering the drug (client refusing to take the medication, difficulty in swallowing, and so forth)

— If the medication was not given, state why. Dispose of the medication according to agency policy.

— The response of the client to the prn drug (decreased pain after receiving an analgesic)

Basic Medication Guidelines

Regardless of a medication's form or the route by which it is administered, certain basic guidelines must be followed. These guidelines are

● Know the system for medication distribution. Cards, Kardex, Medex, computer printout, unit dose, and multiple dose are some of the different systems that may be encountered.

● Check each medication order carefully.

● Be familiar with the following types of medication orders: routine, prn, single, stat, and standing.

● It is advisable to always have a written order from a physician or other authorized practitioner before giving any medication.

● Give only drugs that are ordered by a licensed physician or practitioner authorized to prescribe medications.

● Never give a medication if there is any question about the order.

● Be completely familiar with the drug that you are administering before giving it to your client. You are expected to know the following about any drug that you are to administer:

Safe dosage limit

Adverse reactions

Contraindications

Warnings

Route of administration

Time of administration

Clinical pharmacology

Precautions

● Know the circumstances in which you may be allowed to withhold a drug and not give it to a client. These could occur in conjunction with diagnostic tests, laboratory tests, and/or with surgery.

● Always check the expiration date on the medication label.

● Never give a drug if its normal appearance has been altered in any way (color, structure, consistency, or odor).

● Practice medical asepsis. Wash your hands before and after administering a medication.

- When administering oral medications, stay with the client until you are certain that the medication has been taken.
- Always check for allergies before administering any medication.
- If the client refuses the medication, signify it on the MAR and give a brief explanation in the nurse's notes of why the medicine was not given.

STANDARD PRECAUTIONS

The Centers for Disease Control and Prevention (CDC) recommends a set of infection control guidelines to help protect health care providers, clients, and their visitors from infectious diseases. Standard precautions for infection control should be utilized by all health care professionals for all clients.

Standard precautions combine many of the basic principles of universal precautions with techniques known as **body substance isolation (BSI)**, a system that maintains that personal protective equipment should be worn for contact with all body fluids whether or not blood is visible. Advantages of the new standard precautions are that they include all of the major recommendations of universal precautions and body substance isolation, while incorporating new information intended to protect all clients, all health care providers, and all visitors.

According to the CDC, standard precautions are "designed to reduce the risk of transmission of microorganisms, from both recognized and unrecognized sources of infection in hospitals." Standard precautions apply to

1. Blood
2. All body fluids, secretions, and excretions regardless of whether they contain visible blood
3. Nonintact skin
4. Mucous membranes

To be effective, standard precautions must be practiced conscientiously at all times. Table 14-1 provides a comprehensive review of the standard precautions.

SAFETY MEASURES FOR DRUG ADMINISTRATION

The following are important measures to follow for safety in drug administration:

- Always wash your hands before preparing and administering medications.

- When preparing medications, work in a well-lighted area that is quiet and free of distractions.
- Always observe the "Six Rights."
- Carefully follow the correct procedure for administering controlled substances.
- Give only those medications that you have actually prepared for administration.
- Do not allow someone else to give a medication that you prepared.
- Once you have prepared a medication for administration, do not leave it unattended. Never leave the medication at the bedside when the client is occupied in the shower, special procedures, or out of the room.
- Be careful in transporting the medication to the client.
- Keep all drugs not being administered in a locked storage area (such as the medication cart, medication cabinet, and so forth).
- If the dosage ordered is greater than the safe dosage limit, check the order again. Contact the prescribing physician for verification.
- Do not open unit dose medications until you are at the client's bedside. In this way, if the client refuses the medicine, you have not wasted the medicine, and the client will not be charged for the medicine.
- A product that contains a precipitate should be shaken thoroughly before it is poured. If the product is discolored or contains an unusual precipitate, it should be returned to the pharmacy for replacement.
- When pouring a liquid medicine, hold the measuring device at eye level, and read the correct amount at the lowest point of the **meniscus** (the convex or concave upper surface of a column of liquid in a container). See Figure 14-2.
- Do not contaminate the cap of a bottle while pouring a medication. Place the cap with the rim pointed upward to prevent contamination of that portion that comes into contact with the medication.
- When pouring from a bottle, always place the label in the palm of your hand to avoid defacing the label. Only the pharmacist may replace a damaged or illegible label.
- Do not crush or alter any medication unless you have made sure that you can do so.
- In the event of a medication error, appropriate action should be taken immediately to safeguard the client. Report the error to the proper authority and complete an incident report form.

TABLE 14-1 STANDARD PRECAUTIONS FOR INFECTION CONTROL ISSUED BY THE CDC

Standard Precautions for Infection Control

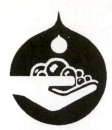

Wash Hands (Plain soap)

Wash after touching **blood, body fluids, secretions, excretions,** and **contaminated items.**

Wash immediately **after gloves are removed** and **between client contacts.**

Avoid transfer of microorganisms to other clients or environments.

Wear Gloves

Wear when touching **blood, body fluids, secretions, excretions,** and **contaminated items.**

Put on **clean** gloves just **before touching mucous membranes** and **nonintact skin.**

Change gloves between tasks and procedures on the same client after contact with material that may contain high concentrations of microorganisms. Remove gloves promptly after use, before touching noncontaminated items and environmental surfaces, and before going to another client, and wash hands immediately to avoid transfer of microorganisms to other clients or environments.

Wear Mask and Eye Protection or Face Shield

Protect mucous membranes of the eyes, nose, and mouth during procedures and client care activities that are likely to generate **splashes** or **sprays** of **blood, body fluids, secretions,** or **excretions.**

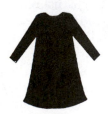

Wear Gown

Protect skin and prevent soiling of clothing during procedures that are likely to generate **splashes** or **sprays** of **blood, body fluids, secretions,** or **excretions.** Remove a soiled gown as promptly as possible and wash hands to avoid transfer of microorganisms to other clients or environments.

Patient Care Equipment

Handle used client care equipment soiled with **blood, body fluids, secretions,** or **excretions** in a manner that prevents skin and mucous membrane exposures, contamination of clothing, and transfer of microorganisms to other clients and environments. Insure that reusable equipment is not used for the care of another client until it has been appropriately cleaned and reprocessed and single use items are properly discarded.

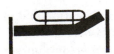

Environmental Control

Follow hospital procedures for routine care, cleaning, and disinfection of environmental surfaces, beds, bedrails, bedside equipment, and other frequently touched surfaces.

(continued)

TABLE 14-1 *(Continued)*

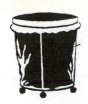

Linen

Handle, transport, and process used linen soiled with **blood, body fluids, secretions,** or **excretions** in a manner that prevents exposures and contamination of clothing, and avoids transfer of microorganisms to other clients and environments.

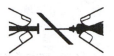

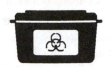

Occupational Health and Bloodborne Pathogens

Prevent injuries when using needles, scalpels, and other sharp instruments or devices; when handling sharp instruments after procedures; when cleaning used instruments; and when disposing of used needles.

Never recap used needles using both hands or any other technique that involves directing the point of a needle toward any part of the body; rather, use either a one-handed "scoop" technique or a mechanical device designed for holding the needle sheath.

Do not remove used needles from disposable syringes by hand, and do not bend, break, or otherwise manipulate used needles by hand. Place used disposable syringes and needles, scalpel blades, and other sharp items in puncture-resistant containers located as close as practical to the area in which the items were used, and place reusable syringes and needles in a puncture-resistant container for transport to the reprocessing area.

Use **resuscitation devices** as an alternative to mouth-to-mouth resuscitation.

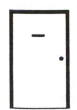

Client Placement

Use a **private room** for a client who contaminates the environment or who does not (or cannot be expected to) assist in maintaining appropriate hygiene or environmental control. Consult Infection Control if a private room is not available.

(Courtesy Brevis Corp.)

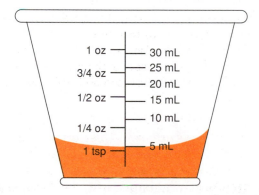

1 oz	30 mL
3/4 oz	25 mL
	20 mL
1/2 oz	15 mL
	10 mL
1/4 oz	
1 tsp	5 mL

FIGURE 14-2 ALWAYS MEASURE THE VOLUME OF A LIQUID MEDICATION AT THE LOWEST LEVEL OF THE MENISCUS. THIS MEDICINE CUP CONTAINS 5 ML OF LIQUID.

● Always keep safety precautions in mind. The U.S. Department of Health and Human Services, Public Health Service, Centers for Disease Control and Prevention recommends the following universal precautions for prevention of HIV and other bloodborne disease transmission in health care settings:

1. All health care workers should routinely use appropriate barrier precautions to prevent skin and mucous membrane exposure when contact with blood or other body fluids of any client is anticipated. Gloves should be worn for touching blood and body fluids, mucous membranes, or

nonintact skin of all clients, for handling items or surfaces soiled with blood or body fluids, and for performing venipuncture and other vascular access procedures. Gloves should be changed after contact with each client. Masks and protective eyewear or face shields should be worn during procedures that are likely to generate droplets of blood or other body fluids to prevent exposure of mucous membranes of the mouth, nose, and eyes. Gowns or aprons should be worn during procedures that are likely to generate splashes of blood or other body fluids.

2. Hands and other skin surfaces should be washed immediately and thoroughly if contaminated with blood or other body fluids. Hands should be washed immediately after gloves are removed.

3. All health care workers should take precautions to prevent injuries caused by needles, scalpels, and other sharp instruments or devices during procedures; when cleaning used instruments; during disposal of used needles; and when handling sharp instruments after procedures. To prevent needlestick injuries, needles should not be recapped, purposely bent or broken by hand, removed from disposable syringes, or otherwise manipulated by hand. After they are used, disposable syringes and needles, scalpel blades, and other sharp items should be placed in puncture-resistant containers for disposal; the puncture-resistant containers should be located as close as practical to the use area. Large-bore reusable needles should be placed in a puncture-resistant container for transport to the reprocessing area.

4. Mouth-to-mouth resuscitation mouthpieces, resuscitation bags, or other ventilation devices should be available for use in areas in which the need for resuscitation is predictable.

5. Health care workers who have exudative lesions or weeping dermatitis should refrain from all direct client care and from handling client care equipment until the condition improves.

6. Pregnant health care workers are not known to be at greater risk of contracting HIV infection than health care workers who are not pregnant; however, if a health care worker develops HIV infection during pregnancy, the infant is at risk of infection resulting from perinatal transmission. Because of this risk, pregnant health care workers should be especially familiar with and strictly adhere to precautions to minimize the risk of HIV transmission.

SAFE STORAGE OF MEDICATIONS

All medications not being administered should be kept in a safe storage place. This place may vary from facility to facility, but there are certain guides and precautions that should be followed.

Guidelines for Safe Storage of Medications

- Ideally, there should be one room designated as the medication room. This room should
  1. Be away from the flow of client traffic
  2. Be well-lighted
  3. Be kept clean, orderly, cool, and dry
  4. Contain a sink and refrigerator
  5. Have enough cabinet space so that internal drugs and external drugs can be kept separate
  6. Have a cabinet, drawer, or metal box equipped with a double lock for controlled substances
  7. Be kept locked when not in use
  8. Have emergency supplies and medications that are readily available when administering any medication to a client. The following drugs should be stored separately from other drugs in their own special place:
     a. epinephrine (Adrenalin)
     b. diphenhydramine HCl (Benadryl)
     c. dopamine HCl (Intropin)
     d. methylprednisolone acetate (Depo-Medrol)
     e. oxygen
     f. naloxone HCl (Narcan)
- Store medications in their original containers. Certain medications must be stored in opaque containers and others in glass containers.
- Refrigerate insulin, sera, vaccines, vitamins, suppositories, and certain liquid antibiotics.
- All medications, supplies, and equipment must be checked on a regular basis.

● When the nurse reconstitutes a powder to a solution, always include on the label the date, amount of diluent added, strength of dilution, time mixed, and your initials.

In a health care setting, such as a physician's office, there are several ways that drugs may be categorized for safe storage.

1. Drugs may be stored according to:

   Preparation: solid, semisolid, and liquid

   Route: oral, parenteral, application to skin, sublingual, transdermal, buccal, rectal, vaginal, inhalation, and instillation

   Therapeutic use: by classification (analgesic, antiemetic, etc.)

   Alphabetical order: generic name, trade or brand name

   Action of drug according to body system: cardiovascular, respiratory, urinary, etc.

2. Pharmaceutical drug samples should be stored according to the policy of the office. In most offices these are kept separate from the other medications.

REACTIONS TO MEDICATIONS

Reactions to medications can be favorable or unfavorable. Usually, the drug used will produce its intended response; however, potentially dangerous reactions can occur. When administering medications, one should make a written report describing the client's responses to the drug. Written documentation is particularly important in those cases that involve an adverse reaction to a medication. Documentation of drug reactions should include the client's name, room number, physician's name, date, time, medication used, and the nature of the reaction.

Do not leave a client who experiences an adverse reaction to a medication. If the reaction appears to be serious, use the call system to get assistance. Do not leave the client alone, even for a moment. Appropriate assessment and action should be taken to reassure the client and to safeguard his or her health. The physician should be notified immediately.

The general procedure that may be used when reporting an adverse drug reaction usually includes these events:

● Report your assessment of the reaction to the supervisor.

● Notify the physician and give a description of the reaction.

● Follow the physician's orders; discontinue the medication.

● Reassess the client's condition. Remain in the client's room.

● Notify the pharmacist, describing the reaction, and giving the room number and the client's identification number. Give the name of the drug administered and the name of the client's physician. Most agencies require that an "Adverse Reaction to Medication" form be filled out, and/or an incident report be completed and sent to the pharmacy.

● You may voluntarily report an adverse event and problem to the FDA through their MED-WATCH program. This program is an initiative designed to educate all health professionals about adverse events and problems and to notify the FDA and/or the manufacturer, as well as to insure that new safety information is rapidly communicated to the medical community, thereby improving client care. The purpose of the MEDWATCH program is to enhance the effectiveness of postmarketing surveillance of medical products as they are used in clinical practice and to rapidly identify significant health hazards associated with these products. The program has four goals.

1. To increase awareness of drug- and device-induced disease

2. To clarify what should (and should not) be reported to the agency

3. To operate a single system for health professionals to make it easier to report adverse events and product problems

4. To provide regular feedback to the health care community about safety issues involving medical products

Adverse events and product problems that occur with vaccines should not be reported to the MEDWATCH program or on the MEDWATCH form, but should be sent to the joint FDA/CDC Vaccine Adverse Event Reporting System (VAERS). To report such an event, one may call 1-800-822-7967 for a copy of the VAERS form.

The FDA MEDWATCH program offers advice about voluntary reporting, and additional information can be found at www.fda.gov/medwatch, or by calling 1-800-FDA-1088. See Figure 14-3 for an example of a MEDWATCH reporting form.

MEDWATCH
HE FDA MEDICAL PRODUCTS REPORTING PROGRAM

For **VOLUNTARY** reporting
by health professionals of adverse
events and product problems

Page ____ of ____

Form Approved: OMB No. 0910-0291 Expires: 7/31/00
See OMB statement on reverse

FDA Use Only

Triage unit
sequence #

A. Patient information

1. **Patient identifier**

In confidence

2. **Age at time
   of event:**
   or
   **Date
   of birth:**

3. **Sex**
   ☐ female
   ☐ male

4. **Weight**
   _____ lbs
   or
   _____ kgs

B. Adverse event or product problem

1. ☐ **Adverse event** and/or ☐ **Product problem** (e.g., defects/malfunctions)

2. **Outcomes attributed to adverse event**
   (check all that apply)
   ☐ death _____
   ☐ life-threatening
   ☐ hospitalization – initial or prolonged

   ☐ disability
   ☐ congenital anomaly
   ☐ required intervention to prevent
     permanent impairment/damage
   ☐ other: _____

3. **Date of
   event**
   (mo/day/yr)

4. **Date of
   this report**
   (mo/day/yr)

5. **Describe event or problem**

6. **Relevant tests/laboratory data,** including dates

7. **Other relevant history, including preexisting medical conditions** (e.g., allergies,
   race, pregnancy, smoking and alcohol use, hepatic/renal dysfunction, etc.)

C. Suspect medication(s)

1. **Name** (give labeled strength & mfr/labeler, if known)
   #1
   #2

2. **Dose, frequency & route used**
   #1
   #2

3. **Therapy dates** (if unknown, give duration)
   from/to (or best estimate)
   #1
   #2

4. **Diagnosis for use** (indication)
   #1
   #2

5. **Event abated after use
   stopped or dose reduced**
   #1 ☐ yes ☐ no ☐ doesn't apply
   #2 ☐ yes ☐ no ☐ doesn't apply

6. **Lot #** (if known)
   #1
   #2

7. **Exp. date** (if known)
   #1
   #2

8. **Event reappeared after
   reintroduction**
   #1 ☐ yes ☐ no ☐ doesn't apply
   #2 ☐ yes ☐ no ☐ doesn't apply

9. **NDC #** (for product problems only)
   ___ – ___ – ___

10. **Concomitant medical products** and therapy dates (exclude treatment of event)

D. Suspect medical device

1. **Brand name**

2. **Type of device**

3. **Manufacturer name & address**

4. **Operator of device**
   ☐ health professional
   ☐ lay user/patient
   ☐ other: _____

5. **Expiration date**
   (mo/day/yr)

6. model # _____
   catalog # _____
   serial # _____
   lot # _____
   other # _____

7. **If implanted, give date**
   (mo/day/yr)

8. **If explanted, give date**
   (mo/day/yr)

9. **Device available for evaluation?** (Do not send to FDA)
   ☐ yes ☐ no ☐ returned to manufacturer on _____
   (mo/day/yr)

10. **Concomitant medical products** and therapy dates (exclude treatment of event)

E. Reporter (see confidentiality section on back)

1. **Name & address**

2. **Health professional?**
   ☐ yes ☐ no

3. **Occupation**

4. **Also reported to**
   ☐ manufacturer
   ☐ user facility
   ☐ distributor

5. **If you do NOT want your identity disclosed to
   the manufacturer, place an " X " in this box.** ☐

PLEASE TYPE OR USE BLACK INK

FDA

Mail to: MEDWATCH
5600 Fishers Lane
Rockville, MD 20852-9787

FAX to:
1-800-FDA-0178

FDA Form 3500

Submission of a report does not constitute an admission that medical personnel or the product caused or contributed to the event.

(continued)

FIGURE 14-3 EXAMPLE OF A MEDWATCH FORM *(Courtesy of MEDWATCH, Food and Drug Administration, Rockville, Maryland)*

ADVICE ABOUT VOLUNTARY REPORTING

Report experiences with:
- medications (drugs or biologics)
- medical devices (including in-vitro diagnostics)
- special nutritional products (dietary supplements, medical foods, infant formulas)
- other products regulated by FDA

Report SERIOUS adverse events. An event is serious when the patient outcome is:
- death
- life-threatening (real risk of dying)
- hospitalization (initial or prolonged)
- disability (significant, persistent or permanent)
- congenital anomaly
- required intervention to prevent permanent impairment or damage

Report even if:
- you're not certain the product caused the event
- you don't have all the details

Report product problems – quality, performance or safety concerns such as:
- suspected contamination
- questionable stability
- defective components
- poor packaging or labeling
- therapeutic failures

How to report:
- just fill in the sections that apply to your report
- use section C for all products except medical devices
- attach additional blank pages if needed
- use a separate form for each patient
- report either to FDA or the manufacturer (or both)

Important numbers:
- 1-800-FDA-0178   to FAX report
- 1-800-FDA-7737   to report by modem
- 1-800-FDA-1088   to report by phone or for more information
- 1-800-822-7967   for a VAERS form for vaccines

If your report involves a serious adverse event with a device and it occurred in a facility outside a doctor's office, that facility may be legally required to report to FDA and/or the manufacturer. Please notify the person in that facility who would handle such reporting.

Confidentiality: The patient's identity is held in strict confidence by FDA and protected to the fullest extent of the law. The reporter's identity, including the identity of a self-reporter, may be shared with the manufacturer unless requested otherwise. However, FDA will not disclose the reporter's identity in response to a request from the public, pursuant to the Freedom of Information Act.

The public reporting burden for this collection of information has been estimated to average 30 minutes per response, including the time for reviewing instructions, searching existing data sources, gathering and maintaining the data needed, and completing and reviewing the collection of information. Send comments regarding this burden estimate or any other aspect of this collection of information, including suggestions for reducing this burden to:

DHHS Reports Clearance Office
Paperwork Reduction Project (0910-0291)
Hubert H. Humphrey Building, Room 531-H
200 Independence Avenue, S.W.
Washington, DC 20201

"An agency may not conduct or sponsor, and a person is not required to respond to, a collection of information unless it displays a currently valid OMB control number."

Please DO NOT
RETURN this form
to this address.

U.S. DEPARTMENT OF HEALTH AND HUMAN SERVICES
Public Health Service ● Food and Drug Administration

FDA Form 3500-back   **Please Use Address Provided Below – Just Fold In Thirds, Tape and Mail**

- -

**Department of
Health and Human Services**
Public Health Service
Food and Drug Administration
Rockville, MD 20857

Official Business
Penalty for Private Use $300

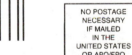

BUSINESS REPLY MAIL
FIRST CLASS MAIL   PERMIT NO. 946   ROCKVILLE, MD

POSTAGE WILL BE PAID BY FOOD AND DRUG ADMINISTRATION

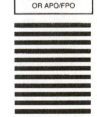

NO POSTAGE
NECESSARY
IF MAILED
IN THE
UNITED STATES
OR APO/FPO

MEDWATCH
**The FDA Medical Products Reporting Program
Food and Drug Administration
5600 Fishers Lane
Rockville, MD 20852-9787**

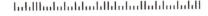

FIGURE 14-3   *(continued)*

Signs of Drug Hypersensitivity

Those who administer medications should always be alert for signs of drug hypersensitivity. Table 14-2 lists the symptoms that can occur when drugs adversely affect certain systems of the body.

Instructing the Client

You should inform your client of any changes that may occur to the body as a result of drug therapy. Certain drugs may cause drowsiness and the client should be so advised. You should also advise the client to avoid consumption of foods and other chemical substances that are known causes of adverse drug interactions, and to follow the physician's prescribed plan for treatment.

MEDICATION ERROR

Medication errors can occur anywhere and at any time during the drug therapy course, from prescribing through transcribing, dispensing, administering, and monitoring. The causes of medication errors are many; for example, lack of product knowledge or training; poor communication; ambiguities in product names, directions for use, medical abbreviations, handwriting, or labeling; job stress; poor procedures or techniques; or client misuse. Any health care worker may be the cause of, or contribute to, an actual or potential error.

It is important to recognize that health care workers can learn from medication errors. By sharing experiences through the nationwide USP Medication Errors Reporting (MER) Program, one can help others to gain an understanding of why errors occur and how to prevent them. To report a medication error, call 1-800-233-7767 to reach a USP health care professional who will take the report and respond to the caller's concerns. See Figure 14-4 for an example of a medication error information report form.

All reports are forwarded to the Food and Drug Administration, the product manufacturer/labeler when appropriate, the Institute for Safe Medication Practices (ISMP), and the USP Divisions of Standards and Information Development. If the reporter wishes to remain anonymous to any of these sources, the USP will act as the intermediary in all correspondence. While including identity is optional, it does allow for appropriate follow-up to discuss the reporter's observations or to provide feedback.

The USP Practitioners' Reporting Network (USP PRN) is a partner in MEDWATCH, the FDA's medical products reporting program. As a partner,

TABLE 14-2   SIGNS OF DRUG HYPERSENSITIVITY

Signs of Drug Hypersensitivity	Body System Affected
Lightheadedness, dizziness, euphoria, headache, vertigo, mental confusion, abnormal temperature	Central nervous system
Nausea, vomiting, diarrhea, constipation, anorexia, gastric irritation, abnormal pain, jaundice, liver dysfunction, hepatitis	Digestive system
Pruritus, rash, alopecia, urticaria (hives), pallor, flushing	Integumentary system
Hypotension, bradycardia, arrhythmias, tachycardia	Cardiovascular system
Blood dyscrasias, petechiae, bone marrow depression, hemorrhage, pancytopenia, purpura	Blood
Hematuria, proteinuria, anuria, urinary frequency, oliguria, impotence, menstrual irregularities, vaginitis	Genitourinary systems
Blurred vision, diplopia, nystagmus	Eye
Tinnitus	Ear
Dry mouth, nasal congestion	Autonomic nervous system
Gynecomastia, menstrual irregularities, Cushingoid state, altered libido	Endocrine system
Muscle weakness, osteoporosis, swelling of joints, pathological fracture of long bones	Musculoskeletal system
Skin eruptions, pruritus, urticaria, anaphylaxis, angioedema, flushing	Multisystem allergic reactions to medications

MEDICATION ERROR INFORMATION REPORT

* REQUIRED Information   ** See MedMARx program for additional choices

	*TYPE OF ERROR	*SEVERITY LEVEL / OUTCOME

*Date of error: _____ (mm/dd/yyyy)

Time (military) of error: _____

*Location where initial error was made: _____

Medication(s) involved: _____

_____

_____

*NODE (Where in the medication process did the <u>initial</u> error occur?)

☐ Prescribing   ☐ Administering

☐ Documenting   ☐ Monitoring

☐ Dispensing

TYPE OF ERROR

☐ Prescribing   ☐ Extra dose

☐ Omission   ☐ Wrong administration technique

☐ Wrong patient   ☐ Wrong dosage form

☐ Wrong time   ☐ Wrong drug preparation

☐ Wrong route   ☐ Other: _____

☐ Improper dose/quantity

   enter dose ordered: _____

   enter dose given: _____

☐ Unauthorized (wrong) drug

   name of medication ordered: _____

   name of medication given: _____

SEVERITY LEVEL / OUTCOME

☐Category A: Circumstances or events that have the capacity to cause error

☐ Category B: An error occurred; medication did not reach the patient

☐ Category C: An error occurred that reached the patient but did not cause patient harm

☐ Category D: An error occurred that resulted in the need for increased patient monitoring but no patient harm

☐ Category E: An error occurred that resulted in the need for treatment or intervention and caused temporary patient harm

☐ Category F: An error occurred that resulted in initial or prolonged hospitalization and caused temporary patient harm

☐ Category G: An error occurred that resulted in permanent patient harm

☐Category H: An error occurred that resulted in a near-death event (e.g., anaphylaxis, cardiac arrest)

☐Category I: An error occurred that resulted in patient death

*Possible cause(s) of error (check all that apply):

☐ Abbreviations
☐ Calculation error
☐ Communication confusing / intimidating / lacking
☐ Computer entry
☐ Decimal point
☐ Diluent wrong
☐ Dispensing device involved
☐ Documentation inaccurate / lacking
☐ Dosage form confusion
☐ Drug distribution system
☐ Equipment design confusing / inadequate for proper use
☐ Failure to activate or properly activate medication
☐ Facsimile of medication order
☐ Handwriting illegible / unclear
☐ Knowledge deficit
☐ Label design
☐ Labeling (your facility) confusing / inaccurate / incomplete
☐ Labeling (manufacturer) confusing / inaccurate / incomplete
☐ Leading zero missing
☐ Measuring device inaccurate/inappropriate
☐ Monitoring inadequate / lacking
☐ Names, brand names look alike
☐ Names, brand names sound alike
☐ Names, brand name / generic name of different products look alike
☐ Names, brand name / generic name of different products sound alike
☐ Names, generic names look alike
☐ Names, generic names sound alike
☐ Non-metric units of measurement (apothecary)
☐ Packaging / container design
☐ Performance deficit, nonspecific (i.e., person trained / expectation not met)
☐ Prefix/ suffix misunderstood / misinterpreted
☐ Preprinted medication order form
☐ Procedure / protocol not followed
☐ Reference manual confusing / inaccurate / unclear / outdated
☐ Similar packaging / labeling
☐ System safeguard(s) inadequate / lacking
☐ Trailing / terminal zero
☐ Transcription inaccurate / omitted
☐ Verbal order confusing / incomplete / misunderstood
☐ Written order confusing / incomplete / misunderstood
☐ **Other: _____

Factor(s) possibly contributing to the error:

☐ Code situation   ☐ Staff, agency/ temp

☐ Cross coverage   ☐ Staff, floating

☐ Distractions   ☐ Staff, inexperienced

☐ Emergency situation   ☐ Staffing, alternative hours

☐ No 24 hour pharmacy   ☐ Staffing, insufficient

☐ No access to patient information   ☐ Workload increase

☐ Poor lighting   ☐ Other: _____

☐ Shift change

Action(s) taken to avoid similar error of this type:

☐ Communication process enhanced

☐ Computer software modified / obtained

☐ Education / training provided

☐ Environment modified

☐ Formulary changed

☐ Informed staff who made the initial error

☐ Informed staff who was also involved in error

☐ Policy / procedure changed

☐ Policy / procedure instituted

☐ Staffing practice / policy modified

☐ None

☐ Other: _____

*Level of staff that made the initial error:

☐ Nurse Anesthetist   ☐ Pharmacy Technician
☐ Nurse Practitioner   ☐ Physician
☐ Nurse, LPN / LVN   ☐ Physician Assistant
☐ Nurse, Registered   ☐ Unit Secretary / Clerk
☐ Pharmacist
☐ **Other: _____

Level of staff also involved in the error (i.e., perpetuated the error):

☐ Nurse Anesthetist   ☐ Pharmacy Technician
☐ Nurse Practitioner   ☐ Physician
☐ Nurse, LPN / LVN   ☐ Physician Assistant
☐ Nurse, Registered   ☐ Unit Secretary / Clerk
☐ Pharmacist
☐ **Other: _____

Level of staff that discovered the error:

☐ Nurse Anesthetist   ☐ Pharmacy Technician
☐ Nurse Practitioner   ☐ Physician
☐ Nurse, LPN / LVN   ☐ Physician Assistant
☐ Nurse, Registered   ☐ Unit Secretary / Clerk
☐ Pharmacist
☐ **Other: _____

Recommendations to avoid similar error:

MEDICATION ERROR INFORMATION REPORT

This document is part of a quality improvement process

CONFIDENTIAL — Not to be included as part of the patient medical record

Patient Name: _____

Medical Record #: _____

Signature of Unit Manager: _____

Risk Management #: _____

(continued)

FIGURE 14-4   MEDICATION ERROR INFORMATION REPORT *(Reprinted with the permission of the United States Pharmacopeia. All rights reserved. © 1999)*

PRODUCT INFORMATION (* REQUIRED Information):

*Generic name:_____

Brand name: _____

Manufacturer: _____

Therapeutic classification: _____

*Dosage form: (e.g., cream, tablet, injection, etc.): _____

Intended route of administration: _____

Strength / Concentration as given on product label: _____

Labeler (if different from manufacturer): _____

Repacker (if different from manufacturer): _____

Compounded ingredients: _____

_____

_____

_____

Type of container: _____

Size of container: _____

PATIENT PROFILE INFORMATION (* REQUIRED Information):

Patient ID: _____

*Patient age: _____ (days, weeks, months, years) circle one

Patient gender: ◻ Male   ◻ Female   ◻ Unavailable

Direct result of the error on the level of care administered to the patient (check all that apply):

◻ Airway established / patient ventilated   ◻ Laboratory tests performed

◻ Antidote administered   ◻ Narcotic antagonist administered

◻ Cardiac defibrillation performed   ◻ Observation initiated / increased

◻ CPR administered   ◻ Oxygen administered

◻ Drug therapy initiated / changed   ◻ Surgery performed

◻ Hospitalization, initial   ◻ Transferred to intensive care

◻ Hospitalization, prolonged 1 - 5 days   ◻ Vital signs monitoring initiated / increased

◻ Hospitalization, prolonged 6 - 10 days   ◻ X-ray / MRI / other diagnostic test performed

◻ Hospitalization, prolonged > 10 days   ◻ None:_____

◻ Other:_____

Details on the direct result of the error on the level of care administered to the patient:

_____

_____

Tests / laboratory data, with dates, if relevant to the error: _____

_____

Other patient history, including pre-existing medical conditions, if relevant to the error:

_____

_____

_____

Concomitant drug therapy, with dates, if relevant to the error:_____

_____

_____

_____

Additional information / details NOT addressed previously (*description of error):

_____

_____

_____

_____

_____

_____

_____

_____

_____

_____

_____

_____

_____

_____

_____

_____

_____

FIGURE 14-4   *(continued)*

USP PRN contributes to the FDA's efforts to protect the public health by helping to identify serious adverse events for the agency. The reported information is shared with the FDA on a daily basis, or immediately if necessary.

> **Note:** For additional information, visit the Practitioners' Reporting Network of the U.S. Pharmacopoeia's Web site at http://www.usp.org/practrep/mer.htm.

A medication error occurs when any of the following actions are taken:

- A drug is given to the wrong client.
- The wrong drug is administered.
- The drug is given via the wrong route.
- The wrong dosage is given.
- The drug is not given at the prescribed time.
- The wrong rate of administration is used.
- A drug that is contraindicated is given.
- A drug is given to which a client is known to be allergic.
- An unordered or unsafe medication is given.
- A drug is given along with an incompatible medication, food, or other substance.
- A drug is contraindicated in the client's current, assessed status.

Medication errors should not happen when personnel follow established procedures; however, honest mistakes will be made periodically. When a medication error occurs, this is the procedure to follow:

1. Recognize that an error has been made.
2. Assess the client's condition and/or reactions to the medication.
3. Report the error immediately to the supervisor.
4. Notify the physician and/or pharmacist of the error.
5. Stay with the client. Follow the physician's order. Observe for signs of difficulty and assess the client for reactions to the medication.
6. Complete a written report. Each health care facility has an established procedure for reporting medication errors.

Ethical and Legal Considerations

Anyone with access to medications may be tempted to use them for personal benefit. To do so is not only unethical, it is illegal. The conversion to personal use of medications intended for another is both unethical and illegal. It is also unethical and illegal to take medicines that belong to your employer, even aspirin, without proper authorization and reimbursement. It can result in suspension or revocation of your license.

Tolerating the misuse of medications may lead to the abuse of more serious drugs such as narcotics and other controlled substances. It is your ethical responsibility to report all incidents of the misuse of medications to your supervisor.

● SELF-ASSESSMENT

Complete the following statements:

Source

p. 104 **1.** On the lines provided, list the five steps of the nursing process.

_____

_____

_____

_____

_____

p. 104 **2.** _____ is the systematic gathering, organizing, and interpretation of data to determine a client's nursing needs.

p. 104 **3.** Supply the missing word or words to complete the following four steps involved in formulating a nursing diagnosis:

- Collect information about the client and establish a _____ .
- Make an _____ of the client's needs, problems, concerns, and human responses.
- _____ of the data to make a diagnostic statement.
- _____ of the sufficiency and accuracy of the data.

p. 106 **4.** Health care professionals who prepare and administer medications are ethically and legally responsible for their actions. Under the law, these individuals are required to be _____, _____, or otherwise _____ by a physician.

p. 106 **5.** By law, those administering medications are expected to be familiar with the effects that drugs might have upon their clients. When there is any question about a medication, the nurse should _____ .

p. 106–108   **6.** On the lines provided, list the "Six Rights" of proper drug administration.

- Right _____
- Right _____
- Right _____
- Right _____
- Right _____
- Right _____

p. 108   **7.** One of the basic guidelines for the administration of medications calls for you to be completely familiar with the drug that is to be administered. Before giving a drug to a client, you are expected to know the following about the medication:

- _____
- _____
- _____
- _____
- _____
- _____
- _____
- _____

p. 109   **8.** The abbreviation BSI stands for _____ .

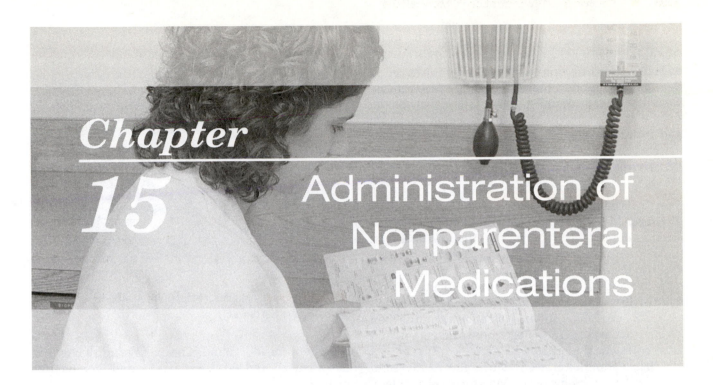

Chapter 15

Administration of Nonparenteral Medications

Chapter Outline

Objectives

Upon completion of this chapter, you should be able to

- Define the key terms
- List three advantages and several disadvantages of the oral route of drug administration
- Prepare and administer oral medications
- Perform an eye instillation
- Perform an ear instillation
- Describe the administration of nasal medications and rectal medications
- Describe a transdermal system
- Give the nurse's responsibility with regard to oxygen administration
- List the symptoms of oxygen toxicity
- Describe the administration of drugs by local application
- Complete the Self-Assessment

Key Terms

application	inunction
buccal medicine	irrigation
canthus	lozenge
enema	nitroglycerin
hypoxemia	ointment
inhalation	oxygen
inhaler	sublingual medicine
insertion	suppository
instillation	transdermal system

INTRODUCTION

Nonparenteral medications are those that are administered by any route other than by injection. In this chapter nonparenteral methods of medication described are: oral, ophthalmic, otic, nasal, rectal, special delivery, by inhalation, by local application, and administration of oxygen.

ORAL MEDICATIONS

The method by which a medicine is to be administered is determined by the condition of the client, the disease or illness, the rate of absorption desired, and the form of the drug available. The most common method of administering a medication is by mouth. Sometimes referred to as the *administration of oral medications*, the use of the oral route when giving a drug offers the safest, most convenient, and most economical method available.

Drugs administered by mouth may be in a solid or a liquid form. Some of the solid forms are tablets, capsules, and caplets. These drugs are usually swallowed with a drink of water.

Not all drugs administered by mouth are swallowed. Although they are oral medications, those drug forms that are not swallowed are referred to as **sublingual** or **buccal medicines**. These terms refer to the route by which the drug is absorbed into the body. Sublingual medications, such as nitroglycerin tablets, are placed under the tongue. Buccal tablets are placed between the cheek and gum and allowed to dissolve. Another solid medication that is allowed to dissolve in the mouth is the **lozenge**, which is used for coughs and sore throats.

Liquid preparations include solutions, suspensions, elixirs, and syrups. These forms of medication are absorbed more rapidly than solid forms. Liquid medications are often artificially colored and flavored to disguise their true appearance and taste. A drug that has an agreeable taste and appearance often has a favorable psychological effect upon the client.

Weight and volume are two means of measuring the amount of medication to be administered. The volume of a liquid medication may be measured in milliliters, cubic centimeters, minims, drams, ounces, and by such household measures as teaspoons. Both solid and liquid forms of drugs can be measured in terms of weight. Dosages may be in micrograms, milligrams, grams, grains, milliequivalents, or units. An example of a drug dosage is Medrol (4 mg), as shown in Figure 15-1.

The amount of medication in the average dose for adults and children is based upon the age and

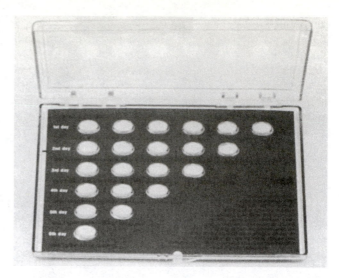

FIGURE 15-1 MEDROL (4 MG) DOSEPAK *(Courtesy of Pharmacia & Upjohn Company)*

weight of the individual. The average adult client is between 20 and 60 years of age and weighs 150 pounds.

Oral medications are easily and economically administered with a high degree of safety. There are, however, several disadvantages associated with the oral route. For instance, the drug may

- Have an objectionable odor
- Have an objectionable taste
- Cause discoloration of the teeth, mouth, and tongue
- Irritate the gastric mucosa
- Be altered by digestive enzymes
- Be poorly absorbed from the digestive system, due to illness or nature of the medication
- Come in a form (tablet, capsule, or caplet) that is too large for the client to swallow
- Be difficult or impossible to take because of nausea and/or vomiting
- Be refused by the client
- Have less predictable effects upon the body when given orally than when given by the parenteral route (by injection)

EQUIPMENT AND SUPPLIES

The equipment and supplies used in the administration of oral medications may include the following items:

- Medication order
- Medication record system

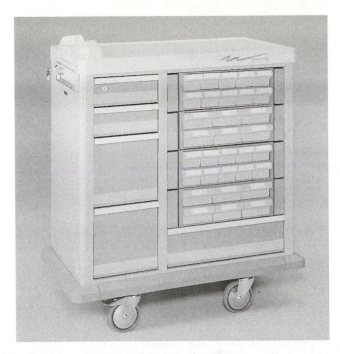

FIGURE 15-2   WATERLOO MEDICATION CART *(Courtesy of Waterloo Healthcare, Cedar Falls, Iowa)*

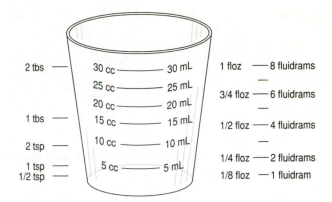

FIGURE 15-3   MEDICINE CUP WITH APPROXIMATE EQUIVALENT MEASURES *(Courtesy of James Russell, Jr.)*

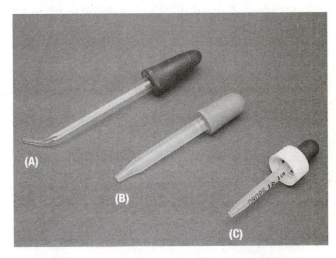

FIGURE 15-4   VARIOUS TYPES OF MEDICINE DROPPERS: (A) GLASS; (B) PLASTIC; (C) PLASTIC CALIBRATED

- Medication cart (Figure 15-2)
- Medication cabinet
- Medication tray
- Medicine cup (plastic, glass, or paper)
- Medicine dropper
- Water cup (plastic, paper)
- Drinking straws
- Syringes
- Tablet crusher
- Other: refrigerator, sink, soap, paper towels, and a pen

Three measuring devices commonly used in the administration of oral medications are the medicine cup, the water cup, and the medicine dropper. The medicine cup (Figure 15-3) comes in various sizes and shapes, depending upon its manufacturer and its intended use. In the illustration provided, note that the cup is calibrated in fluidounces, fluidrams, cubic centimeters (cc), milliliters (ml), teaspoons (tsp), and tablespoons (tbs).

The water cup is a small plastic or paper cup that is disposable. The average water cup holds 3 ounces of liquid. The medicine dropper (Figure 15-4) may be calibrated in milliliters, minims, or drops. Medicine droppers are often provided as a part of the container with many medications. Uncalibrated droppers may be provided when the medicine is ad-

ministered only in drops. The size of the drop varies with the size of the dropper opening, the angle at which it is held, the force exerted on the rubber bulb, and the viscosity of the medication.

It is important that you select the appropriate container for a medication and measure the prescribed dosage accurately. The selection of the container depends upon the physical structure of the medication (solid or liquid), the amount of medication prescribed, the size of the container, and the calibrations on the container.

ADMINISTRATION OF ORAL MEDICATIONS

Earlier chapters of this section provided information on drug sources, standards, dosages, the forms of drugs, and drug actions. Also covered were responsibilities in the administration of medications, and the types of medicine orders. With this background, it is now time to apply this knowledge to the preparation and administration of oral medications.

Before beginning, however, note the following special considerations. Since oral medications may be in solid or liquid form, different procedures are employed, depending upon which form is used. In addition, medications may be supplied in unit dose or multiple dose containers. Thus, different procedural steps are necessary when there is a difference in the way medications are supplied.

Special Considerations

Depending upon the type of medication (liquid or solid) and how supplied (multiple or unit dose), one should adapt Procedure 15-1: Administration of Oral Medications, by adding the following steps at the appropriate point:

Using a Multiple Dose Solid Medication

- Remove the cap from the container in which the medicine is supplied. (Touch only the outside of the cap to avoid contamination.)
- Dispense the prescribed amount of solid medicine into the container's cap. (Do not touch the medication.)
- Transfer the medication from the cap to the disposable paper cup.
- Recap the medication container.
- Dispense only one medication at a time.

Using a Multiple Dose Liquid Medication

- Shake the preparation if it is a precipitate (or if the instructions call for it to be shaken).
- Remove the cap from the medication bottle
- Place the cap, open side up, on a flat surface. (This prevents contamination of the part of the cap that is in contact with the medicine bottle.)
- With the label covered by the palm of your hand (to safeguard the label from becoming stained), pour the liquid medicine into an appropriate measuring device.
- When pouring, always hold the measuring device at eye level. See Figure 15-5.
- When pouring, do not allow the bottle to come into contact with the measuring device.
- Measure the medicine at the lowest level of the meniscus.

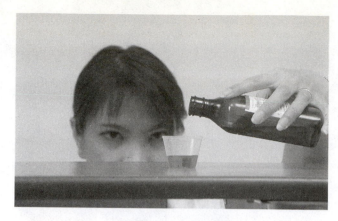

FIGURE 15-5   MEASURE ORAL MEDICATIONS AT EYE LEVEL.

- After pouring, cleanse the bottle, if necessary. (If the label becomes soiled, a pharmacist must relabel the medication.)
- Recap the medication bottle.

Using a Unit Dose Solid or Liquid Medication

- It is best to open a unit dose medication when you are at the client's side. (If the client refuses the medication, an unopened unit dose medication does not have to be discarded.) However, when you have to give $\frac{1}{2}$ tablet, you generally bisect the tablet before entering the client's room and the $\frac{1}{2}$ tablet not given is properly discarded.
- Open the package according to the directions on its label.
- Without touching the medication, place it into the client's hand (or pour it into an appropriate container).

Safety Precautions

Following the administration of an oral medication, the nurse should observe the following safety precautions:

- Return the client to a resting position.
- Be sure the bed's siderails are raised when necessary.
- Check the medication label for the third time.
- Document the procedure correctly.

Aftercare of Equipment

The final steps in the procedure for administering an oral medication involve the disposal or aftercare of equipment and supplies. The nurse should

PROCEDURE 15-1

Administration of Oral Medications

STANDARD PRECAUTIONS:

PURPOSE:

Correctly administer an oral medication after receiving a physician's order and assembling the necessary equipment and supplies.

EQUIPMENT/SUPPLIES

Proper medication
Medicine card
Water, milk, or juice for client

PROCEDURE STEPS:

1. Verify the physician's order.
2. Follow the "Six Rights."
3. Perform medical asepsis handwash.
4. Work in a well-lighted, quiet, clean area.
5. Assemble equipment and supplies.
6. Obtain the correct medication using the medicine card.
7. Compare the medication label with the medicine card (first time).
8. Check the expiration date. (Figure 15-6A)
9. Calculate dosage if necessary.
10. Correctly prepare (a, b, or c) (Figure 15-6B)
    a. Multiple dose solid medication
    b. Unit dose medication
    c. Liquid medication
11. Compare medicine label with medicine card (second time).
12. Return medication to shelf and check label (third time).
13. Properly transport the medicine.
14. Identify the client. Explain the procedure.
15. Assess client. Take vital signs if indicated.
16. Assist client to a comfortable position.
17. Provide water, milk, or juice (unless contraindicated).
18. Administer the medication. Be certain that the client takes the medicine (Figure 15-6C).
19. Provide for the client's safety: Observe the client for any adverse reactions.
20. Document the procedure in the client chart using the medicine card.
21. Care for equipment and supplies according to OSHA guidelines.
22. Wash hands.

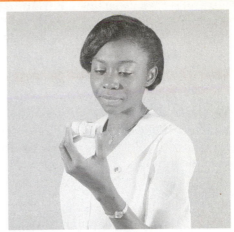

(A)

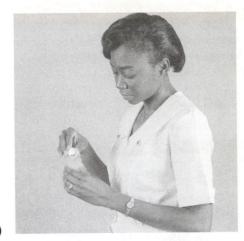

(B)

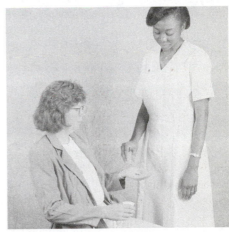

(C)

FIGURE 15-6   (A) NURSE CHECKS FOR RIGHT DRUG, RIGHT DOSE, RIGHT ROUTE, AND EXPIRATION DATE BEFORE POURING MEDICATION. (B) NURSE POURS CAPSULES FROM THE COVER OF THE MEDICINE CONTAINER INTO A MEDICINE CUP PRIOR TO ADMINISTERING THE MEDICINE TO THE CLIENT. (C) NURSE GIVES MEDICATION TO THE CLIENT, MAKING SURE THE CLIENT TAKES THE MEDICINE.

- Properly discard disposable materials
- Return any unused supplies to the designated area
- Clean and return reusable materials to the designated area
- Perform the medical asepsis handwash

Preparing and Administering a Crushed Medicine

Certain clients (pediatric, geriatric, and others) may not be able to swallow a tablet. If the medication is not available in liquid form, one must crush the solid medicine and mix it with either food or a liquid to facilitate administration. Whenever it is necessary to crush a solid medication, the following guidelines should be followed:

1. If you have any questions as to whether a medication should be crushed, ask the pharmacist or the prescribing physician before attempting to crush the medicine.
2. As a general rule, most compressed tablets may be crushed.
3. Buccal or sublingual tablets, sustained-release tablets, and enteric-coated tablets should not be crushed. To do so would alter the effect of these medications. (See Table 15-1.)

TABLE 15-1   TABLETS THAT CANNOT BE CRUSHED OR ALTERED

Check Out This List Before Altering a Drug			
A. Don't crush or alter these common sustained-release, enteric-coated, and sublingual tablets.	Iberet-500 Filmtabs Ilotycin Indocin SR Isordil (Sublingual) Isuprel Glossets	Ritalin SR Roxanol SR Slow-K Sorbitrate SA Sustaire	Slo-bid Gyrocaps Slo-Phyllin Gyrocaps Sudafed SA Temaril Spansules Theobid
Afrinol Repetabs Asbron G Inlay-Tabs Avazyme Azulfidine EN-tabs	Kaon-Cl Kaon-Cl-10 K-Dur Klor-Con Klotrix	Tedral SA Theo-Dur Theolair-SR Trilafon Repetabs	Theo-Dur Sprinkle Thorazine Spansules Tuss-Ornade Spansules
Belladenal-S Bellergal-S bisacodyl Bronkodyl S-R	K-Tab Lithobid	**B.** You can open these sustained-release capsules and carefully mix the contents in a liquid or with a soft food, such as applesauce. Vigorous mixing, however, could alter the rate of release.	Valrelease **C.** Because of the makeup of these miscellaneous drugs, do not crush or alter them.
Chlor-Trimeton Repetabs Choledyl SA Constant-T	Mestinon Timespan Micro-K Extencaps MS Contin		• *Accutane* (liquid-filled capsule). Liquid can irritate mucous membrane.
Diamox Sequels Dimetane Extentabs Dimetapp Extentabs Donnatal Extentabs Donnazyme Drixoral Dulcolax	Nico-Span Nitro-Bid Nitrostat Norflex Pabalate Pancrease Peritrate SA	Artane Sequels Combid Spansules Compazine Spansules Dexedrine Spansules Feosol Spansules	• *Chymoral*. Crushing may interfere with enzymatic activity. • *Feldene*. Powder from this capsule can irritate mucous membrane.
Easprin Ecotrin E-Mycin Eskalith CR	Permitil Chronotab Phazyme-PB Phyllocontin Polaramine Repetab Preludin Repetab Preludin Enduret	Inderal LA Inderide LA Isordil Tembids (capsules)	• *Klorvess* (effervescent tablet). If this tablet is not dissolved before it is given, gastrointestinal upset will occur, and gastrointestinal damage may occur.
Fero-Grad-500 Fero-Gradumet Festal II	Procan SR Pronestyl-SR Quibron-T/SR	Nicobid Nitrostat SR Ornade Spansules	
Hydergine (Sublingual) Iberet Filmtabs	Quinaglute Dura-Tabs Quinidex Extentabs	Pavabid	

(continued)

TABLE 15-1 *(Continued)*

Watch for These Names as a Tip-Off.			
A. These drug manufacturers' names indicate a sustained-release or an enteric-coated form of a drug.	Dura-tab	Lontab	**B.** When attached to a drug name, these terms indicate a sustained-release form of a drug.
	Enduret	Repetab	
	Enseal	Sequel	
	EN-tab	Spansule	
BidCap	Extencap	Tab-in	Bid
Cenule	Extentab	Tembid	Dur
Chronosule	Gradumet	Tempule	Plateau Cap
Chronotab	Granucap	Tentab	SA
D-Lay	Gyrocap	TimeCap	Span
Dospan	Kronocap	Timecelle	SR
Duracap	Lanacap	Timespan	XL

(Courtesy of Springhouse Corporation)

4. When possible, avoid crushing Ecotrin, E-Mycin, and Dulcolax, since these drugs may cause gastric irritation when crushed.

5. As a rule, hard capsules should not be crushed. Some capsules can be pulled apart to allow the dry powder to be removed.

6. Unit dose medications should be crushed in the wrapper prior to opening.

The method used to crush a tablet depends upon the equipment available. A specially designed tablet crusher or a mortar and pestle are the best devices for crushing tablets. When these are not available, one may use two spoons to crush the medicine. Great care must be taken to insure that none of the medication is lost in the crushing process. See Figures 15-7, 15-8, and 15-9.

If the client's diet permits, one may use small amounts of food (applesauce, strained fruit, pudding, ice cream) as a vehicle for administering a crushed medicine. The client should be informed

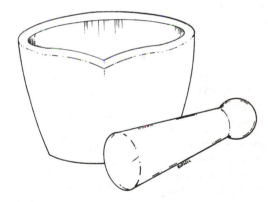

FIGURE 15-8 MORTAR AND PESTLE *(Courtesy of James Russell, Jr.)*

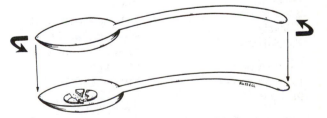

FIGURE 15-9 CRUSHING A TABLET BETWEEN TWO SPOONS *(Courtesy of James Russell, Jr.)*

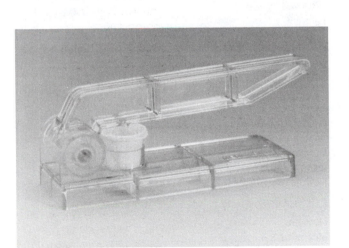

FIGURE 15-7 DELUXE MEDI-CRUSH PILL AND TABLET CRUSHER *(Courtesy of Medi-Crush Company)*

that the prescribed medication is in the food or liquid. The entire amount of food or liquid used as a vehicle must be consumed; this is why small amounts should be used as some clients may not be able to tolerate regular portions.

Using a Syringe to Administer a Liquid Oral Medicine

When a client is unable to take a liquid medicine from a cup or other container, one may use a syringe to administer the medication. Should it become necessary to use this method, be sure that you have the correct amount of medication (milliliters, cubic centimeters, minims, or teaspoons) measured in the appropriate syringe (Figure 15-10).

Safety Precaution: When prepared by the pharmacist, oral preparations in syringes should be brightly labeled as a safety precaution against accidental intramuscular injection.

Devices Used for Administering Oral Medications to a Child

There are various devices that may be used to administer an oral medication to a child. See Figure 15-11. It is essential that you measure the exact prescribed dosage of medication that is to be administered. Note that the spoon has one end for teaspoons and the other end for tablespoons. There are 3 teaspoons to a tablespoon. The calibrated devices are in teaspoons and milliliters. There are 5 milliliters to a teaspoon.

ADMINISTRATION OF OPHTHALMIC MEDICATIONS

Ophthalmic medications are administered by **instillation** (slowly pouring or dropping a liquid into a cavity or onto a surface) or by **application** (the act of applying; to bring into contact with something). When administered properly, ophthalmic medications have a local effect. The rate and extent of absorption into the mucous membranes depends upon the vascularity and the thickness of the membrane. See Procedure 15-2: Performing Eye Instillation.

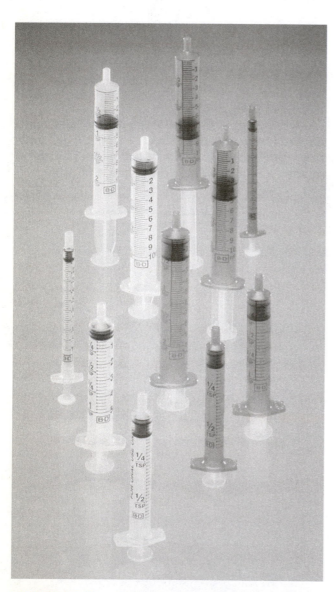

FIGURE 15-10 TYPES OF SYRINGES USED TO ADMINISTER A LIQUID MEDICINE *(Courtesy of Becton, Dickinson and Company)*

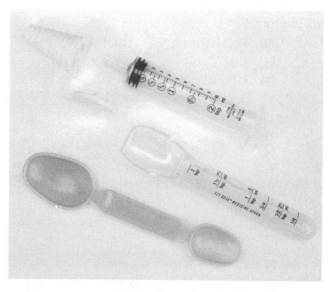

FIGURE 15-11 DEVICES FOR ADMINISTERING ORAL MEDICATIONS TO A CHILD

PROCEDURE 15-2

Performing Eye Instillation

STANDARD PRECAUTIONS:

PURPOSE:

To treat eye infections, soothe irritation, anesthetize, and dilate pupils. Ophthalmic medication is supplied in liquid or ointment form. Use separate medication for each eye, if both are affected.

EQUIPMENT/SUPPLIES:

Sterile eye dropper

Sterile ophthalmic medication as ordered by the physician, either drops or ointment

Sterile cotton balls

Sterile gloves

PROCEDURE STEPS:

1. Wash hands.
2. Assemble supplies.
3. Check medication carefully as ordered by the physician, including expiration date. Read label three times.
4. Identify client.
5. Explain procedure to the client and inform the client that instillation may temporarily blur vision.
6. Position the client in a sitting or lying position.
7. Instruct the client to stare at a fixed spot during instillation of the drops. Put on gloves.
8. Prepare medication using either drops or ointment.
9. Have the client look up to the ceiling and expose the lower conjunctival sac of the affected eye by using fingers over a tissue to pull down lower eyelid (Figure 15-12).
10. Place the number of drops ordered in the center of the lower conjunctival sac or a thin line of ointment in the lower surface of the eyelid being careful not to touch the eyelid, eyeball, or eyelashes with the tip of the medication

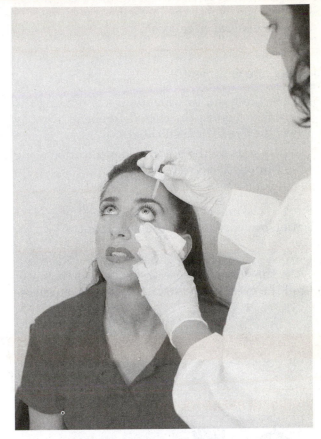

FIGURE 15-12 WHEN INSTILLING MEDICATION INTO THE CLIENT'S EYE, THE CLIENT SHOULD LOOK UP TO THE CEILING AND THE NURSE SHOULD PULL DOWN ON THE LOWER LID. CONTACT WITH THE EYEBALL SHOULD BE AVOIDED.

applicator. Carefully replace dropper in bottle to avoid contamination.

11. Have the client close the eye and roll the eyeball. Movement distributes the medication evenly.
12. Blot excess medication from eyelids with cotton ball from inner to outer **canthus** (the angle at either end of the slit between the eyelids).
13. Dispose of supplies.
14. Remove gloves.
15. Wash hands.
16. Record procedure in client's chart.

> **Safety Precaution:** Ophthalmic medications can cause systemic symptoms if the medicine is allowed to flow into the lacrimal sac, where the medicine is absorbed into the general circulation.

To Apply Eye Ointment:

- Place the hand in which you are holding the ointment against the client's forehead (directly over the eye to be medicated).
- Gently squeeze the prescribed medication along the conjunctival border.

> Start at the inner canthus and spread the medication outward toward the outer canthus.

- Ask the client to close the eyes and to gently roll the eyes around to distribute the ointment.

- Remove any excess ointment with a sterile gauze pad.

> Instruct the client not to rub the eyes, and to remain in the supine position for approximately 5 minutes.

ADMINISTRATION OF OTIC MEDICATIONS

Otic medications are usually administered by instillation. They may be used to treat infection and inflammation, to soften cerumen, to produce a local anesthetic effect, or to immobilize a trapped insect. Ear drops are usually contraindicated if the client has a perforated eardrum, is hypersensitive to any ingredient in its formula, or has certain conditions such as herpes, other viral infections, or systemic fungal infections. See Procedure 15-3: Performing Ear Instillation.

PROCEDURE 15-3

Performing Ear Instillation

STANDARD PRECAUTIONS:

PURPOSE:

To soften impacted cerumen, fight infection with antibiotics, or relieve pain.

EQUIPMENT/SUPPLIES:

Otic medication as prescribed by the physician
Sterile ear dropper
Cotton balls
Gloves

PROCEDURE STEPS:

1. Wash hands and assemble supplies.
2. Identify client.
3. Explain procedure to the client.
4. Position client to either lie on unaffected side or sitting position with head tilted toward unaffected ear to facilitate flow of medication.

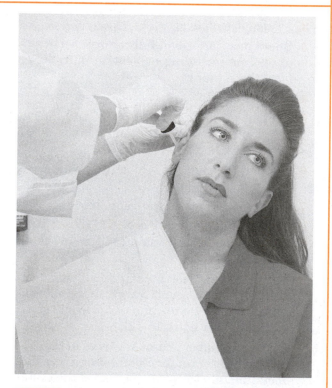

FIGURE 15-13   WHEN INSTILLING DROPS INTO CLIENT'S EAR, HAVE THE CLIENT TILT HEAD SO THAT THE AFFECTED EAR IS UPPERMOST.

(continued)

PROCEDURE 15-3

Performing Ear Instillation *(continued)*

5. Check otic medication three times against the physician's order and check expiration date of the medication. Only otic medication can be used in the ear. Checking the medication three times minimizes medication error.

6. Put on gloves. Draw up the prescribed amount of medication.

7. Gently pull the top of the ear upward and back (adult) or pull earlobe downward and backward (child) (Figure 15-13).

8. Instill prescribed dose of medication (number of drops) into the affected ear by squeezing rubber bulb on dropper.

9. Have the client maintain the position for about 5 minutes to retain medication.

10. When instructed by the physician, insert moistened cotton ball into external ear canal for 15 minutes. Moistened cotton ball will not absorb medication and will help retain medication in ear.

11. Dispose of supplies.

12. Remove gloves.

13. Wash hands.

14. Document procedure.

ADMINISTRATION OF NASAL MEDICATIONS

Nasal medications are usually administered by instillation, spray, or nasal inhaler. They may be used to treat the symptoms of seasonal or perennial rhinitis, and to relieve nasal congestion due to colds and sinusitis. Nose drops, sprays, and inhalers are usually contraindicated in clients who are hypersensitive to any ingredient in their formula. These medications should be used as directed, and one must not exceed the recommended dosage. Continued long-term use of nasal sprays may lead to rebound congestion (swelling and congestion of the nasal mucosa).

Nasal medications are usually best administered by the client. The client should be instructed to clear the nasal passageway before instilling nose drops, or using a spray or inhaler. Caution the client not to use any over-the-counter drugs without advice from his/her physician.

ADMINISTRATION OF RECTAL MEDICATIONS

Rectal medications are usually administered by instillation or insertion. The medication may be in the form of a suppository, ointment, or enema. A **suppository** (a semisolid substance for introduction of medication into the rectum, vagina, or urethra, where it dissolves) may be used as a contact laxative acting directly on the colonic mucosa to produce normal peristalsis throughout the large intestine; as a narcotic analgesic; as a local anesthetic inhibiting pain, burning, and itching; as an anti-inflammatory agent; as an antipyretic agent; as an antiemetic to relieve nausea and vomiting; and as a sedative.

An **enema** is the means of delivering a solution or medication into the rectum and colon. An enema may also be used to cleanse the lower bowel in preparation for radiography, sigmoidoscopy, proctoscopy, endoscopy, surgery, and many other special procedures. The ready-to-use Fleet® enema may be utilized in a hospital, nursing home, extended care facility, home, or physician's office. It is not to be administered to children under 2 years of age or to clients with undiagnosed abdominal pain. See Figures 15-14, 15-15, 15-16, and 15-17.

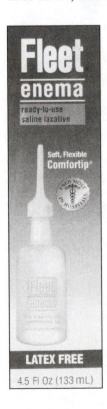

FIGURE 15-14   DISPOSABLE FLEET® READY-TO-USE ENEMA *(Courtesy of Fleet Company, Inc.)*

HOW TO ADMINISTER AN ENEMA

The guiding principles for all forms of therapy, and especially the enema, are effectiveness and safety, proper technique, and consideration of the client's total well-being. When administered properly, the Fleet® Ready-To-Use Enema meets all these requirements with built-in efficiency and convenience.

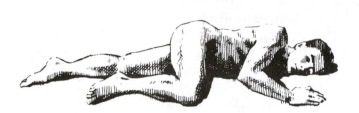

Sims' (left-lateral) Position

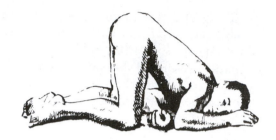

Knee-Chest Position

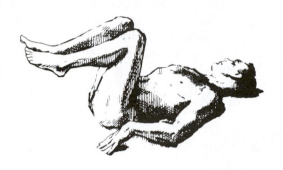

Position for Self-Administration

Child's Position

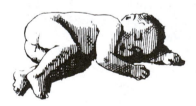

FIGURE 15-15   HOW TO ADMINISTER AN ENEMA *(Courtesy of Fleet Company, Inc.)*

Administration is simple and safe, whether the client is a child or adult, bedridden or ambulatory. Have the client relax by explaining the procedure and insuring privacy. If the client is in bed, put a rubber or plastic sheet or a folded towel under the client to protect the bed. Help the client turn on the left side, knees drawn up. Although not recommended for older persons, the client may find the *Knee-Chest Position* more comfortable. Remove the cover from the tip of the bottle and check to see that the tip's lubrication is adequate. Spread the buttocks. SLOWLY and GENTLY insert the Comfortip® in the direction of the navel. Care during insertion is necessary due to

sensory innervation of the rectum. If there is any resistance when inserting the tip or administering the solution, carefully withdraw the tip and discontinue the procedure. **FORCING THE ENEMA CAN RESULT IN PERFORATION AND/OR ABRASION OF THE RECTUM.** Squeeze SLOWLY until the contents of the bottle are expelled. A small amount (½ ounce) of solution will remain in the bottle. Withdraw the Comfortip® and discard the bottle. Have the client remain in position until a strong urge to defecate is felt, usually within 2 to 5 minutes. It is unnecessary for the client to try and hold the solution for any longer.

The client may wish to administer the enema himself. The simplest procedure is for him to lie on a towel on the bathroom floor, in the bathtub, or on the bed on his back with legs raised. Follow the steps described above. The client stays in whatever position is most comfortable until the urge to evacuate is felt.

In those cases where complications are reported, infants and young children are often involved. **DO NOT ADMINISTER A FLEET® ENEMA TO A CHILD UNDER 2 YEARS OF AGE.** Special care should be exercised in administering any enema to a child. Place the child on the left side, or face down if that seems more comfortable. Spread the buttocks, and SLOWLY and GENTLY insert the prelubricated Comfortip® of Fleet® Enema for Children pointed in the direction of the navel. Remember that care during insertion is necessary due to sensory innervation of the rec-

tum. If there is any resistance when inserting the tip or administering the solution, carefully withdraw the tip and discontinue the procedure. **FORCING THE ENEMA CAN RESULT IN PERFORATION AND/OR ABRASION OF THE RECTUM.** Squeeze SLOWLY and withdraw the Comfortip® when all but ¼ ounce of the solution has been delivered. (The physician may, of course, order a smaller quantity.) Hold the buttocks together until the child appears ready to evacuate, usually within 2 to 5 minutes. Then place the child on a toilet seat or bedpan.

FIGURE 15-15   *(continued)*

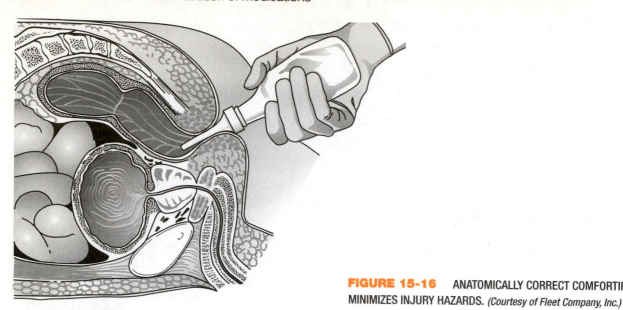

FIGURE 15-16 ANATOMICALLY CORRECT COMFORTIP® MINIMIZES INJURY HAZARDS. *(Courtesy of Fleet Company, Inc.)*

Since colonic peristalsis is induced by increased pressure, it is attainable simply by instilling fluid just past the internal anal sphincter. And the Fleet® Enema Comfortip® does just that, projecting just beyond the internal sphincter and eliminating the possibility of lacerating or perforating the rectal wall or colon. When the sphincter lacks tone, the tapered Comfortip® base serves as an anal plug and prevents rectal leakage.

Used properly, the Fleet® Ready-To-Use Enema is a safe and effective method of cleaning the lower bowel. Used inappropriately, it can cause anatomical injury, significant electrolyte changes, and in rare cases, death. ALWAYS CONSULT THE PROFESSIONAL LABELING OR A PHYSICIANS' DESK REFERENCE BEFORE USING ANY FLEET® BRAND ENEMA.

3-step procedure

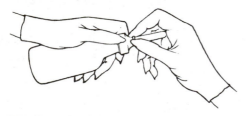

1. Ready to use . . .
   no preparation necessary . . .
   a. Remove protective shield.
   b. Check lubrication.
   c. Apply additional lubrication if necessary.

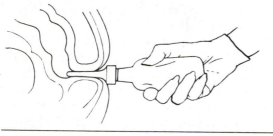

2. Easy to administer . . .
   a. Insert, gently pointing in direction of navel.
   b. Use gentle, slow pressure.
   c. Withdraw if any resistance is met.

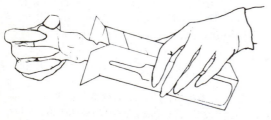

3. Disposable . . .
   a. Replace used enema bottle in original container and discard.
   b. Monitor client's condition.
   c. Evaluate return.

FIGURE 15-17 ADMINISTERING THE FLEET® READY-TO-USE ENEMA *(Courtesy of Fleet Company, Inc.)*

An **ointment** is a semisolid preparation consisting of a drug combined with a base of petroleum jelly or lanolin. These forms are not water soluble; however, some ointments are composed of ingredients that are water soluble. Ointments are generally applied externally to the skin, but certain ointments are prepared for rectal administration. An example is Preparation H® hemorrhoidal ointment that is used to help shrink swelling of hemorrhoidal tissues caused by inflammation and to give prompt, temporary relief in many cases from pain and itching. Before applying, remove the protective cover from the applicator. The applicator must be lubricated before each application and the applicator must be cleansed after each use.

SPECIAL DELIVERY MEDICATIONS

Today, because of technological advances, there are new ways by which a drug can be prepared and delivered to a client. Some of these preparations are known as *special delivery systems* that provide the drug to a targeted area. Others are modified preparations of the conventional form of the drug.

A **transdermal system** is a small adhesive patch or disk that may be applied to the body near the treatment site. A transdermal system generally consists of four layers:

1. An impermeable back that keeps the drug from leaking out of the system
2. A reservoir containing the drug
3. A membrane with tiny holes in it that controls the rate of drug release
4. An adhesive layer or gel that keeps the device in place

The physician will evaluate each client very carefully before prescribing any type of medication. There are warnings, precautions, adverse reactions, and other valuable information supplied by the manufacturer. It is essential that the prescribing physician and staff be totally familiar with all aspects of a drug before it is prescribed for a client.

As a nurse, it may be your responsibility to instruct the client in how to use and apply a transdermal system. It is important to read to the client the instructions that accompany the medication. Each manufacturer of transdermal systems provides this information.

Transdermal systems may be used to administer **nitroglycerin**. Nitroglycerin is a smooth-muscle relaxant with vascular effects manifested predominantly by venous dilatation and pooling. The major beneficial effect of nitroglycerin in angina pectoris is a reduction in myocardial oxygen consumption, secondary to vascular smooth-muscle relaxation with resultant reduction in cardiac preload and afterload. See Figures 15-18 and 15-19.

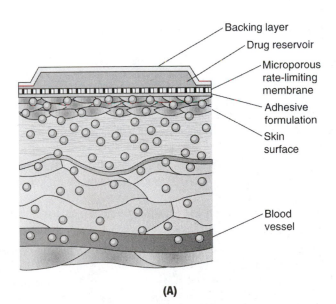

Backing layer
Drug reservoir
Microporous rate-limiting membrane
Adhesive formulation
Skin surface
Blood vessel

(A)

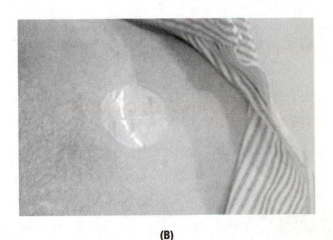

(B)

FIGURE 15-18   (A) THE MULTILAYER UNIT COMPRISING TRANSDERM-NITRO® DELIVERS NITROGLYCERIN INTO THE BLOODSTREAM IN A CONSISTENT, CONTROLLED MANNER FOR 24 HOURS. THE VERY THIN UNIT CONTAINS A BACKING LAYER, A RESERVOIR OF NITROGLYCERIN, A UNIQUE RATE-LIMITING MEMBRANE, AND AN ADHESIVE LAYER THAT HAS A PRIMING DOSE OF NITROGLYCERIN. (B) THE PATCH IS APPLIED TO THE SKIN. *(Courtesy of Geneva Pharmaceuticals)*

How to apply   Transderm-Nitro®nitroglycerine

1. Apply clean gloves.

2. Rotate site and place in area where there is not excessive body hair.

3. Open the package by tearing at the indicated indentations. Carefully pick up the system lengthwise with the tab up, and the clear plastic backing facing you. You should be able to see the white cream containing nitroglycerin. (On very rare occasions, you may find a system without any white medication in it. Do not use it. Simply apply another system.

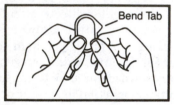

Figure A

4. Firmly bend the tab forward with the thumb (Figure A). With both thumbs, begin to remove the clear plastic backing from the system at the tab (Figure B). Do not

touch the inside of the exposed system, because the adhesive covers the entire surface

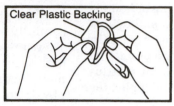

Figure B

5. Continue to remove the clear plastic backing slowly along the length of the system, allowing the system to rest on the outside of your fingers (Figure C).

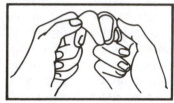

Figure C

6. Place the exposed, adhesive side of the system on the chosen skin site. Press firmly in place with the palm of your hand (Figure D). Once the system is in place, do not test the adhesion by pulling on it.

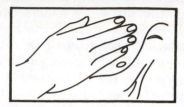

Figure D

7. Remove and discard the system after 24 hours. Place a new system on a different skin site, following steps 1 through 6.

Please note:

Contact with water, as in bathing, swimming, or showering, will not affect the system. In the unlikely event that a system falls off, discard it and put a new one on a different skin site.

Medication can be absorbed through skin; therefore, the nurse must be careful to avoid touching the patch with bare hands.

FIGURE 15-19   HOW TO USE TRANSDERM-NITRO® *(Courtesy of CIBA-GEIGY Pharmaceuticals, Summit, New Jersey)*

ADMINISTERING DRUGS BY INHALATION

The inhalation technique is used for the purpose of providing cold or warm air, usually in the form of medicated steam or aerosol therapy, for the client to breathe at intervals prescribed by the physician. Drugs administered by this method produce either a local or systemic effect and are given by inhalation for the following reasons:

● To provide local treatment for infections of the respiratory tract when these areas can be treated only by vapor. For example, steam

(moist) inhalations are used to relieve inflammation due to colds. The steam may or may not contain a drug.

● To provide systemic treatment for serious respiratory infections. For example, when oxygen is forced under pressure through a nebulizer containing penicillin or another antibiotic, fine particles of the drug are carried into the respiratory tract. The medium is the cold air.

● To supply a medication that can be absorbed into the bloodstream through the lungs, thereby producing a rapid systemic effect. An example is the use of aromatic spirits of ammonia. It is used to elicit reflect stimulation of respiration and as "smelling salts" to stimulate people who have fainted.

Inhalation Methods

The act of drawing breath, vapor, or gas into the lungs is known as **inhalation**. Inhalation therapy may involve the administration of medicines, water vapor, and such gases as oxygen, carbon dioxide, and helium.

An inhaler may be used to deliver medications to the lungs. Medications that utilize an inhaler include bronchodilators, mucolytic agents, and steroids. Inhalers are useful in the delivery of treatment for chronic obstructive pulmonary disease (COPD) and/or reversible obstructive airway disease. An **inhaler** is a small handheld apparatus, usually an aerosol unit, that contains a microcrystalline suspension of medication. See Figure 15-20. When activated, it produces a fine mist or spray containing the medication. This suspension is then drawn into the respiratory tract, settling deep into the lungs and alveoli.

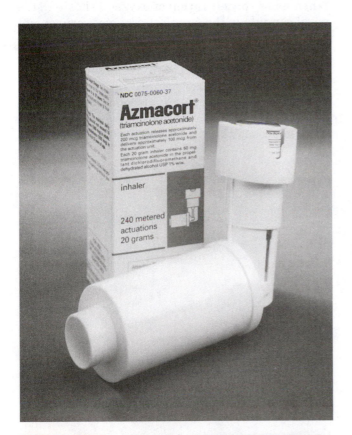

FIGURE 15-20   AZMACORT® (TRIAMCINOLONE ACETONIDE) INHALER, 240 METERED ACTUATIONS, 20 GRAMS *(Courtesy of Aventis Pharmaceuticals)*

Clinical Considerations for the Use of an Inhaler

- Clients should be instructed to follow the physician's order. The prescribed medicine and the type of inhaler to be used will determine the method of administration. The types of inhalers available for use are:
  - Handheld. This type includes nasal and oral inhalers.
  - Nebulizers. For large-volume (heated or cool) delivery, ultrasonic, and side-stream diffusion
  - Intermittent positive-pressure breathing (IPPB) machines
- Clients should be advised to avoid overuse of the inhaler. Tolerance, rebound bronchospasm, and adverse cardiac effects can occur from overuse.
- Clients should be cautioned against the continued use of a metered-dose canister after the stated number of actuations. For example, the Azmacort™ inhaler (in Figure 15-20) should not be used after 240 actuations (pushing the metered-dose canister).
- Clients should be instructed to notify their physician should the prescribed dose of medication fail to produce the desired effect.
- The client should be instructed to perform good oral hygiene, including rinsing the mouth, after each inhalation treatment (to prevent the possible growth of fungi).
- Inhalation therapy may be contraindicated in clients with delicate fluid balance, cardiac arrhythmias, status asthmaticus, and hypersensitivity to the medication.

ADMINISTRATION OF OXYGEN

Oxygen is a colorless, odorless, tasteless gas that is essential for life. When the body does not have an adequate supply of oxygen, a state of **hypoxemia** develops, and irreversible damage to vital organs is possible. When a lack of oxygen threatens a person's survival, supplemental oxygen must be prescribed and administered immediately, and arterial blood gas analysis must be made after oxygen administration has been started. If there is no emergency or life-threatening situation, the arterial blood gas analysis must be made before the physician prescribes the dosage and method of administration. The normal range for oxygen in the arterial blood is 80 to 100 mm Hg (millimeters mercury).

Signs and Symptoms of Hypoxemia

- Anxiety
- Cyanosis
- Pale, cold extremities
- Dyspnea
- Tachycardia
- Increased blood pressure
- Restlessness
- Confusion

Conditions/Diseases That May Require Oxygen Administration

- Apnea
- Carbon monoxide poisoning
- Drowning
- Congestive heart failure
- Chronic obstructive pulmonary disease (COPD)
- Myocardial infarction
- During surgery
- Pulmonary edema
- Pneumonia
- Shock

Dosage

When oxygen is to be administered, dosage is based on individual needs. Since oxygen is a drug, the physician will prescribe the flow rate, concentration, method of delivery, and length of time for administration. Oxygen is ordered as liters per minute (LPM) and as percentage of oxygen concentration (%).

As a nurse, it is your responsibility to follow the physician's order, and to adhere to the guidelines for proper drug administration as listed in Chapter 14. Always assess the client as an individual, explain the procedure, and carefully observe the client for signs of improvement or symptoms of oxygen toxicity.

Oxygen toxicity may develop when 100 percent oxygen is breathed for a prolonged period. As with any other drug, toxicity depends upon dose, time, and the client's response. The higher the dose, the shorter the time required to develop toxicity. Symptoms of oxygen toxicity are substernal pain, nausea, vomiting, malaise, fatigue, numbness, and a tingling of the extremities.

High concentrations of inhaled oxygen cause alveolar collapse, intra-alveolar hemorrhage, hya-line membrane formation, disturbance of the central nervous system, and retrolental fibroplasia in newborns.

> **Safety Precaution:** Apnea can result when giving oxygen at a flow rate greater than 2 liters per minute to COPD clients, especially those with emphysema. The client who has emphysema has difficulty ridding the body of CO_2.

METHODS OF OXYGEN DELIVERY

Many methods are available today for the delivery of oxygen. The more commonly prescribed methods include the use of nasal cannulas and masks. See Figures 15-21 and 15-22. Other methods of delivery involve the use of nasal catheters, isolettes, hoods, and tents.

Nasal Cannula

When a low concentration of oxygen is desired, the nasal cannula is the simplest and most convenient method for the administration of oxygen. See Figure 15-23. Made of plastic, the nasal cannula consists of two hollow prongs through which the oxygen passes, and a strap or other device to secure it to the client's head. The nasal prongs are placed into the client's nostrils. Avoid a direct flow of O_2 against the client's nasal mucosa, as this causes tissue dehydration.

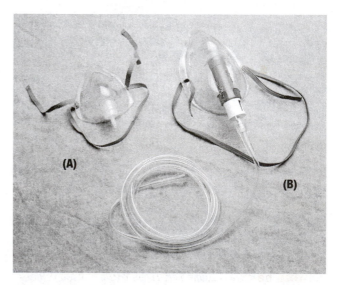

FIGURE 15-21 OXYGEN MASKS (A) WITHOUT TUBING AND (B) WITH TUBING

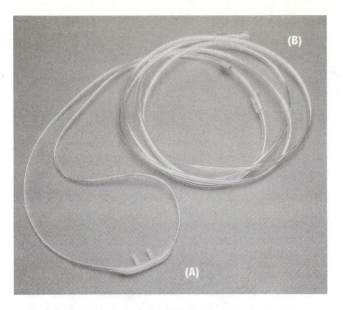

FIGURE 15-22　(A) OXYGEN CANNULA WITH (B) TUBING

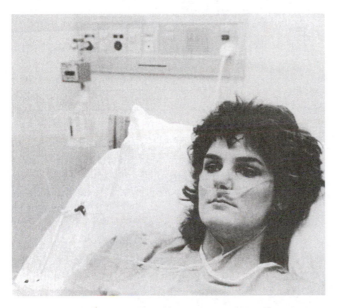

FIGURE 15-23　THE NASAL CANNULA METHOD FOR THE ADMINISTRATION OF OXYGEN

Flow rates greater than 3 to 4 liters per minute require humidification.

Mask

The common types of masks used for inhalation therapy are plastic disposable, partial rebreather, nonrebreather, and Venturi. These devices are employed when the client requires high humidity and a precise amount of oxygen. To be effective, the mask must be fitted snugly to the client.

OXYGEN SAFETY PRECAUTIONS

- Oxygen supports combustion. Thus, there is the danger of a fire being started when oxygen is in use. Extreme caution should be exercised, because ignition can be caused by friction, static electricity, or a lighted cigar or cigarette. When O_2 is being administered, an **OXYGEN IN USE—NO SMOKING** sign should be clearly displayed at the door of the room, and above the client's bed.

- Electrical appliances, such as heating pads, blankets, razors, or other electrical devices should not be used while O_2 is being administered.

- One should use suction machines, x-ray and EKG equipment, and monitors with caution while administering oxygen.

- Check the client's room for safety before initiating O_2 therapy. When possible, replace electrical devices with nonelectric units.

- Explain safety measures to the client, to his or her roommate, and to visitors.

ADMINISTERING DRUGS BY LOCAL APPLICATION

Ointments, lotions, liniments, wet medicated dressings, poultices, and plasters are all applied directly to the skin. Drugs commonly used for local application to the mucous membranes of body cavities are administered by irrigation, instillation, and insertion into body openings.

Application to the Skin

Ointments are applied directly to the skin, or they may be applied as a dressing by spreading the medication on a piece of gauze. When the drug is applied by rubbing it onto the skin, the method is called **inunction**. Ointments may be used to relieve irritations and to treat various skin diseases. Zinc oxide is an example of an ointment used for local application.

Lotions are drugs that are swabbed onto the skin for antiseptic and/or astringent effects. Itching, dryness, and irritations caused by inflammation and diseases of the skin are relieved. Calamine lotion is an example of such a drug.

Liniments are drugs that usually have a counterirritant effect. They are applied by vigorously rubbing them onto the skin of the affected area to relieve soreness in muscles and joints. The psychological effect of massage is an important factor in the application of liniments. Camphor liniment and chloroform liniment are examples.

- Avoid excessive rubbing of counterirritant drugs into skin, as blistering may result.

- When applying ointments and lotions to infected areas, use extreme care not to aggravate the infection. Apply medication as directed. Use disposable gloves to avoid danger of infection to oneself, or if the drug may produce allergic reactions.

Medicated or wet dressings may be used for local treatment of skin disorders; they are gauze sponges, saturated with a drug in solution. The drug may act as an antiseptic or an astringent. Neomycin is an example of a drug that can be prepared as a solution and used as an antiseptic for local application.

> **Safety Precaution:** When medicated wet dressings are applied, the dressings must be changed frequently in order to produce the maximum desired effect.

Application to Body Cavities

Medications are applied to various body cavities to treat inflammation and infection in three ways: (1) **irrigation**, a flushing of the mucous lining with a solution for the purpose of removing secretions and soothing the tissues; (2) **instillation**, the introduction of a drug, usually in liquid form, into a body cavity (eye, ear, nose) for temporary retention; and (3) **insertion**, the placement of a suppository into the rectum or vaginal cavity, or a tablet into the mouth, vagina, or rectum.

Open cavities often treated by irrigation include the nose, mouth, ear, throat, vagina, and rectum. Normal saline and water is a commonly used solution for irrigations of the ear, nose, and throat. Other irrigations (douches) and installations require special strengths of solutions and medications.

The temperature of all irrigations and douches must be moderate, about 39°C to 40°C (102.2°F to 104°F), to avoid burning the client.

Drugs may be inserted rectally or vaginally if a client is likely to become nauseated by oral intake, or if the client is extremely ill or unconscious. Drugs are also given by this method when the physician desires to promote a sustained local action.

● SELF-ASSESSMENT

Write the answer in the space provided or circle true or false as instructed.

Source

p. 122 **1.** Taking a medication by mouth does not always mean that the substance is swallowed. When nitroglycerin tablets are used, the route for this type of oral medication is said to be _____ .

p. 122 **2.** The amount of medication in the average dose for adults and children is based upon the _____ and _____ of the individual.

p. 130 **3.** True or False (circle one) Since ophthalmic medications are intended to have a local effect, the use of these agents will not cause systemic symptoms.

p. 128 **4.** At times a spoon will be used to administer an oral medication. In such cases, you would know that there are _____ milliliters in a teaspoon and _____ teaspoons in a tablespoon.

p. 131, **5.** On the lines provided, write in the three
135   forms of rectal medications given in the text.

(1) _____

(2) _____

(3) _____

p. 138 **6.** Oxygen toxicity may develop when 100 percent oxygen is breathed for a prolonged period of time. As with any other drug, oxygen toxicity will depend upon _____ , _____ , and the client's response.

p. 138 **7.** True or False (circle one) A nasal cannula can best be described as a device for holding the nostrils open in order to facilitate breathing.

p. 139 **8.** When a drug is applied by rubbing it into the skin, the method is called _____ .

p. 140 **9.** On the lines provided, write three terms that describe the methods used to administer drugs by local application to the mucous membranes of body cavities.

(1) _____

(2) _____

(3) _____

p. 140 **10.** On the lines provided, write in the two ingredients commonly used to make a solution that is used in the irrigation of the ear, nose, and throat. _____ and _____

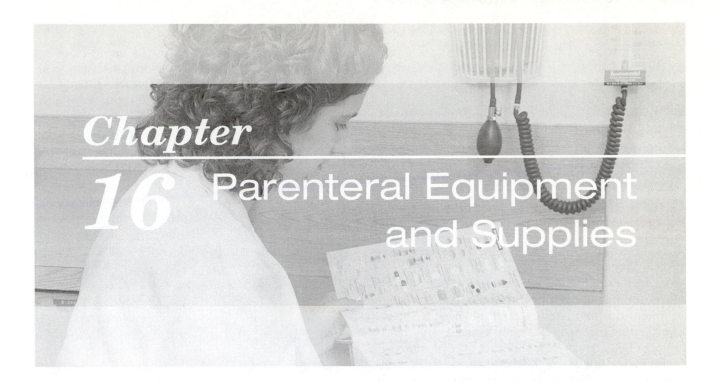

Chapter 16 — Parenteral Equipment and Supplies

Objectives

Upon completion of this chapter, you should be able to

- Define the key terms
- Describe the syringes that are most frequently used for administering parenteral medications
- Describe the component parts of a syringe
- Name the parts of a syringe that must be kept sterile during the preparation and administration of a parenteral medication
- Classify syringes as disposable, nondisposable, or as a combination of these two types
- Explain how to prevent needlestick injuries in health care settings
- Describe various safety design devices
- State the National Institute for Occupational Safety and Health's (NIOSH) recommendations for health care workers
- Give the advantages of using a disposable syringe
- Measure medication in a syringe
- Correctly read the calibrated scales of a 3 cc, 5 cc, Tuberculin, and U-100 insulin syringe
- Describe the component parts of a needle
- Select an appropriate-sized needle and syringe for the following types of injections: intramuscular, subcutaneous, intradermal, and intravenous
- Name the disease commonly transmitted by a contaminated needle/syringe
- Describe how to safely dispose of used needles and syringes
- Demonstrate the procedure for
  — handling a sterile syringe-needle unit
  — loading and unloading a Tubex® Injector
  — removing medication from a vial
  — removing medication from an ampule
  — mixing two medications in one syringe
  — reconstituting a powder medication for administration
- Complete the Self-Assessment

Key Terms

barrel	lumen
bevel	plunger
flange	point
gauge	shaft
hilt	tip
hub	

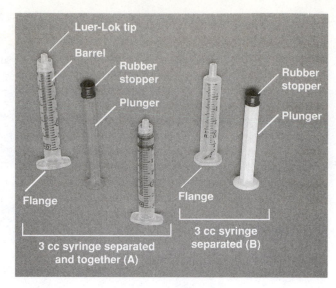

FIGURE 16-1   PARTS OF A SYRINGE

INTRODUCTION

As a nurse or health professional, it may be your responsibility to administer medications by the parenteral route. Thus, you should be familiar with the various types of syringes and needles. A syringe-needle unit is an instrument that is used to inject a liquid substance into the body tissue, vein, artery, joint, or body cavity of a client. It may also be used to remove fluid from the body (aspiration, venipuncture). A syringe alone is used to perform an irrigation (wounds, eyes, and ears) or to administer certain oral medications.

PARTS OF A SYRINGE

The component parts of a syringe consist of a barrel, a plunger, the flange, and the tip. See Figure 16-1. The **barrel** is the part that holds the medication and has graduated markings (calibrations) on its surface for measuring medications. The **plunger** is a movable cylinder, designed for insertion within the barrel. When inserted, the plunger forms a tight-fitting seal against the interior walls of the

barrel and provides the mechanism by which a medication (or other substance) is drawn into or pushed out of the barrel. The **flange** is at the end of the barrel where the plunger is inserted. It forms a rim around the end of the barrel and has appendages against which one places the index and middle fingers when drawing up solution for injection. The flange also prevents the syringe from rolling when laid on a flat surface. The **tip** is the end of the barrel where the needle is attached.

The parts of a syringe that must remain sterile during the preparation and administration of a parenteral medication are the inside of the barrel, the section of the plunger that fits inside the barrel, and the syringe tip to which the needle is to be attached. See Figure 16-2.

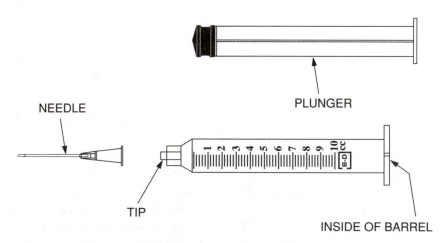

FIGURE 16-2   PARTS OF A NEEDLE AND SYRINGE THAT MUST REMAIN STERILE DURING THE PREPARATION AND ADMINISTRATION OF A MEDICATION

TABLE 16-1   THE MOST FREQUENTLY USED SYRINGES FOR PARENTERAL MEDICATIONS

Type	Size and Calibration	Typical Uses
Hypodermic	3 cc Calibrated 0.1 $\left(\frac{1}{10}\right)$ 15 or 16 minims/cc	Intramuscular and subcutaneous injections
	5 cc Calibrated 0.2 $\left(\frac{2}{10}\right)$ Larger sizes (10 cc, 20 cc, and 60 cc)	Venipuncture, intravenous injection Medical/surgical treatment, aspirations, irrigations, venipunctures, intravenous injections, gavage (tube-to-stomach) feedings
Tuberculin	1 cc Calibrated 0.1 and 0.01 $\left(\frac{1}{10}\right)$ 16 minims/cc $\left(\frac{1}{100}\right)$	To inject minute amounts, for intradermal injections, allergy testing, allergy injections
Insulin	U-100	Insulin administration
Allergist	$\frac{1}{2}$ cc Calibrated 0.01	Allergy skin testing, allergy injections (See Figure 16-3)

CLASSIFICATION OF SYRINGES

Syringes are named according to their sizes and usages. Table 16-1 lists the types, sizes, calibrations, and uses of syringes for the administration of parenteral medications. It is to your advantage to study this table and to memorize the information it contains.

Syringes are classified as disposable, nondisposable, and as combinations of these two types. They may also be classified according to their intended use. In addition to the standard hypodermic syringes that are in general use, there are special-purpose syringes for irrigations and/or oral feedings, tuberculin syringes, insulin syringes, allergist syringes for skin testing, and safety syringes.

Disposable Syringes

Disposable syringes are sterilized, prepackaged, nontoxic, nonpyrogenic, and ready for use. They are available separately or as a syringe-needle unit and are generally enclosed in individual peel-apart packages of durable paper or clear plastic. They are available in sizes from $\frac{1}{2}$ cubic centimeter to 60 cubic centimeters. The 1 cc, 3 cc, 5 cc, and 10 cc syringes are the ones most often used when parenteral medications are administered.

A disposable syringe-needle unit consists of a syringe with an attached needle. See Figure 16-4. The needle is covered by a hard plastic sheath to prevent it from accidentally penetrating the package or sticking the user. The unit may be sealed within a peel-apart package or encased in a rigid plastic container that has been heat sealed to insure sterility. Labeling usually includes the manu-

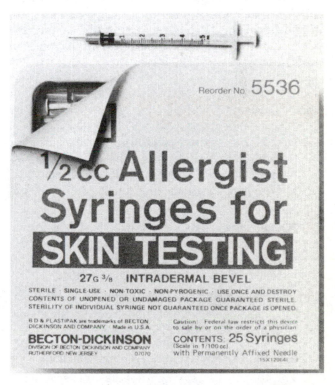

FIGURE 16-3 $\frac{1}{2}$ CC ALLERGIST SYRINGES FOR SKIN TESTING
(Courtesy of Becton, Dickinson and Company)

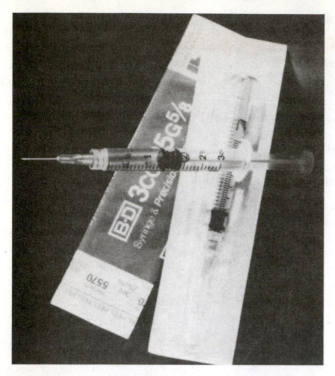

FIGURE 16-4 A DISPOSABLE SYRINGE-NEEDLE UNIT
(Courtesy of Becton, Dickinson and Company)

facturer's name, the type and size of the syringe, the gauge and length of the needle, and a reorder number. Packages are usually color coded for ease of identification. Disposable syringes are generally preferred for the administration of parenteral medications.

Advantages of Using a Disposable Syringe

1. Disposable syringe-needle units are safer for the client and the nurse. The unit is guaranteed to be sterile and the needle comes attached to the syringe, minimizing the possibility of contamination.

2. A wide range of available sizes makes it convenient for the nurse to select a syringe-needle unit that is appropriate for the correct administration of any parenteral medication.

3. The needle in a disposable unit is made of precision-sharpened stainless steel. This allows the nurse to easily penetrate the client's skin and minimizes the sense of pain that accompanies the injection of a needle into the body.

4. The disposable syringe-needle unit saves the nurse time when preparing for the administration of an injection; therefore, it saves money.

5. Once used, the unit is discarded. With correct disposal technique (explained later in this chapter) it is possible to lower the possibility of accidental transfer of diseases such as acquired immunodeficiency syndrome (AIDS) and hepatitis B.

Nondisposable Syringes

Nondisposable syringes are usually made of specially strengthened glass that is resistant to thermal shock. These units, consisting of round glass barrels with individually fitted plungers, are manufactured to exacting specifications.

Nondisposable glass syringes are available in sizes from 1 cubic centimeter to 60 cubic centimeters. These syringes are not often used for the administration of injections. They are used by physicians to perform such special procedures as paracentesis, thoracentesis, thoracotomy, and tracheotomy. They are also used for the administration of medications to clients who have a latex allergy.

Combination Disposable/ Nondisposable Cartridge-Injection Syringes

A cartridge-injection system, such as the Tubex® or Carpuject®, consists of a disposable cartridge-needle unit (Figure 16-5) and a nondisposable cartridge-holder syringe (Figure 16-6). The cartridge-needle unit is factory sealed and sterile and contains a precisely measured unit dose of medicine. The cartridge-holder syringe may be made of durable chrome-plated brass or plastic. These reusable syringes are designed for quick and safe loading and unloading of cartridge-needle units manufactured in various sizes and dosage capacities and containing a wide range of medications.

The combination disposable/nondisposable syringe system is easy to use and convenient. When using this system, be careful to read the label and compare the medication order with the label. For example, the physician orders Demerol 25 mg and the cartridge is 50 mg/cc. You would give $\frac{1}{2}$ cc and properly discard the other $\frac{1}{2}$ cc according to agency policy. You must have another person witness the disposal of the Demerol and cosign with you for the wastage.

PREVENTING NEEDLESTICK INJURIES IN HEALTH CARE SETTINGS

The National Institute for Occupational Safety and Health (NIOSH) requests assistance in preventing

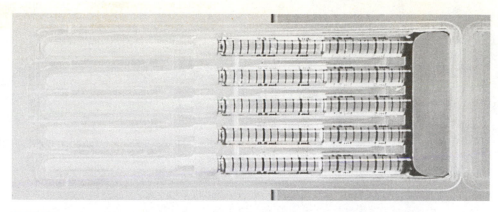

FIGURE 16-5   DISPOSABLE CARTRIDGE-NEEDLE UNITS FOR CARPUJECT *(Courtesy of Sanofi Winthrop Pharmaceuticals)*

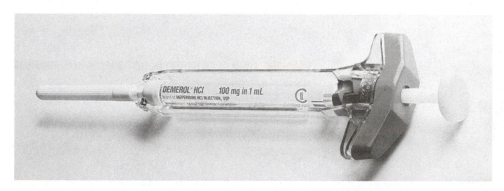

FIGURE 16-6   CARPUJECT STERILE CARTRIDGE-NEEDLE UNIT *(Courtesy of Sanofi Winthrop Pharmaceuticals)*

needlestick injuries among health care workers. These injuries are caused by needles such as hypodermic needles, blood collection needles, intravenous stylets, and needles used to connect parts of IV delivery systems. They can be avoided by eliminating the unnecessary use of needles, using devices with safety features, and promoting education and safe work practices for handling needles and related systems. These measures should be part of a comprehensive program to prevent the transmission of bloodborne pathogens.

> **Safety Precaution:** Health care workers who use or may be exposed to needles are at increased risk of needlestick injury. Such injuries can lead to serious or fatal infections with bloodborne pathogens such as hepatitis B virus, hepatitis C virus, or human immunodeficiency virus (HIV).

Improved engineering controls are often among the most effective approaches to reducing occupational hazards and therefore are an important element of a needlestick prevention program. Such controls include eliminating the unnecessary use of needles and implementing devices with safety features.

Safety Device Designs

An increasing number and variety of needle devices with safety features are now available. Examples of safety device designs are

- Needleless connectors for IV delivery systems (blunt cannula for use with prepierced ports and valved connectors that accept tapered or Luer ends of IV tubing)
- Protected needle IV connectors (the IV connector needle is permanently recessed in a rigid plastic housing that fits over IV ports)
- Needles that retract into a syringe or vacuum tube holder
- Hinged or sliding shield attached to phlebotomy needles, winged-steel needles, and blood gas needles

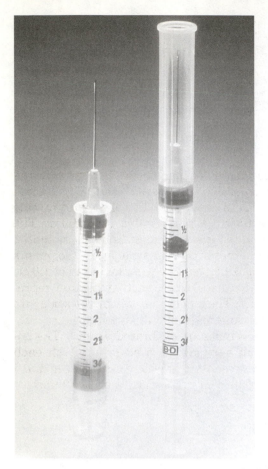

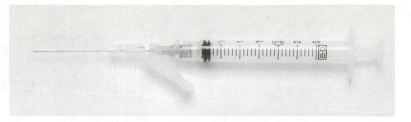

FIGURE 16-8 BD SAFETY GLIDE™ SHIELDING HYPODERMIC NEEDLE—CLOSED
(Courtesy of Becton, Dickinson and Company)

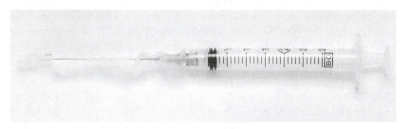

FIGURE 16-9 BD SAFETY GLIDE™ SHIELDING HYPODERMIC NEEDLE—OPEN
(Courtesy of Becton, Dickinson and Company)

FIGURE 16-7 BD SAFETY-LOK™ SLIDING SLEEVE SYRINGE
(Courtesy of Becton, Dickinson and Company)

- Protective encasements to receive an IV stylet as it is withdrawn from the catheter
- Sliding needle shields attached to disposable syringes and vacuum tube holder
- Self-blunting phlebotomy and winged-steel needles (a blunt cannula seated inside the phlebotomy needle is advanced beyond the needle tip before the needle is withdrawn from the vein)
- Retractable finger/heel-stick lancets

See Figures 16-7, 16-8, and 16-9 for examples of safety syringes.

NIOSH's Recommendations for Health Care Workers

Health care workers must be aware of the hazards posed by needlestick injuries and should use safety devices and improved work practices as follows:

- Avoid use of needles where safe and effective alternatives are available.

- Help your employer select and evaluate devices with safety features.
- Use devices with safety features provided by your employer.
- Avoid recapping needles.
- Plan safe handling and disposal before beginning any procedure using needles.
- Dispose of used needle devices promptly in appropriate sharps container.
- Report all needlestick and other sharps-related injuries promptly to insure that you receive appropriate follow-up care.
- Tell your employer about hazards from needles you observe in your work environment.
- Participate in bloodborne pathogen training and follow recommended infection prevention practices, including hepatitis B vaccination.

> **Note:** For additional information about needlestick injuries, call 1-800-356-4674 or visit the NIOSH Web site at www.cdc.gov/niosh.

MEASURING MEDICATION IN A SYRINGE

In order to precisely measure an ordered dose of medication for parenteral administration, you must know how the various syringes used for such therapy are calibrated.

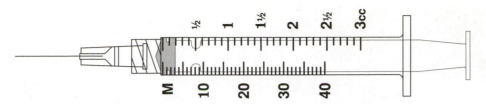

FIGURE 16-10   A 3 CC SYRINGE-NEEDLE UNIT

The 3 cubic centimeter syringe has both a metric (cc) scale and an apothecaries' minim (♏) scale on opposite sides of its barrel. See Figure 16-10. Each small calibration line of the metric scale represents 0.1 ($\frac{1}{10}$) of a cc. The longer graduated lines represent $\frac{1}{2}$, 1, 1$\frac{1}{2}$, 2, 2$\frac{1}{2}$, and 3 cc calibrations. On the apothecaries' scale, each of the small lines equals 1 minim, and the longer graduated lines represent 10, 20, 30, and 40 minim calibrations.

The 5 cubic centimeter syringe is calibrated with a single metric scale. See Figure 16-11. Each small line of this scale represents 0.2 ($\frac{2}{10}$) of a cc. The longer graduated lines represent 1, 2, 3, 4, and 5 cc calibrations. See Figure 16-11.

The tuberculin syringe has both the metric and apothecaries' scales on opposite sides of its barrel. See Figure 16-12. Each small line of the metric scale represents 0.01 ($\frac{1}{100}$) of a cubic centimeter. The longer graduated lines are used to measure tenths of a cc. These lines divide the scale into 10 segments ranging from 0.1 ($\frac{1}{10}$) of a cc to a maximum of 1.0 cc. On the apothecaries' scale, each small line represents $\frac{1}{2}$ minim. The longer lines divide the scale into graduations ranging from 2 to 16 minims.

Insulin syringes are calibrated in units. The Lo-Dose® insulin syringe has a scale in which each small line represents 1 unit, and each longer line 5 units. The scale contains a maximum of 50 units.

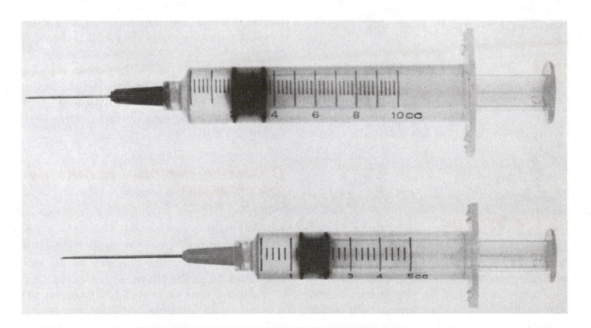

FIGURE 16-11   5 CC AND 10 CC DISPOSABLE SYRINGE-NEEDLE UNITS *(Courtesy of Becton, Dickinson and Company)*

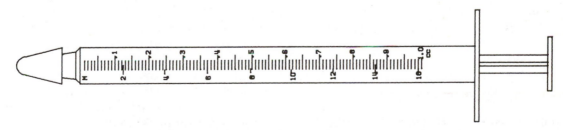

FIGURE 16-12   TUBERCULIN SYRINGE *(Courtesy of James Russell, Jr.)*

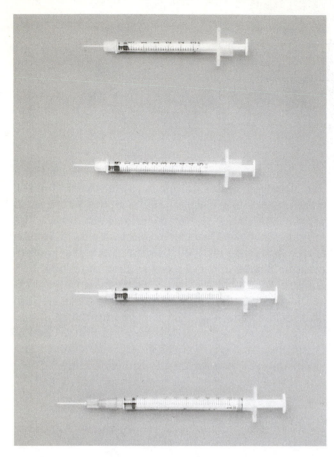

FIGURE 16-13 INSULIN SYRINGES FROM 0.3 CC TO 1 CC
(Courtesy of Becton, Dickinson and Company)

The U-100 insulin syringe has a scale in which each small line represents 2 units, and each longer line 10 units. The scale contains a maximum of 100 units. See Figure 16-13.

Reading the Syringe

The plunger in most disposable syringes has a black rubber suction tip. The slightly pointed face of this rubber tip is designed to line up with the calibrated lines of the scale imprinted on the barrel of the syringe. The back of the rubber suction tip is flat and affixes to the plunger. When reading a syringe, one reads the calibrated scale that directly lines up with the slightly pointed edge of the black rubber tip. See Figure 16-14. Make sure you can correctly read the calibrations on syringes before proceeding to needles.

HYPODERMIC NEEDLES

Both disposable and nondisposable needles are available for use with syringes. Of these, the most frequently used are disposable needles, which are individually packaged in sterile paper or plastic containers. Disposable needles and syringe-needle units are available with a color-coded sheath. The sheath protects the needle and identifies its gauge and length. Needle **gauges** (G) (scale of measurement) range from 16 to 30, and their lengths vary from $\frac{3}{8}$ inch to 2 inches. The needle's gauge is determined by the diameter of the lumen or opening at its beveled tip. The larger the gauge, the smaller the diameter of its lumen. For example, a 30-gauge needle has a much smaller diameter than a 16-gauge needle.

Nondisposable needles are made of high-quality stainless steel. They are equipped with a mounting hub that has a cylindrical opening designed to slip over and lock onto the tip of a syringe, such as a Luer-Lok®.

Parts of a Needle

Figure 16-15 shows the parts of a typical needle used to administer parenteral medications. The **point** is the sharpened end of the needle. The point is formed when the end of the shaft is ground away to form a flat, slanted surface called the **bevel**. The hollow core of the needle, when exposed at the beveled point, forms an oval-shaped opening called the **lumen**. The hollow steel tube through which the medication passes is the **shaft**. The other end of the shaft attaches to the **hub**, which is that part of the needle unit designed to mount onto the syringe. The point at which the shaft attaches to the hub is called the **hilt**.

Selecting the Appropriate Syringe and Needle

The selection of an appropriate syringe and needle for a particular parenteral use involves a number of considerations. Two of the major factors in the selection process are the medication ordered and the age and size of the client.

The amount and viscosity of the medication ordered determines the size of the syringe-needle unit to be selected. Thick, oily medications require a needle with a lumen of 21G to 16G that will permit the flow of such fluids. Thinner medications permit the use of higher gauge needles. The amount of medicine that one may inject into a single site is related to the tissue area selected. For *subcutaneous* tissue, the amount should not exceed 2 cc. Injections into the *deltoid muscle* should not be greater than 2 cc. Other *intramuscular* injections should not exceed 3 cc, unless it can be determined that a larger dose can be safely administered.

Once the amount and consistency of the medication are determined, one must choose the correct

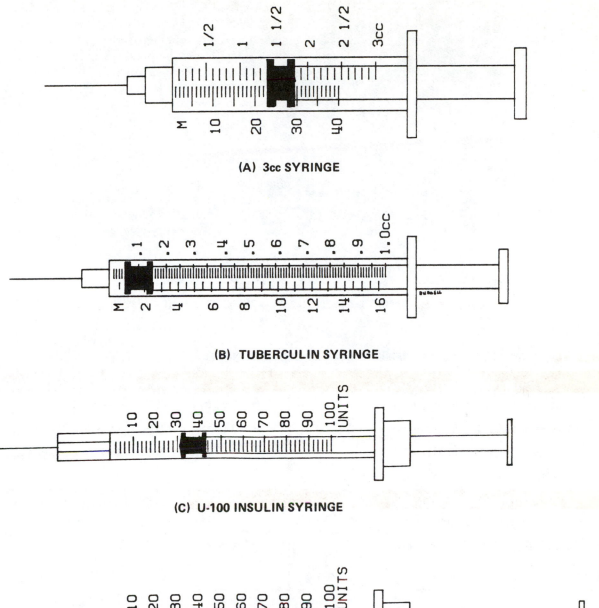

(A) 3cc SYRINGE

(B) TUBERCULIN SYRINGE

(C) U-100 INSULIN SYRINGE

(D) U-100 INSULIN SYRINGE

FIGURE 16-14   READING THE SYRINGE. WHEN READING A SYRINGE, ONE MUST READ THE CALIBRATED SCALE THAT DIRECTLY LINES UP WITH THE SLIGHTLY POINTED EDGE OF THE BLACK RUBBER TIP. (A) READ AT 1.4 CC OR 23 MINIMS. (B) READ AT 0.05 CC. (C) READ AT 32 UNITS. (D) READ AT 64 UNITS. *(Courtesy of James Russell, Jr.)*

site for the injection and the tissue layer into which it will be administered. Table 16-2 shows the syringe-needle combinations that are appropriate for their designated uses.

Another factor to be considered is the age and size of the client. The geriatric and pediatric client may have less subcutaneous or intramuscular tis-

sue per body surface area than the average adult. The size of the syringe-needle unit is related to the depth of penetration permissible in clients of differing ages and sizes.

Always choose a needle with sufficient length to reach the desired tissue level. A large person may require a longer needle to reach the correct body

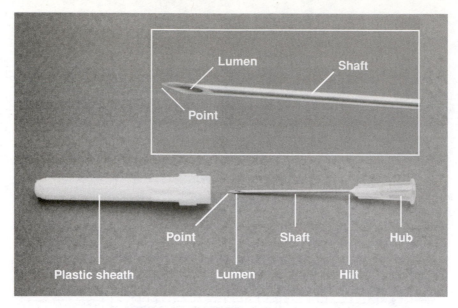

FIGURE 16-15 PARTS OF A NEEDLE USED TO ADMINISTER PARENTERAL MEDICATIONS

TABLE 16-2 SYRINGE-NEEDLE COMBINATIONS FOR VARIOUS PARENTERAL ROUTES

Subcutaneous Injection	Intramuscular Injection
3 cc syringe/25G, $\frac{5}{8}$ inch needle	3 cc syringe/23G, 1 inch needle
3 cc syringe/26G, $\frac{3}{8}$ inch needle	3 cc syringe/22G, $1\frac{1}{2}$ inch needle
3 cc syringe/27G, $\frac{1}{2}$ inch needle	3 cc syringe/21G, $1\frac{1}{2}$ inch to 2 inch needle
U-100 insulin syringe/26G, $\frac{1}{2}$ inch needle	
Intravenous Injection	**Intradermal Injection**
3 cc syringe/22G, 1 inch needle	1 cc syringe/25G, $\frac{5}{8}$ inch needle
5 cc syringe/21G, $1\frac{1}{2}$ inch needle	1 cc syringe/26G, $\frac{3}{8}$ inch needle
	1 cc syringe/27G, $\frac{1}{2}$ inch needle

tissue than would be required for a smaller person. The delivery of medication to the proper tissue level is very important. A concentrated or irritating medication that is intended for deep intramuscular injection could be delivered instead into the subcutaneous tissue of an obese client if one selects a needle that is too short. Such an inappropriate injection may cause a sterile abscess. This unnecessary complication can be avoided by considering the size of the client when choosing the length of the needle.

The Safe Disposal of Needles and Syringes

The careless disposal of used needles and syringes may present a health risk to any person coming into contact with the used equipment. An accidental stick by a contaminated needle could transmit such diseases as hepatitis B, syphilis, Rocky Mountain spotted fever, tuberculosis, malaria, varicella zoster, and acquired immunodeficiency syndrome (AIDS).

Used needles and syringes should be discarded in a rigid, puncture-proof container. Sharps collectors are made of puncture-resistant material. They are designed for infectious waste and have safety lock closures for an extra measure of safety. See Figure 16-16. A sharps collector system eliminates the need to reshield the needle, thereby reducing the risk of an accidental needlestick. Needles are placed point downward, away from the fingers. The disposable inner container is clearly marked and may be incinerated or autoclaved according to agency policy. See Figure 16-17.

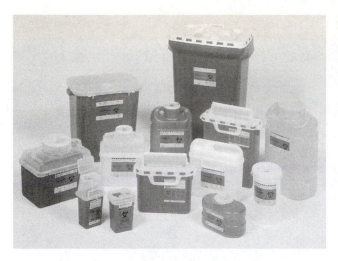

FIGURE 16-16   SHARPS COLLECTORS *(Courtesy of Becton, Dickinson and Company)*

Do not recap the needle after giving the injection. Most needlesticks occur at this time.

PREPARING EQUIPMENT AND SUPPLIES FOR AN INJECTION

An important part of giving a safe injection is preparation of the equipment and supplies. The following information covers the proper procedures to use when handling a sterile syringe-needle unit, using

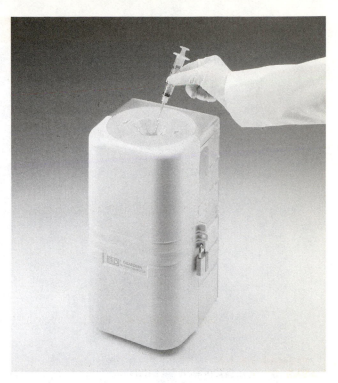

FIGURE 16-17   SHARPS COLLECTOR WITH A DISPOSABLE INNER CONTAINER *(Courtesy of Becton, Dickinson and Company)*

the Tubex Injector, withdrawing medication from a vial and an ampule, mixing two medications in one syringe, and reconstituting a powder medication for administration.

PROCEDURE 16-1

Handling a Sterile Syringe-Needle Unit—Disposable Peel-Back Method

STANDARD PRECAUTIONS:

PURPOSE:

To correctly use a sterile syringe-needle unit—disposable peel-back method

EQUIPMENT/SUPPLIES:

Appropriate syringe-needle package

Disposable gloves

Sharps container

PROCEDURE STEPS:

1. Verify the physician's order.
2. Work in a well-lighted, quiet, clean area.
3. Perform medical asepsis handwash. See Figure 16-18.
4. Put on gloves.
5. Obtain a disposable peel-back package containing a sterile syringe-needle unit.
6. Check the package label to be sure that you have selected the correct size syringe-needle unit for the ordered injection. See Figure 16-19.
7. With the label facing you, open the package by slowly peeling down the outer covering until the plunger and barrel are in view.

(continued)

PROCEDURE 16-1

Handling a Sterile Syringe-Needle Unit—Disposable Peel-Back Method (*continued*)

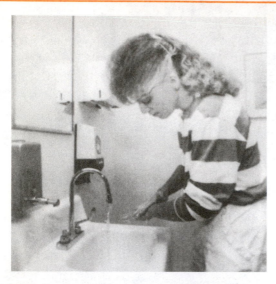

FIGURE 16-18 THE NURSE PERFORMS MEDICAL ASEPSIS HANDWASH.

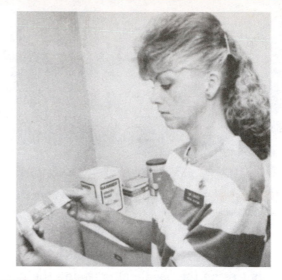

FIGURE 16-19 THE NURSE CHECKS THE SYRINGE-NEEDLE PACKAGE LABEL.

8. Remove the unit from the package by touching only the outside of the barrel.

9. Hold the outside of the barrel between the thumb and index finger with the sheathed needle pointing upward.

10. Use your other hand (thumb and index finger) to touch the end of the plunger. Pull back on the flat end of the plunger to loosen it. Once loosened, push the plunger back to its original position in the barrel of the syringe. Do not touch the plunger's stem as this could contaminate the inside of the syringe.

11. Assure yourself that the needle is firmly attached to the syringe tip by using a clockwise motion to turn the hub of the needle on the syringe tip. Do not turn the hub counterclockwise as this will remove the needle from the syringe.

12. Using your thumb and index finger, loosen the sheath that protects the needle. Once

loosened at the hub, turn the sheath counterclockwise, touching only that part of the sheath that is directly over the hub. Gently loosen the sheath by rocking it from side to side.

13. Remove the sheath using your thumb and index finger to slowly and carefully pull the sheath away from the hub of the needle.

14. To replace the sheath on a needle (that has not been inserted into a client), lay the sheath on a clean surface, being sure that the end into which the needle is going to slide has not come in contact with any surface. Carefully guide the needle into the sheath. Be sure that the needle does not touch the interior of the sheath.

15. Remove gloves and dispose in biohazard waste container.

16. Wash hands.

PROCEDURE 16-2

Loading and Unloading a Tubex® Injector

STANDARD PRECAUTIONS:

PURPOSE:

To correctly use a Tubex® Injector (Figure 16-20)

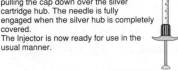

4. Engage the needle-cap assembly by pulling the cap down over the silver cartridge hub. The needle is fully engaged when the silver hub is completely covered.
The Injector is now ready for use in the usual manner.

TUBEX® Injector
NOTE: The TUBEX® Injector is reusable: do not discard.
DIRECTIONS FOR USE:

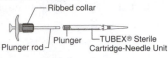
— Ribbed collar
Plunger rod — Plunger — TUBEX® Sterile Cartridge-Needle Unit

To load a TUBEX® Sterile Cartridge-Needle Unit into the TUBEX® Injector

1. Turn the ribbed collar to the "OPEN" position until it stops.

Close   Open

2. Hold the Injector with the open end up and fully insert the TUBEX® Sterile Cartridge-Needle Unit.

Close

Firmly tighten the ribbed collar in the direction of the "CLOSE" arrow.

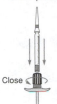

3. Thread the plunger rod into the plunger of the TUBEX® Sterile Cartridge-Needle Unit until slight resistance is felt.

The Injector is now ready for use in the usual manner.

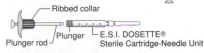
— Ribbed collar
Plunger rod — Plunger — E.S.I. DOSETTE® Sterile Cartridge-Needle Unit

To load an E.S.I. DOSETTE® Sterile Cartridge-Needle Unit into the TUBEX® Injector

Close   Open

1. Turn the ribbed collar to the "OPEN" position until it stops.

2. Hold the Injector with the open end up and fully insert the E.S.I. DOSETTE® Sterile Cartridge-Needle Unit.

Close

Firmly tighten the ribbed collar in the direction of the "CLOSE" arrow.

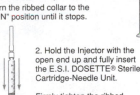

3. Thread the plunger rod into the plunger of the E.S.I. DOSETTE® Sterile Cartridge-Needle Unit until slight resistance is felt.

To administer
Method of administration is the same as with conventional syringe. Remove needle cover by grasping it securely; twist and pull. Introduce needle into client, aspirate by pulling back slightly on the plunger, and inject.

To remove the empty TUBEX® or DOSETTE® Cartridge-Needle Unit and dispose into a vertical needle disposal container

1. Do not recap the needle. Disengage the plunger rod.

2. Hold the Injector, needle down, over a vertical needle disposal container and loosen the ribbed collar. TUBEX® or DOSETTE® Cartridge-Needle Unit will drop into the container.

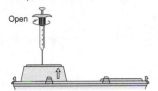
Open

3. Discard the needle cover.

To remove the empty TUBEX® or DOSETTE® Cartridge-Needle Unit and dispose into a horizontal (mailbox) needle disposal container

1. Do not recap the needle. Disengage the plunger rod.

2. Open the horizontal (mailbox) needle disposal container. Insert TUBEX® or DOSETTE® Cartridge-Needle Unit, needle pointing down, halfway into container. Close the container lid on cartridge. Loosen ribbed collar; TUBEX® or DOSETTE® Cartridge-Needle Unit will drop into the container.

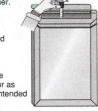

3. Discard the needle cover.

The TUBEX® Injector is reusable and should not be discarded.

Used TUBEX® or DOSETTE® Cartridge-Needle Units should not be employed for successive injections or as multiple dose containers. They are intended to be used only once and discarded.

NOTE: Any graduated markings on TUBEX® or DOSETTE® Sterile Cartridge-Needle Units are to be used only as a guide in mixing, withdrawing, or administering measured doses.

Wyeth-Ayerst does not recommend and will not accept responsibility for the use of any cartridge-needle units other than TUBEX® or E.S.I. DOSETTE® Cartridge-Needle Units in the TUBEX® Injector.

FIGURE 16-20   USING THE TUBEX® INJECTOR. SEE ALSO FIGURE 16-21 FOR DIRECTIONS FOR USE.
(Courtesy of Wyeth Laboratories, Philadelphia, Pennsylvania)

(continued)

PROCEDURE 16-2

Loading and Unloading a Tubex® Injector (*continued*)

EQUIPMENT/SUPPLIES:

Tubex® Injector

Disposable gloves

Sharps container

PROCEDURE STEPS:

1. Verify the physician's order.

2. Work in a well-lighted, quiet, clean area.

3. Perform medical asepsis handwash. Put on gloves.

4. Obtain a Tubex Injector and sterile cartridge-needle unit (Figure 16-21A).

5. Turn the ribbed collar to the "OPEN" position until it stops (Figure 16-21B)

6. Hold the Injector with the open end up, and insert the Tubex sterile cartridge-needle unit (Figure 16-21C)

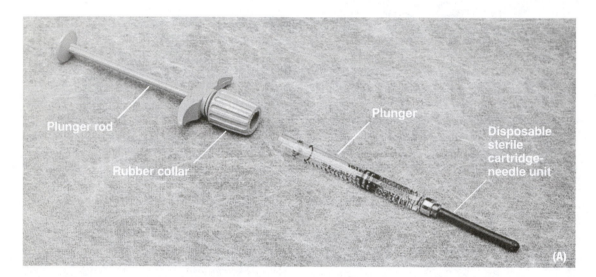

Plunger rod

Rubber collar

Plunger

Disposable sterile cartridge-needle unit

(A)

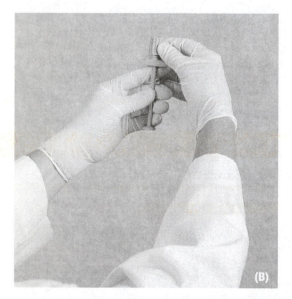

(B)

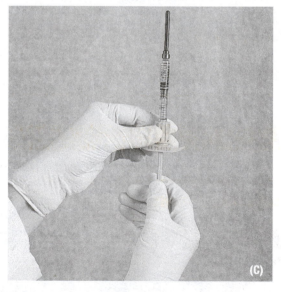

(C)

FIGURE 16-21 (A) TUBEX® INJECTOR. REUSABLE CARTRIDGE HOLDER WITH DISPOSABLE STERILE CARTRIDGE-NEEDLE UNIT. (B) TURN RIBBED COLLAR TO OPEN POSITION. (C) INSERT THE STERILE CARTRIDGE-NEEDLE UNIT INTO THE OPEN END OF THE INJECTOR. THE RIBBED COLLAR IS FIRMLY TIGHTENED. THE PLUNGER OF THE INJECTOR AND THE PLUNGER OF THE CARTRIDGE-NEEDLE UNIT ARE TIGHTENED AND READY FOR USE.

PROCEDURE 16-2

Loading and Unloading a Tubex® Injector (*continued*)

7. Tighten the ribbed collar in the direction of the "CLOSE" arrow.

8. Thread the plunger rod into the plunger of the Tubex sterile cartridge-needle unit until slight resistance is felt.

9. After use, do not recap the needle (Figure 16-21D).

10. Disengage the plunger rod.

11. Hold the Injector, needle down, over a **sharps container** and loosen the ribbed collar (Figure 16-21E).

12. Discard the needle cover.

13. Remove gloves and dispose in **biohazard waste container.**

14. Wash hands.

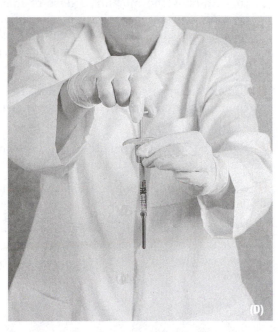
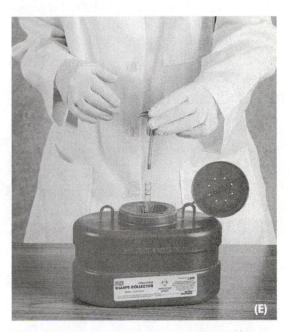

FIGURE 16-21   (D) THE NURSE PREPARES TO DISPOSE OF THE CARTRIDGE-NEEDLE UNIT. THE NEEDLE IS NOT RECAPPED. THE PLUNGER ROD IS DISENGAGED BY UNSCREWING IT. THE RIBBED COLLAR IS LOOSENED. (E) THE NURSE HOLDS THE CARTRIDGE-NEEDLE UNIT OVER A SHARPS CONTAINER AND THE UNIT DROPS INTO THE CONTAINER.

PROCEDURE 16-3

Withdrawing (Aspirating) Medication from a Vial

STANDARD PRECAUTIONS:

PURPOSE:

Medication is supplied in a variety of packaging.

Medication from a vial must be aspirated into a syringe for parenteral injection.

EQUIPMENT/SUPPLIES:

Medication order

Medicine card

Appropriate syringe and needle with **cover**

Vial of medication

Antiseptic wipes or sponges

Disposable gloves

Sharps container

(continued)

PROCEDURE 16-3

Withdrawing (Aspirating) Medication from a Vial (*continued*)

PROCEDURE STEPS:

1. Read the medication order and assemble equipment. Check for the "Six Rights." Read the vial label by holding it next to the medicine card (first time).

2. Wash hands. Apply gloves.

3. Select the proper-sized needle and syringe for the medication and the route (e.g., for subcutaneous injection of insulin, U-100 insulin syringe and 25G, $\frac{5}{8}$ inch needle). If necessary, attach the needle to the syringe.

4. Check the vial label against the medicine card (second time).

5. Remove the metal or plastic cap from the vial. If the vial has been opened previously, clean the rubber stopper by applying a disinfectant wipe in a circular motion (Figure 16-22A).

6. Remove the needle cover—pull it straight off.

7. Inject air into the vial as follows:

   a. Hold the syringe pointed upward at eye level. Pull back the plunger to take in a quantity of air that is equal to the ordered dose of medication.

   b. Hold the vial upright (inverted) according to personal preference. Take care not to touch the rubber stopper.

   c. Insert the needle through the rubber stopper of the vial. Inject the air by pushing in the plunger (Figure 16-22B).

8. Withdraw the medication: Hold the vial and the syringe steady. Pull back on the plunger to withdraw the measured dose of medication. Measure accurately. Keep the tip of the needle below the surface of the liquid; otherwise, air will enter the syringe. Keep syringe at eye level (Figure 16-22C).

9. Check the syringe for air bubbles. Remove them by tapping sharply on the syringe (Figure 16-22D).

10. Remove the needle from the vial. Replace the sterile needle cover (Figure 16-22E).

11. Check the vial label against the medicine card (third time).

12. Place the filled needle and syringe on a medicine tray or cart with an antiseptic wipe and the medicine card. The dose is now ready for injection.

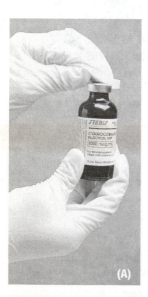
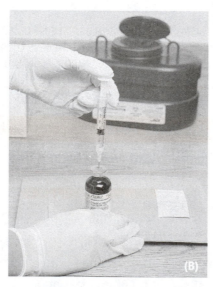
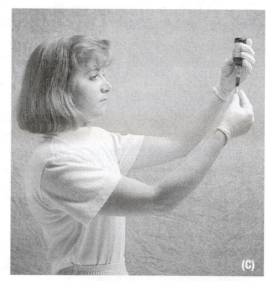

(A)   (B)   (C)

FIGURE 16-22 (A) DISINFECT THE RUBBER STOPPER ON THE MEDICATION VIAL WITH AN ALCOHOL SWAB. (B) KEEPING THE BEVEL OF THE NEEDLE ABOVE THE FLUID LEVEL, INJECT AN AMOUNT OF AIR EQUAL TO THE MEDICATION QUANTITY TO BE WITHDRAWN. (C) HOLD THE SYRINGE POINTED UPWARD AT EYE LEVEL AND WITH THE BEVEL OF THE NEEDLE IN THE MEDICATION. PULL BACK THE PLUNGER AND ASPIRATE THE QUANTITY OF MEDICATION ORDERED.

(continued)

PROCEDURE 16-3

Withdrawing (Aspirating) Medication from a Vial (*continued*)

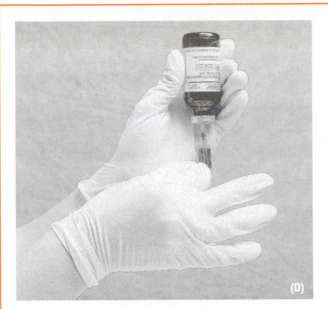
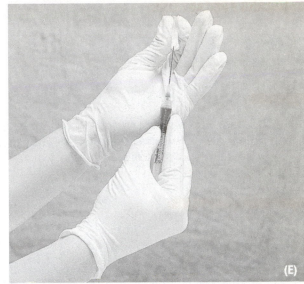

FIGURE 16-22   (D) TAP THE SYRINGE TO ELIMINATE AIR BUBBLES. HOLD THE SYRINGE WHILE TAPPING IT. (E) AFTER THE CORRECT DOSE HAS BEEN WITHDRAWN, RECOVER THE STERILE NEEDLE. PLACE MEDICATION ON A TRAY ALONG WITH A MEDICATION CARD AND AN ALCOHOL SWAB AND SAFELY TRANSPORT TO THE CLIENT.

13. Return multiple dose vial to the proper storage area (cabinet or refrigerator). Dispose of unused medication in a single dose vial according to facility procedure. (Remember, disposal of a controlled substance must be witnessed and the proper forms signed.)

14. Discard used syringe-needle unit immediately after use in a sharps container (Figure 16-23).

15. Remove gloves and dispose in biohazard waste container.

16. Wash hands.

17. Document the procedure.

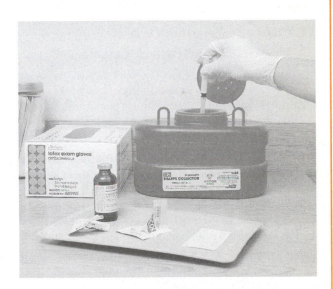

FIGURE 16-23   DISPOSE OF USED SYRINGE-NEEDLE UNIT IN SHARPS CONTAINER.

PROCEDURE 16-4

Withdrawing (Aspirating) Medication from an Ampule

STANDARD PRECAUTIONS:

PURPOSE:

Medication is supplied in a variety of packaging. An ampule is a sterile glass single dose container of liquid medication. It is aspirated into a syringe for parenteral injection.

EQUIPMENT/SUPPLIES:

Medicine tray and medicine card

Ampule of medication

Alcohol wipes

Sterile gauze sponges

Sharps container

Sterile syringe-needle unit

Disposable Gloves

PROCEDURE STEPS:

1. Check the physician's order.
2. Wash hands and gather equipment. Put on gloves.
3. Obtain ampule of medicine. Read label and check medicine card for correct medication, dose, route, and time (first time). Check medication expiration date.
4. Flick ampule of medication (medication will often get "trapped" above the neck of the ampule). A sharp flick of the wrist will help force all of the medication down below the neck of the ampule into the body of the ampule (Figure 16-24A).

   RATIONALE: This is important to insure all medication is available in the body of the ampule in order to calculate the correct dose. If some of the medication remains trapped above the neck in the top of the ampule, some medication will not be available for use and it is possible to give an incorrect dose, especially if the client is to receive the entire contents of the ampule.
5. Thoroughly disinfect the neck with an alcohol swab. Check label (second time).

RATIONALE: The needle will enter the opening of the ampule and wiping the neck of the ampule prior to removal of the top insures disinfection of the neck or opening of the ampule.

6. With a sterile gauze, wipe dry the neck of the ampule. Completely surround the ampule with the gauze and forcefully snap off the top of the ampule by pushing the top away from you (Figure 16-24B).

   RATIONALE: Insures the nurse's safety from possible injury from broken glass. Discard top in sharps container.
7. Place opened ampule down on medicine tray. Check label (third time).
8. With a prepared sterile syringe-needle unit, aspirate the required dose into the syringe (Figure 16-24C). Cover needle with sheath and transport to client on the medicine tray.

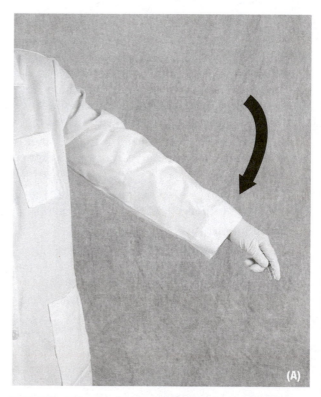

FIGURE 16-24 (A) HOLD AMPULE BY THE TOP AND FORCE ALL THE MEDICATION INTO THE BOTTOM OF THE AMPULE BY A SNAP OF THE ARM AND WRIST.

(continued)

PROCEDURE 16-4

Withdrawing (Aspirating) Medication from an Ampule (*continued*)

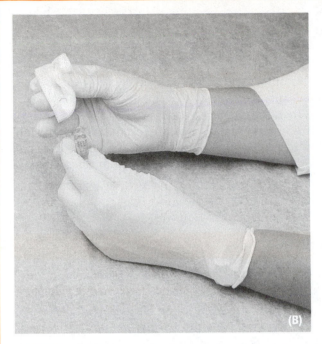 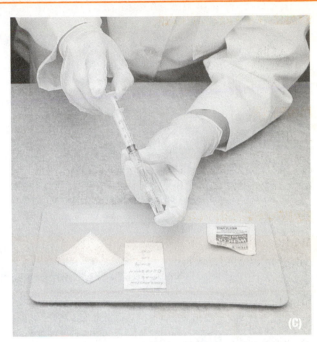

FIGURE 16-24   (B) REMOVE TOP FROM AMPULE. TURN HAND UP AND OUT SIMULTANEOUSLY. (C) ASPIRATE REQUIRED DOSE INTO SYRINGE.

9. Identify the client.
10. Administer the medication.
11. Discard syringe-needle unit into sharps container. Alcohol swabs and gauze are discarded in biohazard waste container.
12. Remove gloves and dispose in biohazard waste container.
13. Wash hands.
14. Document the procedure.

Using a Filter Straw to Remove Medication from an Ampule

A filter straw is a sterile, nonpyrogenic, nontoxic device that may be used to remove medication from an ampule and is available in a peel-open package. It is designed to filter out any small particles of glass that may enter the ampule after breakage of the stem. The filter straw is for single use.

- Compare the medication label with the physician's order.
- Inspect the ampule to see if any of the medicine is trapped in the stem. If necessary, tap the stem gently to cause the trapped medicine to return to the base.
- Cover the stem portion of the ampule with a sterile gauze.

- Exerting firm pressure over the scored portion of the stem, break off the ampule stem by pushing it away from yourself and others.
- Place the base of the ampule on a clean surface. Discard the gauze sponge that contains the broken off stem into an appropriate container.
- Prepare the syringe-needle unit for use. Remove the sheathed needle from the syringe. Place the sheathed needle on the inside of the peel-back syringe-needle wrapper. DO NOT CONTAMINATE.
- Peel open the sterile filter straw package and insert the straw tip onto the syringe tip. Check to make sure that the straw tip is firmly attached to the tip of the syringe. DO NOT CONTAMINATE.

- Slowly insert the filter straw into the opening of the ampule. Keep the tip of the straw immersed in the medication at all times.
- Fill the barrel of the syringe with the ordered amount of medication.
- Carefully remove the filter straw from the ampule.
- Pull back on the plunger of the syringe to insure that all the medication is removed from the filter straw.
- Hold the syringe unit toward the light and make sure that there are no air bubbles. If necessary, correctly remove air bubbles.
- Check to make sure that the amount of medicine in the syringe is the correct dose as ordered.

- Remove the filter straw from the syringe and discard in an appropriate container.
- Place a sterile needle onto the syringe tip.
- Prepare to give the medication to the client.

Mixing Two Medications in One Syringe-Needle Unit

When the physician orders two medications that are to be administered by injection, you may wish to mix the medications in one syringe. First, check with the pharmacist to be sure that the medications are compatible and can be safely mixed in one syringe. See Procedure 16-5.

PROCEDURE 16-5

Mixing Two Medications in One Syringe-Needle Unit

STANDARD PRECAUTIONS:

PURPOSE:

To properly mix two medications in one syringe-needle unit

EQUIPMENT/SUPPLIES:

Medications as ordered by the physician and medicine cards

Appropriately sized syringe-needle units

Sterile needles

Antiseptic wipes

Disposable gloves

Sharps container

PROCEDURE STEPS:

1. Verify the physician's order.
2. Work in a well-lighted, quiet, clean area.
3. Perform medical asepsis handwash and put on gloves.
4. Compare the medication labels with the physician's order.
5. Prepare a syringe-needle unit for use. Check to make sure that the needle is firmly attached to the tip of the syringe.

6. Draw up an amount of air into the syringe that will be equal to the amount of medication that you plan to withdraw from the vial.
7. Cleanse the rubber-stoppered portion of the vial with an antiseptic swab.
8. Place the syringe-needle unit in your dominant hand. Remove the sheath from the needle.
9. Pick up the vial in the other hand. Invert the vial, holding it between your thumb and index finger.
10. With the bevel of the needle toward you, smoothly insert the needle straight into the rubber-stoppered portion of the inverted vial at a 90° angle.
11. Slowly inject the equal amount of air from the barrel of the syringe into the vial.
12. Keeping the needle immersed in the solution, fill the barrel with the ordered amount of medication. Be sure that you do not have any dead air space left in the barrel before you remove the needle from the vial.
13. To remove the needle from the vial, pull the vial away from the needle.
14. Replace the sheath over the needle and secure it to the hub.
15. Hold the syringe-needle unit toward the light and check for air bubbles. If necessary, remove any air bubbles before proceeding to the next step. You must make sure that you have

(continued)

PROCEDURE 16-5

Mixing Two Medications in One Syringe-Needle Unit (*continued*)

the exact amount of ordered medication left in the syringe before removing the ordered medication from the second vial or ampule.

16. Place the above described syringe-needle unit on the medication tray or a clean, dry surface.

17. Compare the second medication label with the physician's order.

18. Open a sterile needle package and prepare to change needles.

19. Remove the needle from the filled syringe. Set the needle aside.

20. Correctly place the opened sterile needle onto the filled syringe.

21. Cleanse the rubber-stoppered portion of the second vial with an antiseptic swab.

22. Place the syringe-needle unit in your dominant hand. Remove the sheath from the needle.

23. Pick up the second vial in the other hand. Invert the vial, holding it between your thumb and index finger.

24. With the bevel of the needle toward you, smoothly insert the needle straight into the rubber-stoppered portion of the inverted vial at a 90° angle.

25. You will not inject air into this vial.

26. Keeping the needle immersed in the solution, fill the barrel with the ordered amount of medication.

27. To remove the needle from the vial, pull the vial away from the needle.

28. Replace the sheath over the needle and secure it to the hub.

29. Hold the syringe-needle unit toward the light and check for air bubbles. If you have air bubbles and have to inject any of the medications that are in the syringe, you will have to discard the filled syringe and start all over.

30. Check to be sure that the total amount of medications in the syringe is the correct total of doses as ordered.

31. Prepare to administer the medication to the client.

PROCEDURE 16-6

Reconstituting a Powder Medication for Administration

STANDARD PRECAUTIONS:

PURPOSE:

Drugs for injection may be supplied in a powdered (dry) form and must be reconstituted to a liquid for injection. A diluent (usually sterile saline) is added to the powder, mixed well, and the appropriate dose drawn up to be administered.

EQUIPMENT/SUPPLIES:

Medication as ordered by the physician and medicine card

Diluent

2 appropriately sized syringe-needle units

Antiseptic swabs

Disposable gloves

Sharps container

PROCEDURE STEPS:

1. Wash hands.

2. Prepare the syringe-needle unit in preparation for reconstituting powder medication (Figure 16-25A).

3. Remove tops from diluent and powder medication containers and wipe with alcohol swabs (Figure 16-25B).

4. Insert the needle of a sterile syringe-needle unit through the rubber stopper on the vial of diluent that has been cleansed with an antiseptic swab. The syringe-needle unit should

(continued)

Reconstituting a Powder Medication for Administration (*continued*)

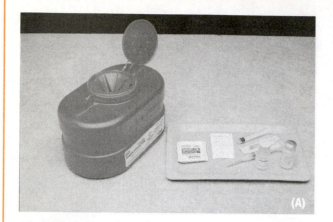
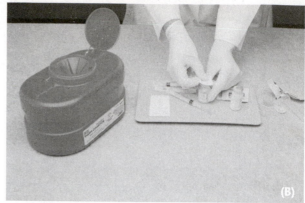
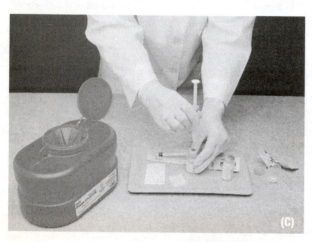
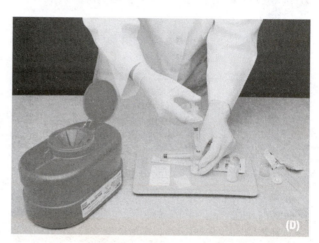

FIGURE 16-25 (A) SUPPLIES FOR RECONSTITUTING POWDER MEDICATION. (B) REMOVE TOPS FROM DILUENT AND POWDERED MEDICATION. WIPE TOP OF EACH WITH AN ALCOHOL SWAB. (C) PREPARE TO INJECT AIR IN AN EQUAL AMOUNT TO DILUENT BEING REMOVED FROM THE VIAL. (D) INJECT AIR INTO THE VIAL.

have an amount of air in it equal to the amount of diluent to be withdrawn (Figures 16-25 C and D).

5. Withdraw the appropriate amount of diluent to be added to the power medication (Figure 16-25 E and F). Cover the sterile needle on the syringe containing appropriate amount of diluent.

6. Add this liquid to the power medication that has been cleansed with an antiseptic swab (Figure 16-25G).

7. Remove needle and syringe from vial with powder medication and diluent and discard into sharps container (Figure 16-25H).

8. Roll the vial between the palms of the hands to completely mix together the powder and diluent (Figure 16-25I). Label the multiple dose vial with the dilution or strength of the medication prepared, the date and time, your initials, and the expiration date.

9. With a second sterile syringe and needle, withdraw the desired amount of medication (Figure 16-25J).

10. Flick away any air bubbles that cling to side of syringe (Figure 16-25K).

11. The medicine tray with reconstituted medication is ready for transport to the client (Figure 16-25L).

(continued)

PROCEDURE 16-6

Reconstituting a Powder Medication for Administration (*continued*)

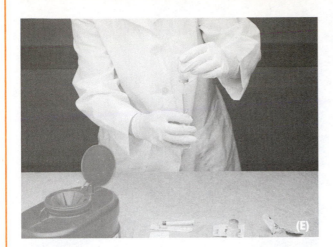

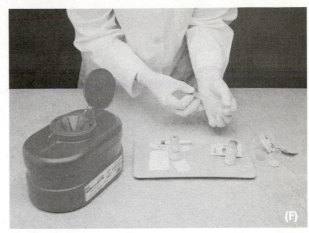

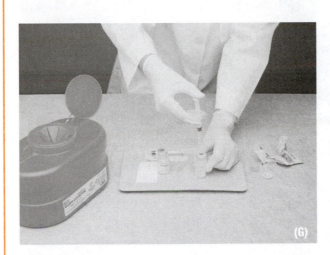

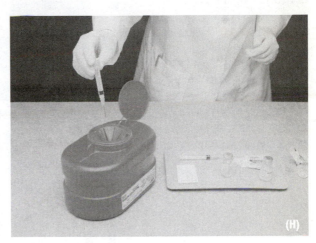

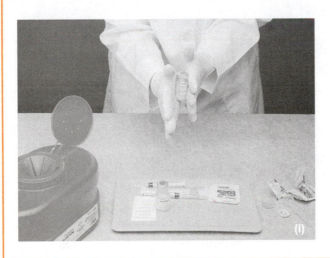

FIGURE 16-25   (E) PREPARE TO SEPARATE VIAL FROM SYRINGE-NEEDLE UNIT AFTER WITHDRAWING DILUENT. (F) COVER THE STERILE NEEDLE ON THE SYRINGE CONTAINING DILUENT. (G) INJECT DILUENT INTO VIAL CONTAINING POWDERED MEDICATION. BEFORE INJECTING, TOP OF VIAL SHOULD BE CLEANSED AGAIN WITH AN ALCOHOL SWAB. (H) DISCARD SYRINGE-NEEDLE UNIT AFTER MIXING. (I) ROLL VIAL OF POWDERED MEDICATION WITH DILUENT BETWEEN PALMS OF HANDS TO MIX WELL. LABEL VIAL WITH DATE, AMOUNT OF DILUENT ADDED, STRENGTH OF DILUTION, TIME MIXED, YOUR INITIALS, AND EXPIRATION DATE.

(continued)

PROCEDURE 16-6

Reconstituting a Powder Medication for Administration (*continued*)

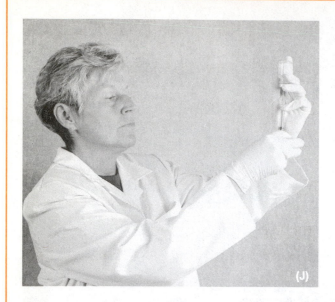

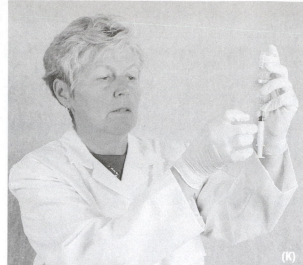

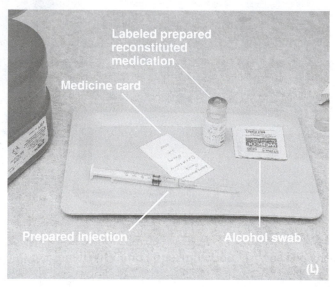

FIGURE 16-25 (J) USE A SECOND STERILE SYRINGE-NEEDLE UNIT TO DRAW UP THE PRESCRIBED DOSE OF MEDICATION ORDERED BY THE PHYSICIAN. (K) FLICK AWAY ANY AIR BUBBLES THAT CLING TO THE SIDE OF THE SYRINGE. (L) MEDICINE TRAY SHOWS PREPARED INJECTION READY FOR TRANSPORT TO CLIENT. LABELED, RECONSTITUTED MEDICATION WILL BE PLACED ON THE SHELF OR IN THE REFRIGERATOR ACCORDING TO THE MANUFACTURER'S INSTRUCTIONS.

Labeled prepared reconstituted medication

Medicine card

Prepared injection

Alcohol swab

● SELF-ASSESSMENT

Write the answer in the space provided or circle true or false as instructed.

Source

p. 142 **1.** During the preparation and administration of a parenteral medication, the following three parts of a syringe must remain sterile: (1) _____ (2) _____ (3) _____

p. 143 **2.** Table 16-1 lists four types of syringes. In addition to the standard hypodermic syringe, what are the remaining three special-purpose types? (1) _____ (2) _____ (3) _____

p. 143 **3.** The 1 cc, _____, _____, and _____ sizes of disposable syringe-needle units are the ones most often used when parenteral medications are administered.

p. 144 **4.** Nondisposable glass syringes are not often used to inject medications; however, they can become the syringe of choice for those clients who have _____.

p. 144 **5.** True or False (circle one) The physician orders Demerol 25 mg. Your equipment is a combination disposable/nondisposable syringe system and a Demerol 50 mg/cc cartridge-needle unit. You would give $\frac{1}{2}$ cc and properly discard the remaining $\frac{1}{2}$ cc according to agency policy.

p. 147 **6.** On the U-100 insulin syringe, each small line represents _____ and each long line is a measure of _____.

p. 148 **7.** You are about to administer an injection and must choose between a 16-gauge needle and a 30-gauge needle. Needle gauge is determined by the diameter of its lumen (opening at the beveled tip). Which needle has the smaller diameter? _____

p. 148 **8.** True or False (circle one) The amount and viscosity of the medication ordered determines the size of the syringe-needle unit to be selected. You would choose among the highest-gauged needles for use with a thick, oily medication.

p. 151 **9.** True or False (circle one) As a safety precaution, you should always replace the sheath over the needle after administering an injection and before disposal in a rigid, puncture-proof container.

p. 139 **10.** After breaking open the stem of an ampule, what equipment may you use in combination with your syringe-needle unit to remove the medication? _____

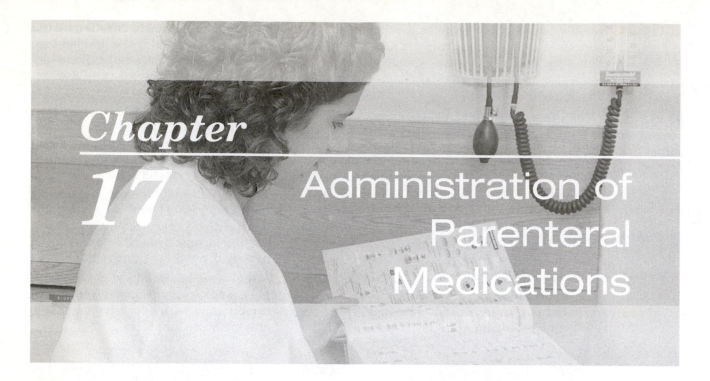

Chapter 17

Administration of Parenteral Medications

Chapter Outline

Objectives

Upon completion of this chapter, you should be able to

- Define the key terms
- Give five advantages of the parenteral route of drug administration
- Give eight disadvantages (possible dangers and complications) associated with the administration of parenteral medications
- List the basic guidelines for administering an injection
- Explain why it is important to do a client assessment prior to the administration of an injection
- Select the correct sites for a subcutaneous, an intramuscular, and an intradermal injection
- Mark the correct site for an intramuscular injection
- Prepare a client for an injection
- Demonstrate the proper procedure to be used when giving a subcutaneous, an intramuscular, and an intradermal injection
- Describe the Z-track method of intramuscular injection
- Give the special considerations to be observed when administering insulin and heparin
- Complete the Self-Assessment

Key Terms

aspirate   taut

palpate   wheal

rapport

INTRODUCTION

The parenteral route of drug administration offers an effective mode of delivering medication to a client when a rapid and direct result is desired. Injected drugs are absorbed directly into the bloodstream; therefore, they manifest their medicinal effects within minutes. Absorption also depends on the client's physical state, especially his or her circulatory status, and the route of administration.

- Intravenous: produces most rapid effect
- Intramuscular: produces next most rapid effect
- Subcutaneous: produces effect slowest of all three methods

ADVANTAGES OF THE PARENTERAL ROUTE

There are certain situations in which the use of the parenteral route for the administration of medications is indicated because it offers definite advantages over other possible routes. The following are three major advantages offered by the parenteral route:

- It provides an effective route for the delivery of a drug when the client's physical or mental state would make other routes (oral, sublingual, buccal, and so forth) difficult or impossible, for example, an unconscious client.
- Drugs that are administered by injection are not altered by gastric acids, nor do they cause irritation to the client's digestive system. In that parenteral medications do not enter the digestive system, there is no possibility that the drug will be lost as a result of vomiting. For example, insulin is made of amino acids and would be digested.
- The parenteral route provides a method of delivering a precise dose to a targeted area of the body. For example, a physician may give an intra-articular injection (within the joint) or an intrathecal injection (within the spinal canal) to deliver a medication to a target area.

DISADVANTAGES OF THE PARENTERAL ROUTE

A number of complications and dangers can occur when the parenteral route is used to administer medications. It is the nurse's responsibility to know how to administer injections safely, accurately, and with proper technique. Some of the possible disadvantages of the parenteral route are:

- The client may have an allergic reaction to the injected medication. An allergic response may range from mild to severe, and could be fatal. Allergic reactions to medications can occur immediately or manifest themselves after considerable delay.
- With the introduction of the hypodermic needle and the medication (two foreign substances) into the client, there is the possibility for introduction of microorganisms. This can occur as a result of incorrect preparation of equipment and/or the use of poor technique by the nurse.
- An injection can do injury to tissue, nerves, veins, and other vessels.
- The possibility of a needle breaking off from the hilt while still in the client could result from defective equipment or improper injection technique.
- Failure to **aspirate** (to pull back on the plunger in order to ascertain that the needle is not in a blood vessel) during the injection process may cause a subcutaneous or an intramuscular medication to be given intravenously.
- A medication intended for intramuscular injection could be given into subcutaneous tissue, which could possibly cause a sterile abscess.
- The needle can strike a bone in a geriatric, pediatric, or extremely thin person, as a result of improper selection of syringe-needle unit.
- Intravenous injection can traumatize a vein and possibly cause a hematoma, phlebitis, or tissue damage.

PREPARING THE CLIENT FOR AN INJECTION

When explaining the injection procedure, you must take into account the client's age, physical and mental condition, level of understanding, any hearing or visual impairments, and differences in language spoken or understood. Select an appropriate means to communicate your procedural plan. Explain the purpose of the injection and the desired effect that it should have on the client. An informed client will usually be more cooperative, relaxed, and agreeable. See Figure 17-1.

Establish **rapport** (a feeling of trust and understanding between the client and those providing health care) with the client by being courteous and professional. Give the client the opportunity to ask questions about the procedure. When possible, allow the client to expose the intended injection site. Involving the client in the procedure generally

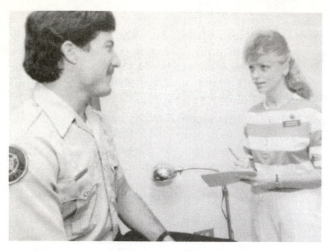

FIGURE 17-1 THE NURSE EXPLAINS THE INJECTION PROCEDURE TO THE CLIENT.

assures cooperation and relieves anxiety. Drape the client appropriately and be sure that the client is in a comfortable position. Ask the client to relax the site to be used for the injection.

When ready, inform the client that he or she will feel a slight stick or stinging sensation when the needle is inserted. Never tell a client that the injection will not hurt. This is especially true for the pediatric client and those who have received numerous injections. An injection that is given using correct technique will cause a minimum of discomfort to the client, and should only require a few seconds of time. The nurse must remember that frequently the pain stems from the medication and not the puncture of the needle.

Immediately following the administration of the injection, correctly document the procedural process that was used.

CLIENT ASSESSMENT

Before administering any medication, you must carefully assess the client's condition. Your assessment should include, but is not limited to, the following conditions:

- Age: Is the medication and route suitable for the client at a particular stage in life? During infancy, early childhood, and old age, a smaller dose of medication may be required.
- Physical condition: One must consider potential problems associated with the client's physical condition. Female clients during pregnancy or while breastfeeding should not be given certain medications. Males suffering from hemophilia

require special considerations to counter bleeding following an injection. Apply pressure for 5 to 10 minutes and make sure bleeding has stopped.

- Body size: The amount of medication given, and the size of the needle used is directly related to the size of the client. Pediatric and geriatric clients usually have less subcutaneous and/or muscular tissue per body surface area than the average adult. Small, thin clients usually require less medication, and a shorter needle may be used to reach the appropriate tissue level. On the other hand, the large or obese client may require more medication than the average adult and a longer needle to reach the appropriate tissue level.
- Sex: One must consider differences that are related to the sex of the client.
  — Muscular build: Male clients are generally more muscular than female clients. Always inspect and **palpate** (examine by means of touch) muscle tissue with this in mind when determining the appropriate needle length to reach muscle tissue.
  — Skin texture: Male clients usually have tougher skin than females. A young person's skin usually has more tone than that of an older person. Slightly more force is required to penetrate skin that is tough or lacking in tone.
- Injection site: Always inspect and palpate the skin before administering an injection. The following body areas should be avoided when choosing the site for an injection:
  — any type of skin lesion
  — burned areas
  — inflamed areas
  — previous injection sites
  — any traumatized area
  — scar tissue (vaccination, keloid)
  — moles, warts, birthmarks, tumors, lumps, hard nodules
  — nerves, large blood vessels, bones
  — cyanotic areas
  — edematous areas
  — paralyzed areas

SITE SELECTION

The selection of a proper site for a subcutaneous, intramuscular, or intradermal injection and the correct angle of insertion for each will assure that the

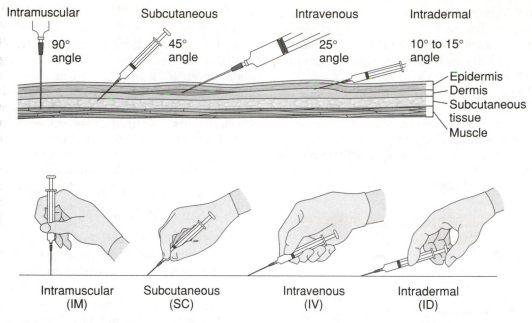

FIGURE 17-2   ANGLES OF INSERTION FOR INTRAMUSCULAR, SUBCUTANEOUS, AND INTRADERMAL INJECTION

medication is delivered to the correct tissue type. See Figure 17-2.

A *subcutaneous injection* is given at an angle of 45°, just below the surface of the skin wherever there is subcutaneous tissue. The shaded areas in Figure 17-3 are usually used for subcutaneous injections because they are located away from bones, joints, nerves, and large blood vessels.

An *intramuscular injection* is given at a 90° angle (refer again to Figure 17-2), passing through

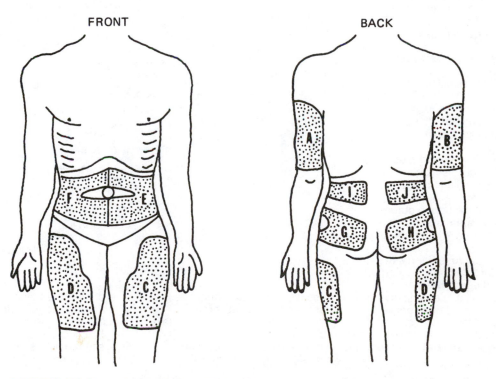

FIGURE 17-3   SUBCUTANEOUS INJECTION SITES *(Courtesy of Becton, Dickinson and Company. Adapted by James Russell, Sr.)*

the skin and subcutaneous tissue and penetrating deep into muscle tissue.

Body areas normally used for intramuscular injections are the dorsogluteal area, ventrogluteal area, deltoid muscle, and vastus lateralis.

Intradermal injections are given at an angle between 10° and 15° within the epidermal layer of skin. The body areas used for intradermal injections are the inner forearm and the middle of the back because the skin is thin and there is very little hair at these sites.

MARKING THE CORRECT SITE FOR INTRAMUSCULAR INJECTION

To give a safe injection, it is necessary that you become familiar with the anatomical structures associated with the injection site. With knowledge of where such structures are located, you will be able to mark injection sites that avoid bones, nerves, and large blood vessels.

The *dorsogluteal* is the traditional location for giving most (adult) deep intramuscular injections. See Figure 17-4. Commonly referred to as the upper outer quadrant of the buttocks, this description can be easily misinterpreted and result in an injection into an inappropriate area. To locate the correct site for a dorsogluteal injection, locate the *posterior iliac spine* and place a small X on this spot. Then, locate the *greater trochanter of the femur* and mark this spot. Draw (or imagine) a diagonal line between the two locations. The area above and outside this line, but several inches below the iliac crest, is the correct location of the dorsogluteal site.

> **Safety Precaution:** Extreme caution should be used when giving intramuscular injections in the dorsogluteal area. Improper site selection can result in damage to the sciatic nerve or injection into the superior gluteal artery or vein. This site is contraindicated for infants and is used only as a site of last resort in children. The muscle mass may be degenerated in the elderly, the nonwalking, or the emaciated client.

The *ventrogluteal site* can generally accommodate the majority of medications ordered for intramuscular injection. It may be used for individuals

- Volume of drug administered
  Usual: 1.0 ml to 4.0 ml
  Maximum   5.0 ml
- Needle size frequently used
  18G to 23G. 1¼ in. to 3 in.
  (greater length needed for very obese individuals)
- Acceptable client position
  prone
- Angle of injection
  90° angle to flat surface upon which prone client is lying
- Advantages of site
  large muscle mass accommodates deep IM/Z-track injections
  injection not visible to client
- Disadvantages of site
  boundaries of the upper, outer quadrant are often arbitrarily selected and may exceed margin of safety
  danger of injury to major nerves and vascular structures if incorrect site or technique is used
  subcutaneous fat in area is often very thick; an injection intended for muscle may in fact be subcutaneous
  should a hypersensitivity reaction occur a tourniquet cannot be applied to delay absorption
  difficult area in which to maintain proper antisepsis
  should abscesses develop, incision and drainage are complicated by proximity of large nerves and vascular structures
- Additional considerations
  IM injection using the dorsogluteal site requires strict adherence to proper anatomical site location

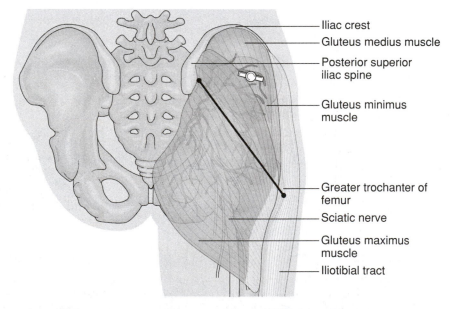

Iliac crest
Gluteus medius muscle
Posterior superior iliac spine
Gluteus minimus muscle
Greater trochanter of femur
Sciatic nerve
Gluteus maximus muscle
Iliotibial tract

FIGURE 17-4 THE DORSOGLUTEAL SITE—ADULT *(Courtesy of Wyeth Laboratories, Philadelphia, Pennsylvania)*

- Volume of drug administered
  Usual: 1.0 ml to 4.0 ml
  Maximum   5.0 ml
- Needle size frequently used
  18G to 23G. 1¼ in. to 3 in.
- Acceptable client position
  supine, lateral
- Angle of injection
  angle the needle slightly toward the
  iliac crest
- Advantages of site
  relatively free of major nerves and
  vascular branches
  well localized by bony anatomical
  landmarks
  thinner layer of subcutaneous fat
  than dorsogluteal site
  sufficient muscle mass for deep
  IM/Z-track injections
  readily accessible from several
  client positions
- Disadvantages of site
  should hypersensitivity reaction
  occur, a tourniquet cannot be
  applied to delay absorption
  health professional's unfamiliarity
  with site
- Additional considerations
  serves as alternative to
  dorsogluteal and vastus lateralis
  for deep IM/Z-track injections

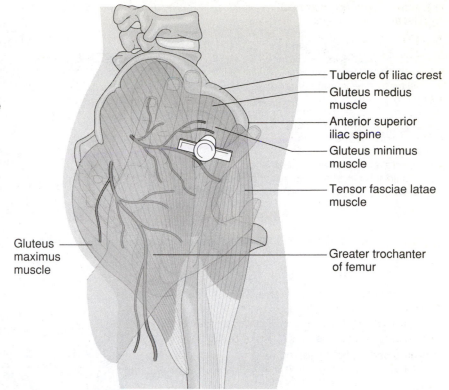

FIGURE 17-5   THE VENTROGLUTEAL SITE—ADULT *(Courtesy of Wyeth Laboratories, Philadelphia, Pennsylvania)*

from infancy to adulthood. The ventrogluteal site is relatively free of major nerves and vessels, thereby making it a choice site for IM injections. To locate the ventrogluteal injection site, palpate to find the *greater trochanter*, the *anterior superior iliac spine*, and the *bony ridge of the iliac crest*. See Figure 17-5. With these three locations identified, place the palm of your hand against the greater trochanter with the tip of your index finger on the anterior superior iliac spine. Then spread your middle finger as far from the index finger as possible. Place an X in the center of the triangle formed by the middle and index fingers to mark the correct injection site.

The *deltoid muscle* is a small but adequate site for certain intramuscular injections. These IM preparations include vaccines, narcotics, sedatives, and vitamin preparations. The site should not be used for an infant. To locate the deltoid injection site, place your fingers on the shoulder and find the *acromion* (lateral triangular projection of the spine of the scapula forming the point of the shoulder) and the *deltoid tuberosity* that lies lateral to the

side of the arm, opposite the axilla. See Figure 17-6. The correct injection site is 1 to 2 inches (about the width of three fingers) below the acromion.

> **Safety Precaution:** Do not inject medicine into the upper or lower aspects of the deltoid muscle. Care should be taken to avoid brachial and axillary nerves and blood vessels, the radial nerve, the acromion, and the humerus.

The *vastus lateralis* is the preferred site for intramuscular injections in infants and children. It is also used for IM injections in adults. This site generally accommodates the majority of IM injections ordered, and is a relatively safe site as the nerves and vessels supplying the area are not generally endangered. The vastus lateralis is a part of the quadriceps femoris muscle located on the anterolateral aspect of the thigh. The correct injection site is relative to the age of the client. For infants and children, the site lies below the greater trochanter

- Volume of drug administered
  Usual: 0.5 ml
  Maximum   2.0 ml
- Needle size frequently used
  23G to 25G. ⅝ in. to 1½ in.
- Acceptable client position
  sitting, prone, supine, lateral
- Angle of injection
  90° angle to skin surface (or angled very slightly
  upward toward acromion)
- Advantages of site
  easily accessible
  general client acceptance of site
  should a hypersensitivity reaction occur a
  tourniquet may be applied above injection site

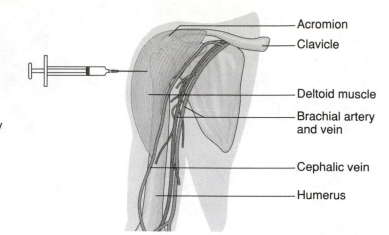

- Acromion
- Clavicle
- Deltoid muscle
- Brachial artery and vein
- Cephalic vein
- Humerus

FIGURE 17-6   THE DELTOID SITE—ADULT *(Courtesy of Wyeth Laboratories, Philadelphia, Pennsylvania)*

- Volume of drug administered
  Usual: ≤ 0.5 ml (infants);
                      1.0 ml (pediatric)
  Maximum   1.0 ml (infants);
                      2.0 ml (pediatric)
- Needle size frequently used
  22G to 25G. ⅝ in to 1 in.
- Acceptable client position
  supine, sitting
- Angle of injection
  45° angle to the frontal, sagittal,
  and horizontal planes of the thigh
  (directed toward the knee)
- Advantages of site
  relatively large muscle mass at
  birth
  suitable site for infants
  surface area provides sufficient
  space for several injections
  free of major nerves and vascular
  branches

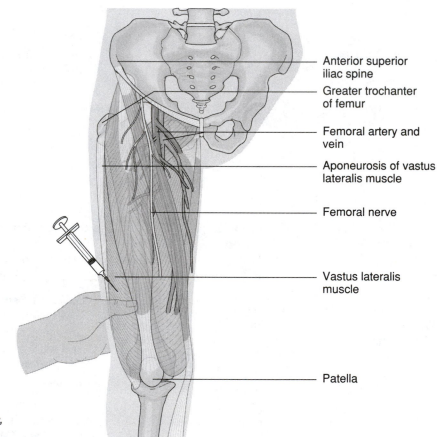

- Anterior superior iliac spine
- Greater trochanter of femur
- Femoral artery and vein
- Aponeurosis of vastus lateralis muscle
- Femoral nerve
- Vastus lateralis muscle
- Patella

FIGURE 17-7   THE VASTUS LATERALIS
SITE—PEDIATRIC *(Courtesy of Wyeth Laboratories,
Philadelphia, Pennsylvania)*

of the femur and within the upper lateral quadrant of the thigh. See Figure 17-7.

For the adult client, the correct injection site is within the middle third of the muscle. See Figure 17-8.

Safety Precaution: The muscle mass is likely to be degenerated in the elderly, the nonwalking, and in emaciated clients.

- Volume of drug administered
  Usual: 1.0 to 4 ml
  Maximum   5.0 ml
- Needle size frequently used
  20G to 23G. 1¼ in. to 1½ in.
- Acceptable client position supine, sitting
- Angle of injection
  90° angle to skin surface (for small or thin adults the technique used for pediatric injections may be preferable)
- Advantages of site
  large muscle mass can tolerate relatively large quantities of medication
  surface area provides sufficient space for several injections
  free of major nerves and vascular branches

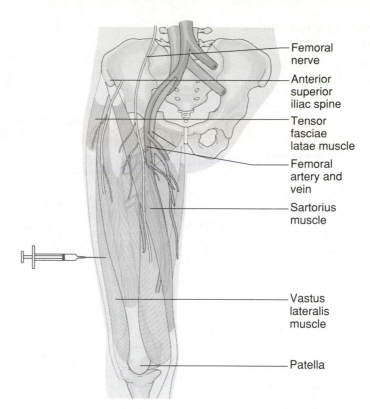

FIGURE 17-8   THE VASTUS LATERALIS SITE—ADULT *(Courtesy of Wyeth Laboratories, Philadelphia, Pennsylvania)*

BASIC GUIDELINES FOR THE ADMINISTRATION OF INJECTIONS

Regardless of the type of injection, there are basic guidelines that you must follow to safeguard the client. These guidelines are given next, according to the sequence of the events to which they relate.

1. The nurse should follow the Basic Medication Guidelines listed in Chapter 14.
2. Adhere to the "Six Rights" of proper drug administration.
3. Always evaluate each client as an individual.
4. Select a syringe-needle unit that is the appropriate size for the proper administration of a parenteral medication.
5. Correctly prepare the appropriate parenteral equipment and supplies for use. Put on gloves.
6. Select the correct site for the intended injection.
7. Prepare the client properly for the injection.
8. For subcutaneous and intramuscular injections, use a smooth, quick, dart-like motion to insert the needle into the client's skin. Use the correct angle of insertion (45° or 90°) for the injection. Once the needle is inserted, gently pull back on the plunger (aspirate) to insure that the needle

is not in a blood vessel. Do not aspirate if you are administering heparin or insulin.

> **Safety Precaution:** If blood appears in the syringe upon aspiration, smoothly withdraw the needle, properly discard the used unit, and prepare another injection for administration. Repeat the above steps.

9. Inject the medication slowly into the client.
10. With a quick, smooth motion, remove the needle from the injection site. Cover the injection site with a dry, sterile cotton swab and gently massage the site.

> **Safety Precaution:** Do not massage the site when administering insulin, iron dextran, or heparin.

11. Remove the cotton swab and check for bleeding. If bruising occurs, apply ice to the injection site. Remove gloves.
12. Observe the client for any signs of hypersensitivity.
13. Take precautions to insure the client's safety.

14. Follow documentation procedures to record the administration of the medication.

15. Properly discard the used equipment and supplies.

16. Before leaving the room, make sure that the client is given proper instructions and feels all right.

17. Correctly document the procedure.

PROCEDURE 17-1

Administration of Subcutaneous, Intramuscular, and/or Intradermal Injections

STANDARD PRECAUTIONS:

PURPOSE:

To properly administer subcutaneous, intramuscular, and/or intradermal injections

EQUIPMENT/SUPPLIES:

Medication as ordered by the physician and medicine card

Appropriately sized syringe-needle unit

Antiseptic wipes

Disposable gloves

Sharps container

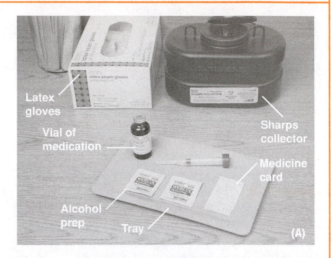

PROCEDURE STEPS:

1. Verify the physician's order. Make out medicine card, taking information from physician's order sheet from client record.

2. Follow the "Six Rights."

3. Perform medical asepsis handwash. Adhere to OSHA (Occupational Safety and Health Administration) guidelines.

4. Work in a well-lighted, quiet, clean area.

5. Obtain the appropriate syringe-needle unit and alcohol swab.

6. Obtain the correct medication.

7. Compare the medication label with the medicine card (first time).

8. Check expiration date on medicine.

9. Calculate dosage, if necessary.

10. Prepare syringe-needle unit for use (Figure 17-9A–E).

11. Withdraw medication from container.

12. Compare medicine label with the medicine card (second time).

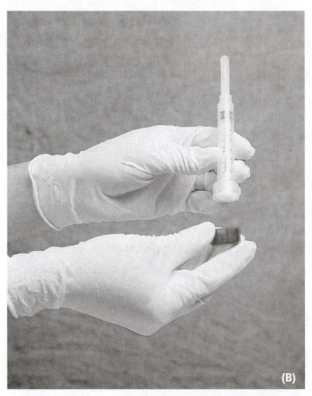

FIGURE 17-9   PREPARING THE SYRINGE-NEEDLE UNIT FOR USE. (A) ASSEMBLE THE EQUIPMENT AND SUPPLIES NEEDED TO DRAW UP MEDICATION FROM A VIAL. (B) REMOVE THE CAP FROM THE COVER OF THE STERILE SYRINGE-NEEDLE UNIT.

(continued)

PROCEDURE 17-1

Administration of Subcutaneous, Intramuscular, and/or Intradermal Injections (*continued*)

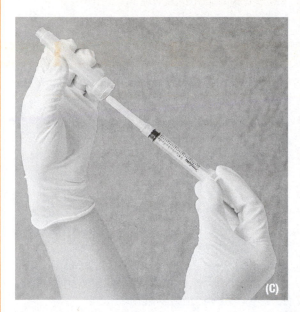
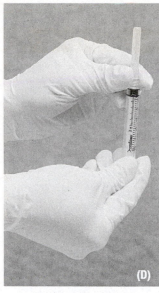
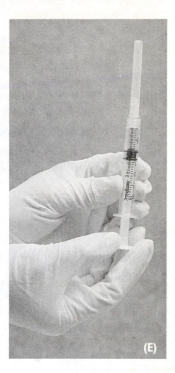

FIGURE 17-9   (C) PULL THE SLEEVE OF THE COVER OFF AND REMOVE THE SYRINGE-NEEDLE UNIT. (D) SECURE THE NEEDLE BY TWISTING IT CLOCKWISE. (E) PULL THE PLUNGER TO CHECK FOR EASE FOR GLIDING OPERATION.

13. Place filled syringe-needle unit on the medicine tray with medicine card. Check the medication label with the medicine card (third time).

14. Correctly transport the medicine to the client.

15. Identify the client. Explain the procedure.

16. Assess the client. Put on gloves.

17. Prepare the client for the injection (drape, position, allay apprehension).

18. Select an appropriate injection site. Follow a rotating schedule if appropriate.

19. Cleanse the injection site with a sterile antiseptic swab. Use a circular motion, working from the center out to about 2 inches beyond the planned injection site.

20. Allow the skin to dry.

21. Administer the injection (aspirate to be certain needle is not in a blood vessel). Immediately dispose of syringe-needle unit in a puncture-proof container.

22. Massage injection site unless contraindicated (insulin, iron dextran, heparin).

23. Observe the client for signs of difficulty.

24. Inspect the injection site for bleeding; apply Band-Aid if necessary.

25. Properly dispose of used equipment and supplies. Remove gloves.

26. Perform medical asepsis handwash.

27. Correctly document the procedure.

Procedure to follow should the nurse sustain an accidental needlestick after the injection:

- Thoroughly wash the site where the stick occurred with soap and water.

- Cleanse the skin with an antiseptic.

- Report the incident.

- Document the incident and retain a copy for yourself.

- Obtain medical attention. Be tested for HBV and HIV.

- Fill out appropriate OSHA paperwork (200 form).

PROCEDURE 17-2

Administering a Subcutaneous Injection

STANDARD PRECAUTIONS:

PURPOSE:

To properly administer a subcutaneous injection after receiving a physician's order and assembling the necessary equipment and supplies

EQUIPMENT/SUPPLIES:

Medication ordered by physician

Medicine card

Appropriately sized needle-syringe unit

Antiseptic wipe

Disposable gloves

Sharps container

PROCEDURE STEPS:

1. Verify the physician's order. Make out a medicine card.
2. Follow the "Six Rights."
3. Perform medical asepsis handwash. Adhere to OSHA guidelines.
4. Work in a well-lighted, quiet, clean area.
5. Obtain the appropriate equipment and supplies.
6. Obtain the correct medication.
7. Compare the medication label with the medicine card (first time).
8. Check expiration date on medicine.
9. Calculate dosage, if necessary.
10. Correctly prepare the parenteral medication.
11. Compare medication label with the medicine card (second time).
12. Replace medication in appropriate area (shelf, refrigerator). Compare the medication label (third time).
13. Correctly transport the medicine to the client.
14. Identify the client. Explain the procedure.
15. Assess the client. Put on gloves.
16. Prepare the client for the injection (drape, position, allay apprehension).
17. Select an appropriate injection site.
18. Correctly cleanse the site using a circular motion starting with the injection site and moving outward to a 2 inch diameter. Allow skin to dry.
19. Remove needle guard.
20. Grasp skin to form a 1 inch fold.
21. Insert needle quickly at a 45° angle (Figure 17-10).
22. Aspirate to be certain needle is not in a blood vessel.
23. Slowly inject the medicine.
24. Correctly remove the needle and syringe.
25. Immediately dispose of needle and syringe in a sharps container.
26. Cover site. Massage (unless contraindicated, as with insulin, iron dextran, and heparin).
27. Remove gloves and wash hands.
28. Provide for client's safety.
29. Document the procedure.

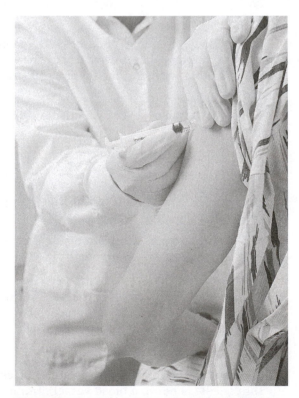

FIGURE 17-10   INSERT NEEDLE AT 45° ANGLE INTO UPPER ARM.

PROCEDURE 17-3

Administering an Intramuscular Injection

STANDARD PRECAUTIONS:

PURPOSE:

To properly administer an intramuscular injection after receiving a physician's order and assembling the necessary equipment and supplies

EQUIPMENT/SUPPLIES:

Medication ordered by physician with medication card

Appropriately sized syringe-needle unit

Antiseptic wipe

Disposable gloves

Sharps container

PROCEDURE STEPS:

1. Verify the physician's order. Make out a medicine card.
2. Follow the "Six Rights."
3. Perform medical asepsis handwash. Adhere to OSHA guidelines.
4. Work in a well-lighted, quiet, clean area.
5. Obtain the appropriate equipment and supplies.
6. Obtain the correct medication.
7. Compare the medication label with the medicine card (first time).
8. Check expiration date.
9. Calculate dosage, if necessary.
10. Correctly prepare the parenteral medication.
11. Compare medicine label with the medicine card (second time).
12. Replace medication on appropriate shelf and compare medication label with medicine card (third time).
13. Correctly transport the medicine to the client.
14. Identify the client. Explain the procedure.
15. Assess the client. Put on gloves.
16. Prepare the client for the injection (drape, position, allay apprehension).
17. Select an appropriate injection site.

18. Correctly cleanse the site using a circular motion and covering a 2 inch diameter. Allow the skin to dry.
19. Remove needle guard.
20. Stretch the skin **taut**, pulling it tight.
21. Using a dart-like motion, insert needle to the hub at a 90° angle (Figure 17-11).
22. Release the skin.
23. Aspirate to check for blood.
24. Slowly inject the medicine.
25. Correctly remove the needle and syringe.
26. Immediately dispose of needle and syringe in a sharps container.
27. Cover site. Massage (unless contraindicated, as with insulin, iron dextran, and heparin).
28. Dispose of equipment. Remove gloves.
29. Wash hands.
30. Observe the client for signs of difficulty.
31. Provide for client's safety.
32. Document the procedure.

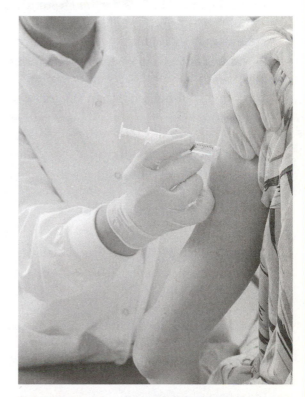

FIGURE 17-11   USING DELTOID AREA OF UPPER ARM, INSERT NEEDLE TO THE HUB AT A 90° ANGLE.

PROCEDURE 17-4

Administering an Intradermal Injection

STANDARD PRECAUTIONS:

PURPOSE:

To properly administer an intradermal injection after receiving a physician's order and assembling the necessary equipment and supplies

EQUIPMENT/SUPPLIES:

Medication as ordered by physician with medication card

Appropriately sized syringe-needle unit

Antiseptic wipe

Disposable gloves

Sharps container

PROCEDURE STEPS:

1. Verify the physician's order. Make out a medicine card.
2. Follow the "Six Rights."
3. Perform medical asepsis handwash. Adhere to OSHA guidelines.
4. Work in a well-lighted, quiet, clean area.
5. Obtain the appropriate equipment and supplies.
6. Obtain the correct medication.
7. Compare the medication label with the medicine card (first time).
8. Check expiration date.
9. Calculate dosage, if necessary.
10. Correctly prepare the parenteral medication.
11. Compare medication label with the medicine card (second time).
12. Replace medication on appropriate shelf and compare medication label with medicine card (third time).
13. Correctly transport the medicine to the client.
14. Identify the client. Explain the procedure.
15. Assess the client. Put on gloves.
16. Prepare the client for the injection (drape, position, allay apprehension).
17. Select an appropriate injection site (Figure 17-12A).
18. Correctly cleanse the site using a circular motion and covering a 2 inch diameter. Allow the skin to dry.
19. Remove needle guard.
20. Pull the skin tissue taut.
21. Carefully insert the needle at a 10° to 15° angle, bevel upward to about $\frac{1}{8}$ inch. Do not aspirate.
22. Steadily inject the medicine (Figure 17-12B). Produce a **wheal**, or slight elevation of the skin.
23. Correctly remove the needle.

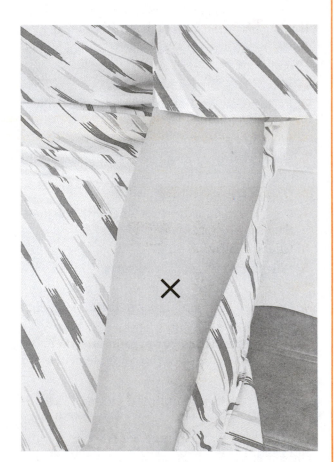

FIGURE 17-12A AN INTRADERMAL INJECTION IS ADMINISTERED AT A SITE ON THE FOREARM.

(continued)

PROCEDURE 17-4

Administering an Intradermal Injection (*continued*)

24. Immediately dispose of needle and syringe in a sharps container.
25. Cover site. Do not massage. Dispose of equipment. Remove gloves.
26. Wash hands.
27. Observe the client for signs of difficulty.
28. Provide for client's safety.
29. Document the procedure.

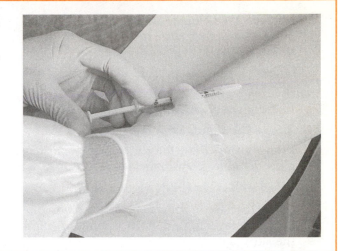

FIGURE 17-12B   STEADILY INJECT THE MEDICINE.

Z-TRACK METHOD OF INTRAMUSCULAR INJECTION

The Z-track method of injection is used for administering medications that can be irritating to or may stain subcutaneous tissue. This method may also be used to decrease pain that can be caused by certain medications and to reduce the possibility of necrosis occurring in soft tissue. Iron dextran and hydroxyzine HCl/hydroxyzine pamoate are examples of medications administered by this method.

The Z-track method involves pulling the skin in such a way that the needle track is sealed off after the injection. The recommended site for the injection is the dorsogluteal area.

PROCEDURE 17-5

Z-Track Intramuscular Injection Technique

STANDARD PRECAUTIONS:

PURPOSE:

To properly administer a Z-track intramuscular injection after receiving a physician's order and assembling the necessary equipment and supplies

EQUIPMENT/SUPPLIES:

Medication ordered by physician and medicine card

Appropriately sized syringe-needle unit

Antiseptic wipe

Disposable gloves

Sharps container

PROCEDURE STEPS:

1. Verify the physician's order. Make out a medicine card.
2. Follow the "Six Rights."
3. Perform medical asepsis handwash. Adhere to OSHA guidelines.
4. Work in a well-lighted, quiet, clean area.
5. Obtain the appropriate equipment and supplies.
6. Obtain the correct medication.
7. Compare the medication label with the medicine card (first time).
8. Check expiration date.
9. Calculate dosage, if necessary.
10. Correctly prepare the parenteral medication.
11. Compare medicine label with the medicine card (second time).

(continued)

PROCEDURE 17-5

Z-Track Intramuscular Injection Technique (*continued*)

12. Replace medication on shelf and compare medication label with medicine card (third time).
13. Correctly transport the medicine to the client.
14. Identify the client. Explain the procedure.
15. Assess the client. Put on gloves.
16. Prepare the client for the injection (drape, position, allay apprehension).
17. Select an appropriate injection site.
18. Correctly cleanse the site using a circular motion and covering a 2 inch diameter. Allow the skin to dry.
19. Remove needle guard.
20. Pull the skin laterally $1\frac{1}{2}$ inches away from the injection site.
21. Insert needle quickly, using a dart-like motion at a 90° angle. Maintain Z position.
22. Aspirate to check for blood.
23. Slowly inject medication.
24. Wait 10 seconds before removing needle to allow medication to begin to be absorbed.
25. Remove needle and syringe at same angle of insertion.
26. Release traction of the Z position in order to seal off the needle track. This prevents medication from reaching the subcutaneous tissues and the surface of the skin.
27. Immediately dispose of needle-syringe unit in a sharps container.
28. Cover site. Do not massage.
29. Remove gloves.
30. Wash hands.
31. Observe client for signs of difficulty.
32. Provide for client safety.
33. Document the procedure.

SPECIAL CONSIDERATIONS FOR THE ADMINISTRATION OF INSULIN AND HEPARIN

Drugs administered through the subcutaneous route are absorbed primarily by the capillaries, thus providing slower, more sustained action by the drug. Drugs recommended for subcutaneous injection should be nonirritating aqueous solutions and suspensions. Examples of drugs that are administered subcutaneously include narcotics, vitamin B_{12}, epinephrine, certain vaccines, insulin, and heparin.

Safety Precaution: When injecting insulin, the following special considerations should be observed:

- Be sure that you have selected the correct insulin for administration.
- Slowly and gently roll the bottle of insulin between the palms of your hands to evenly mix the components of the drug.
- Never shake the bottle.
- Draw up the ordered dosage of insulin using the insulin syringe. Have another nurse verify the dosage.

- Using a site-rotation system, select an appropriate site. Insulin injection sites must be rotated to prevent tissue damage and the accumulation of unabsorbed medication. More than 250 different sites are identified in the *Becton-Dickinson and Company Injection Log* for the administration of insulin. Always record the site that was used. (See Figure 17-13.)
- Do not massage the injection site.
- When mixing two insulins in one syringe, always make sure that they are compatible. An example of two compatible insulins that may be mixed are NPH and Regular. *To mix two insulins in one syringe, draw up the Regular insulin first and then draw up the NPH or other compatible insulin.*
- Always follow the physician's order and your institution's policy when mixing insulins.

Safety Precaution: When injecting heparin, the following special considerations should be observed:

- Have another nurse verify the dosage.
- Administer heparin in the lower abdominal sub-

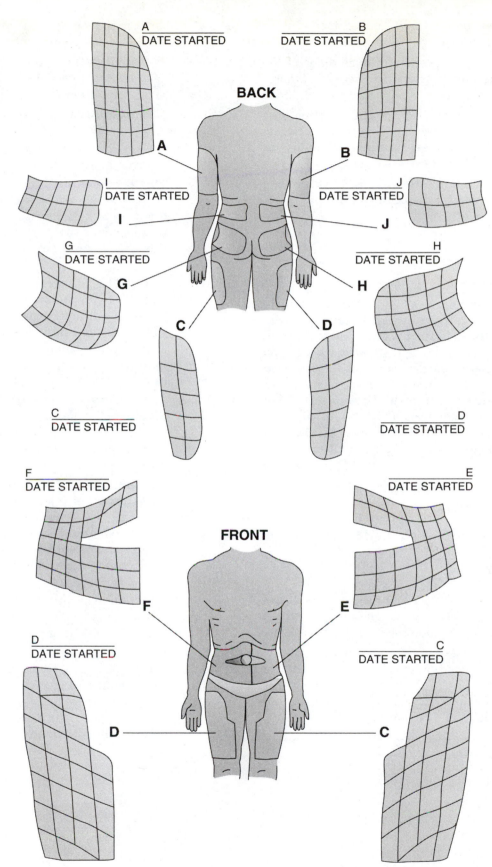

FIGURE 17-13   INJECTION LOG *(Courtesy of Becton, Dickinson and Company)*

cutaneous tissue (fat fold). Stay 2 inches away from the umbilicus.

- Rotate the injection site to reduce the possibility of tissue damage. Heparin can cause damage to skin tissue.

- Do not aspirate or massage the injection site. Aspiration may cause bleeding into the tissue. Massage may cause localized bleeding or bruising.

- Apply ice to the injection site before cleansing and after injecting heparin to minimize local bleeding and bruising.

INJECTION LOG

The body map in Figure 17-13 is designed to help the client record his/her insulin injections. Write down the date that you start using an area. Place an X in the space on the map to show which site you used. One suggested pattern for using the map is to rotate your injections in one area for one week or until you have used each site in the area once. Then move to another body area. This system will help you rotate insulin injection sites over the 12 body areas and avoid using any one area or site too often.

● SELF-ASSESSMENT

Write the answer in the space provided or circle true or false as instructed.

Source

p. 167   **1.** Of the three parenteral routes of administration given in the text, which offers the slowest rate of absorption? _____

p. 168   **2.** Prior to administering an injection, you must assess the client's condition. List the five conditions mentioned in the text that should be part of your assessment: (1) _____ (2) _____ (3) _____ (4) _____ (5) _____

p. 169   **3.** Write in the correct angle of insertion for each of the following types of injections:
- Intradermal injections are best given at an angle between _____ and _____.
- A subcutaneous injection is best given at an angle of _____.
- An intramuscular injection is best given at an angle of _____.

p. 170   **4.** This text mentions the inner forearm and the middle of the back as good sites for intradermal injections. What two reasons make these areas good sites for this type of injection? (1) _____ (2) _____

p. 170   **5.** True or False (circle one) The dorsogluteal site (upper outer quadrant of the buttocks) rather than the ventrogluteal site is the preferred location for giving deep intramuscular injections to adults, infants, children, and the elderly because of its low risk to safety.

p. 171   **6.** An adequate site for the intramuscular injection of a vaccine to an adult would be the _____; however, this site should not be used when administering a vaccine to an infant.

p. 173   **7.** According to basic guidelines for the administration of injections, as listed in the text, _____ in the syringe upon aspiration would cause you to discontinue your procedure and prepare another injection for administration.

p. 179   **8.** The _____ method of injection is recommended for use when irritating medications or those that might stain subcutaneous tissue are to be administered.

p. 180   **9.** You may be asked to mix two types of insulin in one syringe. An example of two compatible insulins are _____ and _____. To mix these types in one syringe, the first to be drawn up would be _____.

Section 4

DRUGS AND RELATED SUBSTANCES

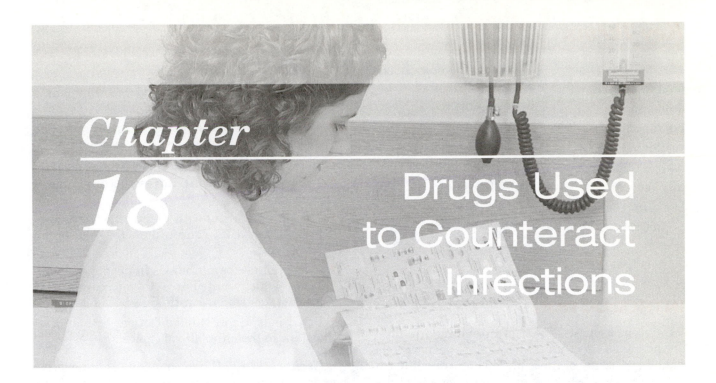

Chapter 18

Drugs Used to Counteract Infections

Chapter Outline

Objectives
Key Terms
Introduction
Deadly Infections
Treatment of Infectious Diseases
Major Antibiotic Groupings
Macrolides
Quinolones
Monobactams
Oxazolidinones
Streptogramins
Miscellaneous Antibiotics
Anthelmintics
Antiprotozoal Agents
Antiseptics and Disinfectants
Self-Assessment
Web Activity

Objectives

Upon completion of this chapter, you should be able to

- Define the key terms
- Describe infection
- List the danger signs of a serious infection
- Describe ways a person may minimize his/her risk of developing a serious infection
- List some of the diseases caused by bacteria
- List the characteristics of an effective antibiotic
- Describe three adverse reactions that may occur with the administration of an antibiotic
- Explain how the overuse of antibiotics has helped cause drug-resistant strains of bacteria
- State the actions, uses, contraindications, adverse reactions, dosage and route, nursing considerations, client's instruction, and special considerations for selected antibiotics
- Complete the Spot Check on major antibiotic groupings
- List the emergency supplies and medications that should be readily available when administering any drug to a client
- State the usual dosage, adverse reactions, and special considerations for selected anthelmintics and antiprotozoal agents
- Describe antiseptics and disinfectants
- Complete the Self-Assessment
- Visit indicated Web sites for additional information on drugs used to counteract infections

Key Terms

anaphylactic shock

antibiotics

antiseptics

bactericidal

bacteriostatic

campylobacteriosis

disinfectants

Escherichia coli

germicides

Group B Streptococcus (GBS)

helminthiasis

infection

microorganisms

oliguria

pathogenic

proteinuria

salmonellosis

INTRODUCTION

We live in a virtual "sea" of **microorganisms**—organisms so tiny that they cannot be seen with the naked eye. Many of these organisms are not harmful to humans, whereas others are agents of disease. Infectious diseases are the fourth largest cause of death in humans. Approximately 50 percent of all infectious diseases are virus related. Other agents that cause infectious diseases are bacteria, fungi, protozoa, rickettsia, and helminths.

Infection is the process or state whereby a **pathogenic** (disease-producing) agent invades the body or a body part, multiplies, and produces injury. Infection occurs when certain factors or conditions exist. The conditions that determine whether a pathogenic agent enters the body, multiplies, and produces disease may vary with the type of invading organism and the susceptibility of the individual.

Infectious diseases are the world's number one killer, claiming 13 million lives annually. According to Dr. James Hughes, director of the National Center for Infectious Diseases at the Centers for Disease Control and Prevention, "the microbes are challenging us in ways we wouldn't have imagined 10 years ago and for which we're not prepared."

Bacteria and viruses multiply quickly and can therefore evolve rapidly into more aggressive strains. The deadly diseases caused by microbes appearing in the last quarter-century include Legionnaires' disease, toxic shock syndrome, AIDS, rodent-borne hantaviruses, the airborne Ebola virus, Lyme disease, bovine spongiform encephalopathy (a fatal brain disease in England caught from eating "mad cows"), West Nile encephalitis, and new drug-resistant tuberculosis strains in many cities. Also, there are other drug-resistant organisms that are causing much concern.

The experts cite numerous factors for the emergence and reemergence of deadly microorganisms, including the following:

- Increased international travel and shipment of food
- Unprecedented population growth cramming people together in unsanitary conditions
- Changes in how food is grown and handled
- Decaying public health infrastructure in many areas
- More people living with immune systems suppressed by AIDS, cancer, diabetes, and organ transplants
- Increased use of antibiotics in people and livestock, which contributes to microorganisms growing resistant to antibiotics
- Potentially deadly staph infections becoming resistant to the antibiotic of choice

Escherichia coli is a common gram-negative bacterium found in normal human bacterial flora; however, some strains can cause severe and life-threatening diarrhea. Recently there has been a worldwide increase in disease caused by strain 0157:H7. Contaminated ground beef has been incriminated as the major mode of transmission. Eating meat that is rare or inadequately cooked is the most common way of getting the infection. Fresh fruits and vegetables may also become contaminated with *E. coli*. Person-to-person transmission can occur if infected people do not wash their hands after using the bathroom. When a fecal accident occurs, usually by an infant or a child with diarrhea, a swimming pool, hot tub, or other water facility can become contaminated with *E. coli*.

While infection with this strain results in diarrhea, it can cause hemorrhagic colitis and hemolytic uremic syndrome (HUS), which is the leading cause of acute renal failure in children under the age of 4. Persons developing HUS have a mortality rate of 3 to 10 percent.

Salmonellosis is a common bacterial infection caused by any of more than 2000 strains of *Salmonella*. These bacteria infect the intestinal tract and occasionally the blood. Salmonellosis is typically a foodborne illness acquired from contaminated raw poultry, eggs, or unpasturized milk and cheese products, but all foods, including vegetables, may become contaminated. Food may also become contaminated by the hands of an infected food handler. *Salmonella* may be found in the feces of some pets, especially those with diarrhea, and people can become infected if they do not wash their hands after contact with these pets. Reptiles (turtles, iguanas, other lizards, snakes) are particularly likely to harbor *Salmonella*, and people should wash their hands after handling a reptile.

Most persons infected with *Salmonella* develop diarrhea, fever, and abdominal cramps 12 to 72 hours after infection. The illness usually lasts 4 to 7 days, and people recover without treatment. However, in some cases the diarrhea may be so severe that the client needs to be hospitalized. The elderly, infants, and those with impaired immune systems are more likely to have a severe illness.

Every year approximately 40,000 cases of salmonellosis are reported in the United States. Because many milder cases are not diagnosed or reported, the actual number of infections may be 20 or more times greater. Salmonellosis is more common in the summer than winter. Children are the most likely to get it. It is estimated that approximately 1000 people die each year with acute salmonellosis.

Campylobacteriosis is an infectious disease caused by bacteria of the genus *Campylobacter*. It is the most common bacterial cause of diarrheal illness in the United States. *Campylobacter* occurs widely as part of the normal flora of many warm-blooded animals including chickens and turkeys. In addition, the organism occurs in raw water and raw milk. In humans, transmission is via contaminated food, water, or milk. The main route is thought to be either undercooking of poultry or cross-contamination from raw to ready-to-eat food. Over 10,000 cases are reported to the Centers for Disease Control and Prevention (CDC) each year. Many more cases go undiagnosed or unreported, and campylobacteriosis is estimated to affect over 2 million people every year, or 1 percent of the population. It occurs more frequently in the summer months than in the winter.

Most people who become ill with campylobacteriosis get diarrhea, cramping, abdominal pain, and fever within 2 to 5 days after exposure to the organism. The diarrhea may be bloody and can be accompanied by nausea and vomiting. The illness typically lasts 1 week. Some who are infected may not have any symptoms at all. In people with compromised immune systems, *Campylobacter* occasionally spreads to the bloodstream and causes a serious life-threatening infection.

Group B streptococcus (GBS) is a bacterium that causes illness in newborns, pregnant women, the elderly, and adults with other illnesses, such as diabetes or liver disease. GBS is the most common cause of life-threatening infections in newborns.

GBS is the most common cause of sepsis and meningitis in newborns. It is a frequent cause of newborn pneumonia and is more common than better-known newborn problems such as rubella, congenital syphilis, and spina bifida.

Approximately one out of every 100 to 200 babies whose mothers carry GBS develops signs and symptoms of GBS disease. Three-fourths of the cases of GBS disease among newborns occur in the first week of life, and most of these cases are apparent a few hours after birth. Sepsis, pneumonia, and meningitis are the most common problems.

Most GBS disease in newborns can be prevented by giving certain pregnant women antibiotics intravenously during labor. In fact, any pregnant woman who previously had a baby with GBS disease or who has a urinary tract infection caused by GBS should receive antibiotics during labor. Penicillin is very effective at preventing GBS disease in the newborn and is generally safe.

DEADLY INFECTIONS

The reports of "deadly, flesh eating bacteria" caused much concern in the summer of 1994. The infections, known as necrotizing fasciitis were fatal to 10 of the 11 people infected. It was determined that the infections were caused by a virulent strain of Group A streptococcus bacterium.

In the United States, the Centers for Disease Control and Prevention estimate that of the 10,000 to 15,000 serious Group A streptococcus infections, only 500 to 1,000 of them result in necrotizing fasciitis. About 30 percent of the clients die of it, primarily because they were not treated with antibiotics soon enough.

There are approximately 70 known strains of Group A streptococcus. In its various forms it can cause sore throats, scarlet fever, rheumatic fever, impetigo, and toxic shock syndrome. Moderate fever and chills are rarely serious, but some symptoms could signal infection with a life-threatening strain of Group A streptococcus, because this strain of bacteria emits a powerful fever-producing substance. One of the hallmarks of virulent strep A is the speed with which it attacks. The infection can become quite serious, anywhere from a day to a week.

Minimize Your Risk of Developing a Serious Infection

- Practice good hygiene: Wash your hands frequently.
- Have at least five servings of fruits and vegetables daily.
- Don't smoke.
- Reduce stress.
- Exercise regularly.

- Get a proper amount of sleep. This is usually 6–8 hours in a given 24-hour time period.
- Keep immunizations current.
- Drink at least 8 glasses of water daily.
- Keep a positive attitude.
- Don't share food or drink with another person.
- Keep fingers away from your mouth, nose, and eyes.

Know the danger signs and seek medical attention *immediately* if any of the following conditions exist:

- Sudden onset of high fever (adult fever of 102°F or higher), violent chills, or confusion
- Infection that seems to be spreading
- Injury that becomes extremely painful
- Injury that rapidly enlarges, especially if there is a high fever
- Redness and blistering of the skin
- Pain in muscles
- Enlarged lymph nodes under the arm
- Increased pain in the incision after a surgical procedure
- Patient with chickenpox (on or beyond the fourth day of pox eruption): fever of 101°F or higher, vomiting, lethargy and painful or swollen areas of the body, inflammation that has spread beyond the area of the chickenpox sores
- Pregnant women with flu-like symptoms

TREATMENT OF INFECTIOUS DISEASES

Antibiotics are used to treat infectious diseases in plants, animals, and humans. They may be natural or synthetic substances that inhibit the growth of or destroy microorganisms, especially bacteria.

Bacteria may be described as gram-positive, gram-negative, or acid-fast. Gram-positive bacteria retain the gentian violet stain in Gram's method of staining. Gram-negative bacteria do not retain the stain and take the color of the counterstain. Acid-fast bacteria, when stained with certain dyes, retain the stain even when treated with an acid.

Gram-positive, gram-negative, and acid-fast bacteria cause a variety of infectious diseases. Gonorrhea, syphilis, tuberculosis, pneumonia, chlamydia, rheumatic fever, scarlet fever, meningitis, strep throat, and salmonellosis are some of the diseases caused by bacteria.

Many antibiotics may be effective against gram-positive bacteria, gram-negative bacteria, or both.

Antibiotics may be classified as broad-spectrum, narrow-spectrum, and/or extended-spectrum.

Classification of Antibiotics

- *Broad-spectrum* antibiotics are effective against many different kinds of microorganisms. Amoxicillin, tetracycline, and cephalosporins are examples of broad-spectrum antibiotics. See Figures 18-1 and 18-2.
- *Narrow-spectrum* antibiotics are effective against limited types of microorganisms. Penicillin G is an example of a narrow-spectrum antibiotic.
- *Extended-spectrum* antibiotics are those for which the antimicrobial activity is extended to include *Pseudomonas, Enterobacter,* and *Proteus* species. Carbenicillin indanyl sodium (Geocillin) is an example of an extended-spectrum antibiotic.

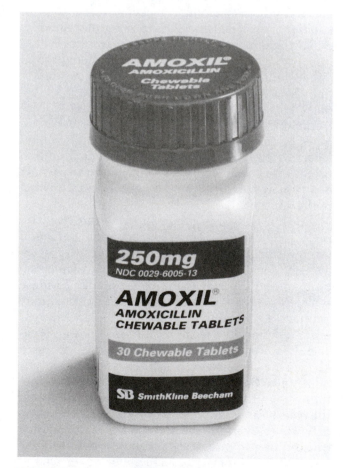

FIGURE 18-1 AMOXIL (AMOXICILLIN) CHEWABLE TABLETS, 250 MG *(Courtesy of SmithKline Beecham)*

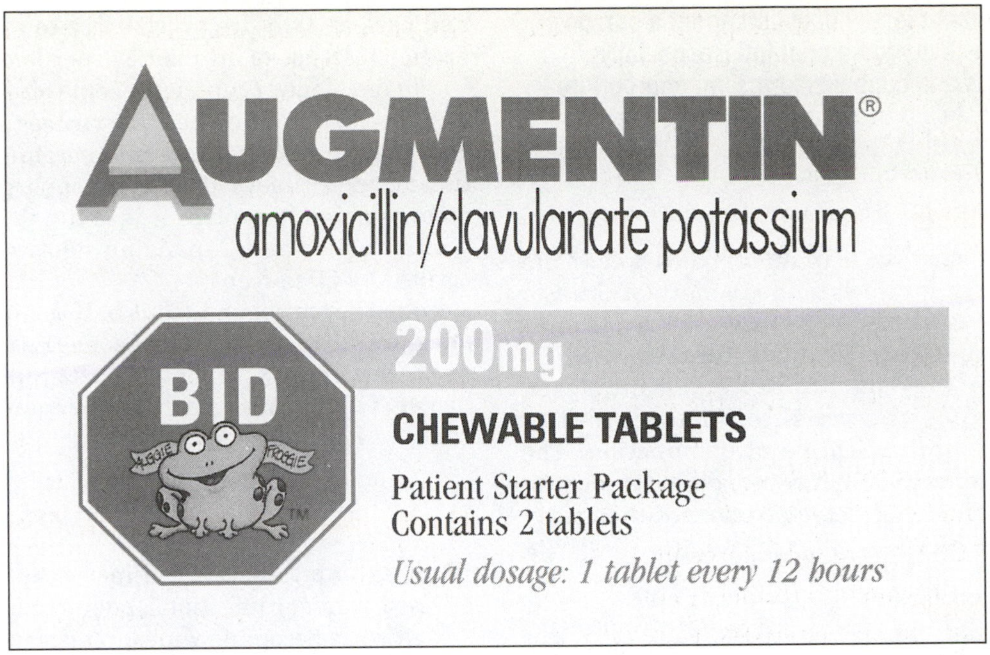

AUGMENTIN®
amoxicillin/clavulanate potassium

200mg

BID

CHEWABLE TABLETS

Patient Starter Package
Contains 2 tablets

Usual dosage: 1 tablet every 12 hours

FIGURE 18-2   AUGMENTIN (AMOXICILLIN/CLAVULANATE POTASSIUM) CHEWABLE TABLETS CLIENT STARTER PACKAGE, 200 MG *(Courtesy of SmithKline Beecham)*

Administering Antibiotics

Before administering any antibiotic, ask the client if he or she is allergic to any drug. If the client has an allergy or sensitivity to any antibiotic or other drug, this information is reported to the physician and recorded in red on the client's permanent record. An antibiotic is never administered to a client when there is an allergy to the drug.

Safety Precaution: To determine the type of invading organism, a culture and sensitivity test is ordered. This test should be performed as soon as possible to guarantee that the appropriate antibiotic is prescribed for the client.

Characteristics of an Effective Antibiotic

The characteristics of an effective antibiotic are (1) it must be harmless to the blood, the liver, the bone marrow, and the kidneys; (2) it must be low in causing toxicity to the body; (3) it must be effective against the invading microorganism; and (4) it must be more beneficial than harmful.

Adverse Reactions

Antibiotics may cause certain harmful effects to occur within the body of some clients. The adverse effect of an antibiotic may manifest itself in the following ways.

Hypersensitivity

Reactions may range from an allergic response to anaphylactic shock. The symptoms of an allergic response may include urticaria, skin eruptions (especially rash), fever, headache, nausea, vomiting, and diarrhea.

Note: A person may develop an allergy at any time; therefore, after giving an antibiotic always assess the client for at least 30 minutes.

Anaphylactic shock is a severe allergic reaction, usually to a substance to which the person has become sensitized. The symptoms of anaphylaxis are: facial or laryngeal edema, dyspnea, cyanosis, circulatory collapse, and convulsions. *Death may occur if emergency treatment is not initiated.* Such treatment consists of the administration of a vasopressor agent (epinephrine, Adrenalin), corticosteroids, oxygen, diphenhydramine (Benadryl), and dopamine (Intropin).

Note: If there is any question about a person's hypersensitivity to an antibiotic, especially penicillins and cephalosporins, an appropriate skin test should be performed before the initiation of drug therapy.

Organ Toxicity

This condition may occur when high doses of an antibiotic are used for an extended length of time, or when the client has impaired liver or renal function. The symptoms of liver dysfunction may include pain in the right upper quadrant, fever, nausea, vomiting, and jaundice. Changes in liver function tests are indicative of dysfunction. The symptoms of renal dysfunction are oliguria and proteinuria. These may be detected through changes in renal function tests.

Superinfection

This condition may occur when there is overgrowth of a resistant strain of bacteria, fungi, or yeast. The symptoms may include black tongue, sore mouth, perianal infection and itching, foul-smelling vaginal discharge, loose stools, sudden fever, and cough.

Overuse of Antibiotics

Drug-Resistant Strains of Bacteria

In recent years, certain strains of bacteria have become increasingly resistant to drugs such as penicillin, erythromycin, vancomycin, and tetracycline. Experts blame the problem on the overuse of antibiotics, which kills the weakest bacteria and leaves the strongest to become more powerful. Drug-resistant organisms develop when a genetic mutation enables one or two bacteria to survive out of the millions in an infected person. The new strain multiplies and spreads, eventually replacing the older, less lethal type. It is noted that all organisms have "survival-of-the-fittest" type mechanisms. The emergence of drug-resistant strains of bacteria could become a public health threat. Drug-resistant bacteria can be spread by human contact from one person to another.

The World Health Organization warns that increasingly drug-resistant infections are threatening to make once-treatable diseases incurable. Scientists have been urging action for years to fight the growing problem of infections becoming impervious to treatment.

Bacteria, parasites, and viruses all naturally evolve to fight treatment. Organisms exposed to drugs that do not kill them become stronger, are able to withstand subsequent treatment attempts, and pass on that drug resistance to their next generation. Misuse of antibiotics speeds this process.

In developed countries, people often overuse antibiotics, demanding them for viruses such as colds. The body always harbors microorganisms, so each unneeded antibiotic dose is an opportunity for microorganisms to evolve. It is estimated that in the United States and Canada antibiotics are overprescribed by 50 percent.

Another problem is that half the world's antibiotics are used on the farm, sometimes to treat illness, but mostly to help healthy animals grow bigger. This encourages drug-resistant microorganisms, which cause food poisoning.

Examples of Antibiotic Overuse

1. Sharp and unexpected increases in penicillin-resistant ear infections, pneumonia, and meningitis are becoming widespread, especially in day care centers, and this is causing great concern in the medical community. Researchers at the Centers for Disease Control and Prevention say the cause of the alarming rise in penicillin resistance among the most common community-acquired diseases appears to be overuse of antibiotics. Without more restrained use of antibiotics, the scientists say, penicillin and other drugs will become increasingly useless in treating the germs that cause 24.5 million trips to the doctor's office for childhood ear infections, as many as 570,000 cases of pneumonia among older individuals and as many as 4000 cases of meningitis.

   Evidence gathered by the CDC in day care centers and public health clinics in Tennessee and Kentucky showed that up to 60 percent of the streptococcal infections in some groups of children were resistant to penicillin and more than half were resistant to other antibiotics.

2. Many of the reported tuberculosis cases are resistant to at least one of the major drugs used to treat the disease. Aggressive intervention will be needed to prevent the spread of a new, potentially untreatable strain of tuberculosis throughout the United States. After 30 years of decline, TB rates are rising again. Most of the 26,000 TB cases a year still respond to drugs, but some new strains are resistant to drugs and are virtually untreatable.

3. One of the most dramatic examples of the diminishing effectiveness of antibiotics is vancomycin-resistant enterococci, or VRE. Because VRE are immune to all available antibiotics, they kill half of those they infect, usually the very old or very ill. In response to an increase in

nosocomial infections with VRE, the Centers for Disease Control and Prevention has issued guidelines to help check their spread.

4. Gonorrhea was once easily curable with penicillin and tetracycline. Today, these drugs are not effective against gonorrhea.

5. Malaria, the mosquito-spread infection that kills a million people a year, is resistant to the top medication 80 percent of the time.

6. Some 5000 Americans may have suffered longer-lasting food poisoning in 1998 from drug-resistant germs in chicken.

7. Annually, 88,000 Americans die of nosocomial infections, many of which are resistant to at least one antibiotic, complicating treatment attempts.

8. Some strains of *Staphylococcus aureus* are showing signs of resistance to vancomycin.

The following is a summary of the CDC's recommendation for hospitals.

Education

Staff should be taught about VRE epidemiology and the need for stringent control.

Detection and Reporting

Early detection and reporting are essential. Clients who are at high risk, such as those who are critically ill, should be regularly screened for the presence of VRE infection. Bodily secretions such as urine, feces, or isolates from wound sites should be tested for VRE. Positive findings should be reported and proper treatment and isolation measures initiated immediately.

Infection Control

VRE-infected clients should be put into isolation rooms. Staff should follow isolation techniques carefully. Clients should remain in isolation until at least three cultures, taken at least a week apart, are negative.

Prudent Vancomycin Use

To help decrease the emergence of VRE and other drug-resistant organisms, vancomycin should be used only when appropriate, for example, when antibiotic-associated colitis does not respond to metronidazole.

MAJOR ANTIBIOTIC GROUPINGS

Antibiotics may be grouped when they have a similar action and usage. The major antibiotic group-

ings described in this section are: penicillins, cephalosporins, tetracyclines, and aminoglycosides.

Penicillins

Penicillin was discovered in 1928 by Sir Alexander Fleming, a British bacteriologist. Today, the penicillins consist of a group of natural and semisynthetic agents that are active against gram-positive and gram-negative cocci and bacilli. Penicillin may be either the natural product of such molds as *Penicillium notatum* and *Penicillium chrysogenum*, or a semisynthetic derivative of the *Penicillium* molds. See Figure 18-3.

Actions

The penicillins act by interfering with cell wall synthesis among newly formed bacterial cells. Unable to develop rigid cell walls when affected by penicillin, the rapidly developing cells die as a result of an increase in the flow of fluid into the cell.

Uses

There are a number of penicillins, each with a similar effect on bacterial cells, yet differing in stabil-

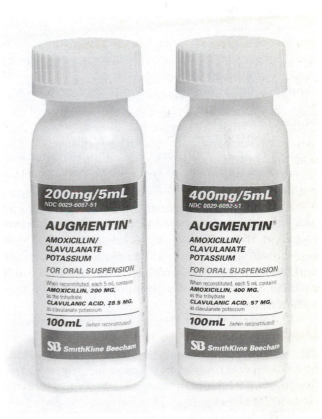

FIGURE 18-3 AUGMENTIN (AMOXICILLIN/CLAVULANATE POTASSIUM) FOR ORAL SUSPENSION, 200 MG/5 ML, 400 MG/5 ML *(Courtesy of SmithKline Beecham)*

ity and absorption rate when introduced into the body. Physicians, after an analysis of the factors associated with a disease, choose among the types of penicillins for the variety most effective against the invading microorganisms.

Some diseases for which a physician might prescribe a penicillin are pneumonia, gonorrhea, syphilis, meningitis, diphtheria, sinusitis, bronchitis, acute osteomyelitis, otitis media, and infections caused by *Staphylococci, Streptococci, Escherichia coli*, and *Salmonella* bacteria.

Contraindications

Penicillins are contraindicated in clients who are known to be allergic or hypersensitive to any of its varieties or to any of the cephalosporins. Those known to be sensitive to either of these groups of drugs should wear a Medic Alert bracelet or other identification warning of this condition.

> **Safety Precaution:** A client's drug allergy must be noted in red on the chart.

Adverse Reactions

The most common adverse reaction to penicillins is an allergic one. This reaction may be an immediate anaphylactic response requiring emergency treatment, or a delayed response whereupon the client must discontinue the medication and seek medical attention. Other adverse reactions may include nausea, vomiting, diarrhea, fever, chills, rash, itching, and signs of superinfection.

With intramuscular administration, there may be pain at the site of injection, inflammation, sterile abscess, phlebitis, and thrombophlebitis.

Dosage and Route

The dosage and route of administration is determined by the physician and will vary with the type of penicillin prescribed. Table 18-1 lists some of the frequently used penicillins, the average adult and children's dosages, and the usual route of administration.

Nursing Considerations

The nurse should treat each client as an individual and take a careful history of allergies. It is very important to determine if the client has an allergy to penicillins or cephalosporins before either of these groups of drugs is prescribed.

It is recommended that certain emergency supplies and medications be readily available when administering any drug to a client, especially peni-

cillins or cephalosporins. The recommended emergency supplies and medications are

- Epinephrine (Adrenalin)
- Diphenhydramine (Benadryl)
- Corticosteroids
- Blood pressure equipment
- Oxygen
- Dopamine (Vasopressor), (Intropin)
- IV infusion materials
- Oral airways
- Cardiac support system

Clients' Instruction

Instruct clients to report any signs of an adverse reaction and to take their medication as prescribed until all of the drug has been taken. It is most important that the client understand this, as many times, once the client starts to feel better, he or she may discontinue taking the antibiotic and a relapse can occur. Caution clients against taking any medication unless it is prescribed for them. Instruct clients that the prescribed medication is for them and they should not allow anyone else to take their medication.

Special Considerations

- Oral doses should be taken on an empty stomach, 1 hour before or 2 hours after a meal.
- It is best to take the medication with 8 ounces of water and should not be taken with soft drinks, fruit juices, or wine, as the acid in these products can destroy the drug.
- Administration with erythromycin or a tetracycline may diminish effectiveness.
- Probenecid (Benemid) decreases renal elimination and may cause higher blood levels and longer duration of action of penicillins.

Penicillinase-Resistant Penicillin

Penicillinase-resistant penicillin is a group of penicillins that was developed because some organisms are resistant to penicillin. These drugs are effective against most gram-positive and gram-negative aerobes and a few gram-positive and gram-negative anaerobic bacteria. See Table 18-2.

Cephalosporins

The cephalosporins are semisynthetic broad-spectrum antibiotics derived from cephalosporin C, which is obtained from the fungus *Cephalosporium*.

TABLE 18-1 SELECTED PENICILLINS, ROUTES, AND DOSAGES

Generic Name	Trade Name	Route(s)	Usual Dosage(s)	
amoxicillin	Amoxil Wymox	Oral	*Adults:* *Children:*	250–500 mg every 8 hours (Under 20 kg) 20–40 mg/kg daily in divided doses every 8 hours
ampicillin	Omnipen	Oral	*Adults:* *Children:*	250–500 mg every 6 hours 50–100 mg/kg daily in divided doses every 6 hours
bacampicillin	Spectrobid	Oral	*Adults:* *Children:*	400 mg every 12 hours (Under 25 kg) 25–50 mg/kg/day in 2 divided doses every 12 hours
carbenicillin indanyl sodium	Geocillin	Oral	*Adults:*	1–2 tablets qid
penicillin G benzathine	Bicillin L-A	IM	*Adults:* *Children:* *Neonates:*	1.2 million units as a single dose 300,000–1.2 million units as a single dose 50,000 units/kg as a single dose
penicillin G potassium	Pentids	Oral	*Adults:* *Children:*	200,000–500,000 units every 6–8 hours 25,000–90,000 units/kg daily in 3–6 divided doses
	Pfizerpen	IM, IV	*Adults:*	2–20 million units daily
penicillin G procaine, aqueous	Pfizerpen A.S.	IM	*Adults and Children:* *Newborns:*	600,000–1.2 million units/day in 1 or 2 doses for 10–14 days 50,000 units/kg as a single dose
penicillin V potassium	Pen-Vee K	Oral	*Adults:* *Children under 12:*	125–500 mg qid 25–50 mg/kg/day in 3–4 divided doses
piperacillin sodium	Pipracil	IM IV	*Adults:* *Adults:*	2–8 g daily in 2–4 divided doses 6–18 g daily in 2–6 divided doses
ticarcillin disodium clavulanate potassium	Timentin	IV	*Adults:* *Gyn Infections:*	3.1 g every 4–6 hours Moderate: 200 mg/kg/day in divided doses every 6 hours Severe: 300 mg/kg/day in divided doses every 4 hours Clients weighing less than 60 kg: 200–300 mg/kg/day in divided doses every 4–6 hours

They are chemically and pharmacologically related to the penicillins.

Cephalosporins are classified into three generations.

- First-generation cephalosporins tend to have the greatest *bacteriostatic* or *bactericidal* activity against gram-positive and several gram-negative organisms, and are generally susceptible to being inactivated by *beta-lactamase* enzymes produced by some bacteria.

Examples: cefadroxil (Duricef)
cefazolin (Ancef, Kefzol, Zolicef)
cephalexin (Biocef, Keflex, Keftab)
cephalothin (Keflin)
cephapirin (Cefadyl)
cephradine (Velosef)

- Second-generation cephalosporins have a broader spectrum of activity against gram-negative organisms and a slightly more diminished

TABLE 18-2 SELECTED PENICILLINASE-RESISTANT PENICILLINS

Generic Name	Trade Name	Route(s)	Usual Dosage(s)	
cloxacillin	Cloxapen Tegopen	Oral	*Adults:*	250–500 mg every 6 hours
			Children:	(Up to 20 kg) 12.5–25 mg/kg every 6 hours; under 20 kg 50–100 mg/kg/day in 4 divided doses every 6 hours
dicloxacillin	Dynapen	Oral	*Adults:*	125–250 mg every 6 hours
			Children:	(Under 40 kg) 12.5–25 mg/kg/day in divided doses every 6 hours
mezlocillin sodium	Mezlin	IM, IV	*Adults:*	200–300 mg/kg/day in 4–6 divided doses
			Children:	150–300 mg/kg/day in 2–6 divided doses
nafcillin	Unipen	Oral	*Adults:*	250 mg: 1 g every 4–6 hours
			Children:	Neonates: 10 mg/kg every 6–8 hours
			Older Children:	25–50 mg/kg/day in 4 divided doses every 6 hours
oxacillin	Bactocill Prostaphlin	Oral	*Adults:*	500 mg: 1 g every 4–6 hours
			Children:	(Under 40 kg) 50–100 mg/kg/day in 4 equally divided doses

activity against gram-positive organisms than first-generation cephalosporins. *Haemophilus influenzae* is especially sensitive to second-generation cephalosporins.

Examples: cefaclor (Ceclor)
cefamandole (Mandol)
cefmetazole (Zefazone)
cefonicid (Monocid)
cefotetan (Cefotan)
cefoxitin (Mefoxin)
cefprozil (Cefzil)
cefuroxime (Ceftin, Kefurox, Zinacef)
loracarbef (Lorabid)

● Third-generation cephalosporins have even a broader spectrum of activity against such gram-negative organisms as *Escherichia coli (E. coli)*, *Klebsiella* species, *Proteus mirabilis* and possibly *Proteus vulgaris*, *Providencia rettgeri* and *Morganella morganii*, streptococcus, staphylococcus, *Neisseria gonorrhoeae*, and *Haemophilus influenzae*. The third-generation drugs are resistant to the defensive beta-lactamase enzymes that some bacteria secrete.

Examples: cefepime (Maxipime)
cefixime (Suprax)
cefoperazone (Cefobid)
cefotaxime (Claforan)
cefpodoxime (Vantin)
ceftazidime (Ceptaz, Fortaz, Tazicef, Tazidime)
ceftibuten (Cedax)
ceftizoxime (Cefizox)
ceftriaxone (Rocephin)

Actions

The cephalosporins, like penicillins, act by inhibiting bacterial cell wall synthesis, thereby promoting the death of developing microorganisms.

Uses

Cephalosporins are indicated in the treatment of mild to severe respiratory infections, especially those caused by *Haemophilus influenzae* organisms resistant to penicillins. They may also be prescribed for otitis media, skin and soft tissue infections, septicemia, gastrointestinal infections, genitourinary tract infections, meningitis, and bone and joint infections.

Contraindications

Hypersensitivity to cephalosporins and/or penicillin may result in an allergic reaction. Cephalosporins should be used with caution in clients with impaired renal function and a history of colitis.

TABLE 18-3   SELECTED CEPHALOSPORINS, ROUTES, AND DOSAGES

Generic Name	Trade Name	Route(s)	Usual Dosage(s)	
cefaclor	Ceclor	Oral	*Adults:*	250–500 mg every 8 hours, not to exceed 4 g daily
			Children:	(1 month and older) 20–40 mg/kg daily in divided doses every 8 hours, not to exceed 1 g daily
cefadroxil	Duricef	Oral	*Adults:*	500 mg capsules or 1 g tablets in single or two divided doses
			Children:	30 mg/kg per day in divided doses every 12 hours
cefamandole	Mandol	IM, IV	*Adults:*	500 mg to 1 g every 4–8 hours
			Children:	(1 month and older) 12.5–25 mg/kg every 4 hours
cefazolin sodium	Ancef Kefzol	IM, IV	*Adults:*	250 mg to 1 g every 6, 8, or 12 hours
			Children:	25–50 mg/kg/day divided into 3–4 equal doses
cefixime	Suprax	Oral	*Adults:*	400 mg daily or 200 mg every 12 hours
			Children:	(Under 50 kg) 8 mg/kg/day or 4 mg/kg every 12 hours
cefonicid	Monocid	IM, IV	*Adults:*	1 g once a day every 24 hours
cefotaxime	Claforan	IM, IV	*Adults:*	1–2 g every 8 to 12 hours
			Children:	50–180 mg/kg divided into 4–6 equal doses
cefotetan	Cefotan	IM, IV	*Adults:*	1–2 g every 12 hours for 5–10 days
cefoxitin sodium	Mefoxin	IM, IV	*Adults:*	1–2 g every 6–8 hours
			Children:	3 months and older 80–160 mg/kg/day divided into 4–6 doses
cefpodoxime	Vantin	Oral	*Adults:*	200–400 mg every 12 hours
			Children:	100 mg/kg/day, maximum 400 mg/day
ceftazidime	Fortaz	IM, IV	*Adults:*	250 mg to 2 g every 8–12 hours
			Children:	30–50 mg/kg every 8 hours
ceftizoxime sodium	Cefizox	IM, IV	*Adults:*	1–2 g every 8–12 hours
			Children:	6 months and older 50 mg/kg every 6–8 hours
ceftriaxone sodium	Rocephin	IM, IV	*Adults:*	1–2 g once a day, or divided doses every 12 hours
			Children:	50–100 mg/kg in divided doses every 12 hours (not to exceed 4 g)
cefuroxime	Kefurox	IM, IV	*Adults:*	750 mg to 1.5 g every 8 hours
			Children:	50–100 mg/kg/day every 6–8 hours in equally divided doses
	Ceftin	Oral	*Adults:*	250–500 mg every 12 hours
			Children:	20 mg/kg/day in 2 divided doses, not to exceed 500 mg total dose/day, for 10 days
cephalexin	Keflex	Oral	*Adults:*	250 mg every 6 hours or 500 mg every 12 hours
			Children:	25–50 mg/kg in 4 divided doses
cephalothin sodium	Ceporacin Keflin	IM, IV	*Adults:*	1–2 g every 4–6 hours
			Children:	13.3–26.6 mg/kg every 4 hours
cephapirin	Cefadyl	IM, IV	*Adults:*	500 mg–1 g every 4–6 hours
			Children:	(Over 3 months) 40–80 mg/kg/day in four equally divided doses

Adverse Reactions

Mild to severe allergic reaction, rash, itching, diarrhea, dizziness, headache, dyspepsia, and abdominal pain may result.

Dosage and Route

The dosage and route of administration is determined by the physician. See Table 18-3 for selected cephalosporins.

Nursing Considerations

Take a careful history of allergies. Clients who are allergic to penicillins are likely to be allergic to cephalosporins. Keep emergency drugs on hand.

Clients' Instruction

Advise the client to report any signs of hypersensitivity. Instruct the client to continue the medication as prescribed until all of the drug has been taken.

Instruct the client to avoid the use of alcohol with certain cephalosporins, such as Mandol (cefamandole) and Cefizox (ceftizoxime). Inform the client that over-the-counter medications such as certain mouthwashes and cough preparations may contain alcohol.

Special Considerations

- Oral doses may be taken on a full or empty stomach. They may be taken with food, or tablets can be crushed and mixed with food.
- Administration with probenecid (Benemid) may increase and prolong plasma levels of cephalosporin.
- Administration with erythromycin and/or tetracycline may interfere with cephalosporin's bactericidal action.
- Diabetics should know that this medicine may cause false test results with some urine sugar tests. Diabetics should check with their physician before changing diet or dosage of diabetes medicine.
- Avoid alcohol consumption during the use of certain cephalosporins, such as Mandol (cefamandole) and Cefizox (ceftizoxime). Cephalosporins may interact with acute alcohol consumption and produce a disulfiram-like (Antabuse-like) reaction, which is a severe hypersensitivity to alcohol. Symptoms that may occur are flushing, chest pain, palpitations, tachycardia, hypotension, syncope (fainting), and arrhythmias.

Tetracyclines

Tetracyclines are primarily **bacteriostatic** (inhibiting or retarding bacterial growth) and are active against a wide range of gram-negative and gram-positive microorganisms. There are both natural and semisynthetic tetracyclines, which are derived from various species of *Streptomyces*. The tetracycline drugs exhibit similarities in their range of antimicrobial activity. (See Figures 18-1 and 18-2.)

Actions

The tetracyclines are thought to exert their effect on microorganisms by inhibiting protein synthesis in the bacterial cell.

Uses

Tetracyclines are indicated in the treatment of rickettsial disease, respiratory infections, venereal diseases, acne, and amebiasis.

Contraindications

Tetracyclines are contraindicated in clients with renal and liver impairment, during pregnancy and lactation, and in children 8 years of age and younger. These drugs cause permanent discoloration of tooth enamel and a predisposition to cavities among children with developing teeth.

Adverse Reactions

Nausea, vomiting, diarrhea, colitis, anorexia, photosensitivity, permanent discoloration of deciduous teeth, and overgrowth of fungi (candidiasis or moniliasis).

Dosage and Route

The dosage and route of administration is determined by the physician. See Table 18-4.

Nursing Considerations

The nurse should be familiar with the signs of hypersensitivity and superinfection. Advise the client about such signs. Instruct the client to report any signs of hypersensitivity and/or superinfection to the physician.

Tetracyclines should be given on an empty stomach (1 hour before meals or 2 hours after meals) with a full glass of water. The drug expiration date should always be checked before administration. Renal injury (Fanconi-like syndrome) and other problems may result from the use of outdated tetracyclines.

Clients' Instruction

Advise clients to avoid direct or artificial sunlight, as they are more sensitive to it and may suffer a sunburn. Instruct clients to not eat dairy products or take antacids, laxatives, or iron supplements within 1 to 2 hours of taking tetracycline.

TABLE 18-4   SELECTED TETRACYCLINES, ROUTES, AND DOSAGES

Generic Name	Trade Name	Route(s)	Usual Dosage(s)	
demeclocycline hydrochloride	Declomycin DMCT	Oral	*Adults:*	150 mg every 6 hours
			Children:	3–6 mg/lb daily in 2–4 divided doses
doxycycline	Doryx Doxy-Caps Vibramycin Vibra-Tabs	Oral	*Adults:*	100 mg every 12 hours on first day, then 100 mg once daily
			Children:	2 mg/kg for 2 doses every 12 hours, then 2.3–4.4 mg/kg once daily
minocycline hydrochloride	Minocin	Oral	*Adults:*	200 mg initially followed by 100 mg every 12 hours
			Children:	Above 8 years of age, 4 mg/kg initially followed by 2 mg/kg every 12 hours
tetracycline hydrochloride	Achromycin Sumycin Panmycin	Oral	*Adults:*	250 mg every 6 hours or 500 mg twice a day
			Children:	25–50 mg/kg daily in 4 divided doses

Special Considerations

- Oral doses should be taken on an empty stomach, 1 hour before or 2 hours after a meal.
- It is best to take with 8 ounces of water and should not be taken with milk or any dairy product. Alkaline products can interact with tetracycline and make it less effective.
- Administration with calcium or magnesium supplements, antacids and/or iron may reduce tetracycline absorption.
- Store away from light, heat, humidity, or cold.

Aminoglycosides

The aminoglycosides include any of a group of **bactericidal** (killing or destruction of bacteria) antibiotics derived from various species of microbes from the genus *Streptomyces*. The aminoglycosides are broad-spectrum antibiotics, the best known of which is streptomycin.

Actions

The aminoglycosides act by interfering with the synthesis of bacterial cell protein, thereby promoting the death of the affected microorganism.

Uses

Aminoglycosides are indicated in the treatment of diseases caused by gram-negative microorganisms. They may be used to treat active tuberculosis, plague, subacute bacterial endocarditis, *Haemophilus in-* *fluenzae*, pneumonia, peritonitis, respiratory tract infections, urinary tract infections, and infections caused by *Escherichia coli*.

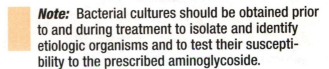

Note: Bacterial cultures should be obtained prior to and during treatment to isolate and identify etiologic organisms and to test their susceptibility to the prescribed aminoglycoside.

Contraindications

Hypersensitivity to drugs of the aminoglycosides. These drugs are contraindicated in clients with labyrinthine disease, myasthenia gravis, and those who are pregnant and/or lactating. Cautious use in clients with impaired renal function, the elderly, infants, and children. Aminoglycosides should not be given concurrently with potent diuretics such as ethacrynic acid and furosemide. Ototoxicity may be enhanced by these diuretics.

Adverse Reactions

Aminoglycosides can cause irreversible damage to the auditory branch of the eighth cranial nerve (acoustic). Factors contributing to this side effect include the drug, the client's condition, the dose, the length of therapy, and the client's renal function. Other adverse reactions may include skin rashes, pruritus, stomatitis, headache, muscular weakness, and nephrotoxicity with signs of oliguria and proteinuria. Clients may experience vertigo, tinnitus, dizziness, ataxia, nausea, and vomiting.

Dosage and Route

The dosage and route of administration is prescribed by the physician. See Table 18-5.

Nursing Considerations

Observe for signs of ototoxicity (nausea, vomiting, tinnitus, vertigo, and acute loss of hearing). Monitor clients with impaired renal function for signs of oliguria and proteinuria by recording the intake and output volume, and by urinalysis.

Clients' Instruction

Advise the client to drink plenty of fluids. Instruct the client to report any signs of hypersensitivity. Clients with tuberculosis should be advised that drug therapy is only a part of their long-term treatment and must be combined with proper diet and adequate rest.

Special Considerations

- Because of the potential toxicity associated with aminoglycosides, clients should be under close clinical observation. The major toxic effects are the action on the auditory and vestibular branches of the eighth nerve and the renal tubules. The client should be instructed to observe for signs of ototoxicity and/or nephrotoxicity.

- Signs of ototoxicity: Nausea, vomiting, tinnitus (ringing sound in the ear), vertigo, acute loss of hearing.

- Signs of nephrotoxicity: **Oliguria** (decreased amount of urine formation) and **proteinuria** (presence of protein [albumin] in the urine).

- The client should be encouraged to drink plenty of liquids (eight glasses of water a day) to reduce the development of nephrotoxicity.

- Administration with anesthetics and/or muscle relaxants could cause neuromuscular blockade and respiratory paralysis.

- Administration with other drugs that could cause ototoxicity and/or nephrotoxicity should be avoided. This is particularly true of polymyxin B, bacitracin, colistin, amphotericin B, cisplatin, vancomycin, potent diuretics, and all other aminoglycosides.

TABLE 18-5 SELECTED AMINOGLYCOSIDES

Generic Name	Trade Name	Route(s)	Usual Dosage(s)	
amikacin	Amikin	IM, IV	*Adults:*	15 mg/kg/day divided into 2 or 3 equal doses
gentamicin sulfate	Garamycin	IM, IV	*Adults:*	3 mg/kg/day in 3 divided doses every 8 hours
			Children:	6–7.5 mg/kg/day (2–2.25 mg/kg every 8 hours)
kanamycin	Kantrex	Oral	*Adults:*	1–8 g daily in 4 divided doses
			Children:	50 mg/kg daily in 4–6 divided doses every 6 hours
		IM	*Adults and Children:*	15 mg/kg in 2–4 divided doses
		IV	*Adults and Children:*	Not to exceed 15 mg/kg body weight daily in 2–3 divided doses
netilmicin	Netromycin	IM, IV	*Adults:*	With normal renal function: complicated urinary tract infections: 3.0–4.0 mg/kg/day Serious systemic infections: 4.0–6.5 mg/kg/day Dosage for clients with impaired renal function must be individualized.
streptomycin sulfate	Streptomycin	IM	*Adults:*	1–2 g daily (15–25 mg/kg). 500 mg to 1 g every 12 hours
			Children:	20–40 mg/kg daily in 2 divided doses
tobramycin sulfate	Nebcin Tobrex	IM, IV	*Adults:*	3 mg/kg daily in 3 equal doses every 8 hours
			Children:	2–2.5 mg/kg every 8 hours

● SPOT CHECK

For each of the antibiotic groupings given, list several aspects of client instruction and several special considerations.

Major Antibiotic Groupings	Client Instruction	Special Considerations
Penicillins		
Cephalosporins		
Tetracyclines		
Aminoglycosides		

MACROLIDES

Macrolide antibiotics include the erythromycins, azithromycin (Zithromax), and clarithromycin (Biaxin). These drugs exert their antimicrobial action by binding to the bacterial 50S ribosomal subunit, thereby inhibiting protein synthesis. Numerous erythromycin preparations exist today. See Table 18-6.

Azithromycin (Zithromax) and clarithromycin (Biaxin) are also described in this section.

Erythromycin

Erythromycin is produced by a strain of bacteria (*Streptomyces erythraeus*) and belongs to the

TABLE 18-6   SELECTED ERYTHROMYCINS

Generic Name	Trade Name	Route	Usual Dosage	
erythromycin base	E-Mycin Ery-Tab	Oral	*Adults:* 250–500 mg every 6 hours	*Children:* 30–50 mg/kg/day in 3–4 divided doses
erythromycin estolate	Ilosone	Oral	*Adults:* 250–500 mg every 6 hours	*Children:* 30–50 mg/kg/day in 3–4 divided doses
erythromycin ethylsuccinate	EES EryPed	Oral	*Adults:* 250 mg every 6 hours	*Children:* 30–50 mg/kg/day in 3–4 divided doses
erythromycin gluceptate	Ilotycin	IV infusion	*Adults:* 200–500 mg (up to 1 g) q 6 hours	*Children:* 3.75–5 mg/kg q 6 hours
erythromycin lactobionate	Erythrocin	IV infusion	*Adults:* 200–500 mg (up to 1 g) q 6 hours	*Children:* 3.75–5 mg/kg q 6 hours
erythromycin stearate	Erythrocin	Oral	*Adults:* 250–500 mg every 6 hours	*Children:* 30–50 mg/kg/day in 3–4 divided doses

macrolide group of antibiotics. Depending upon the concentration of the drug and the nature of the microorganism against which it is used, erythromycin can be bacteriostatic or bactericidal.

Actions

Erythromycin works by inhibiting protein synthesis in susceptible bacteria.

Uses

Erythromycin is a broad-spectrum antibiotic, similar to penicillin, and is often used against penicillin-resistant microorganisms. It is also indicated for clients who are allergic to penicillin. Infections for which erythromycin might be prescribed include penumococcal and diplococcal pneumonia, pelvic inflammatory disease, *Neisseria gonorrhoeae*, Legionnaires' disease, upper and lower respiratory tract infections, and infections of the skin and soft tissues.

Contraindications

Caution should be used when administering this drug to clients with liver dysfunction. Its safe use in pregnancy has not been established.

Adverse Reactions

Erythromycin may cause nausea, vomiting, diarrhea, and abdominal discomfort when given orally. Hypersensitivity reactions include urticaria, skin eruptions, and fever. Superinfection by nonsusceptible bacteria, yeasts, or fungi may occur. When applied topically, burning, tenderness, dryness or oiliness, pruritus, and erythema may occur.

Dosage and Route

Dosage and route is prescribed by the physician. See Table 18-6.

Nursing Considerations

Observe the client for signs of hypersensitivity. Monitor liver function tests. Give on an empty stomach (1 hour before or 2 hours after meals). Enteric-coated tablets may be given without regard to meals.

Clients' Instruction

The client should be instructed to follow the complete course of therapy, to avoid taking the drug with fruit juices, and to report such signs of hepatotoxicity as jaundice and abdominal cramps.

Azithromycin—Zithromax

Actions

Zithromax is an azalide, a subclass of a macrolide antibiotic. It acts by binding to the 50S ribosomal subunit of susceptible microorganisms and thus interferes with microbial protein synthesis.

Uses

Indicated for the treatment of individuals older than 6 years of age with mild to moderate infections caused by susceptible strains of the designated microorganisms in lower respiratory infections due to *Haemophilus influenzae, Moraxella catarrhalis,* or *Streptococcus pneumoniae.* As an alternative to first-line drug therapy in the treatment of upper respiratory infections such as streptococcal pharyngitis/tonsillitis. Zithromax is often effective in the eradication of susceptible strains of *Streptococcus pyogenes* from the nasopharynx. It is also used in the treatment of uncomplicated skin and skin structure infections due to *Staphylococcus aureus*, *Streptococcus pyogenes*, or *Streptococcus agalactiae*. It may be used in the treatment of nongonococcal urethritis and cervicitis due to *Chlamydia trachomatis*.

Contraindications

Zithromax is contraindicated in clients with known hypersensitivity to azithromycin, erythromycin, or any macrolide antibiotic.

Adverse Reactions

Most side effects are related to the gastrointestinal tract: nausea, vomiting, diarrhea, or abdominal pain. Rare but potentially serious side effects are angioedema and cholestatic jaundice. Other side effects include dizziness, headache, somnolence, fatigue, and vertigo.

Dosage and Route

Zithromax is given orally in capsules or in an oral suspension. Dosage is 500 mg as a single dose on the first day, then 250 mg once daily on days 2–5 for a total dose of 1.5 grams.

Nursing Considerations

Observe the client for signs of hypersensitivity. Medication should be administered at least 1 hour before a meal or at least 2 hours after a meal. Because some strains of bacteria are resistant to Zithromax, susceptibility tests should be performed before and during treatment.

Clients' Instruction

The client should be instructed to follow the complete course of therapy and to avoid the use of aluminum- or magnesium-containing antacids when taking Zithromax.

Clarithromycin—Biaxin

Actions

Clarithromycin inhibits protein synthesis at the level of the 50S bacterial ribosome. It exerts bacteriostatic action against susceptible bacteria.

Uses

The drug is used to treat upper respiratory tract infections including streptococcal pharyngitis and sinusitis and lower respiratory tract infections in-cluding bronchitis and pneumonia. It is effective in the treatment (with ethambutol) and prevention of disseminated *Mycobacterium avium* complex (MAC). Otitis media, sinusitis, pharyngitis, and skin and skin structure infections in children are treated with clarithromycin. The drug is also part of a combination regimen (with a gastric acid pump inhibitor and amoxicillin or with ranitidine bismuth citrate) for ulcer disease due to *Helicobacter pylori*. It is recommended for endocarditis prophylaxis in preventing bacterial infection during certain cardiac, dental, respiratory, gastrointestinal tract, and genitourinary tract procedures.

Contraindications

Hypersensitivity to clarithromycin, erythromycin, or other macrolide anti-infectives. Pregnancy and lactation unless no alternatives are available. Use cautiously in severe liver and/or renal impairment.

Adverse Reactions

Side effects include headache, pseudomembranous colitis, abdominal pain/discomfort, abnormal taste, diarrhea, dyspepsia, and nausea.

Dosage and Route

Oral, adults: bronchitis/pneumonia/skin and soft tissue infections: 250 mg every 12 hours. Bronchitis/sinusitis/disseminated MAC/*H. pylori*: 500 mg every 12 hours. Endocarditis prophylaxis: 500 mg 1 hour before procedure. *Oral, children:* most infections: 7.5 mg/kg every 12 hours (up to 500 mg/dose for MAC). Endocarditis prophylaxis: 15 mg/kg 1 hour before procedure.

Nursing Considerations

Assess client for infection at beginning of and throughout therapy. Obtain specimens for culture and sensitivity prior to initiating therapy. First dose may be given before receiving results. Administer around the clock, without regard to meals. Food slows but does not decrease the extent of absorption. Shake suspension well before administration. Do not administer within 4 hours of zidovudine.

Clients' Instruction

Instruct the client to take the medication around the clock and to finish the drug completely as directed, even if feeling better. Missed doses should be taken as soon as possible, unless it is almost time for the next dose. Do not double doses. Advise that medication should not be shared with anyone. Advise to report signs of superinfection and fever and diarrhea to health care provider. Caution client taking zidovudine that clarithromycin and zidovudine must be taken at least 4 hours apart. Advise the client to notify health care provider if symptoms do not improve within a few days.

QUINOLONES

Quinolones are synthetic broad-spectrum antibiotics/anti-infectives that have a rapid bactericidal action against most gram-negative and many gram-positive bacteria. They alter deoxyribonucleic acid (DNA) by interfering with DNA gyrase, an enzyme that is necessary for the duplication, transcription, and repair of bacterial DNA. Since humans do not have this enzyme, their cells are not affected.

These drugs are indicated for treatment of susceptible strains of designated microorganisms that cause a wide range of mild to moderate genitourinary tract infections, including cystitis, urinary tract infection, prostatitis, and sexually transmitted diseases: gonorrhea and chlamydia, upper respiratory infections, infectious diarrhea, ophthalmic infections, bone and joint infections, for dental work, gum and tooth infections.

Examples of quinolones are ciprofloxacin (Cipro), enoxacin (Penetrex), gatifloxacin (Tequin), levofloxacin (Levaquin), lomefloxacin (Maxaquin), moxifloxacin (Avelox), norfloxacin (Noroxin), and ofloxacin (Floxin).

Certain adverse reactions are common to the quinolones and others are drug specific. For dosage and route and selected adverse reactions, see Table 18-7.

MONOBACTAMS

Monobactams are synthetic antibiotics that contain a cyclic beta-lactam structure. They are bactericidal against gram-negative aerobic pathogens. Aztreonam (Azactam) is the most widely known monobactam. It acts by inhibiting cell wall synthesis due to a high affinity of the drug for penicillin-binding protein 3; this results in cell lysis and death.

Aztreonam—Azactam

Actions

Azactam is the first member of a new class of antibiotics classified as monobactams. It is a totally synthetic bactericidal antibiotic with activity against a wide spectrum of gram-negative aerobic pathogens.

TABLE 18-7   SELECTED QUINOLONES

Medication	Usual Dosage	Adverse Reactions
ciprofloxacin (Cipro)	Oral: *Adults:* 250–500 mg every 12 hours for 1–2 weeks IV: *Adults:* 400 mg every 12 hours	Nausea, diarrhea, vomiting, rash, headache, tremors, abdominal pain, dry/painful mouth, Stevens-Johnson syndrome
enoxacin (Penetrex)	Oral: *Adults:* 200–400 mg every 12 hours for 1–2 weeks	Anorexia, bloody stools, gastritis, stomatitis, anxiety, tremors, Stevens-Johnson syndrome
gatifloxacin (Tequin)	IV: *Adults:* 400 mg once daily for 7–10 days	Tremors, confusion, hallucinations, vertigo, abdominal pain, glossitis, stomatitis, Stevens-Johnson syndrome
levofloxacin (Levaquin)	Oral, IV: *Adults:* 250–500 mg every 24 hours	Nausea, vomiting, diarrhea, dry or painful mouth, headache, dizziness, photosensitivity, cardiovascular collapse
lomefloxacin (Maxaquin)	Oral: *Adults:* 400 mg daily for 10–14 days	Confusion, tremor, vertigo, anxiety, anorexia, coma, bad taste in mouth, dysphagia, tongue discoloration, cardiovascular collapse
moxifloxacin (Avelox)	Oral: *Adults:* 400 mg every 24 hours for 10 days	Anaphylaxis after the first dose, cardiovascular collapse, loss of consciousness, vertigo, dysphagia
norfloxacin (Noroxin)	Oral: *Adults:* 400 mg every 12 hours for 72 hours	Nausea, vomiting, diarrhea, dry or painful mouth, headache, dizziness, photosensitivity, cardiovascular collapse
ofloxacin (Floxin)	Oral, IV: *Adults:* 300–400 mg every 12 hours for 10 days	Nausea, vomiting, diarrhea, abdominal pain, headache, dizziness, anxiety, hypertension, photosensitivity, rash

Uses

Azactam is indicated for the treatment of infections caused by susceptible gram-negative microorganisms: urinary tract, lower respiratory tract, skin and skin structure, intra-abdominal, gynecologic infections, and septicemia.

Contraindications

Azactam is contraindicated in clients with known allergy to this antibiotic.

Adverse Reactions

Phlebitis/thrombophlebitis following IV administration, and discomfort/swelling at the injection site following IM administration. Diarrhea, nausea and/or vomiting, skin rash, anaphylaxis, pancytopenia, abdominal cramps, purpura, hypotension, weakness, headache, fever, and malaise.

Dosage and Route

Dosage and route of administration should be determined by susceptibility of the causitive organisms, severity and site of infection, and the condition of the client. For urinary tract infection IM, IV: 500 mg or 1 g every 8–12 hours; IM, IV: moderately severe systemic infection 1 g or 2 g every 8–12 hours; IM, IV: severe systemic or life-threatening infections 2 g every 6–8 hours.

Nursing Considerations

The nurse should obtain a history of hypersensitivity to any antibiotic or other drug. It is important to relay this information to the physician. Antibiotics should be given with caution to any client who has had some form of allergy to drugs.

Clients' Instruction

Advise the client to report any signs of superinfection (black tongue, sore mouth, perianal infection and itching, foul-smelling vaginal discharge, loose stools, sudden fever, cough) immediately. Instruct the client that a taste alteration may be experienced during IV therapy and to report if eating becomes significantly impaired.

OXAZOLIDINONES

Oxazolidinones are a new class of antibiotics that act by inhibiting the formation of the ribosomal initiation complex, a unique site not overlapping other ribosomally active antimicrobials. Linezolid (Zyvox) is the first of this class and the first entirely new type of antibiotic in 35 years. It attacks bacteria by stopping protein production at an early point in the process, and thus works differently from any other antibiotic. Without protein production, bacteria cannot multiply and they die.

Linezolid (Zyvox) has primary activity against all gram-positive organisms. It is approved for the treatment of adult clients with vancomycin-resistant *Enterococcus faecium* (VREF) infections by indicated bacteria, nosocomial pneumonia, complicated and uncomplicated skin and skin structure infections, and community-acquired pneumonia. It is mainly intended for hospital or institutional care settings. Due to concerns about inappropriate use of antibiotics leading to an increase in resistant organisms, prescribers should carefully consider alternatives before initiating treatment with Zyvox in the outpatient setting.

The most common adverse reactions to the drug are diarrhea, headache, nausea, and vomiting. The most important laboratory test change was a decrease in platelet counts. It is available in 400 mg and 600 mg tablets, oral suspension of 100 mg/5 ml, and intravenous bags of 200 mg/100 ml, 400 mg/200 ml, and 600 mg/300 ml. Interactions of Zyvox with other drugs include over-the-counter cold remedies that contain pseudoephedrine or phenylpropanolamine, with a risk of increasing blood pressure. Clients receiving Zyvox should inform their physicians if they are taking such medications.

STREPTOGRAMINS

Streptogramins is a distinct class of antibacterials. Synercid (quinupristin/dalfopristin) IV is the first injectable antibiotic approved by the U.S. Food and Drug Administration (FDA) to treat bloodstream infections due to vancomycin-resistant *Enterococcus faecium* (VREF) and skin and skin structure infections (SSSI) caused by methicillin-susceptible *Staphylococcus aureus* or *Streptococcus pyogenes*.

The two distinct antibiotic agents that form Synercid, quinupristin and dalfopristin, work synergistically to inhibit or destroy susceptible bacteria through a two-pronged attack on protein synthesis. The most common adverse reactions are inflammation and pain at the infusion site. Other adverse reactions are arthralgia, myalgia, nausea, vomiting, diarrhea, constipation, dyspepsia, oral moniliasis, pancreatitis, stomatitis, headache, anxiety, confusion, dizziness, insomnia, thrombophlebitis, palpitation, rash, pruritus, urticaria, hematuria, dyspnea, allergic reaction, chest pain, fever, infection, superinfection, and pseudomembranous colitis (antibiotic-associated colitis).

The recommended dosage for the treatment of vancomysin-resistant *Enterococcus faecium* infections is IV infusion 7.5 mg/kg every 8 hours, with the duration of treatment determined by the site and severity of the infection. The recommended dosage for the treatment of complicated skin and skin structure infections is IV infusion 7.5 mg/kg every 12 hours for a period of at least 7 days.

Although quinupristin and dalfopristin are the first streptogramins to be approved for human use in the United States, other agents in this class (pristinamycin, virginiamycin) have also been developed. The use of the new drugs is contraindicated in clients with known hypersensitivity to any of these agents.

MISCELLANEOUS ANTIBIOTICS

Table 18-8 lists miscellaneous antibiotics. Only the basic drug information is provided. Before administering any of these drugs, you should refer to the *Physicians' Desk Reference* or the Delmar's *Nurse's Drug Handbook* for more detailed information.

TABLE 18-8 MISCELLANEOUS ANTIBIOTICS/ANTIBACTERIALS

Medication	Usual Dosage			Adverse Reactions
chloramphenicol (Ak chlor)	*Oral and IV:*		50 mg/kg/day every 6 hours in divided doses	Bone marrow depression, blood dyscrasias, headache, confusion, nausea, vomiting, diarrhea, stomatitis, hypersensitivity, superinfection
clindamycin HCl (Cleocin)	*Oral:*	*Adults:*	150–450 mg every 6 hours with 8 ounces of water	Diarrhea, rash, GI upset, jaundice, anaphylaxis, renal dysfunction
		Children:	8–20 mg/kg/day in 3–4 divided doses	
	IM, IV:	*Adults:*	1.2–2.7 g/day in 2–4 equal divided doses	
		Children:	20–40 mg/kg/day in 3–4 equal divided doses	
imipenem cilastatin (Primaxin)	*IV:*	*Adults:*	250 mg–1 g every 6–8 hours not to exceed 50 mg/kg/day or 4 g/day	Nausea, diarrhea, confusion, myoclonus, seizures, superinfection
lincomycin HCl (Lincocin)	*Oral:*	*Adults:*	500 mg every 6–8 hours	Nausea, vomiting, diarrhea, hypersensitivity, superinfection, hematopoietic changes
		Children:	Over 1 month old, 30–60 mg/kg/day in 3–4 divided doses	
	IM:	*Adults:*	600 mg once or twice daily	
		Children:	Over 1 month old, 10 mg/kg once or twice daily	
	IV:	*Adults:*	600–1000 mg every 8–12 hours	
		Children:	Over 1 month old, 10–20 mg/kg/day	
metronidazole HCl (Flagyl)	*Oral:*	7.5 mg/kg every 6 hours		Nausea, vomiting, diarrhea, skin rash, seizures, peripheral neuropathy
	IV:	Initially 15 mg/kg infused over 1 hour as a loading dose; thereafter 7.5 mg/kg infused over 1 hour every 6 hours		
polymyxin B bacitracin neomycin (Neosporin)	*Ointment or Cream:*	Apply a thin layer to the area 2–5 times a day		Ototoxicity, nephrotoxicity, hypersensitivity to neomycin

(continued)

TABLE 18-8 *(Continued)*

Medication	Usual Dosage			Adverse Reactions
spectinomycin HCl (Trobicin)	*IM:*	*Adults:*	2 g	Urticaria, dizziness, nausea, chills, fever, insomnia
vancomycin HCl (Vancocin HCl)	*Oral:*	*Adults:*	500 mg every 6 hours or 1000 mg every 12 hours	Nausea, chills, fever, urticaria, macular rashes, eosinophilia, hypersensitivity
		Children:	10 mg/kg every 6 hours	
	IV:	*Adults:*	500 mg every 6 hours or 1000 mg every 12 hours	
		Children:	10 mg/kg every 6 hours or 20 mg/kg every 12 hours	

ANTHELMINTICS

Helminthiasis is a condition in which there is an intestinal infestation by parasitic worms. Infections of this type are a major cause of disease in many areas of the world and have been associated with unsanitary living conditions. Although most commonly found in the developing countries, worm infestations can occur in any society. The helminths that infest humans belong to the phyla *Platyhelminthes* (flatworms), *Acanthocephala* (spiny-headed worms), *Nemathelminthes* (threadworms or roundworms), or *Annelida* (segmented worms). The roundworms, pinworms, hookworms, and other *Nemathelminthes* of class *Nematoda* are the organisms responsible for the most common helminthic diseases worldwide and in the United States. The flatworms causing parasitic diseases are tapeworms and flukes. Most of these intestinal parasites can be eliminated by therapy with the appropriate anthelmintic. See Table 18-9.

TABLE 18-9 ANTHELMINTICS

Medication	Infected by	Usual Dosage	Adverse Reactions
ivermectin (Stromectol)	Strongyloidiasis (roundworm)	*Oral:* single dose to provide about 200 mcg/kg 15–24 kg 0.5 tab 25–35 kg 1 tab 36–50 kg 1.5 tab 51–65 kg 2 tab 66–79 kg 2.5 tab	Diarrhea, nausea, vomiting, anorexia, constipation, abdominal pain, dizziness, tremor, vertigo, pruritus, rash, fatigue
	Onchocerciasis (filarial worm)	*Oral:* single dose to provide about 150 mcg/kg 15–25 kg 0.5 tab 26–44 kg 1 tab 45–64 kg 1.5 tab 65–84 kg 2 tab	Mazzotti reaction: pruritus, edema, papular and pustular or frank urticarial rash, fever, inguinal lymph node enlargement and tenderness, axillary lymph node enlargement and tenderness, arthralgia, synovitis, cervical lymph node enlargement and tenderness Ophthalmic: limbitis, punctate opacity, abnormal sensations in the eyes Miscellaneous: tachycardia, orthostatic hypotension, headache, myalgia

(continued)

TABLE 18-9   *(Continued)*

Medication	Infected by	Usual Dosage	Adverse Reactions
mebendazole (Vermox)	Roundworm, hookworm, whipworm, pinworm	*Oral:* 100 mg twice/day (morning and evening) for 3 consecutive days *Oral:* 100 mg as a single dose	Diarrhea, fever, dizziness, transient abdominal pain
praziquantel (Biltricide)	Blood fluke	*Oral:* 60 mg/kg in 3 divided doses at 4–6 hour intervals for one day	Abdominal pain, nausea, anorexia, dizziness, headache, malaise, drowsiness, pruritus, urticaria, fever
	Other flukes	*Oral:* 75 mg/kg in 3 doses at 4–6 hour intervals for one day	
	Tapeworms	*Oral:* 10–20 mg/kg as a single dose	
pyrantel pamoate (Antiminth)	Pinworm, roundworm	*Oral:* 11 mg/kg (5 mg/lb) in a single dose (maximum total dose 1 g)	Dizziness, drowsiness, headache, anorexia, nausea, abdominal distention, rash
thiabendazole (Mintezol)	Roundworm, pinworm, hookworm, threadworm	*Oral* (Client less than 150 lb): 10–25 mg/kg in 2 doses per day; (client over 150 lb): 1.5 g in 2 doses per day	Hypotension, bradycardia, anorexia, nausea, vomiting, jaundice, cholestasis, liver damage, headache, blurred vision, malodor of urine, seizures

Special Considerations

- With infections of pinworm and threadworm, all members of the family must be treated.
- An accurate body weight is taken before drug therapy is initiated.
- Antiminth and Vermox may be taken with food. Mintezol is usually given after meals.
- The client's close contacts are examined and treated when necessary.
- Client education includes ways to avoid reinfestation. Beef and pork should be thoroughly cooked to prevent the possibility of tapeworms. Avoid walking barefoot in areas where hookworms are endemic. Thoroughly wash fruits and vegetables before eating to prevent the possibility of roundworms. Instruct client in proper hygienic measures especially handwashing procedure before meals and after using the bathroom.

ANTIPROTOZOAL AGENTS

Protozoa rival worms as the world's leading cause of disease, and although there has been great improvement in worldwide sanitation, developing countries continue to have a high incidence of parasitic disease. Travel and military service often expose Americans to such protozoal diseases as malaria, giardiasis, trichomoniasis, and amebiasis. Worldwide, malaria is the most common cause of infectious disease. Although not widespread in the United States, the organisms that cause this disease are becoming increasingly resistant to the drugs used in treating the disease. Antiprotozoal agents are listed in Table 18-10.

Trichomoniasis is primarily a disease of the vagina, although it can be present in the male urethra and the rectum of either sex. Infection by *Trichomonas vaginalis* is characterized by a thin, yellow, malodorous discharge and pruritus. Giardiasis is caused by the flagellate *Giardia lamblia* that inhabit the small intestine. Many hosts are asymptomatic to the organism, which is increasingly found in the United States as a result of travel to and from other countries. Amebiasis is caused by *Entamoeba histolytica* and is transmitted by ingestion of mature cysts. Colonies develop in the intestinal tract, causing diarrhea and abdominal pain in many infected by the organism.

Pneumocystis carinii pneumonia (PCP) is an opportunistic infection that is prevalent in AIDS clients. It is caused by a protozoan, and, if not treated, the mortality rate is high. See Table 18-10 for selected drugs that are used to treat this condition.

TABLE 18-10   ANTIPROTOZOAL AGENTS

Medication	Disease	Usual Dosage	Adverse Reactions
atovaquone (Mepron)	mild to moderate *Pneumocystis carinii* pneumonia (PCP)	*Oral (Adults):* 750 mg twice daily for 21 days	Headache, insomnia, cough, diarrhea, nausea, vomiting, rash fever
chloroquine (Aralen)	Malaria	*IM (Adults):* 160–200 mg of base repeated in 6 hours if necessary (maximum, 800 mg [base] in the first 24 hours) *IM (Children):* 5 mg base/kg repeated in 6 hours (maximum, 10 mg base/kg/24 hours)	Fatigue, irritability, psychoses, nightmares, heart block, hypotension, eczema, vomiting, abdominal cramps, visual disturbances
chloroquine phosphate (Aralen Phosphate)	Malaria	*Oral (Adults):* 600 mg of base, then 300 mg of base at 6, 24, and 48 hours	Same as above
	Amebiasis (hepatic)	*Oral (Adults):* 600 mg of base daily for 2 days, then 300 mg base/day for 2–3 weeks	
hydroxy-chloroquine sulfate (Plaquenil)	Malaria	*Oral (Adults):* 800 mg followed by 400 mg after 6–8 hours, then 400 mg on each of the next 2 days for a total of 2 g	GI distress, visual disturbances, retinopathy, vertigo, nerve deafness, tinnitus
metronidazole (Flagyl)	Amebiasis, trichomoniasis, giardiasis	*Oral* (Trichomoniasis): 2 g in a single or divided dose (1 day therapy) *Oral* (Amebiasis) *(Adult):* 500–750 mg 3 times/day for 5–10 days *(Children):* 35–50 mg/kg/day in 3 doses for 10 days *Oral* (Giardiasis): *Adult:* 250 mg 3 times/day for 7 days	Rash, flushing, headache, vertigo, confusion, insomnia, depression, polyuria, cystitis, nausea, vomiting, anorexia, abdominal cramps, dry mouth, bitter taste, leukopenia
paromomycin sulfate (Humatin)	Amebiasis	*Oral:* 25–35 mg/kg divided in 3 doses for 5–10 days	Headache, vertigo, abdominal cramps, diarrhea, nausea, ototoxicity, nephrotoxicity
pentamidine (Pentam 300)	*Pneumocystis carinii* pneumonia (PCP)	*IV (Adults and Children):* 4 mg/kg/day for 14–21 days	Anxiety, headache, dizziness, arrhythmias, hypotension, abdominal pain, pancreatitis, chills, anorexia, nephrotoxicity, hypoglycemia, anaphylaxis, Stevens-Johnson syndrome
primaquine phosphate	Malaria	*Oral:* 15 mg of base daily for 14 days	Hemolytic anemia in clients with G6PD deficiency, nausea
trimetrexate (NeuTrexin)	*Pneumocystis carinii* pneumonia (PCP)	*IV (Adults):* 1.2 mg/kg/day for 21 days. Concurrent administration of leucovorin 20 mg/m^2 oral or IV every 6 hours for 24 days, with the first dose given IV prior to first dose of trimetrexate	Confusion, fatigue, increased AST/ALT, nausea, vomiting, rash, pruritus, hypocalcemia, hyponatremia, neutropenia, thrombocytopenia, anemia, fever

Special Considerations

- Clients on long-term drug therapy for malaria should have periodic blood cell counts, liver function tests, and vision and hearing tests.

- Hemolytic reactions may occur in dark-skinned persons taking primaquine phosphate. Clients should be instructed to report any evidence of bleeding (blood in urine; nosebleed).

- Most antimalarial drugs are given before or after meals to prevent gastrointestinal distress.

- Clients with amebiasis and trichomonal infections need to know the nature of their condition and its mode of transmission. Education should include proper hygienic methods.

- For treatment of trichomoniasis to be effective both male and female sexual partners must be treated simultaneously.

- Clients taking metronidazole should be instructed to avoid the use of alcohol as it may cause nausea, vomiting, headache, and abdominal cramps. Also, the urine may turn reddish brown.

ANTISEPTICS AND DISINFECTANTS

Antiseptics are substances that prevent or inhibit the growth of microorganisms. The process by which growth is inhibited is called bacteriostatic action. Antiseptics are generally applied to the surface of living tissue. Due to their lack of potency, they do little or no damage to surrounding tissue.

Disinfectants are substances, usually of chemical origin, that kill vegetative forms of microorganisms. They are described as having a bactericidal action due to their destruction of bacteria. Disinfectants rapidly kill microorganisms on the surfaces to which they are applied, and are used on walls, floors, bed linens, furniture, and bathroom fixtures. *Fungicides* are closely related agents with the ability to kill fungi and their spores. **Germicides** are agents that kill or destroy microorganisms. These agents are of sufficient strength to cause harm to living tissues; therefore, they are usually applied to inanimate objects.

Phenol was the first antiseptic. Other antiseptics are compared with phenol to measure their effectiveness; this measure is known as the phenol coefficient (P/C). Many antiseptics contain phenol and related compounds (see Table 18-11).

Alcohol may be used as an antiseptic or as a germicide depending upon the type used and its strength. Ethyl alcohol (70 percent solution) is often used as an antiseptic for minor injuries, and to prepare the skin for injections. Used full strength, isopropyl alcohol is a germicide for the disinfection of instruments. It may also be used in a 70 percent solution for the disinfection of oral thermometers.

Tincture of iodine contains 2 percent iodine and 2.4 percent sodium iodide diluted in 50 percent ethyl alcohol. It may be used as a disinfectant for the skin, and as a germicide. Adding 3 drops of tincture of iodine to a quart of water will kill amebas and bacteria within 30 minutes, and the water will still be palatable.

The effectiveness of an antiseptic or a disinfectant depends upon the following factors:

- The strength of the solution
- The temperature of the solution
- The time of exposure
- The ionization rate of the substance used

Table 18-11 lists antiseptics and disinfectants that are in general use. Note that the brand or trade name for these products is shown in parentheses.

TABLE 18-11 ANTISEPTICS AND DISINFECTANTS

Substance	Strength	Action	Comments
alcohol		Antiseptic	For external use only. Used to prepare the skin for injections, venipuncture, and IV therapy.
Ethyl	70% solution		
Isopropyl (rubbing)	full strength	Germicide	Flammable
benzalkonium	1:750	Antiseptic	On intact skin, mucous membranes, superficial injury
chloride	1:2000–1:5000		
(Zephiran)	1:5000		Vaginal douching
	1:5000–1:10,000		Wet dressings
	1:2000–1:20,000		Irrigations of the eye, body cavities
			Infected wounds

(continued)

TABLE 18-11   *(Continued)*

Substance	Strength	Action	Comments
chlorhexidine gluconate (Hibiclens)	4%	Antiseptic Antimicrobial	Skin cleanser. Surgical scrub, health care personnel handwash. For clients' preoperative showering and bathing, client preoperative skin preparation, skin wound cleanser, and general skin cleanser
chlorhexidine gluconate (Hibistat Towelette)	0.5%	Germicidal Handwipe	Germidical hand rinse. Use for hand hygiene on physically clean hands. It is used in those situations where hands are physically clean but in need of degerming, when routine handwashing is not convenient or desirable.
gentian violet	1:100–1:1000	Antiseptic Fungicide Dye	Used on skin and mucous membrane for fungus infections (thrush, impetigo)
green soap (solution or tincture)	1:10	Antiseptic	Handwash; used to wash thermometers
hexachlorophene (pHisoHex) (WescoHex) (Septi-Soft) (Septisol)	3% topical emulsion, liquid soap, lotions, ointments, and shampoos	Bacteriostatic against gram-positive bacteria on the skin	Not used for bathing infants. Rinse skin after use. May produce erythema, dryness, and scaling on clients with sensitive skin
hydrogen peroxide	3% (diluted with 1–4 parts water)	Antiseptic	Cleans wounds of pus, dead tissue. Deteriorates upon standing. Store in a cool, dark place.
iodine (solution or tincture) (Wescodyne) (Betadine)	2% 1–1½% iodine and detergent	Antiseptic Fungicide Germicide	Used on small wounds and abrasions. *Check for allergies.* Used as a surgical prep to reduce number of organisms on the skin and reduce the chance of infection. Hand rinse
phenolics (Cresol) (Lysol) (Amphyl) (Staphene)	2%–5% ½% 2½%	Disinfectant Antiseptic Disinfectant	On contaminated objects: linens, basins, bedpans. Action not affected by organic material As a footbath for athlete's foot; prolonged use may be injurious to tissues.
silver nitrate	1% (ophthalmic solution) 1:1000 1:10,000	Antiseptic	Prevents gonorrheal conjunctivitis in newborns Astringent Bladder irrigations
sodium hypochlorite (household bleach)	1:10 1:100	Germicide	HIV (AIDS) inactivator Use on contaminated surfaces.

● SELF-ASSESSMENT

Write the answer in the space provided or circle true or false as instructed.

Source
p. 186   **1.** The text lists six types of microorganisms that cause infectious diseases. Viruses and bacteria are two; the other four are

(1) _____ ,

(2) _____ ,

(3) _____ , and

(4) _____ .

p. 186– **2.** The text names three strains of bacteria
187   that can cause diarrheal illnesses. Give the name of each strain.

(1) _____

(2) _____

(3) _____

p. 188 **3.** Amoxicillin, tetracycline, and the cephalosporins are broad-spectrum antibiotics. Briefly define the term broad-spectrum antibiotic. _____

_____

_____

_____

p. 189 **4.** The characteristics of an effective antibiotic are that it must be (1) harmless to the blood, the liver, the bone marrow, and the kidneys; (2) low in causing toxicity to the body; (3) effective against the invading microorganism; and (4)

_____

_____

p. 189 **5.** True or False (circle one) The difference between an allergic response to an antibiotic agent and anaphylaxis is the severity of symptoms exhibited by the client.

p. 191 **6.** The group of drugs known as the penicillins act against gram-positive and gram-negative cocci and bacilli by

_____ .

p. 193– **7.** The group of drugs known as the
194 cephalosporins are classified into three generations. Complete the following statements:

● Cefaclor (Celecor) is an example of a

_____
generation cephalosporin.

● Cefprozil (Cefzil) is an example of a

_____
generation cephalosporin.

● Cephalothin (Keflin) is an example of a _____
generation cephalosporin.

● Cefoperazone (Cefobid) is an example of a _____
generation cephalosporin.

p. 196 **8.** The group of drugs known as the tetracyclines are thought to exert their effect on microorganisms by _____ .

p. 197 **9.** The group of drugs known as aminoglycosides have been associated with irreversible damage to the _____ .

p. 199 **10.** The erythromycins belong to a group of drugs known as _____ .

p. 202 **11.** The drug _____
is a synthetic bactericidal antibiotic belonging in the classification known as monobactams.

● WEB ACTIVITY

Visit the following Web sites for additional information on drugs used to counteract infections:

http://www.pslgroup.com

http://www.merck.com

http://www.discoveryhealth.com

http://www.medicinenet.com

http://pharmacotherapy.medscape.com

http://www.onhealth.com

http://www.fda.gov/bbs/topics

http://www.cdc.gov

http://www.niaid.nih.gov

http://www.health.msn.com

http://www.fhsu.edu/nursing.html

http://www.intelihealth.com

http://www.ortho-mcneil.com

http://www.aegis.com

http://www.wadsworth.org

http://www.micromedex.com

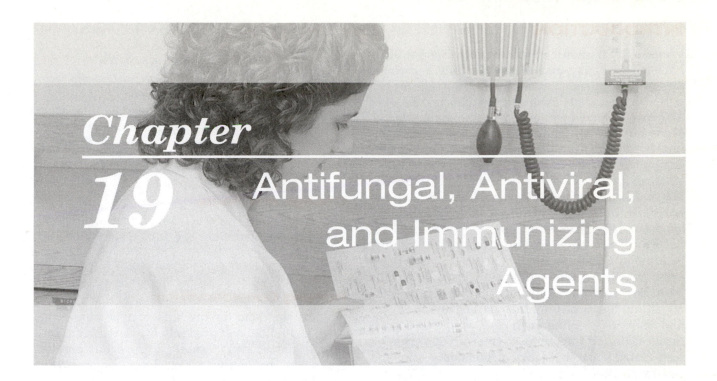

Chapter

19

Antifungal, Antiviral, and Immunizing Agents

Chapter Outline

Objectives
Key Terms
Introduction
Antifungal Agents
Antiviral Agents
Antiretroviral Agents
Immunization
Self-Assessment
Web Activity

Objectives

Upon completion of this chapter, you should be able to

- Define the key terms

- State the actions, uses, contraindications, adverse reactions, dosages, routes, nursing considerations, and clients' instruction of selected antifungal and antiviral agents

- Describe three classifications of antiretroviral drugs

- Describe highly active antiretroviral therapy (HAART)

- Differentiate between active and passive immunization

- State the general recommendations of immunization

- Describe the conditions when a live, attenuated-virus vaccine should not be given

- Define *vaccine, toxoid, immune globulin, specific immune globulin,* and *antitoxin*

- State who should be immunized against vaccine-preventable diseases

- Describe the immunization schedule given in this chapter

- Complete the Spot Check on childhood immunizations

- Complete the Self-Assessment

- Visit indicated Web sites for additional information on antifungal, antiviral, and immunizing agents

Key Terms

active immunization
fungi
human immunodeficiency
 virus (HIV)
immunity

immunization
passive
 immunization
virus

INTRODUCTION

Viruses are parasitic in nature and are minute organisms that may invade normal cells and cause disease. They depend upon the invaded cells for nutrition, metabolism, and reproduction. To date, over 300 viruses have been isolated from animal hosts. Many of these viruses are considered to be harmless, but others are the cause of approximately half of all infectious diseases. The common cold (coryza), smallpox, yellow fever, most childhood diseases, herpes, influenza, Epstein-Barr syndrome, rabies, hepatitis B, and AIDS (acquired immunodeficiency syndrome) are virus infections.

Fungi are plant-like organisms that also depend upon a host for their existence. These organisms, which include molds and yeasts, may be parasitic, or grow in dead and decaying organic matter. Many forms of fungi are pathogenic to plants and animals, causing such diseases as histoplasmosis, *Candida* infections, cryptococcosis, athlete's foot, tinea, blastomycosis, coccidioidomycosis, and aspergillosis.

ANTIFUNGAL AGENTS

Antifungal agents are synthetic drugs that destroy or inhibit the growth of fungi. They are also effective against yeast (Candida).

Characteristics and Uses

Actions

Antifungal agents act by exerting fungistatic or fungicidal action on both resting and growing cells. They bind to certain sterols of the cell membrane, thus allowing leakage of essential intracellular compounds that results in death of the cell. They are not effective against bacteria, rickettsiae, or viruses.

Uses

Antifungal agents are used for systemic, skin, and mucous membrane fungal infections. Some diseases for which a physician may prescribe an antifungal agent are histoplasmosis, Candida infections of the skin, mucous membrane, intestines, and vagina, cryptococcosis, athlete's foot, tinea (ringworm) infections, blastomycosis, coccidioidomycosis, and aspergillosis.

Contraindications

Hypersensitivity to antifungal agents. Contraindicated in clients with bone marrow depression or renal function impairment. Safe use of some agents during pregnancy and lactation has not been established.

Adverse Reactions

Nausea, vomiting, diarrhea, headache, vertigo, muscle pain, tinnitus, anemia, leukopenia, and hypersensitive reactions such as pruritus, urticaria, rash, fever, and anaphylaxis.

Dosage and Route

The dosage and route of administration is determined by the physician. See Table 19-1 for selected antifungal agents.

Nursing Considerations

Observe the client for any signs of hypersensitivity. Care should be exercised when inserting an antifungal agent intravaginally. To prevent possible spread of the disease, wear latex gloves. When applying a cream, lotion or ointment to the candidal lesions, wear latex gloves, use an appropriate applicator, and do not contaminate the medication container. The applicator must be thoroughly washed, if not disposable, before and after use.

Clients' Instruction

Instruct the client in the importance of following the prescribed medication regimen. Clients with vaginal infections should also be advised that fungus or yeast infections are easily spread. Some physicians prefer that the client refrain from sexual intercourse while the infection is being treated. Inform the client that her infection can be spread through sexual intercourse and that her partner could become infected, and then possibly reinfect her. It is highly recommended that a protective device, such as a condom, be used during sexual intercourse and that the client and her partner be treated at the same time to prevent the possibility of reinfection.

Female clients with Candida infections should be instructed in correct handwashing procedure, proper personal hygiene (drying the genital area after bathing, showering, or swimming; wiping from front to back after a bowel movement so that the organisms from the rectum will not be spread to the vagina), and wearing natural (cotton) underclothes. They should also avoid using heavily fragranced products such as soaps, bubble baths, toilet paper, and feminine hygiene sprays, as these products contain ingredients that can worsen any local irritation.

TABLE 19-1   SELECTED ANTIFUNGAL AGENTS

Medication	Usual Dosage	Adverse Reactions
amphotericin B (Fungizone)	*Cream, lotion, ointment:* applied liberally to the candidal lesions 2–4 times a day	No evidence of systemic toxicity; may have a "drying" effect on some skin, local irritation, erythema, pruritus or burning
clotrimazole (Lotrimin) (Mycelex)	*Cream, lotion, solution:* Gently massage sufficient medication into the affected and surrounding skin areas twice a day, in the morning and evening.	Erythema, stinging, blistering, peeling, edema, pruritus, urticaria, burning and general irritation of the skin
fluconazole (Diflucan)	*Oral:* 200 mg on the first day, then 100 mg once a day for 2–4 weeks *IV:* maximum rate of 200 mg/hour given as a continuous infusion	Nausea, headache, skin rash, vomiting, abdominal pain, diarrhea
flucytosine (Ancobon)	*Oral:* 50–150 mg/kg/day at 6-hour intervals	Nausea, vomiting, diarrhea, rash, anemia, leukopenia, thrombopenia, elevated hepatic enzymes

griseofulvin (Grifulvin V)	*Oral: Adults:* 500 mg daily dose
	  Children: 5 mg/lb body weight, per day:
	    30–50 lb 125–250 mg,
	    over 50 lb 250–500 mg
		Hypersensitivity, skin rashes, urticaria, oral thrush, nausea, vomiting, epigastric distress, diarrhea, headache, fatigue, dizziness

itraconazole (Sporanox)	*Oral:* 2–5 mg/kg/day with maximum dose of 100–400 mg/day	Nausea, vomiting, headache, increased liver transaminase, hypokalemia

ketoconazole (Nizoral)	*Oral: Adults:* 200 mg (1 tab);
	    400 mg (2 tab) once daily
	  Children: Over 2 years of age:
	    3.3–6.6 mg/kg daily dose
		Anaphylaxis (rare cases), hypersensitivity, nausea, vomiting, abdominal pain, pruritus, headache, fever, diarrhea, gynecomastia, impotence, oligospermia

miconazole nitrate (Monistat) (See Figure 19-1)	*Vaginal Suppository:* one 100 mg suppository inserted intravaginally once daily at bedtime for 7 nights *Vaginal Cream:* 1 full applicator intravaginally once daily at bedtime for 7 nights	Vulvovaginal burning, itching or irritation, cramping, headache, hives, skin rash
nystatin (Mycostatin)	*Oral:* 500,000–1,000,000 units (1–2 tabs) tid *Suspension:* *Adults and Children:* 4–6 ml qid (400,000–600,000 units) *Infants:* 2 ml qid (200,000 units) *Vaginal Tabs:* 100,000 units (1 tab) daily for 2 weeks	Virtually nontoxic—large oral doses have occasionally produced diarrhea, nausea, and vomiting

terbinafine (Lamisil)	*Oral:* Fingernail onychomycosis:
	  250 mg tab, once daily for 6 weeks
	  Toenail onychomycosis: 250 mg tab, once daily for 12 weeks
		Diarrhea, dyspepsia, abdominal pain, liver test abnormalities, rash, urticaria, pruritus, taste disturbances

terconazole (Terazol)	*Vaginal Cream:* 1 applicatorful (5 g) of 0.4% cream at bedtime for 7 nights *Vaginal Suppository:* 1 suppository (80 mg) at bedtime for 3 nights	Headache, local irritation, sensitization, vulvovaginal burning, hypersensitivity reactions, body pain

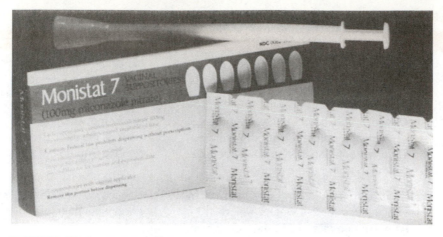

FIGURE 19-1   MONISTAT™ 7 *(Courtesy of Ortho Pharmaceutical Corporation)*

ANTIVIRAL AGENTS

Antiviral agents are synthetic drugs that have been developed to combat specific viral diseases. Viruses are responsible for many diseases, such as the common cold (coryza), influenza, genital herpes, herpes zoster, and acquired immunodeficiency syndrome (AIDS). In the United States, several antiviral drugs are employed in the treatment of specific viral diseases. Details on these drugs follow. (*Note:* The generic drug name is listed first, followed by the trade name in parentheses.)

Acyclovir (Zovirax)

Actions

Interferes with viral DNA synthesis.

Uses

Treatment for initial episodes and the management of recurrent episodes of genital herpes in certain clients. It is not a cure for genital herpes.

Contraindications

In clients who develop hypersensitivity or intolerance to the components of the formulation. Not used during pregnancy. Cautious use during lactation.

Adverse Reactions

Nausea, vomiting, diarrhea, dizziness, anorexia, fatigue, edema, skin rash, leg pain, inguinal adenopathy, confusion, and headache.

Dosage and Route

For genital herpes:

Oral: Initial: 200 mg cap every 4 hours for total of 5 caps daily for 10 days (total of 50 caps)

Recurrent disease: one 200 mg cap tid for up to 6 months

Ointment: Apply sufficient quantity to adequately cover all lesions every 3 hours, 6 times a day for 7 days.

> **Safety Precaution:** A finger cot or latex glove should be used when applying Zovirax to prevent autoinoculation of other body sites and transmission of infection to other persons.

Nursing Considerations

The nurse should observe the client for any signs of hypersensitivity, nausea, and vomiting. Care should be exercised when applying Zovirax to lesions.

Clients' Instruction

The client should be informed that genital herpes is a sexually transmitted disease, and that intercourse should be avoided when lesions are visible because of the risk of infecting one's sexual partner. Advise the female client to contact her physician if sufficient relief is not obtained, if there are any adverse reactions, if she becomes pregnant or plans to become pregnant, or if she has any questions.

Famciclovir (Famvir)

Actions

Prevents viral replication by inhibition of DNA synthesis.

Uses

Indicated for the management of acute herpes zoster (shingles) and recurrent herpes genitalis in immunocompetent clients.

Contraindications

In clients with known hypersensitivity to the product.

Adverse Reactions

Headache, nausea, diarrhea, and fatigue.

Dosage and Route

Herpes zoster: 500 mg every 8 hours for 7 days; herpes genitalis: 125 mg twice daily for 5 days. See Figure 19-2.

Nursing Considerations

For best results treatment should begin as soon as herpes zoster is diagnosed. Treatment is most effective if started within 48 hours of rash onset. In clients with reduced renal function, dosage reduction is recommended.

Clients' Instruction

Famvir may be taken without regard to meals. Advise client to report any adverse reactions to his/her physician.

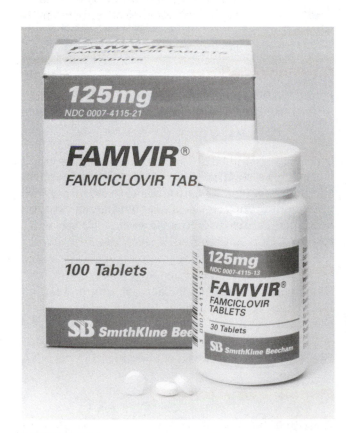

FIGURE 19-2   FAMVIR® (FAMCICLOVIR) *(Courtesy of SmithKline Beecham)*

Amantadine Hydrochloride (Symmetrel)

Actions

Antiviral activity against influenza A is not completely understood. The mode of action appears to be prevention of the release of infectious viral nucleic acid into the host cell.

Uses

Influenza A virus respiratory tract illness prevention and treatment. Also used in Parkinson's disease/syndrome and drug-induced extrapyramidal reactions.

Contraindications

In clients with known hypersensitivity to the drug. Not used during pregnancy. Cautious use during lactation.

Adverse Reactions

Depression, congestive heart failure, orthostatic hypotensive episodes, psychosis, urinary retention, drowsiness, and dizziness.

Dosage and Route

For influenza A virus:

Oral: Adults: 200 mg daily dose (two 100 mg caps) or 4 tsp of syrup

Children: 1–9 years of age: 100 mg twice a day (one 100 mg cap) or 2 tsp bid

Nursing Considerations

Medication should be taken after meals. Client assessment includes observing for signs of hypersensitivity and adverse reactions.

Clients' Instruction

Instruct the client not to stand or change positions too quickly, as orthostatic hypotensive episodes may occur. With these episodes the client would feel faint as the blood pressure drops suddenly.

Rimantadine (Flumadine)

Actions

Antiviral activity against influenza A virus.

Uses

In adults, rimantadine is indicated for the prevention and treatment of illness caused by various strains of influenza A virus. In children, it is only approved for prevention.

Contraindications

Known hypersensitivity to rimantadine or other drugs of the adamantane class such as amantadine (Symadine, Symmetrel).

Adverse Reactions

Nausea, vomiting, nervousness, insomnia, and dizziness.

Dosage and Route

Oral: Adults: 100 mg twice a day

For geriatric clients or anyone with kidney failure or severe liver problems, the dose is reduced to 100 mg once a day.

Children: 10 years or older 100 mg twice a day

1–9 years: 5 mg/kg, but not exceeding 150 mg

Nursing Considerations

For prevention, one should start on medication as early as possible after a community outbreak of influenza A. For additional prophylaxis after vaccination, medication may be taken for 2 to 4 weeks.

Clients' Instruction

Advise client to report any adverse reactions to his/her physician. Inform the geriatric client that he/she may experience gastrointestinal problems, insomnia, and nervousness.

Trifluridine (Viroptic ophthalmic solution 1%)

Actions

Antiviral activity against herpes simplex virus, types 1 and 2 and vaccinia virus. Some strains of *Adenovirus* are also inhibited in vitro.

Uses

Topical treatment of epithelial keratitis caused by herpes simplex virus, types 1 and 2. Treatment of primary keratoconjunctivitis.

Contraindications

In clients who develop hypersensitivity reactions or chemical intolerance to trifluridine. Not used during pregnancy or lactation.

Adverse Reactions

Mild burning or stinging upon instillation; hypersensitivity.

Dosage and Route

Ophthalmic: Instill 1 drop onto cornea of affected eye every 2 hours. Maximum daily dose 9 drops until corneal ulcer has completely re-epithelialized.

Nursing Considerations

Use aseptic technique when instilling eye drops.

Clients' Instruction

Instruct the client to follow the recommended dosage and not to exceed the number of drops prescribed. Aseptic technique should be used when instilling eye drops. Instruct the client in the proper instillation of eye drops.

Ribavirin (Virazole)

Actions

Antiviral inhibitory activity in vitro against respiratory syncytial virus, influenza virus, and herpes simplex virus. The mechanism of action is unknown.

Uses

Ribavirin aerosol is indicated in the treatment of carefully selected hospitalized infants and young children with severe lower respiratory tract infections due to respiratory syncytial virus (RSV).

Contraindications

In women or girls who are or may become pregnant during exposure to the drug. Ribavirin may cause fetal harm.

Adverse Reactions

Chronic obstructive lung disease, dyspnea, chest soreness, worsening of respiratory status, bacterial pneumonia, pneumothorax, apnea, ventilator dependence, cardiac arrest, hypotension, and digitalis toxicity.

Dosage and Route

Ribavirin is lyophilized for aerosol administration. Before use, read the Viratek Small Particle Aerosol Generator (SPAG) Model SPAG-2 Operations Manual thoroughly for small-particle aerosol generator operating instructions.

Penciclovir (Denavir)

Actions

Antiviral activity against herpes viruses type 1 (HSV-1) and type 2 (HSV-2). Penciclovir penetrates into the infected cells to block the multiplying of the virus that causes the cold sore.

Uses

In adults, penciclovir cream is indicated for the treatment of recurrent herpes labialis (cold sores).

Contraindications

Contraindicated in clients with known hypersensitivity to any of the components of the product.

Adverse Reactions

Headache, application site reaction, hypesthesia, local anesthesia, taste perversion, pruritus, pain, rash, allergic reaction.

Dosage and Route

Apply every 2 hours during waking hours for a period of 4 days. Treatment should be started as early as possible (during the prodrome or when lesions appear).

Nursing Considerations

Denavir should be used only on herpes labialis on the lips and face. It is not indicated for internal use on mucous membranes inside the mouth, nose, genital or rectal areas.

Clients' Instruction

Instruct client to wash hands thoroughly before application and to avoid application in or near the eyes, since it may cause irritation.

Oseltamivir Phosphate (Tamiflu)

Actions

Antiviral activity against influenza A and B viruses.

Uses

In adults who have been symptomatic for no more than 2 days, oseltamivir is indicated for the treatment of uncomplicated acute illness due to influenza A or B infection.

Contraindications

Contraindicated in clients with known hypersensitivity to any of the components of the product.

Adverse Reactions

Nausea and vomiting.

Dosage and Route

The recommended oral dose is 75 mg twice daily for 5 days. Treatment should begin within 2 days of onset of symptoms of influenza. It may be taken with or without food. However, when taken with food, tolerability may be enhanced in some clients.

Nursing Considerations

Tamiflu is not a substitute for a flu shot. Clients should continue receiving an annual flu shot according to guidelines on immunization practices.

Clients' Instruction

Instruct client to begin treatment with Tamiflu as soon as flu symptoms first appear. Inform the client to take any missed doses as soon as he/she remembers, except if it is within 2 hours of the next scheduled dose, and then continue to take Tamiflu at the prescribed times.

Zanamivir (Relenza)

Actions

Antiviral activity against influenza A and B viruses.

Uses

In adults and adolescents 12 years and older who have been symptomatic for no more than 2 days, zanamivir is indicated for the treatment of uncomplicated acute illness due to influenza virus A or B infection.

Contraindications

Contraindicated in clients with known hypersensitivity to any of the components of the product.

Adverse Reactions

Diarrhea, nausea, nasal signs and symptoms, headache.

Dosage and Route

Taken twice daily for 5 days. Clients inhale Relenza orally using a handheld breath-activated device called a Diskhaler. When the client takes a breath, Relenza is delivered directly to the surface of the respiratory tract, the primary site of infection where the influenza virus replicates.

Nursing Considerations

Relenza is not a substitute for a flu shot. Clients should continue receiving an annual flu shot according to guidelines on immunization practices.

Clients' Instruction

Instruct client to begin treatment with Relenza as soon as possible from the first appearance of flu symptoms. Instruct the client in the proper use of the inhaler, including a demonstration whenever possible.

ANTIRETROVIRAL AGENTS

The **human immunodeficiency virus (HIV)** is a retrovirus that causes acquired immunodeficiency syndrome (AIDS). Two human immunodeficiency viruses: HIV-1 and HIV-2, have been identified. Both cause AIDS, but infection with HIV-2 has been primarily limited to Africa and Europe.

The human immunodeficiency virus (HIV) uses an enzyme called reverse transcriptase to convert its viral RNA to viral DNA, using the host cell DNA to do so. The viral DNA then becomes incorporated into the host cell DNA. The change in DNA prevents the cell from functioning normally; it can only create more virus. Eventually, the cell ruptures, releasing more HIV into the bloodstream.

Since 1987 the Food and Drug Administration has approved a number of antiretroviral drugs. The first group of drugs used to treat HIV infection, nucleoside reverse transcriptase inhibitors (NRTIs), interrupt an early stage of virus replication. Drugs in this class may slow the spread of HIV infection in the body and delay the onset of opportunistic infections. They do not prevent transmission of HIV to other individuals.

- Nucleoside reverse transcriptase inhibitors (NRTIs) include zidovudine (Retrovir or AZT); didanosine (Videx or ddI, zalcitabine (HIVID or ddC), stavudine (Zerit), lamivudine (Epivir or 3TC), and abacavir (Ziagen). Combivir is a combination drug that contains both lamivudine and zidovudine. See Table 19-2.

The second class of drugs used in the treatment of HIV infection are called nonnucleoside reverse transcriptase inhibitors (NNRTIs). These drugs inhibit HIV production by binding directly to reverse transcriptase and preventing the conversion of RNA to DNA.

- Nonnucleoside reverse transcriptase inhibitors (NNRTIs) include nevirapine (Viramune), delavirdine (Rescriptor), and efavirenz (Sustiva). See Table 19-3.

The third class of drugs used in the treatment of HIV infection are protease inhibitors (PIs). These drugs interrupt virus replication at a later step in its life cycle. Once the HIV DNA enters the nucleus of the CD4+T cell and inserts itself into the cell's DNA, it instructs the cell to make many copies of the original virus. Protease inhibitors prevent HIV from being successfully assembled and released from infected CD4+T cells.

- Protease inhibitors (PIs) include saquinavir (Invirase, Fortovase), ritonavir (Norvir), indinavir (Crixivan), nelfinavir (Viracept), and amprenavir (Agenerase). See Table 19-4.

Another treatment approach is highly active antiretroviral therapy (HAART). This is a combination of three drugs that include two nucleoside analogues and one protease inhibitor.

So far, the combination HAART treatment is the closest thing medical science has to an effective therapy. The key to its success in some clients lies

TABLE 19-2 NUCLEOSIDE REVERSE TRANSCRIPTASE INHIBITORS

Medication	Usual Dosage	Adverse Reactions
abacavir (Ziagen)	300 mg twice daily	Hypersensitivity reaction, malaise, fever, rash, GI disturbances
didanosine, ddI (Videx)	400 mg once daily or 200 mg twice daily on empty stomach	Peripheral neuropathy, pancreatitis
lamivudine, 3TC (Epivir)	150 mg twice daily	Nausea, headache, fatigue, diarrhea, neuropathy, neutropenia, anemia
stavudine (Zerit)	40 mg twice daily	Peripheral neuropathy, pancreatitis
zalcitabine, ddC (Hivid)	0.75 mg 3 times daily	Peripheral neuropathy, pancreatitis, oral ulcers
zidovudine, AZT (Retrovir)	100 mg every 4 hours	Nausea, headache, fatigue, anemia, neutropenia, neuropathy, myopathy
zidovudine/lamivudine (Combivir)	1 tablet twice daily	Nausea, headache, fatigue, diarrhea, neuropathy, neutropenia, anemia

TABLE 19-3 NONNUCLEOSIDE REVERSE TRANSCRIPTASE INHIBITORS

Medication	Usual Dosage	Adverse Reactions
delavirdine (Rescriptor)	400 mg 3 times daily	Transient rash
efavirenz (Sustiva)	600 mg once daily initially at bedtime	Initial dizziness, insomnia, transient rash
nevirapine (Viramune)	200 mg once daily for 2 weeks, then 200 mg twice daily	Transient rash, hepatitis

in the ability of the drug combination to disrupt HIV at different stages in its replication. Reverse transcriptase inhibitors, which usually make up two drugs in the HAART regimen, restrain an enzyme crucial to an early stage of HIV duplication. Protease inhibitors hold back another enzyme that functions near the end of the HIV replication process. The combination can be prescribed to those newly infected with the virus, as well as AIDS clients. Although HAART treatment is effective, there are some concerns that experts see as drawbacks to the therapy, including the following:

- Treatment is not a cure for AIDS.
- Following successful treatment, the HIV virus may not be detectable in the blood. Experts generally feel that the virus is still present, lurking in hiding spots such as the lymph nodes, brain, testes, and retina.

- Due to the improved sense of well-being and the incorrect belief that lower viral load means the virus will not be transmitted, there has been a lapse in certain prevention practices. This is dangerous because infected people, even with diminished viral counts, can spread the virus.

- Combination therapy is very expensive and requires a more complicated treatment regimen. If not taken on a strict regimen, protease inhibitors can result in the emergence of HIV strains that are resistant to treatment.

TABLE 19-4 PROTEASE INHIBITORS

Medication	Usual Dosage	Adverse Reactions
amprenavir (Agenerase)	1200 mg twice daily with or without food	Rash, diarrhea, nausea, vomiting, taste disorders, pruritus, depression
indinavir (Crixivan)	800 mg every 8 hours on empty stomach or with snack containing <2 g of fat	Kidney stones in 6–8%; good hydration essential. Occasional nausea and GI upset
nelfinavir (Viracept)	750 mg 3 times daily with food	Diarrhea common, which may respond to Ultrase MT20 enzyme preparations or calcium supplementation; occasional nausea
ritonavir (Norvir)	600 mg twice daily; start with 300 mg twice daily and increase to full dose over 10 days	Nausea, diarrhea, numb lips for up to 5 weeks; occasional hepatitis
saquinavir hard gel cap (Invirase)	600 mg 3 times daily with fatty meals	Diarrhea, abdominal discomfort, nausea
saquinavir soft gel cap (Fortovase)	1200 mg 3 times daily with taken within 2 hours of a full meal—fat-containing food (>28 g)	Diarrhea, abdominal discomfort, nausea

- Viral load can "rebound" to high levels if clients discontinue part or all of the triple therapy regimen.
- AIDS treatment may interact with many commonly prescribed drugs.
- AIDS drugs may prompt onset of diabetes or a worsening of existing diabetes and hyperglycemia, along with increased bleeding in people with hemophilia types A or B.
- Some clients on triple therapy have experienced a type of weight redistribution where face and limbs become thin while the breasts, stomach, or neck enlarges.
- Clients who experience fat redistribution could increase their risk for cardiovascular complications such as strokes or heart attacks.

Antiretroviral drugs do not cure people of HIV infection or AIDS. They all have adverse reactions that can be severe. Each client must be monitored carefully, and blood tests should be done regularly to watch for signs of neutropenia and anemia. Triglycerides should be monitored to look for signs of pancreatitis (abdominal pain, nausea, vomiting); this is particularly important in children taking 3TC. Since peripheral neuropathy may occur, the client should be taught to report tingling, weakness, numbness, and possible pain in the extremities. If these signs occur, the drug should be stopped immediately.

Antiretroviral drugs are intended for oral administration and the client must take the medication exactly as prescribed. This means dosing around the clock, even though it may interrupt normal sleep. Advise clients not to share the medication and not to exceed the recommended dose.

Since FDA approval of newer antiretroviral drugs, the number of deaths from AIDS has decreased dramatically in the United States. Between 1996 and 1997, 44 percent fewer AIDS clients died, and the rate of AIDS hospitalizations and complications also declined. As more clients take advantage of the new combination therapies, there is hope that all clients with AIDS will have the chance to live longer and healthier lives.

IMMUNIZATION

Immunity is the state of being protected from or resistant to a particular disease due to the development of antibodies. The mechanisms of immunity involve an *antigen-antibody* response. When an antigen enters the body, complex activities are set into motion. These activities involve chemical and mechanical forces that defend and protect the body's cells and tissues. Antibodies are formed and released from plasma cells, after which they enter the body fluids where they react with the invading antigen.

The mechanisms of immunity are basic to the body's ability to

- Protect itself against specific infectious microorganisms
- Defend body cells and tissues that are invaded by foreign substances
- Accept or reject another's blood or organ (blood transfusion or organ transplant)
- Protect itself against cancer and immunodeficiency disease

Note: The following portion of this unit is adapted from materials printed by the U.S. Department of Health and Human Services, Public Health Service, Centers for Disease Control and Prevention, Atlanta, GA 30333.

Immunization is the process of inducing or providing immunity artificially by administering an immunobiologic (immunizing agent). Immunization can be active or passive.

- **Active immunization** denotes the production of antibodies in response to the administration of a vaccine or toxoid.
- **Passive immunization** denotes the provision of temporary immunity by the administration of preformed antitoxins or antibodies. Three types of immunobiologics are used for passive immunization.
  1. Pooled human IG (immune globulin)
  2. Specific IG preparations
  3. Antitoxin

General Recommendation for Immunization

Recommendations for immunization of infants, children, and adults are based on facts about immunobiologics and scientific knowledge about the principles of active and passive immunization, and on judgments by public health officials and specialists in clinical and preventive medicine. Benefits and risks are associated with the use of all products—no vaccine is completely safe or completely effective. The benefits range from partial to complete protection from the consequences of disease, and the risks range from common, trivial, and inconvenient side effects to rare, severe, and life-threatening conditions.

Thus, recommendations on immunization practices balance scientific evidence of benefits, costs, and risks to achieve optimal levels of protection against infectious or communicable diseases. These recommendations may apply only in the United States, as epidemiological circumstances and vaccines may differ in other countries.

Immunobiologics

The specific nature and content of immunobiologics may differ. When immunobiologics against the same infectious agents are produced by different manufacturers, active and inert ingredients among the various products may differ. Practitioners are urged to become familiar with the constituents of the products they use. The constituents of immunobiologics are explained here.

Suspending Fluid

This frequently is as simple as sterile water or saline, but it may be a complex fluid containing small amounts of proteins or other constituents derived from the medium, or biologic system in which the vaccine is produced (serum proteins, egg antigens, cell culture–derived antigens).

Preservatives, Stabilizers, Antibiotics

These components of vaccines are used to inhibit or prevent bacterial growth in viral culture or the final product, or to stabilize the antigen. They include such material as mercurials and specific antibiotics. Allergic reactions may occur if the recipient is sensitive to one of these additives.

Adjuvants

An aluminum compound is used in some vaccines to enhance the immune response to vaccines containing inactivated microorganisms or their products; for example, toxoids and hepatitis B virus vaccine. Vaccines with such adjuvants must be injected deeply in muscle masses, since subcutaneous or intracutaneous administration may cause local irritation, inflammation, granuloma formation, or necrosis.

Immunizing Agents

Immunobiologics include vaccines, toxoids, and antibody-containing preparations from human or animal donors, including globulins and antitoxins.

Vaccine

A suspension of attenuated live or killed microorganisms (bacteria, viruses, or rickettsiae), or fractions thereof, administered to induce immunity and thereby prevent infectious disease.

Toxoid

A modified bacterial toxin that has been rendered nontoxic but that retains the ability to stimulate the formation of antitoxin.

Immune Globulin (IG)

A sterile solution containing antibody from human blood. It is a 15–18 percent protein obtained by cold ethanol fractionation of large pools of blood plasma. It is primarily indicated for routine maintenance of certain immunodeficient persons, and for passive immunization against measles and hepatitis A.

Specific Immune Globulin

Special preparations obtained from donor pools preselected for a high antibody content against a specific disease. For example: Hepatitis B Immune Globulin (HBIG), Varicella Zoster Immune Globulin (VZIG), Rabies Immune Globulin (RIG), Tetanus Immune Globulin (TIG), and RhoGam.

Antitoxin

A solution of antibodies derived from the serum of animals immunized with specific antigens (diphtheria, tetanus) used to achieve passive immunity or to effect a treatment. May produce many adverse effects, some life-threatening. Use with discretion (e.g., black widow spider antitoxin and rattlesnake antitoxin).

Route and Site Selection

The route and selection of site for each immunobiologic is predetermined; therefore, those administering injectable immunobiologics must follow the recommended route and site.

Route

There is a recommended route of administration for each immunobiologic. To avoid unnecessary local or systemic effects and/or to insure optimal efficacy, the practitioner should not deviate from the recommended route of administration.

Site

Injectable immunobiologics should be administered in an area where there is minimal opportunity for local, neural, vascular, or tissue injury. Subcutaneous injections are usually administered into the thigh of infants and in the deltoid area of older children and adults. Intradermal injections are generally given on the volar surface of the forearms, except for human diploid cell rabies vaccine, where reactions are less severe when given in the deltoid area.

Intramuscular Injections

Preferred sites for intramuscular injections are the anterolateral aspect of the upper thigh and the deltoid muscle of the upper arm. In most infants, the anterolateral aspect of the thigh provides the largest muscle mass and therefore is the preferred site. In older children, the deltoid mass is of sufficient size for intramuscular injection. An individual decision must be made for each child, based on the volume of the injected material and the size of the muscle into which it is to be injected. In adults, the deltoid is generally used for routine intramuscular vaccine administration.

The upper, outer quadrant of the gluteal region should be used only for the largest volumes of injection or when multiple doses need to be given, such as when large doses of IG must be administered. The site selected should be well into the upper, outer mass of the gluteus maximus and away from the central region of the buttocks.

Hypersensitivity to Vaccine Components

Vaccine antigens produced in systems or with substrates containing allergenic substances (e.g., antigens derived from growing microorganisms in embryonated chicken eggs) may cause hypersensitivity reactions. These reactions may include anaphylaxis when the final vaccine contains a substantial amount of the allergen. Yellow fever vaccine is such an antigen. Vaccines with such characteristics should not be given to persons with known hypersensitivity to components of the substrates.

Screening persons by history of ability or inability to eat eggs without adverse effects is a reasonable way to identify those possibly at risk from receiving measles, mumps, and influenza vaccine. Individuals with anaphylactic hypersensitivity to eggs (hives, swelling of the mouth and throat, difficulty breathing, hypotension, or shock) should not be given these vaccines.

Those administering vaccines should carefully review the information provided with the package insert and ascertain whether the client is hypersensitive to any of its components. The physician must carefully evaluate each client with known hypersensitivity before administering the vaccine.

Altered Immunocompetence

Virus replication after administration of live attenuated-virus vaccines may be enhanced in persons with immunodeficiency diseases, and in those with suppressed capability for immune response, as oc-

curs with leukemia, lymphoma, generalized malignancy, or therapy with corticosteroids, alkylating agents, antimetabolites, or radiation. Clients with such conditions should not be given live attenuated-virus vaccines. Also, because of the possibility of familial immunodeficiency, live attenuated-virus vaccines should not be given to a member of a household in which there is family history of congenital or hereditary immunodeficiency, until the immune competence of the potential recipient is known.

Severe Febrile Illnesses

Minor illnesses, such as mild upper respiratory infections, should not cause postponement of vaccine administration. However, immunization of persons with severe febrile illnesses should generally be deferred until they have recovered.

Immunization During Pregnancy

On the grounds of a theoretical risk to the developing fetus, live attenuated-virus vaccines are not generally given to pregnant women or to those likely to become pregnant within 3 months after receiving vaccine(s). With some of these vaccines, particularly rubella, measles, and mumps, pregnancy is a contraindication.

There is no convincing evidence of risk to the fetus from immunization of pregnant women using inactivated virus vaccines, bacterial vaccines, or toxoids. Tetanus and diphtheria toxoid (Td) should be given to inadequately immunized pregnant women because it affords protection against neonatal tetanus.

Adverse Events Following Immunization

Modern vaccines are extremely safe and effective, but not completely so. Adverse events following immunization have been reported with all vaccines. To improve knowledge about adverse reactions, all temporarily associated events severe enough to require the recipient to seek medical attention should be evaluated and reported in detail to local or state health officials and to the vaccine manufacturer.

Immunization Schedules

Immunization schedules are recommended by the CDC's Advisory Committee on Immunization Practices (ACIP), the American Academy of Pediatrics (AAP), and the American Academy of Family Physicians (AAFP). These schedules are updated on a regular basis and recommendations for an immunization may change yearly. Detailed recommendations about the use of vaccines are available from the manufacturers' package inserts, the current Red Book, or ACIP statements on specific vaccines.

> **Note:** When giving vaccines to infants and children, the nurse must get a signed consent from the parent or guardian. The nurse must also document on the client's record the lot number of the vaccine used.

The widespread and successful implementation of childhood immunization programs has greatly reduced the occurrence of many vaccine-preventable diseases. However, successful childhood immunization alone will not necessarily eliminate specific disease problems. A substantial proportion of the remaining morbidity and mortality from vaccine-preventable disease now occurs in older adolescents and adults. Persons who escaped natural infection or were not immunized with vaccines and toxoids against diphtheria, tetanus, measles, mumps, rubella, and poliomyelitis may be at risk of these diseases and their complications.

To further reduce the unnecessary occurrence of these vaccine-preventable diseases, all those who provide health care to older adolescents and adults should provide immunizations as a routine part of their practice. In addition, the epidemiology of other vaccine-preventable diseases (e.g., hepatitis B, rabies, influenza, and pneumococcal disease) indicates that individuals who have special health problems are at increased risk of these illnesses and should be immunized. Travelers to some countries may be at increased risk of exposure to vaccine-preventable diseases and should be immunized. Several factors need to be considered before any client is vaccinated. These include

- The susceptibility of the client
- The risk of exposure to the disease
- The risk from the disease
- The benefits and risks from the immunizing agent

Physicians should maintain detailed information about previous vaccinations received by each individual, including type of vaccination, date of receipt, and adverse events, if any, following vaccination. Information should also include the person's history of vaccine-preventable illnesses, occupation, and lifestyle. After the administration of any immunobiologic, the client should be given written documentation of its receipt and information on which vaccines or toxoids will be needed in the future.

The immunization schedule in Table 19-5 applies generally to individuals in the indicated groups. For more detailed information on immunobiologics, and before administering any immunizing agent, refer to an appropriate source of information regarding indications, side effects, adverse reactions, precautions, contraindications, dosages, and route of administration.

TABLE 19-5   IMMUNIZATIONS FOR CHILDREN AND ADULTS

Vaccine (Brand Name)	Route and Dosage	Schedule
Diphtheria, Tetanus Toxoids, and Acellular Pertussis Adsorbed (DTaP) Vaccine (Infanrix—see Figure 19-3)	IM: 0.5 ml	2, 4, 6, and 15–18 months Booster: 4–6 years
Haemophilus b Conjugate (Meningococcal Protein Conjugate) Liquid Vaccine (PedvaxHIB—see Figures 19-4, 19-5, and 19-6)	IM: 0.5 ml	Given in a 2-dose primary regimen before 12 months of age, usually at 2 and 4 months Booster: 12–15 months of age but not earlier than 2 months after the second dose
Haemophilus b Conjugate (Meningococcal Protein Conjugate) and Hepatitis B (Recombinant) Vaccine (COMVAX—see Figures 19-7, 19-8, and 19-9)	IM: 0.5 ml	2, 4, and 12–15 months of age

(continued)

TABLE 19-5 IMMUNIZATIONS FOR CHILDREN AND ADULTS (*Continued*)

Vaccine (Brand Name)	Route and Dosage	Schedule
Poliovirus-IPV (inactivated poliovirus) Vaccine	SC: 0.5 ml	2, 4, 6 and 15–18 months Booster: 4–6 years
Measles, Mumps, and Rubella Virus Vaccine Live (M-M-R II) (See Figures 19-10, 19-11, and 19-12)	SC: 0.5 ml	Primary: 12–15 months Booster: 4–6 years

Hepatitis B Vaccine (Recombinant) (Recombivax HB—see Figures 19-13 through 19-17)	Infants, Children and Adolescents 0–19 years
	  IM: 5 mcg (0.5 ml)
	Adults: 20 years+
	  IM: 10 mcg (1 ml)
	Adolescents 11–15 years
	  IM: 10 mcg (1 ml)
	
	Predialysis and Dialysis Clients
	  IM: 40 mcg (1 ml)
		Regimen consists of 3 doses:
		initial dose, then 1 month later, and then 6 months from initial dose
		
		Regimen consists of 2 doses:
		initial dose, then second dose 4–6 months later
		Regimen consists of 3 doses:
		initial dose, then 1 month later, and then 6 months from initial dose

Hepatitis B Vaccine (Recombinant) (Engerix-B—see Figure 19-18)	Pediatric/Adolescents
	  IM: 10 mcg (0.5 ml)
	Adults
	  IM: 20 mcg (1 ml)
		Regimen consists of 3 doses:
		initial dose, then 1 month later, and then 6 months from initial dose

Hepatitis A Vaccine (Inactivated) (VAQTA—see Figures 19-19 through 19-22)	Pediatric/Adolescents
	  IM: 25 U (0.5 ml)
	Adults
	  IM: 50 U (1 ml)
		Single dose at elected date
		Booster: 6–18 months later
		Single dose at elected date
		Booster: 6 months later

Hepatitis A Vaccine, Inactivated (HAVRIX—see Figure 19-23)	Children and Adolescents 2–18 years
	  IM: 360 EL. U (0.5 ml)
	
	Adults
	  IM: 1440 EL. U (1 ml)
		Regimen consists of 2 doses:
		second dose given 1 month after primary dose
		Booster: 6–12 months after primary dose
		Regimen consists of 1 dose.
		Booster: 6–12 months after primary dose

Pneumococcal Vaccine Polyvalent (PNEUMOVAX 23—see Figures 19-24 through 19-27)	Children and Adults IM: 0.5 ml	Single dose given to high-risk children over 2 years of age, all high-risk adults, and adults at age 50 and again at age 65
Pneumococcal 7-valent Conjugate Vaccine (Prevnar)	Infants and Toddlers IM: 0.5 ml	Regimen consists of 3 doses given at approximately 2-month intervals, followed by a fourth dose at 12–15 months of age. The customary age for the first dose is 2 months of age, but it can be given as young as 6 weeks of age.

Varicella Virus Vaccine Live (VARIVAX—see Figures 19-28 through 19-29)	Children 12 months to 12 years
	  SC: 0.5 ml
	Adolescents and Adults
	  SC: 0.5 ml
		Single dose of 0.5 ml
		
		Regimen consists of 2 doses:
		primary dose and second dose 4–8 weeks later

(continued)

TABLE 19-5   *(Continued)*

Vaccine (Brand Name)	Route and Dosage	Schedule
Influenza Type A and Type B	Children 6 months or older and Adults IM: 0.5 ml	Given during the fall of the year, usually in early October. Single dose given to adults and children with chronic heart or lung disorders; clients in nursing homes or chronic care facilities; individuals with diabetes, kidney disease, and other chronic diseases. May be given as a preventive measure to those who wish to receive the vaccine.
Lyme Disease Vaccine (Recombinant) (LYMErix— see Figure 19-30)	15–70 years old IM: 0.5 ml (30 mcg)	Regimen consists of 3 doses given at 0, 1, and 12 months before the onset of Lyme disease season.

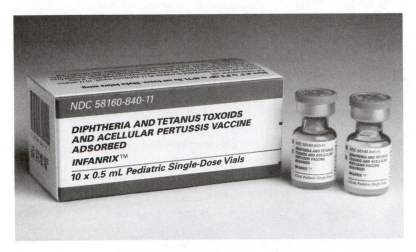

FIGURE 19-3   INFANRIX™ (DIPHTHERIA AND TETANUS TOXOIDS AND ACELLULAR PERTUSSIS VACCINE ADSORBED) *(Courtesy of SmithKline Beecham)*

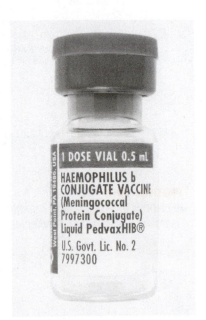

FIGURE 19-4   1 DOSE VIAL 0.5 ML HAEMOPHILUS B CONJUGATE VACCINE (MENINGOCOCCAL PROTEIN CONJUGATE) LIQUID PEDVAXHIB® *(Courtesy of Merck & Co., Inc.)*

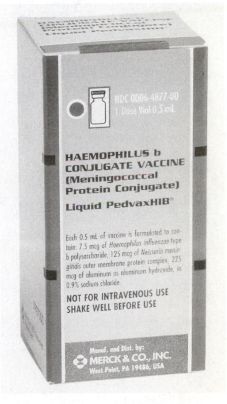

FIGURE 19-5   1 DOSE VIAL 0.5 ML PACKAGE HAEMOPHILUS B CONJUGATE VACCINE (MENINGOCOCCAL PROTEIN CONJUGATE) LIQUID PEDVAXHIB® *(Courtesy of Merck & Co., Inc.)*

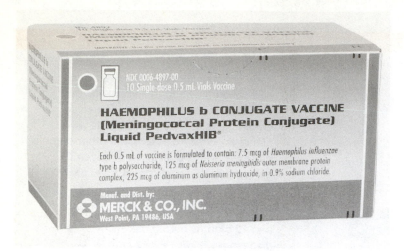

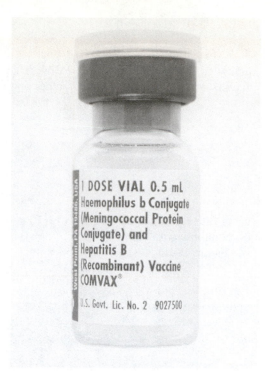

FIGURE 19-6 1 DOSE VIAL 0.5 ML—10 SINGLE DOSE PACKAGE
HAEMOPHILUS B CONJUGATE VACCINE (MENINGOCOCCAL PROTEIN CONJUGATE)
LIQUID PEDVAXHIB® *(Courtesy of Merck & Co., Inc.)*

FIGURE 19-7 1 DOSE VIAL 0.5 ML
HAEMOPHILUS B CONJUGATE (MENINGOCOCCAL
PROTEIN CONJUGATE) AND HEPATITIS B
(RECOMBINANT) VACCINE COMVAX® *(Courtesy of
Merck & Co., Inc.)*

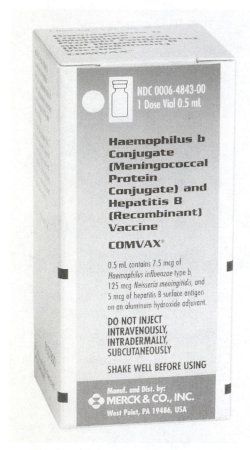

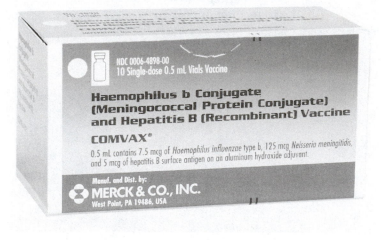

FIGURE 19-9 1 DOSE VIAL 0.5 ML—10 SINGLE DOSE PACKAGE
HAEMOPHILUS B CONJUGATE (MENINGOCOCCAL PROTEIN CONJUGATE) AND
HEPATITIS B (RECOMBINANT) VACCINE COMVAX® *(Courtesy of Merck & Co., Inc.)*

FIGURE 19-8 1 DOSE VIAL 0.5 ML PACKAGE
HAEMOPHILUS B CONJUGATE (MENINGOCOCCAL
PROTEIN CONJUGATE) AND HEPATITIS B
(RECOMBINANT) VACCINE COMVAX® *(Courtesy of
Merck & Co., Inc.)*

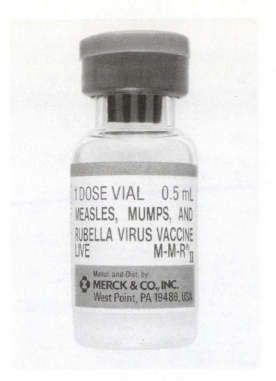

FIGURE 19-10   1 DOSE VIAL 0.5 ML MEASLES, MUMPS, AND RUBELLA VIRUS VACCINE LIVE M-M-R® II *(Courtesy of Merck & Co., Inc.)*

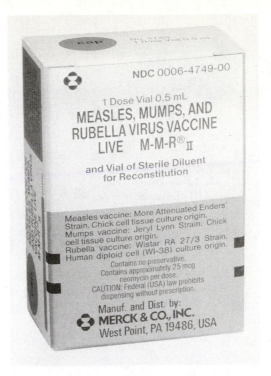

FIGURE 19-11   1 DOSE VIAL 0.5 ML PACKAGE MEASLES, MUMPS, AND RUBELLA VIRUS VACCINE LIVE M-M-R® II *(Courtesy of Merck & Co., Inc.)*

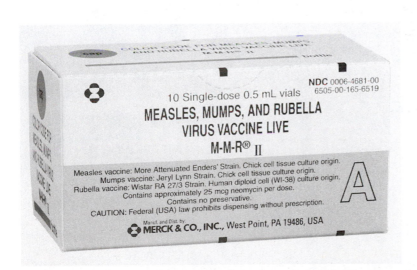

FIGURE 19-12   1 DOSE VIAL 0.5 ML–10 SINGLE DOSE PACKAGE MEASLES, MUMPS, AND RUBELLA VIRUS VACCINE LIVE M-M-R® II *(Courtesy of Merck & Co., Inc.)*

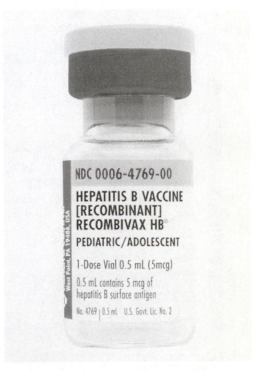

FIGURE 19-13   PEDIATRIC/ADOLESCENT 1 DOSE VIAL 0.5 ML (5 MCG) HEPATITIS B VACCINE (RECOMBINANT) RECOMBIVAX HB® *(Courtesy of Merck & Co., Inc.)*

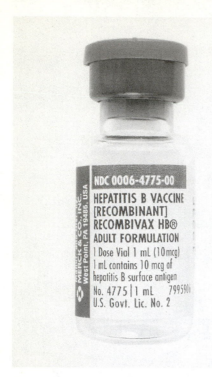

FIGURE 19-14 ADULT FORMULATION 1 DOSE VIAL 1 ML (10 MCG) HEPATITIS B VACCINE (RECOMBINANT) RECOMBIVAX HB® *(Courtesy of Merck & Co., Inc.)*

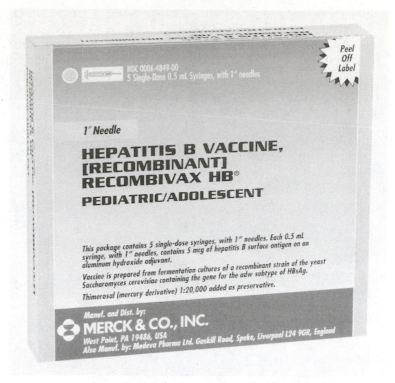

FIGURE 19-15 PEDIATRIC/ADOLESCENT 5 SINGLE-DOSE 0.5 ML SYRINGES WITH 1 IN. NEEDLES HEPATITIS B VACCINE (RECOMBINANT) RECOMBIVAX HB® *(Courtesy of Merck & Co., Inc.)*

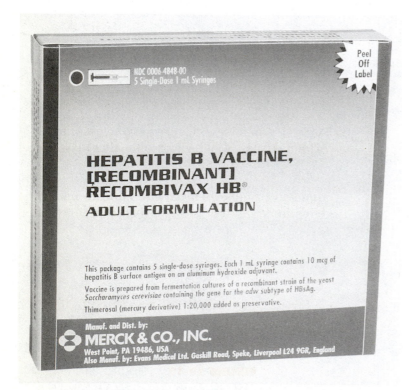

FIGURE 19-16 ADULT FORMULATION 5 SINGLE-DOSE 1 ML SYRINGES HEPATITIS B VACCINE (RECOMBINANT) RECOMBIVAX HB® *(Courtesy of Merck & Co., Inc.)*

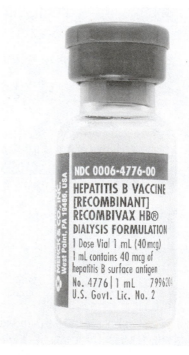

FIGURE 19-17 DIALYSIS FORMULATION 1 DOSE VIAL 1 ML (40 MCG) HEPATITIS B VACCINE (RECOMBINANT) RECOMBIVAX HB® *(Courtesy of Merck & Co., Inc.)*

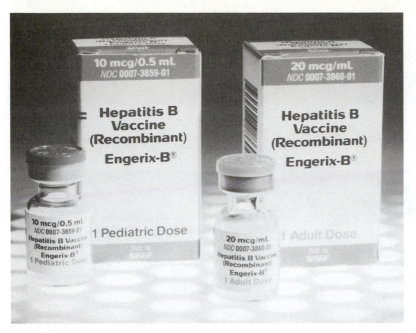

FIGURE 19-18   ENGERIX-B® HEPATITIS B VACCINE (RECOMBINANT) *(Courtesy of SmithKline Beecham)*

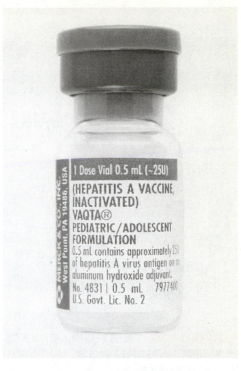

FIGURE 19-19   PEDIATRIC/ADOLESCENT FORMULATION 1 DOSE VIAL 0.5 ML HEPATITIS A VACCINE (INACTIVATED) VAQTA® *(Courtesy of Merck & Co., Inc.)*

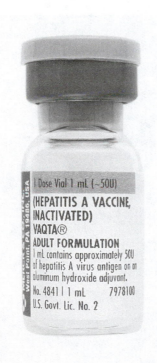

FIGURE 19-20   ADULT FORMULATION 1 DOSE VIAL 1 ML HEPATITIS A VACCINE (INACTIVATED) VAQTA® *(Courtesy of Merck & Co., Inc.)*

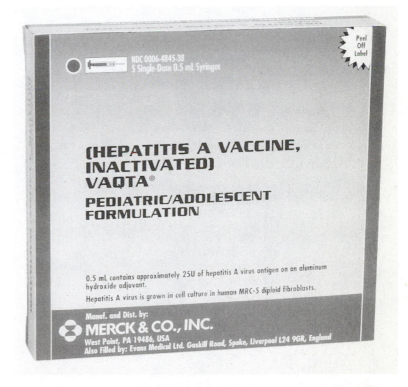

FIGURE 19-21   PEDIATRIC/ADOLESCENT FORMULATION 5 SINGLE-DOSE 0.5 ML SYRINGES HEPATITIS A VACCINE (INACTIVATED) VAQTA® *(Courtesy of Merck & Co., Inc.)*

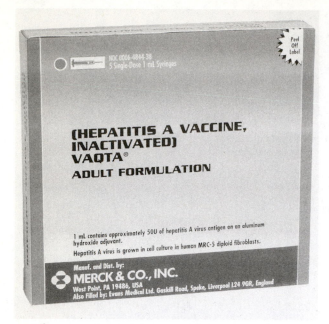

FIGURE 19-22 ADULT FORMULATION 5 SINGLE-DOSE 1 ML SYRINGES HEPATITIS A VACCINE (INACTIVATED) VAQTA® *(Courtesy of Merck & Co., Inc.)*

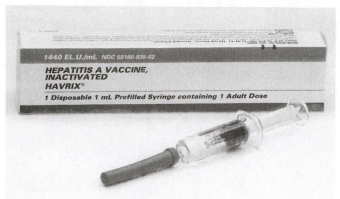

FIGURE 19-23 HEPATITIS A VACCINE, INACTIVATED, HAVRIX® 1 DISPOSABLE 1 ML PREFILLED SYRINGE CONTAINING 1 ADULT DOSE *(Courtesy of SmithKline Beecham)*

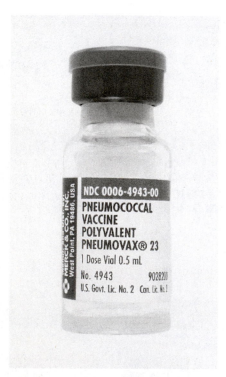

FIGURE 19-24 1 DOSE VIAL 0.5 ML PNEUMOCOCCAL VACCINE POLYVALENT PNEUMOVAX® 23 *(Courtesy of Merck & Co., Inc.)*

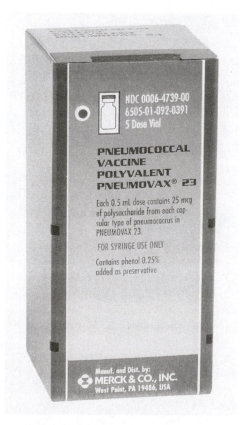

FIGURE 19-25 5 DOSE VIAL PNEUMOCOCCAL VACCINE POLYVALENT PNEUMOVAX® 23 *(Courtesy of Merck & Co., Inc.)*

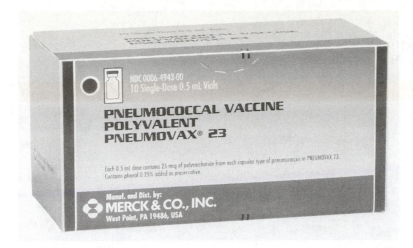

FIGURE 19-26   10 SINGLE-DOSE 0.5 ML VIALS PNEUMOCOCCAL VACCINE POLYVALENT PNEUMOVAX® 23 *(Courtesy of Merck & Co., Inc.)*

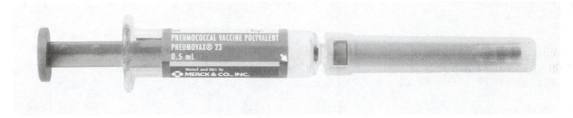

FIGURE 19-27   PREFILLED SYRINGE 0.5 ML PNEUMOCOCCAL VACCINE POLYVALENT PNEUMOVAX®23 *(Courtesy of Merck & Co., Inc.)*

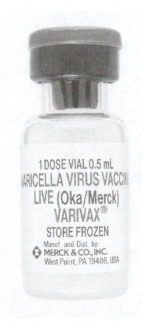

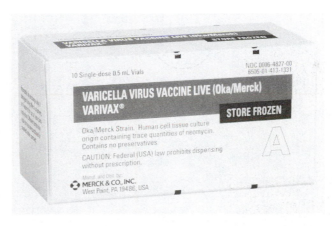

FIGURE 19-29

10 SINGLE-DOSE PACKAGE VARICELLA VIRUS VACCINE LIVE (OKA/MERCK) VARIVAX® *(Courtesy of Merck & Co., Inc.)*

FIGURE 19-28   1 DOSE VIAL 0.5 ML VARICELLA VIRUS VACCINE LIVE (OKA/MERCK) VARIVAX® *(Courtesy of Merck & Co., Inc.)*

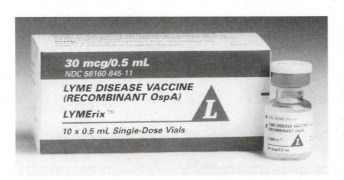

FIGURE 19-30

10 0.5 ML SINGLE-DOSE VIALS LYME DISEASE VACCINE (RECOMBINANT OSPA) LYMERIX™ *(Courtesy of SmithKline Beecham)*

● SPOT CHECK

For childhood immunizations there are routinely recommended ages and a range of acceptable ages. For each of the vaccines listed, give the appropriate information that relates to age/ages.

Vaccine	Schedule

Hepatitis B   Doses
  Hep B-1
  Hep B-2
  Hep B-3	

Diphtheria, Tetanus, Pertussis (DTaP)	
Haemophilus b Conjugate	
Poliovirus Vaccine (IPV)	
Measles, Mumps, Rubella (MMR)	

● SELF-ASSESSMENT

Write the answer in the space provided or circle true or false as instructed.

Source

p. 212　**1.** Describe fungi. _____

p. 213　**2.** Monistat 7 is an antifungal agent used _____ for 7 nights.

p. 214　**3.** The antiviral drug acyclovir (Zovirax) is used in the treatment and management of _____; however, it is not a cure for the condition.

p. 215　**4.** The antiviral drug amantadine hydrochloride (Symmetrel) is used in the treatment and management of _____. The adult oral daily dose of Symmetrel in capsule form is _____.

p. 217　**5.** True or False (circle one) Denavir is prescribed for the recurrent treatment of herpes labialis and can be used on the genital and rectal mucosa.

p. 218　**6.** On the lines provided, write the full names of the following abbreviations for antiretroviral agents used in the treatment of HIV:

- NRTIs _____
- NNRTs _____
- PIs _____

p. 219　**7.** True or False (circle one) Thus far, highly active antiretroviral therapy (HAART) is the closest thing medical science has to an effective HIV therapy, as it has been known to successfully rid the body of the HIV virus.

p. 220　**8.** In as few words as possible, tell the major difference between

- Active immunization _____
- Passive immunization _____

p. 222　**9.** True or False (circle one) There is no convincing evidence of risk to the fetus from immunization of pregnant women using inactivated virus vaccines or toxoids.

p. 223　**10.** True or False (circle one) When giving vaccines to infants and children, the nurse must obtain a signed consent from the parent or guardian.

● WEB ACTIVITY

Visit the following Web sites for additional information on antifungal, antiviral, and immunizing agents:

http://www.sb.com

http://www.vaccinesbynet.com

http://www.pslgroup.com

http://www.discoveryhealth.com

http://www.medicinenet.com

http://pharmacotherapy.medscape.com

http://www.onhealth.com

http://www.fda.gov/oashi/aids/virals.html

http://www.cdc.gov

http://www.health.msn.com

http://www.intelihealth.com

http://www.nih.gov/nia

http://www.uic.edc/depts/matec/nahof.html

http://www.pharminfo.com

http://www.aidsinfonyc.org

http://www.docguide.com

http://www.hivatis.org

http://www.aegis.com

http://www.thebody.com

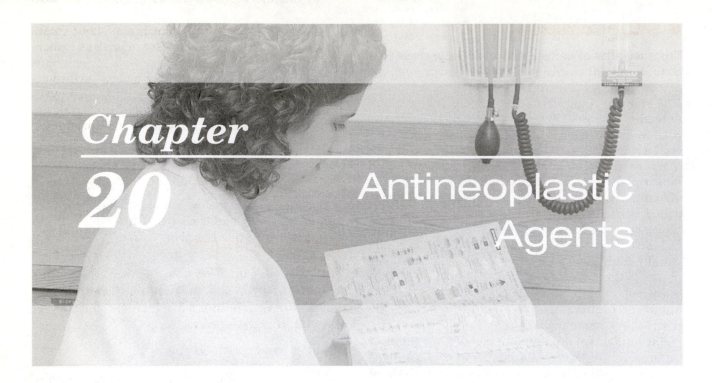

Chapter 20

Antineoplastic Agents

Chapter Outline

Objectives
Key Terms
Introduction
Chemotherapy with Antineoplastic Agents
Care of Chemotherapy Clients
Classification of Antineoplastic Agents
Combination Chemotherapy
Other Forms of Treatment for Cancer
Self-Assessment
Web Activity

Objectives

Upon completion of this chapter, you should be able to

- Define the key terms
- State when chemotherapy is the treatment of choice for cancer
- List the normal cells that have the greatest sensitivity to destruction from antineoplastic agents
- State the aim of chemotherapy
- State who should prepare and administer antineoplastic agents

- Describe examples of adverse reactions associated with antineoplastic agents
- List and give the normal ranges of laboratory tests performed to establish a client's baseline before initiation of chemotherapy
- Explain the care of chemotherapy clients
- Describe the classifications of antineoplastic agents
- Complete the Spot Check on the classification of antineoplastic agents
- Give examples of combination chemotherapy agents
- Describe other forms of treatment for cancer
- Complete the Self-Assessment
- Visit indicated Web sites for additional information on antineoplastic agents

Key Terms

alopecia	exacerbation
anorexia	metastasis
carcinogenic	mutagenic
chemotherapy	petechiae
cytotoxic	remission
dedifferentiation	stomatitis
epistaxis	

INTRODUCTION

The incidence of cancer is five times greater now than it was 100 years ago. Cancer will strike one out of every four Americans, according to recent statistics from the American Cancer Society. With early detection, followed by immediate treatment, the cure rate for cancer is now one in every two.

In cancer, there is an abnormal process wherein a cell or group of cells undergoes change and no longer carries on normal cell functions. This failure of immature cells to develop specialized functions is called **dedifferentiation**. It is believed that this process involves a disturbance in the deoxyribonucleic acid (DNA) of the affected cells. Malignant cells usually multiply rapidly, forming a mass of abnormal cells that enlarges, ulcerates, and sheds malignant cells to surrounding tissues. This process, known as **metastasis**, destroys the normal cells, with the malignant cells taking their places. Microscopic analysis of a malignant cell reveals a loss of differentiation, anaplasia, nuclei of various sizes that are hyperchromatic, and cells in the process of rapid and disorderly division.

Oncologists have identified numerous factors that play a role in the development of cancer. These factors are environmental, hereditary, and biological. Over 200 forms of cancer have been identified.

The treatment of cancer may be any one or a combination of surgery, chemotherapy, radiation therapy, or immunotherapy. The treatment of choice depends upon the type of cancer, its location, its invasive process, and the client's state of health.

CHEMOTHERAPY WITH ANTINEOPLASTIC AGENTS

Chemotherapy (the treatment of disease by using chemical agents, such as cancer drugs that destroy cancer cells) may be the treatment of choice when the cancer is disseminated and cannot be removed surgically. It is also used when a tumor fails to respond to radiation therapy, and is used in combination with other forms of therapy.

Antineoplastic (anticancer) agents do injury to individual cells, interfere with their vital functions, and kill or destroy malignant cells. In rendering cancerous cells harmless, certain normal cells may be destroyed. The normal cells with the greatest sensitivity to destruction are the hematopoietic cells, epithelial cells, and hair follicles.

The plan of treatment for clients undergoing chemotherapy is individualized. The aim of chemotherapy is to put the client in **remission** (the time when the symptoms of a disease process are lessened) so that life may continue without **exacerbation** (the time when a disease process is most severe) of symptoms.

Antineoplastic agents are potentially hazardous and fatal complications can occur. Most are **cytotoxic** (destructive to cells), **mutagenic** (causing genetic mutations), and **carcinogenic** (producing cancer).

Toxicities and Adverse Reactions

Toxicities and adverse reactions vary with the antineoplastic agent and each individual client. Some examples of adverse reactions follow.

Gastrointestinal

Anorexia (loss of appetite), nausea, vomiting, mucositis, **stomatitis** (inflammation of the mouth), colitis, and liver dysfunction.

Hematopoietic

Bone marrow depression/suppression, anemia, leukopenia, thrombocytopenia, and pancytopenia.

Secondary Neoplasia

May increase incidence of a second malignant tumor.

Genitourinary

Sterile hemorrhagic cystitis, hyperuricemia, and renal failure.

Gonadal Suppression

Amenorrhea, azoospermia.

Integument

Alopecia (loss of hair), skin and fingernails may become darker, rash, maculopapular skin eruption.

Pulmonary

Interstitial pulmonary fibrosis.

Cardiac

Acute left ventricular failure, arrhythmias, cardiomyopathy.

Respiratory

Dyspnea.

Immunosuppressive Activity

May predispose client to bacterial, viral (herpes zoster), or fungal infection.

Chromosomal Abnormalities

Mutagenic.

Teratogenic Effects

May cause fetal harm in pregnancy. Women of childbearing potential should be advised to avoid becoming pregnant.

Extravasation

Injection into subcutaneous tissues results in a painful inflammation. The area usually becomes indurated and sloughing of tissue may occur.

Client Evaluation

The physician carefully evaluates each client and determines an exact diagnosis. A plan of treatment is prescribed. When chemotherapy is the treatment regimen or part of the treatment regimen, certain laboratory tests are performed to determine the client's baseline data before the initiation of therapy.

Tests	Normal Ranges
● Platelet Count	Approximately 150,000–450,000 thrombocytes per cubic millimeter of blood
● White Blood Cell Count (WBC)	Approximately 5,000–10,000 leukocytes per cubic millimeter of blood
● Hemoglobin	Adult female: 12–16 g/100 milliliters of blood
	Adult male: 14–18 g/100 milliliters of blood
	Children: varies with age
● Hematocrit	Adult female: 37–47%
	Adult male: 40–54%
	Children: varies with age from 35–49%
	Newborn: 49–54%
● Differential	Neutrophils 40–60% Eosinophils 1–3% Basophils 0.5–1% Lymphocytes 20–40% Monocytes 4–8%

● Liver and kidney function and creatinine clearance tests should be performed before beginning therapy.

During chemotherapy, these laboratory tests must be evaluated very carefully. When there is a deviation from normal, the physician is notified. At this time, the physician will evaluate the results of the test and determine the course of action to take.

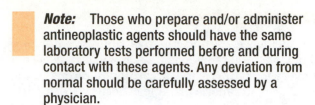

Note: Those who prepare and/or administer antineoplastic agents should have the same laboratory tests performed before and during contact with these agents. Any deviation from normal should be carefully assessed by a physician.

Dosage

The dosage of antineoplastic agents is individualized for each client. It is based upon body surface area or kilogram of body weight. The physician will order the chemotherapy regimen, giving the client's name, the agent or agents to use, the dose, route, rate, and time for administration. Those preparing and administering these agents should have a second qualified person check and verify the order and their preparation of the drug or drugs.

CARE OF CHEMOTHERAPY CLIENTS

Assess the client's understanding of the disease process and the prescribed treatment regimen. Encourage the client to express his or her emotional feelings about the disease and the treatment. Encourage the client to ask questions and provide appropriate answers. Follow the proper protocol for preparing and/or administering antineoplastic agents.

Assess and monitor:

- Laboratory test results
- Intravenous infusion site/sites for extravasation, thrombosis, or phlebitis
- Signs of adverse reactions
- Client's response to treatment

During chemotherapy, force fluids (1, $1\frac{1}{2}$, or 2 liters per day), unless otherwise ordered or contraindicated. Administer antiemetics and analgesics as ordered. If the client's nausea, vomiting, and pain are not controlled by the prescribed dose, notify the physician. A more satisfactory regimen should be initiated.

Protect the client from infection:

- Perform medical asepsis handwash.
- Maintain a clean environment.
- Administer antibiotics as ordered.
- Educate the client, family, and visitors about the spread of infectious diseases.
- When neutropenia is present, limit entry to the client's room, and restrict fresh flowers and fruit.

Provide for nutritional needs:

- Encourage the client to eat and take sufficient liquids.
- Assist the client in selecting foods of choice from the menu.
- Assist the client with eating as necessary.
- Cater to the client's dietary needs. Provide small frequent feedings.

Additional measures are as follows:

- Monitor fluid and electrolyte balance.
- Record intake and output.
- Provide good mouth care. Keep the client's mucous membranes moist. Apply lip balm as ordered. Should stomatitis occur, check with the physician for a plan of treatment.

Note: Over-the-counter mouthwashes usually contain alcohol that may be irritating to the mucosa. Lemon glycerine swabs can irritate the mucous membranes. One teaspoon of baking soda dissolved in one cup (8 ounces) of water or a mixture of one cup of hydrogen peroxide and two cups of water are soothing mixtures. Apply with special oral care sponges (Toothettes) or a soft-bristled toothbrush. For severe mucositis, a saline solution rinse may be used at least six times a day. Other rinses that are helpful are a 1:4 mixture of dyclonine (local anesthetic agent) and sterile water; triple mixture of equal parts 2 percent viscous lidocaine, diphenhydramine HCl elixir, and Mylanta-II.

- Encourage the client to eat moist foods.
- Encourage the client to drink plenty of fluids. Sucking on ice chips and sugarless hard candy helps to moisten the mouth.
- Advise the client to avoid spicy, hot, and acidic foods and beverages.
- Advise the client not to smoke.
- Provide emotional support.

Clients' Instruction

Client instruction encompasses a wide scope of factors. The client needs to understand the disease process and the treatment regimen. With regard to chemotherapy, the client needs to know about possible adverse reactions and what he or she can do to lessen the side effects. Inform and teach each client about the medication regimen.

Most antineoplastic agents cause nausea and vomiting. To lessen the severity of nausea and vomiting, advise the client to

- Avoid hot, spicy, greasy, and acidic foods and beverages
- Avoid unpleasant odors
- Eat small, frequent meals
- Take a prescribed antiemetic before chemotherapy
- Suck on ice chips and/or sugarless hard candy
- Refrain from smoking

Teach the client to be alert for the following signs of infection, and to report such signs to the attending physician:

- An elevated body temperature
- Sneezing, coughing, and malaise
- Pain, heat, redness, and swelling

Teach the client to be consciously alert for the following signs of bleeding and to report such signs to the attending physician:

- Excessive bruising
- Nosebleed (**epistaxis**), rectal bleeding, abnormal vaginal bleeding, and bleeding gums
- Small, purplish, hemorrhagic spots on the skin (**petechiae**)

One of the most dreaded adverse reactions to chemotherapy is alopecia, the loss of hair. Suggest that the client temporarily wear a wig or some other form of scalp cover. Usually, the hair will begin to grow back after the effects of chemotherapy are eliminated from the client's body. The new hair may be even darker than the hair that was lost.

Nausea and vomiting can be well controlled with three relatively new drugs administered at the time of chemotherapy: Zofran (ondansetron), Kytril (granisetron), and Anzemet (dolasetron). The dose of these medications will be different for each client. The information that follows includes the average oral doses of medications that may prevent the nausea and vomiting associated with chemotherapy.

Ondansetron (Zofran)
Uses

To prevent the nausea and vomiting that may occur after treatment with chemotherapy or radiation, or after surgery.

Dosage and Route

For prevention of nausea and vomiting after anti-cancer medicine. For adults and children 12 years of age and older, the oral dosage (tablets) is as follows: At first, the dose is 8 mg taken 30 minutes before the anticancer medicine is given. The 8 mg is taken again 8 hours after the first dose. Then the dose is 8 mg every 12 hours for 1 to 2 days. For children 4 to 12 years old, at first the dose is 4 mg taken 30 minutes before the anticancer medicine is given. The 4 mg dose is taken again 4 to 8 hours after the first dose. Then the dose is 4 mg every 8 hours for 1 to 2 days. For children up to 4 years old, the dose must be determined by the client's physician.

Note: Instruct the client that if he/she vomits within 30 minutes after taking this medicine that the same amount of medicine should be taken again. If vomiting continues, the client should check with his/her physician for further instructions. If the client misses a dose of this medicine and he/she does not feel nauseous, the missed dose should be skipped and the client should go back to the regular dosing schedule. If he/she misses a dose of this medicine and he/she feels nauseous or vomits, the missed dose should be taken as soon as possible.

Granisetron (Kytril)

Uses

To prevent the nausea and vomiting that may occur after treatment with chemotherapy or radiation.

Dosage and Route

For prevention of nausea and vomiting after anti-cancer medicine. For adults and teenagers, the oral dosage (tablets) is usually 1 mg taken up to 1 hour before the anticancer medicine. The 1 mg dose is taken again 12 hours after the first dose.

Dolasetron (Anzemet)

Uses

To prevent and treat the nausea and vomiting that may occur after treatment with anticancer medicines or after surgery.

Dosage and Route

For prevention of nausea and vomiting after anti-cancer medicine. For adults the oral dosage (tablets) is 100 mg given within 1 hour before the anticancer medicine is given. For children 2 to 16 years old, 1.8 mg/kg of body weight, the dose is given within 1 hour before the anticancer medicine is given. The dose generally is not greater than 100 mg.

CLASSIFICATIONS OF ANTINEOPLASTIC AGENTS

Antineoplastic agents prevent the development, growth, or proliferation of malignant cells. The primary classifications of antineoplastic agents are discussed next.

Alkylating Agents

Alkylating agents are chemical compounds that cause chromosome breakage and prevent the formation of new DNA, thereby interfering with cell division. They affect all rapidly proliferating cells and often cause toxicity to the hematopoietic system. Bone marrow depression/suppression, anemia, leukopenia, thrombocytopenia, and pancytopenia may occur. Most alkylating agents disrupt cells within the gastrointestinal tract, thereby producing nausea and vomiting.

Examples:
busulfan (Myleran)
chlorambucil (Leukeran)
cisplatin (Platinol)
cyclophosphamide (Cytoxan)
dacarbazine (DTIC-Dome)
ifosfamide (Ifex)
mechlorethamine HCl (Mustargen)
melphalan (Alkeran)
procarbazine (Matulane)
temozolomide (Temodar)
thiotepa (Thioplex)

Nitrosureas

Nitrosureas act in a similar way to alkylating agents. They inhibit enzymes that are needed for DNA repair. These agents are able to travel to the brain, so they are used to treat brain tumors, as well as non-Hodgkin's lymphomas, multiple myeloma, and malignant melanoma.

Examples:
carmustine (BiCNU)
lomustine (CeeNU)

Antimetabolites

Antimetabolites are substances that interfere with the metabolic process of the cell, thus preventing cell reproduction. They act only on dividing cells, and are most effective in treating rapidly proliferating malignant cells. These agents often cause toxicity to the hematopoietic system. Bone marrow depression/suppression, anemia, leukopenia, thrombocytopenia, and pancytopenia may occur. They also cause nausea and vomiting.

Examples:

cytarabine (Cytosar)

fluorouracil (5-FU)

hydroxyurea (Hydrea)

mercaptopurine (Purinethol)

methotrexate (Rheumatrex)

capecitabine (Xeloda)

Antitumor Antibiotics

Certain antibiotics have an antineoplastic effect. These antibodies are derived from species of microorganisms and are not to be confused with antibiotics that are used in the treatment of infections. Their action is not known, but it appears they act by interfering with one or more stages of RNA and/or DNA synthesis. They interfere with the malignant cell's ability to grow and reproduce. These antibiotics cause toxicity.

Examples:

bleomycin sulfate (Blenoxane)

dactinomycin (Cosmegen)

daunorubicin (Cerubidine)

daunorubicin citrate liposomal (DaunoXome)

doxorubicin HCl liposomal (Doxil)

doxorubicin HCl (Adriamycin)

epirubicin HCl (Ellence)

mitomycin (Mutamycin)

plicamycin (Mithracin)

valrubicin (Valstar)

Mitotic Inhibitors

Mitotic inhibitors are plant alkaloids and natural products that can inhibit mitosis or inhibit enzymes that prevent protein synthesis, which is needed for cell reproduction. They are phase cycle specific and work during the mitosis (M) phase.

Examples:

docetaxel (Taxotere)

etoposide (VePesid)

paclitaxel (Taxol)

vinblastine (Velban)

vincristine (Oncovin)

vinorelbine (Navelbine)

Enzyme Inhibitors

Camptosar (irinotecan) is an enzyme inhibitor that interferes with DNA synthesis by inhibiting the enzyme topoisomerase I. Irinotecan is a derivative of camptothecin. Camptothecins interact specifically with the enzyme topoisomerase I, which relieves torsional strain in DNA by inducing reversible single-strain breaks. It is used in metastatic carcinoma of the colon or rectum in those whose disease has recurred or progressed following 5-fluorouracil therapy. See Figure 20-1.

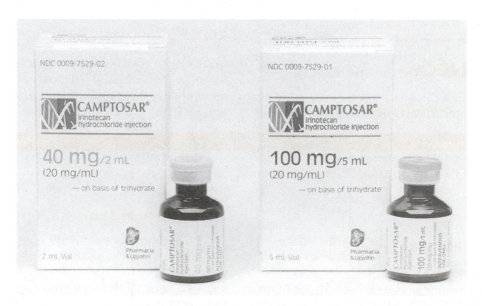

FIGURE 20-1   CAMPTOSAR® (IRINOTECAN HYDROCHLORIDE INJECTION) 40 MG/2 ML (20 MG/ML), 100 MG/5 ML (20 MG/ML) *(Courtesy Pharmacia & Upjohn)*

Hormones

Hormones are used to treat endocrine-related tumors (carcinoma of the breast, prostate, endometrium, ovary, kidney, and thyroid) and nonendocrine malignant neoplasms (leukemia, lymphomas). They have been used in antineoplastic therapy because they are capable of suppressing the growth of certain tissues of the body without exerting cytotoxic action.

Corticosteroids (prednisone and prednisolone) are used in conjunction with antineoplastic agents in the treatment of acute lymphoblastic leukemia and malignant lymphomas. Corticosteroids produce a wide variety of adverse reactions after extended use, such as Cushingoid features, edema, hypertension, heart failure, potassium loss, paper-thin skin, euphoria, and poor wound healing.

The following are examples of the different types of hormones used in antineoplastic therapy and some of the more common adverse reactions:

Hormones	*Adverse Reactions*
Estrogens conjugated estrogens (Premarin)	Edema, nausea, anorexia, changes in libido, breast tenderness, abdominal cramps, dizziness, irritability, and urinary frequency when used for prostatic carcinoma gynecomastia and impotence
Androgens testolactone (Teslac)	Fluid retention, masculinization with clitoral enlargement, hirsutism, deepening of the voice, increased libido, acne, alopecia, and erythrocythemia
Progestins medroxyprogesterone acetate (Depo-Provera) megestrol acetate (Megace)	Anorexia, fluid retention, and pain at site of injection
Antiestrogen tamoxifen citrate (Nolvadex)	Nausea, vomiting, hot flashes, vaginal bleeding or discharge
Gonadotropin-releasing hormone agonist leuprolide (Lupron) (see Figure 20-2)	Dizziness, headache, syncope, blurred vision, angina, anorexia, dysuria, nausea, vomiting, prostate pain
Adrenal corticosteroids prednisone prednisolone	Cushingoid features, edema, hypertension, heart failure, potassium loss, paper-thin skin, euphoria, and poor wound healing

● SPOT CHECK

For each of the classifications of antineoplastic agents given, list several examples of drugs and their action. Give the major toxicity of each classification.

Classification	Action	Major Toxicity
Alkylating Agents		

(continued)

Classification	Action	Major Toxicity
Antimetabolites		
Antitumor Antibiotics		
Mitotic Inhibitors		
Hormones		

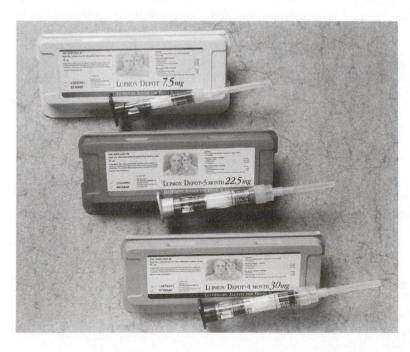

FIGURE 20-2   LUPRON DEPOT® (LEUPROLIDE ACETATE) 7.5 MG, 22.5 MG, 30 MG *(Courtesy of TAP Pharmaceutical Products Inc.)*

COMBINATION CHEMOTHERAPY

The combination of certain antineoplastic agents has proven to be effective in treating acute leukemia; Hodgkin's disease; non-Hodgkin's lymphoma; carcinoma of the breast, testis, and ovary; childhood neuroblastoma; Wilm's tumor; and osteogenic sarcoma. The physician who prescribes combination chemotherapy weighs the anticipated benefits against the possible additive toxic effects of the drugs. The following are some examples of combination chemotherapy:

CEF	cyclophosphamide (Cytoxan)
	epirubicin (Ellence)
	5-fluorouracil (5-FU)
CFPT	cyclophosphamide (Cytoxan)
	5-fluorouracil (5-FU)
	prednisone
	tamoxifen (Nolvadex)
COPE	cyclophosphamide (Cytoxan)
	vincristine (Oncovin)
	cisplatin (Platinol)
	etoposide (VePesid)
ECF	epirubicin (Ellence)
	cisplatin (Platinol)
	5-fluorouracil (5-FU)
TPE	paclitaxel (Taxol)
	cisplatin (Platinol)
	etoposide (VePesid)

Miscellaneous Antineoplastic Agents

Miscellaneous antineoplastic agents are used in the treatment of various types of cancer. The following are examples of antineoplastic agents:

- Asparaginase (Elspar) is used as part of combination chemotherapy in the treatment of acute lymphocytic leukemia (ALL). It acts as a catalyst in the conversion of asparagine (an amino acid) to aspartic acid and ammonia. It depletes asparagine in leukemia cells, thereby causing their death.

- Aldesleukin (interleukin-2, IL-2, Proleukin) modified recombinant interleukin is a genetically engineered immune-boosting drug that stimulates the immune system to produce more lymphocytes.

- Altretamine (Hexalen) is used in the management of ovarian cancer that has been unresponsive to treatment with other antineoplastic agents. Its mechanism of action is unknown, but it may disrupt DNA and RNA synthesis, thereby causing death of rapidly replicating cells, particularly malignant cells.

- Interferon alfa-2a recombinant (Roferon-A) is a genetically engineered immune system activator. It has antineoplastic, antiviral, and antiproliferative activity. It strengthens the body's immune system and helps it fight cancer cells. It is used in the treatment of hairy cell leukemia, AIDS-associated Kaposi's sarcoma, and chronic myelogenous leukemia.

- Interferon alfa-2b recombinant (α-2-interferon, Intron A) is a genetically engineered immune system activator. It has antineoplastic, antiviral, and antiproliferative activity. It strengthens the body's immune system and helps it fight cancer cells. It is used in the treatment of hairy cell leukemia, malignant melanoma, AIDS-associated Kaposi's sarcoma, condylomata acuminata, chronic hepatitis non-A, non-B/C.

- Interferon alfa-n3, human (Alferon N) is from pooled human leukocytes. It has antineoplastic, antiviral, and antiproliferative activity. It is used in the treatment of condylomata acuminata.

- Levamisole (Ergamisol) restores depressed immune function including formation of antibodies, T-cell response, phagocytosis, and chemotaxis. There is enhanced immunologic response to presence of tumor when used in conjunction with fluorouracil. It is used as adjunctive therapy following surgery of Dukes' C colorectal carcinoma (with fluorouracil).

- Denileukin diftitox (Ontak) is a recombinant DNA-derived cytotoxic protein produced in an *Escherichia coli* expression system. It is a fusion protein that directs diphtheria toxin to cells that express the CD25 component of the IL-2 receptor. Malignant cells expressing one or more of the subunits of the IL-2 receptor are found in certain leukemias and lymphomas, including cutaneous T-cell lymphoma. It is a highly toxic compound, and the more serious toxicities decrease with continued exposure to the agent.

- Filgrastim (Neupogen) is a human granulocyte colony-stimulating factor (G-CSF) produced by recombinant DNA technology and approved to fight infection in clients receiving chemotherapeutic agents that commonly cause severe neutropenia with fever.

- Sargramostim (Leukine) is a recombinant granulocyte-macrophage colony-stimulating factor (GM-CSF) used to treat clients with Hodgkin's disease, non-Hodgkin's lymphoma, and acute lymphoblastic leukemia who undergo autologous bone marrow transplantation.

OTHER FORMS OF TREATMENT FOR CANCER

Treatment for cancer may be one or a combination of chemotherapy, surgery, radiation therapy, immunotherapy, and other forms of treatment that have emerged from scientific investigation and the advent of genetic engineering.

Surgery

Surgery may be the treatment of choice when the tumor is small and localized and the surrounding tissue is accessible for removal. The aim of surgery is the removal of all cancerous tissue plus some of the surrounding normal tissue. Surgery may also be used to alleviate some of the complications of cancer, such as the obstruction of an area caused by the enlargement of a tumor.

Radiation Therapy

Radiation therapy is the treatment of disease by the use of ionizing radiation. The aim of this treatment is to deliver a precise, calculated dose of radiation to diseased tissue, such as a tumor, causing the least possible damage to surrounding normal tissue. Malignant cells are more sensitive to radiation than normal cells. They seem less able to repair themselves; therefore, radiation is frequently used in cancer treatment as either a curative or a palliative mode of therapy.

Immunotherapy

Immunotherapy is the treatment of disease by stimulation of the body's immune system. It may be used as an adjuvant to other types of treatment. Immunotherapy, sometimes called biological therapy, biotherapy, or biological response modifier therapy, uses the body's own immune defense system to attack cancer. Once the body's immune system has recognized cancer cells by their foreign substances (antigens), it can send immune cells to destroy the cancer. It can also manufacture antibodies that attach themselves to the antigens of the cancer cells and help the immune system destroy the targeted invader.

Cancer Treatment of the Future

Over the years, the development and use of chemotherapy drugs have resulted in the successful treatment of many individuals with cancer. Yet, some cancers still recur. There are several innovative uses of chemotherapy and other agents that hold even more promise for controlling cancer. These include novel approaches to targeting drugs more specifically at the cancer cells (such as attaching drugs to monoclonal antibodies or packaging them inside liposomes) to produce fewer adverse reactions, transplanting hematopoietic stem cells, and overcoming multidrug resistance. New drugs including new combinations of chemotherapy drugs and new delivery techniques hold significant promise for controlling cancer and improving quality of life.

With the identification of gene sequencing and the announcement of the mapping of the human genome, the future of cancer therapy will be focused at the chromosomal level. Therapies will be targeted at preventing disease, identifying genetic abnormalities, and developing agents that will trick tumor cells into self-destruction without causing any toxicity for the client.

● SELF-ASSESSMENT

Write the answer in the space provided or circle true or false as instructed.

Source

p. 235   1. The treatment of cancer may involve any one or a combination of the following four therapies: (1) _____, (2) _____, (3) _____, (4) _____.

p. 235   2. Normal cells may be destroyed as a result of cancer therapies. The normal cells with the greatest sensitivity to destruction are _____ cells, hair follicles, and _____ cells.

p. 236   3. A white blood cell count is done and the results show 8000 leukocytes per cubic millimeter of blood. Is this count in the low, normal, or high range? _____

p. 236   4. An adult female has a hemoglobin count of 8 g/100 milliliters of blood. Is this count in the low, normal, or high range? _____

p. 237   5. Alopecia can be a dreaded adverse reaction to chemotherapy. In a few words, define the term *alopecia*. _____

p. 237   6. The text mentions three relatively new drugs used to prevent the nausea and vomiting that may occur after treatment with chemotherapy. Give the generic name for each of these drugs. (1) _____, (2) _____, (3) _____

p. 238   **7.** True or False (circle one) If the client vomits within 30 minutes after taking the antinausea drug ondansetron, he or she should take a second dose consisting of the same amount of medicine.

p. 238–240   **8.** On the lines provided, write in the primary classifications of antineoplastic agents. _____ _____ _____ _____ _____ _____ _____

p. 242   **9.** In the abbreviations CEF, CFPT, and COPE, what chemotherapeutic agent does the letter C represent? _____

p. 243   **10.** True or False (circle one) Malignant cells are more sensitive to radiation than normal cells and they seem more able to repair themselves.

● **WEB ACTIVITY**

Visit the following Web sites for additional information on antineoplastic agents:

http://www.cancernetwork.com
http://www.cancer.org
http://www.pslgroup.com
http://www.discoveryhealth.com
http://www.medicinenet.com
http://pharmacotherapy.medscape.com
http://www.onhealth.com
http://www.fda.gov/oashi/aids/virals.html
http://www.cdc.gov
http://www.intelihealth.com
http://www.nih.gov/nia
http://www.pharminfo.com
http://www.docguide.com
http://www.medscape.com
http://www.mayohealth.org

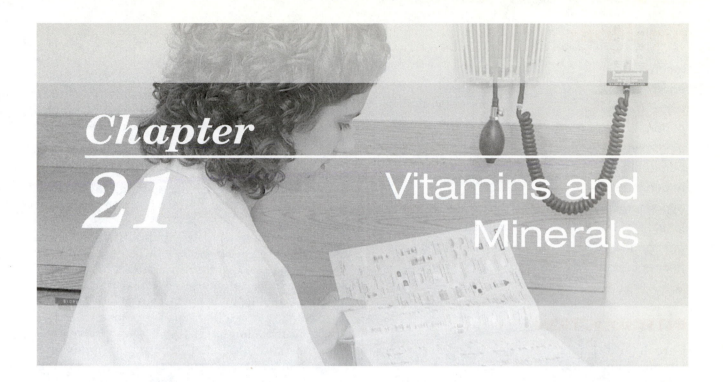

Chapter 21

Vitamins and Minerals

Chapter Outline

Objectives

Upon completion of this chapter, you should be able to

- Define the key terms

- Explain how many health problems could be prevented by proper nutrition

- Give four examples of when a body may require additional nutrients

- List the six food groups that make up the Food Guide Pyramid

- Describe antioxidants

- Describe phytochemicals

- Differentiate between fat-soluble and water-soluble vitamins

- Give the functions, food sources, USRDA, and indications of deficiency of selected vitamins and minerals

- State the symptoms of hypervitaminosis for vitamins A, D, and E

- Describe the importance of cations and anions in electrolyte balance

- Complete the Spot Check on selected vitamins and minerals

- Complete the Self-Assessment

- Visit indicated Web sites for additional information on vitamins and minerals

245

Key Terms

anion

antioxidants

avitaminosis

cation

electrolytes

homeostasis

hypervitaminosis

hypovitaminosis

ions

macromineral

micromineral

minerals

National Research
Council (NRC)

phytochemical

RDA (Recommended
Daily Allowance)

United States
Recommended
Daily Allowance
(USRDA)

vitamins

INTRODUCTION

Carbohydrates, fats, proteins, water, electrolytes, vitamins, and minerals are nutrients that are essential for life. Carbohydrates and fats furnish heat and energy. Proteins provide energy and build and repair body tissues. Water and electrolytes are essential for maintaining the body's acid-base balance. Vitamins, minerals, and water help regulate such body processes as circulation, respiration, digestion, and elimination.

At least four of the ten leading causes of death in the United States (heart disease, cancer, stroke, and diabetes) are directly related to a person's eating habits. It is now noted that many health problems could be prevented by proper nutrition. For example, atherosclerosis can begin in early childhood and this process can be halted if healthy changes in diet and lifestyle are initiated and followed. The gradual bone thinning that results in osteoporosis can be prevented if enough calcium is consumed throughout life.

The U.S. Food and Drug Administration ordered that most breads, flour, pasta, and other food from grains be fortified with folic acid. It is recommended that women of childbearing age and children over 4 years of age consume 0.4 mg of folic acid daily. There is strong evidence that folic acid reduces homocysteine, a chemical associated with high risk of heart attacks and strokes. When pregnant women consume too little folic acid, infants may have malformations of the spinal cord such as spina bifida and/or anencephaly.

Diabetes in the United States rose by about 6 percent in 1999 in what the government called dramatic evidence of an unfolding epidemic. The rise is blamed largely on obesity. The obesity rate increased to nearly one in five Americans. Nearly 30 percent of clients diagnosed as overweight in the past years have been 35 years of age or younger. The number of overweight children between 6 and 17 years of age has risen 22 percent since the 1960s. Less than 30 percent of American children eat the recommended five servings of fruits and vegetables per day, and many young people do not get enough physical exercise to burn the calories that they consume. Obesity is associated with increased risks of high blood pressure, heart disease, high cholesterol, stroke, diabetes, cancer, gallbladder disease, arthritis, sleep disturbances, complications in pregnancy, and early death.

Good nutrition involves balance, variety, and moderation. High-fat foods can be balanced with low-fat foods and calorie intake can be offset by enough activity to maintain normal weight. Good nutrition should be a part of an overall healthy lifestyle. Other healthy considerations include a program of regular exercise, not using tobacco products, drinking alcohol in moderation, managing stress, and limiting the intake of caffeinated beverages and exposure to environmental hazards.

THE FOOD GUIDE PYRAMID

Through proper selection of foods from the Food Guide Pyramid (Figure 21-1), most healthy adults can receive the nutrients essential for life, but there are times that a body may require additional nutrients; for example, during the various stages of growth and development, pregnancy, breast-feeding, surgery, disease processes, and aging. Also, teenagers with irregular eating habits, vegetarians, dieters, and people who avoid entire food groups may need a multivitamin and mineral supplement. Smokers may have lower vitamin C levels in their blood than nonsmokers and may benefit from supplementation of up to 500 mg of vitamin C a day.

People with deficiency diseases or absorption disorders may need therapeutic doses of nutrients prescribed by a physician that may be two to ten times the **RDA (Recommended Daily Allowance)**. The RDA is the nutrient level of intake that is considered by the **National Research Council (NRC)** and Nutrition Board to be adequate for most healthy individuals. People who take prescription medications that interfere with nutrients or who abuse alcohol or other drugs may also need a supplement. Women may need to supplement calcium to help prevent osteoporosis and those who bleed excessively during menstruation may need to take a multivitamin and mineral supplement that contains iron.

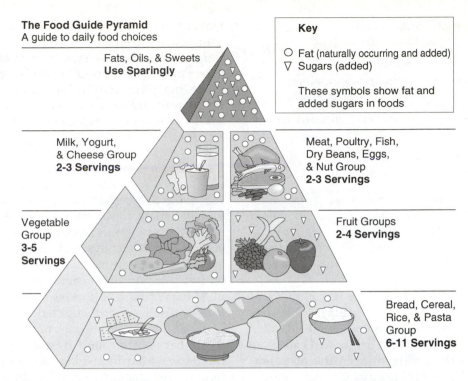

The Food Guide Pyramid
A guide to daily food choices

Fats, Oils, & Sweets
Use Sparingly

Key
○ Fat (naturally occurring and added)
▽ Sugars (added)

These symbols show fat and
added sugars in foods

Milk, Yogurt,
& Cheese Group
2-3 Servings

Meat, Poultry, Fish,
Dry Beans, Eggs,
& Nut Group
2-3 Servings

Vegetable
Group
**3-5
Servings**

Fruit Groups
2-4 Servings

Bread, Cereal,
Rice, & Pasta
Group
6-11 Servings

FIGURE 21-1   THE FOOD GUIDE PYRAMID *(Courtesy of U.S. Department of Agriculture)*

Additional nutrients are generally prescribed as a vitamin and/or mineral supplement by a physician. It is important for the client to understand that the prescribed nutrient is a drug and should be used as such.

ANTIOXIDANTS

Antioxidants are chemical substances that neutralize free radicals, the highly reactive and unstable molecules that can cause significant cellular damage. The body makes antioxidants and antioxidants are found in various foods, herbs, and nutritional supplements. Vitamins C, E, and beta carotene are known as antioxidant vitamins.

Vitamin C is found in many fruits and vegetables, including oranges, grapefruit, strawberries, broccoli, kale, and tomatoes. Vitamin E is found in nuts, certain vegetable oils, and leafy greens. Beta carotene is found in dark green leafy vegetables such as spinach, and in yellow-orange fruits and vegetables such as cantaloupes, peaches, carrots, and sweet potatoes. Tea leaves also contain antioxidants called polyphenols, which can prevent damage to DNA.

Antioxidants help to protect the body's cells. The billions of cells in the body are continually exposed to free radicals that are produced through normal bodily processes, as well as external sources such as air pollution and tobacco smoke. It is believed that this cellular damage, along with other factors, may lead to aging and the development of chronic diseases such as cancer, cataracts, and heart disease.

PHYTOCHEMICALS

A **phytochemical** is any one of a hundred natural chemical substances present in plants. Many have nutritional value; others are protective (antioxidants) or cause cell damage (free radicals). Garlic, soybeans, licorice root, broccoli, carrots, and tomatoes are just a few of the many foods that have been analyzed by scientists who are exploring how phytochemicals might help prevent cancer and other diseases. It is believed that some may keep cancer cells from forming or attaching to healthy cells. They may also help offset some of the damage that cause cancers by toxins, such as cigarette smoke and pollutants. Some of the phytochemicals that have been linked with disease prevention include

- Capsaicin found in peppers
- Coumarins in citrus fruit and tomatoes
- Flavonoids in citrus fruit, tomatoes, berries, peppers, and carrots

- Indoles in broccoli and cabbage
- Isothiocyanates in broccoli, cabbage, mustard, and horseradish
- Lycopene in tomatoes and red grapefruit
- Allyl sulfide in garlic, onions, and chives
- Triterpenoids in licorice root and citrus fruit

VITAMINS

Vitamins are organic substances that are essential for normal metabolism, growth, and development of the human body. They are complex chemical substances that may be obtained naturally from plants, animals, and sunshine, or they may be made commercially.

Vitamins may be classified as fat-soluble and water-soluble (see Table 21-1). The fat-soluble vitamins are A, D, E, and K. The water-soluble vitamins are thiamine (B_1), riboflavin (B_2), niacin (nicotinic acid), pyridoxin (B_6), folic acid, cyanocobalamin (B_{12}), biotin, and C (ascorbic acid).

The fat-soluble vitamins are stored in adipose tissue and the liver. The water-soluble vitamins are not stored in the body. They are essential to health and need to be replaced on a daily basis. The **United States Recommended Daily Allowance (USRDA)** (the accepted amount of a substance, especially vitamins and minerals, that a person needs each day) for each vitamin is given in Table 21-1. When an individual follows these recommended allowances, conditions such as **avitaminosis** (a deficiency disease due to a lack of vitamins in the diet), **hypovitaminosis** (a condition due to a lack of vitamins, especially from an inadequate diet), and **hypervitaminosis** (a condition caused by an excessive amount of vitamins, especially from the taking of too many vitamin pills) can be prevented.

Some of the commonly prescribed vitamin products are Theragran, Centrum, Citracal, B–C–Bid, Therabid, Vicon–C, Vicon Forte, Vita-plus H, Nico–400, Os-Cal Forte, cyanocobalamin—vitamin B_{12} (Redisol, Rubramin), folic acid (Folvite), folinic acid (Leucovorin), and vitamin K (Aqua MEPHYTON).

The U.S. Food and Drug Administration has ordered that most breads, flour, pasta, and other food from grains be fortified with folic acid. Folic acid is a trace B vitamin found in citrus fruits and dark, leafy vegetables such as spinach and lettuce. It is also available in multiple vitamin supplements. The U.S. Recommended Daily Allowance for children under 4 years of age is 0.2 mg, and for the child over 4 years of age, 0.4 mg. Women of childbearing age should consume 0.4 mg of folic acid daily, but it is estimated that most women consume about half that amount. Folic acid is required to make DNA, the genetic building blocks of life. When pregnant women consume too little folic acid, infants may have malformations of the spinal cord such as spina bifida and/or anencephaly. In addition to improving the lives of children, folic acid may reduce the possibility of heart attacks and strokes.

MINERALS

Minerals are nonorganic substances that are essential constituents of all body cells. While each mineral plays a unique role, collectively they support the body's enzyme systems and keep blood and other body fluids balanced and healthy. Minerals, the major components of bones, also help regulate blood pressure and heart muscle contraction, heal wounds, and conduct nerve impulses. See Table 21-2.

Minerals are found in a variety of foods and there is no scientific evidence that consuming more than the recommended amount of a mineral has any health benefit. Overdosing on minerals can be toxic or can interfere with the function of other minerals. For example, too much zinc can interfere with the absorption of calcium, and too much iron can interfere with the absorption of zinc.

Electrolytes

The body's weight is 60 to 70 percent water. All cells are bathed by an aqueous solution that brings nourishment to the cells and removes wastes. Electrolytes (acids, bases, and salts) are suspended in this solution. **Electrolytes** are particles that result from disintegration of compounds. They are found dissolved in body fluids as **ions** that carry electrical charges. **Cation** is an ion with a positive charge of electricity. **Anion** is an ion with a negative charge of electricity. Cations and anions are involved in metabolic activities and are essential to the normal function of all cells. The normal fluid state in which positive and negative ions are in balance is called **homeostasis**.

The chief cations and anions are

Cations		Anions	
Na^+	Sodium	Cl^-	Chloride
K^+	Potassium	HCO_3^-	Carbonate
Ca^{++}	Calcium	HCO_4^-	Phosphate
Mg^{++}	Magnesium	SO_4^-	Sulfate

Selected minerals and their functions, food sources, RDA, indications of deficiency and toxicity are described in Table 21-2. Minerals are excreted

TABLE 21-1 VITAMINS

Vitamin and Function	Food Sources	USRDA	Indications of Deficiency	Hypervitaminosis
A Important for healthy mucous membranes, skin, epithelial cells, development of bones and teeth, and for vision in dim light	Dairy products, fish liver oils, animal liver, green and yellow vegetables	5,000 IU	Retarded growth, susceptibility to disease, skin lesions, and night blindness	Anorexia, loss of hair, pain in long bones, fragility of bones, dry skin, pruritus, enlarged liver and spleen
D Aids in the proper use of calcium and phosphorus in the body	Ultraviolet rays, dairy products and commercial foods that contain supplemental vitamin D (milk and cereals) and fish liver oils	400 IU	*Childhood:* Rickets *Adults:* Osteomalacia, muscle spasms, and spontaneous fractures	Demineralization (softening) of bone, hypercalcemia, calcium deposits in soft tissue, hypertension, diarrhea, and deafness
E May promote normal reproduction, and helps in the formation of muscles and red blood cells	Leafy green vegetables, wheat germ, margarine	30 IU	Edema, ataxia, absence of reflexes	Not definitely known. Large doses may destroy vitamin K in the intestine.
K Essential in the formation of prothrombin in the liver, which is necessary for normal blood clotting	Dairy products, leafy green vegetables, cauliflower, soybeans, liver, peas, potatoes, and tomatoes		Poor blood clotting, even hemorrhage	
C Important for maintenance of bones, teeth, and small blood vessels. Prevents scurvy and promotes healing of wounds and formation of protein collagen. Aids in the absorption of calcium. May help in preventing the common cold	Citrus fruits, tomatoes, melons, fresh berries, raw vegetables, and sweet potatoes	60 mg	Fatigue, irritability, fleeting joint pain, tendency to bruise, and small petechiae under the tongue	
B₁ Essential for the release of energy from carbohydrates and nerve conduction	Yeast, wheat germ, lean meats, pork, dried beans and peas, dairy products, poultry, eggs, dark green vegetables, and whole-grain enriched foods	1.5 mg	Beriberi, malaise, polyneuritis, numbness and tingling in the extremities	

(continued)

TABLE 21-1 VITAMINS (Continued)

Vitamin and Function	Food Sources	USRDA	Indications of Deficiency	Hypervitaminosis
B₂ Essential for cellular oxidation and the storage of energy. Helps maintain the skin and mucous membranes	Organ meats, lean meats, milk, green vegetables, eggs, poultry, and yeast	1.7 mg	Skin and lip lesions, seborrheic dermatitis, inflamed tongue, lack of vigor, and ocular changes	
Niacin Important for cellular respiration, glycolysis, and lipid synthesis	Liver, lean meats, fish, poultry, whole grain, and enriched flour and cereals	20 mg	Pellagra, dermatitis, irritability, dizziness, skin and mucous membrane lesions	
B₅ Aids in the metabolism of foods. Also helps the work of certain hormones and chemicals in the nervous system	Whole and enriched grain products, dried beans and peas, legumes, dairy products, eggs, organ meats, lean meats, poultry, dark green vegetables, and fish	10 mg	Not known	
B₆ Necessary for the metabolism of amino acids and fatty acids. Also aids in the production of red blood cells	Muscle meats, liver, yeast, molasses, and whole-grain cereals	2 mg	Skin lesions, anemia, hypochromic anemia, insomnia, numbness in extremities	
B₁₂ Vital for the production of red blood cells and genetic material. Helps the nervous system function properly	Liver, kidney, milk, fish, and muscle meats	6 mcg	Anemias, sore tongue, dyspepsia, breathlessness	
Folic Acid Necessary for the synthesis of amino acids, DNA, and formation of red blood cells	Liver, yeast, green leafy vegetables, and most food groups	0.4 mg	Fatigue, sore tongue, low red blood cell count, and macrocytic anemia	
Biotin Regulates amino acid and fatty acid metabolism	Liver, kidney, egg yolk, yeast, nuts, legumes, and cauliflower	0.3 mg	Dermatitis, glossitis, anorexia, and muscle pain	

TABLE 21-2 MINERALS

Minerals and Function	Food Sources	RDA	Indications of Deficiency	Toxicity
Sodium (Na) Chief cation in the extracellular fluid. Important for maintaining acid-base balance, regulating osmotic pressure in cells and body fluids, controlling fluid volume in the body. Helps in maintaining normal heart action, regulating muscle and nerve irritability	Meats, sardines, cheese, green olives, table salt, baking soda, baking powder, milk, eggs, beets, spinach, and is added to many foods such as nuts, potato chips, soups, butter, breads, cakes, sauces, salad dressings, and cereals	1100–3300 mg	Hyponatremia, loss of weight, weakness, cramps, "salt hunger," and nervous disorders	Hypernatremia, confusion, and coma
Potassium (K) Chief cation in the intracellular fluid. Helps maintain the acid-base balance. Important in nerve impulse conduction and muscle tissue excitability	Cereals, dried peas and beans, fresh vegetables, fresh or dried fruits (especially bananas, prunes, and raisins), sunflower seeds, nuts, meats, molasses, oranges, and orange juice	50–150 mEq	Hypokalemia, muscle weakness, thirst, dizziness, mental confusion, and arrhythmias	Hyperkalemia, confusion, and coma
Calcium (Ca) Plays a key role in blood clotting and lactation. Helps in maintaining acid-base balance. Activates enzymes. Needed for proper functioning of the nerves and muscles. Maintains cell membrane permeability. In combination with phosphorus helps form strong bones and teeth	Dairy products, beans, cauliflower, egg yolk, molasses, leafy green vegetables, tofu, sardines, clams, and oysters	800–1200 mg	Hypocalcemia, brittle bones, poor development of bones and teeth, rickets, tetany, excessive bleeding, and irritability	Hypercalcemia, gastrointestinal atony, renal stones or failure, psychosis, drowsiness, and lethargy
Magnesium (Mg) Important in maintaining muscle and nerve irritability. Helps regulate body temperature, aids in bone and tooth development. Activates certain enzymes	Widely distributed in foods, especially whole grains, fruits, milk, nuts, vegetables, seafoods, foods, and meats	400 mg	Hypomagnesemia, tetany, muscle tremor and weakness, mental confusion, depression, and ataxia	Hypermagnesemia, respiratory failure, and cardiac disturbances

(continued)

TABLE 21-2 MINERALS (Continued)

Minerals and Function	Food Sources	RDA	Indications of Deficiency	Toxicity
Phosphorus (P) Needed for metabolism of fats, carbohydrates, and proteins. Helps the body extract energy from foods. Important for healthy bones, teeth, and tissues. Helps maintain acid-base balance	Dairy products, eggs, fish, poultry, meats, dried peas and beans, whole grain cereals and nuts	800–1200 mg	Hypophosphatemia, irritability, weakness, retarded growth, poor tooth and bone development, rickets, anorexia, malaise, and pain in bones	Hyperphosphatemia
Iron (Fe) Essential to hemoglobin formation. Component of proteins in the blood and muscle	Liver, soybean flour, muscle meats, dried fruits, egg yolk, enriched breads and cereals, potatoes, dark green leafy vegetables	18 mg	Anemia, dizziness, weakness, fatigue, loss of weight, pallor, spoon-shaped nails, poor resistance to infection, and anorexia	Hemochromatosis
Iodine (I) Important in the development and functioning of the thyroid gland, formation of thyroxine (T_4) and triiodothyronine (T_3). Aids in the prevention of goiter	Seafood, iodized salt	150 mg	Simple goiter, cretinism	Occasional myxedema
Copper (Cu) Helps iron form blood cells and aids in enzyme activity. Helps the central nervous system function properly	Liver, nuts, shellfish, kidney, fruits, and dried peas and beans	2 mg	Anemia	Hepatolenticular degeneration
Zinc (Zn) Aids in enzyme activity, wound healing, and growth	Meats, liver, eggs, and seafood	15 mg	Retarded growth, hypogonadism, anorexia, impaired wound healing, night blindness, and white spots on nails	

daily from the body; therefore, it is most important to replace them through a well-balanced diet.

Minerals may be grouped as macrominerals and microminerals. **Macrominerals** are magnesium, sodium, potassium, chlorine, and sulfur. **Micro-** **minerals** are minerals that are required in small amounts. They are also known as trace elements. This group includes iron, copper, iodine, manganese, zinc, fluorine, cobalt, chromium, tin, selenium, vanadium, silicon, nickel, and molybdenum.

● SPOT CHECK

Vitamins and minerals are very important nutrients that are needed for proper functioning of the human body. For each selected vitamin and mineral, provide the function and USRDA.

Vitamin/Mineral	Function	USRDA
Vitamin A		
Vitamin D		
Vitamin E		
Vitamin C		

(continued)

Vitamin/Mineral	Function	USRDA
Folic Acid		
Sodium		
Potassium		

● SELF-ASSESSMENT

Write the answer in the space provided or circle true or false as instructed.

Source

p. 246   1. Water, vitamins, and minerals help regulate the following body processes: _____, _____, _____, and _____.

p. 246   2. Folic acid is added to many breads, pastas, and food products from grain because there is evidence that it causes a reduction in levels of homocysteine. This is important because homocysteine has been associated with _____.

p. 247   3. Antioxidants are important in the neutralization of free radicals that can cause damage at the cellular level. _____, _____, and _____ are known as antioxidant vitamins.

p. 248   4. _____-soluble and water-soluble are the two classifications of vitamins given in this chapter. Identify the first classification and list four vitamins that belong to it. (1) _____ (2) _____ (3) _____ (4) _____

p. 247   5. True or False (circle one) A phytochemical is any one of a hundred natural chemical substances present in plants.

p. 248   6. In a few words, explain why it is necessary to replace water-soluble vitamins on a daily basis. _____

p. 248   7. _____ is a condition caused by excessive levels of vitamins in the body and may occur when a person ingests large doses of vitamins.

p. 248   8. True or False (circle one) There is no scientific evidence that overconsumption of minerals has any health detriment.

p. 248   **9.** _____ are particles resulting from the disintegration of compounds and are found in body fluids as charged ions.

p. 248   **10.** Name the four chief cations given in this chapter. (1) _____ (2) _____ (3) _____ (4) _____

● WEB ACTIVITY

Visit the following Web sites for additional information on vitamins and minerals:

http://www.pslgroup.com

http://www.discoveryhealth.com

http://www.medicinenet.com

http://pharmacotherapy.medscape.com

http://www.onhealth.com

http://www.intelihealth.com

http://www.pharminfo.com

http://www.docguide.com

http://www.medscape.com

http://www.mayohealth.org

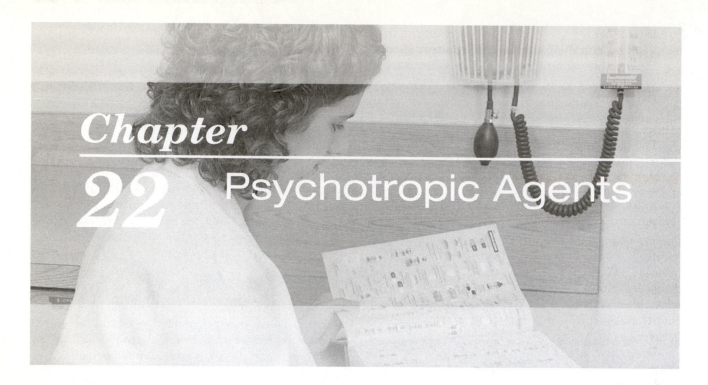

Chapter 22 Psychotropic Agents

Chapter Outline

Objectives
Key Terms
Introduction
Antianxiety Agents
Antidepressant Agents
Antimanic Agent(s)
Antipsychotic Agents
Self-Assessment
Web Activity

- List the foods and beverages a person should avoid when taking monoamine oxidase inhibitors
- List the early symptoms of lithium intoxication
- Complete the Spot Check on psychotropic agents
- Complete the Self-Assessment
- Visit indicated Web sites for additional information on psychotropic agents

Objectives

Upon completion of this chapter, you should be able to

- Define the key terms
- Describe four classifications of psychotropic drugs
- State the actions, uses, contraindications, adverse reactions, dosages, routes, nursing considerations, and clients' instruction of selected antianxiety, antidepressant, antipsychotic, and antimanic agents
- List the symptoms of marked elevation of blood pressure

Key Terms

affective disorder
akathisia
anxiety
bipolar disorder
dystonia
limbic system

mood
neuroleptics
phenothiazine
pseudo-parkinsonism
tardive dyskinesia

INTRODUCTION

Health is defined by the World Health Organization as a state of complete physical, mental, and social well-being. When a deviation from normal occurs in any of these states, a process known as disease, illness, or disorder generally appears.

Mental health may be defined as a state of well-being of the mind. When there is a disturbance in the functioning of the mind, a state of emotional and/or mental disorder may appear. The exact cause of mental illness is not known. Contributing factors may include genetics, environment, biochemical changes in the brain, and certain drugs.

The treatment of emotional and/or mental disorders encompasses a wide scope of factors. In this chapter, emphasis is given to the four classifications of drugs that are prescribed to reduce and control symptoms of emotional disturbances.

The physician determines a diagnosis and then prescribes a plan of treatment. This plan has to be carefully monitored on a continuous basis to determine the effectiveness of the program. Psychotropic drugs are usually only a part of the prescribed treatment plan. The dosage is individualized for each client and is carefully evaluated for maximum effectiveness.

Drugs that affect psychic function, behavior, or experience are called *psychotropic*. These drugs may be classified as

- *Antianxiety (anxiolytic) agents:* drugs that counteract or relieve anxiety
- *Antidepressant agents:* drugs that elevate a person's mood
- *Antimanic agents:* drugs used to treat the manic phase of bipolar disorder
- *Antipsychotic (neuroleptic) agents:* drugs that modify psychotic behavior

Psychotropic drugs are among the most frequently prescribed medications in the United States. It should be noted that some of these drugs can cause physical and/or psychological dependence.

ANTIANXIETY AGENTS

Antianxiety agents are chemical substances that counteract or relieve anxiety. They are indicated when anxiety interferes with a person's ability to function properly. **Anxiety** is a feeling of uneasiness, apprehension, worry, or dread. It is an involuntary or reflex reaction of the body to stress. The signs and symptoms of anxiety vary with the cause and an individual's response to the distressing situation. The physiologic signs may include palpitation, heart pain, nausea, anorexia, dyspepsia, constriction of the throat, muscle tension, pressure about the head, and cold, sweaty, tremulous hands. The psychological symptoms may include feelings of nervousness, apprehension, tension, inadequacy, indecisiveness, and insomnia.

Benzodiazepines

Benzodiazepines are a group of drugs with similar chemical structure and pharmaceutical activity. They are the most widely prescribed drugs for the treatment of anxiety.

Actions

The precise mechanism of action of the benzodiazepines is not known. They appear to exert their primary action on the **limbic system** (a group of brain structures including the hippocampus that is activated by motivated behavior and arousal). Benzodiazepines suppress the response to conflict or aggression in animals.

Uses

Benzodiazepines are used for the management of anxiety disorders, for the short-term relief of symptoms of anxiety, withdrawal symptoms of acute alcoholism, and preoperative apprehension and anxiety.

Contraindications

Hypersensitivity to benzodiazepines.

Adverse Reactions

Drowsiness, daytime sedation, ataxia, dizziness, fatigue, muscle weakness, dryness of the mouth, nausea, vomiting, increased irritability, insomnia, hyperactivity, blood dyscrasias.

Dosage and Route

The dosage and route of administration is determined by the physician. The dosage is individualized for each client and regulated according to the effectiveness of the medication. See Table 22-1 for selected benzodiazepines.

Nursing Considerations

Observe the client for any signs of hypersensitivity. Note the effectiveness of the drug. Are the signs and symptoms improved? Observe for adverse reactions. Be especially aware of possible signs of blood dyscrasias such as a sore throat, fever, purpura, jaundice, excessive and progressive weakness. Report any adverse reactions to the proper authority or to the physician.

During hospitalization, provide for safety measures, monitor vital signs, and record intake and output when indicated. In geriatric and/or debilitated clients, be especially aware of signs of confusion, drowsiness, and ataxia. Provide adequate protection.

TABLE 22-1 SELECTED BENZODIAZEPINES

Generic Name	Trade Name	Route	Usual Dosage		
alprazolam	Xanax	Oral	*Adults:*	0.25–2 mg tid	
			Geriatric or Debilitated Clients:		
				0.25 mg bid or tid	
chlordiazepoxide HCl	Librium	Oral	*Adults:*	Mild and moderate anxiety: 5–10 mg tid or qid	
				Severe anxiety: 20–25 mg tid or qid	
			Geriatric or Debilitated Clients:		
				5 mg 2–4 times daily	
			Children:	6–12 years old	
				5 mg 2–4 times daily. May be increased in some children to 10 mg 2–4 times daily.	
clonazepam	Klonopin	Oral	*Adults:*	0.5 mg tid. May be increased by 0.5–1 mg every 3rd day. Total daily maintenance dose should not exceed 20 mg.	
			Panic Disorder:	0.125 mg bid. Increase after 3 days toward target dose of 1 mg/day.	
			Children:	Up to 10 years old or 30 kg. Initial dose of 0.01–0.03 mg/kg/day (not to exceed 0.05 mg/kg/day) given in 2–3 equally divided doses; increase by no more than 0.25–0.5 mg every 3rd day until therapeutic blood levels are reached (not to exceed 0.2 mg/kg/day).	
clorazepate	Tranxene	Oral	*Adults:*	15–60 mg daily in 2–4 divided doses	
			Geriatric or Debilitated Clients:		
				7.5–15 mg daily in 2–4 divided doses	
diazepam	Valium	Oral	*Adults:*	2–10 mg 2–4 times daily	
			Geriatric or Debilitated Clients:		
				2–2.5 mg 1–2 times daily	
			Children:	6 months and older	
				1–2.5 mg 2–4 times daily	
lorazepam	Ativan	Oral	*Adults:*	1–3 mg daily in 2–3 divided doses	
			Geriatric or Debilitated Clients:		
				0.5–2 mg/day in 2–3 divided doses	
oxazepam	Serax	Oral	*Adults:*	Mild and moderate anxiety: 10–30 mg tid or qid	
			Geriatric or Debilitated Clients:		
				10 mg tid	

Clients' Instruction

Inform the client that benzodiazepines may impair mental and/or physical abilities; therefore, one should not operate machinery or drive a motor vehicle while on these medications. Teach the client that alcohol and/or other central nervous system depressants have an additive effect and should not be used while on these medications. Teach the client that smoking may enhance the metabolism of benzodiazepines and larger doses may be needed to maintain a sedative effect. Advise the client who smokes to discuss this matter with his/her physician.

Inform the client that physical dependence may occur. Withdrawal symptoms will be similar to those produced by dependence on alcohol or barbiturates. Insomnia, anxiety, irritability, headache, muscle tremor, weakness, anorexia, nausea, and vomiting are symptoms of withdrawal from an addictive substance. Instruct the client to take the medication as ordered. If the prescribed dosage does not produce the desired results, the client should notify his/her physician. *One should not stop taking the drug abruptly.*

Benzodiazepines should be kept out of the reach of children or those who may have a tendency to abuse drugs.

> **Safety Precaution:** Benzodiazepines have been used in suicide attempts. When taken in large amounts and mixed with alcohol or other central nervous system depressants, the effects may be fatal.

The client should be advised to inform his or her physician about

- All over-the-counter drugs being taken
- Any plans to become pregnant
- Being pregnant
- Presently breast-feeding
- All other prescription medication being taken
- Consumption of alcohol

ANTIDEPRESSANT AGENTS

Antidepressant agents are chemical substances that relieve the symptoms of depression. They are indicated when depression interferes with a person's ability to function properly. The signs and symptoms of depression vary with the cause and each individual. Most individuals experience some form of depression during their lifetimes. When the feelings of depression occur every day and persist for weeks, a severe depressive illness may be present. This form of depression is called an affective disorder.

An **affective disorder** is characterized by a disturbance of mood, accompanied by a manic or depressive syndrome. This syndrome is not caused by any other physical or mental disorder. **Mood** is a pervasive and sustained emotion that may play a key role in an individual's perception of the world. With depression there is generally a loss of interest in food, sex, work, family, friends, and hobbies, among others. Feelings of helplessness, worthlessness, and guilt prevail with this form of depression. Suicide is often contemplated or attempted.

There are various forms of depression. Depression is one of the most common illnesses in America today. It is estimated that 18 million Americans are affected by clinical depression every year. Twenty-five percent of all women and 13 percent of men suffer at least one episode of serious depression during their lifetimes. It is estimated that 20 percent to 40 percent of older adults experience depressive symptoms, with the highest rates of depression found among those who are medically ill or in long-term care. Depression is not something that occurs normally as a result of aging or illness. In three out of ten depressed older adults, the depression is related to treatable physical illness or adverse effects of medications. For others, it is a recurring and disabling illness that is unrelated to any other health problem or medications.

When depression lasts more than a few weeks and gets in the way of living, it is more than a mood. It is an illness that needs to be treated by a professional. The symptoms of clinical depression include a deep sense of sadness, a noticeable change in appetite or sleep patterns, a loss of interest in pleasurable activities, fatigue or loss of energy, a feeling of worthlessness, recurrent thoughts of death or suicide, plus other possible symptoms.

Clinical Depression Test

If the client answers yes to five or more of the following questions and if the symptoms described have been present nearly every day for 2 weeks or more, he/she should seek professional assistance:

- Are there persistent feelings of sadness, emptiness, pessimism, or anxiety?
- Are there feelings of helplessness, hopelessness, guilt, or worthlessness?
- Is it difficult to make decisions, concentrate, or remember?
- Is there loss of interest or pleasure in everyday activities?
- Is there loss of drive or energy?
- Is there a significant change in sleep patterns (insomnia, early-morning waking, oversleeping)?
- Is there a significant change in appetite or weight change when not dieting?
- Are there symptoms such as headache, stomachache, backache, or chronic aches and pains of the joints and muscles? Sometimes depressive disorders masquerade as chronic physical symptoms that do not respond to treatment.
- Are there feelings of restlessness or irritability?
- Is there a significant change in smoking and drinking habits?
- Are there thoughts about death or suicide?

Antidepressant agents may be categorized in the following groups:

- *Selective serotonin reuptake inhibitors (SSRIs).* Drugs in this group specifically block reabsorption of serotonin. The most widely known are fluoxetine (Prozac), sertraline (Zoloft), paroxetine (Paxil), and fluvoxamine (Luvox).

- *Serotonin nonselective reuptake inhibitors (SNRIs).* Venlafaxine (Effexor) is a fairly new antidepressant that inhibits the reuptake of both serotonin and norepinephrine.

- *Tricyclic antidepressants (TCAs).* Drugs in this group raise the level of norepinephrine and serotonin in the brain by slowing the rate at which they are reabsorbed by nerve cells. There are many examples including imipramine (Tofranil), amitriptyline (Elavil), and nortriptyline (Pamelor).

- *Monamine oxidase inhibitors (MAOIs).* Drugs in this group work by blocking the breakdown of two potent neurotransmitters—norepinephrine and serotonin—and allowing them to bathe the nerve endings for an extended length of time. There are many examples including phenelzine (Nardil) and tranylcypromine (Parnate).

- *Lithium carbonate.* Although this is not a group of drugs, there are various lithium medications that control mood disorders by directly affecting internal nerve cell processes in all the neurotransmitter systems. Lithium is best known as an antimanic drug used in the treatment of bipolar disorder.

- *Miscellaneous drugs.* Nefazodone (Serzone) is a synthetically derived phenylpiperazine antidepressant with a mechanism of action distinct from those of other currently available antidepressants. It selectively blocks postsynaptic serotonin (5-hydroxytryptamine; 5-HT) 5-HT2A receptors (polymorphism gene implicated in bipolar disorder and harm avoidance personality trait) and moderately inhibits serotonin and norepinephrine reuptake.

Selective Serotonin Reuptake Inhibitors (SSRIs)

Selective serotonin reuptake inhibitors (SSRIs) are the result of research for drugs as effective as tricyclic antidepressants but with fewer safety and tolerability problems. SSRIs selectively inhibit serotonin reuptake and result in a potentiation of serotonergic neurotransmission. They are structurally diverse with variations in their pharmacodynamic and pharmacokinetic profiles.

Actions

Specifically block reabsorption of serotonin. Inhibit neuronal reuptake of serotonin in the central nervous system (CNS), thus potentiating the activity of serotonin.

Uses

SSRIs are used for the treatment of depression, social anxiety disorder, obsessive-compulsive disorder (OCD), and panic disorder.

Contraindications

Hypersensitivity. Concurrent MAO inhibitor therapy (may result in potentially fatal reactions).

Adverse Reactions

Anxiety, dizziness, drowsiness, headache, insomnia, weakness, agitation, amnesia, confusion, constipation, diarrhea, dry mouth, nausea, sweating, tremor, ejaculatory disturbances, decreased libido, genital disorders, weight gain, weight loss, chills, fever.

Dosage and Route

The dosage and route is determined by the physician. The dosage is individualized for each client and regulated according to the effectiveness of the medication. See Table 22-2.

Nursing Considerations

Observe the client for any signs of hypersensitivity. Note the effectiveness of the drug. Are the symptoms improved? Observe for adverse reactions and report them to the proper authority or to the physician. Monitor appetite and nutrition intake. Weigh weekly. Note weight gain and/or loss. Evaluate the client for history of drug abuse and be aware of the possibility of misuse or abuse. Be alert to the possibility of suicide.

Clients' Instruction

Inform the client that SSRIs may impair mental and/or physical abilities; therefore, he/she should not operate machinery or drive a motor vehicle. Advise the client to inform the physician if he/she is taking or plans to take any prescription or over-the-counter medication or alcohol. The client should advise the physician if she becomes pregnant or intends to become pregnant or if she is breast-feeding an infant.

Instruct the client to take the medication as ordered. Inform the client to keep the medication out of the reach of children.

TABLE 22-2   SELECTIVE SEROTONIN REUPTAKE INHIBITORS (SSRIs)

Generic Name	Trade Name	Route	Usual Dosage	
fluoxetine	Prozac	Oral	*Adults:*	Initially 20 mg/day in the morning. May be increased if needed after several weeks. Doses greater than 20 mg/day are given in 2 divided doses (morning and noon). Maximum dose is 80 mg/day.
			Geriatric:	Initially 10 mg/day in the morning. May be increased, but should not exceed 60 mg/day.
fluvoxamine	Luvox	Oral	*Adults:*	Initially 50 mg daily at bedtime. May be increased by 50 mg every 4–7 days until desired effect is achieved. If daily dose is 100 mg or greater, give in 2 equally divided doses or give a larger dose at bedtime (not to exceed 300 mg/day).
			Children:	8–17 years old: 25 mg at bedtime. May be increased by 25 mg/day every 4–7 days (not to exceed 200 mg/day).
paroxetine (See Figure 22-1)	Paxil	Oral	*Depression:*	
			Adults:	20 mg as a single dose in the morning. May be increased by 10 mg/day at weekly intervals (not to exceed 50 mg/day).
			Geriatric:	Initially 10 mg/day. May be slowly increased (not to exceed 40 mg/day).
			Obsessive-Compulsive Disorder:	
			Adults:	Initially 20 mg/day. May be increased by 10 mg/day every week up to 40 mg (range 40–60 mg/day).
			Panic Disorder:	
			Adults:	Initially 10 mg/day. May be increased by 10 mg/day every week up to 40 mg/kg (not to exceed 60 mg/day).
sertraline	Zoloft	Oral	*Depression/Obsessive-Compulsive Disorder:*	
			Adults:	Initially 50 mg/day as a single dose in the morning or evening. After several weeks may be increased at weekly intervals up to 200 mg/day, depending on response.
			Obsessive-Compulsive Disorder:	
			Children:	13–17 years old: 50 mg once daily; 6 to 12 years old: 25 mg once daily
			Panic Disorder:	
			Adults:	Initially 25 mg/day. May be increased after 1 week to 50 mg/day.

Inform the client to report any adverse reactions to this medication, especially a rash or hives.

Encourage the client to seek medical attention if symptoms do not improve.

Safety Precaution: With the combined administration of MAOIs and tricyclics, at least 14 days should elapse between discontinuation of an MAO inhibitor and initiation of treatment with SSRIs.

Serotonin Nonselective Reuptake Inhibitors (SNRIs)

Serotonin nonselective reuptake inhibitors (SNRIs)—venlafaxine (Effexor)—is a structurally novel antidepressant for oral administration. It inhibits the reuptake of both serotonin and norepinephrine.

Venlafaxine HCl (Effexor)

Effexor is a structurally novel antidepressant for oral administration. It is chemically unrelated to

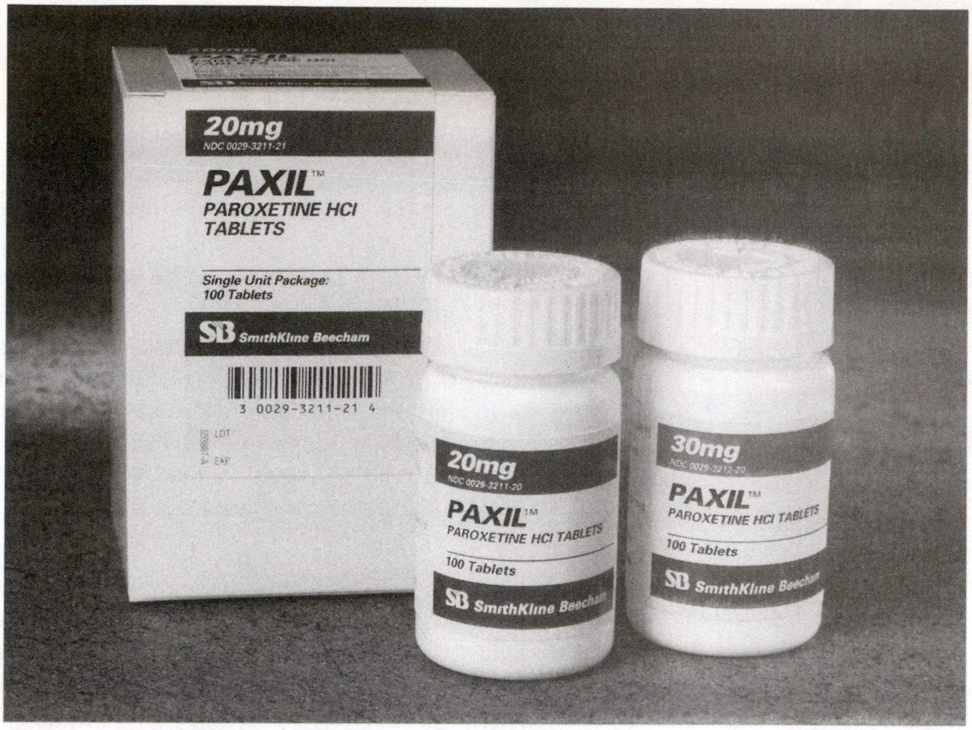

FIGURE 22-1 PAXIL™ (PAROXETINE HCL) TABLETS 20 MG, 30 MG *(Courtesy of SmithKline Beecham)*

tricyclic, tetracyclic, or other available antidepressant agents.

Actions

It is believed that venlafaxine potentiates neurotransmitter activity of the central nervous system. Preclinical studies have shown that it inhibits serotonin and norepinephrine reuptake and is a weak inhibitor of dopamine reuptake.

Uses

Indicated for the treatment of depression.

Contraindications

Hypersensitivity to venlafaxine.

Adverse Reactions

General weakness, sweating, nausea, constipation, anorexia, vomiting, sleepiness, dry mouth, dizziness, nervousness, anxiety, tremor, blurred vision, abnormal ejaculation or orgasm in men, and impotence.

Dosage and Route

Effexor is an oral antidepressant drug and the dosage is prescribed by the physician. The recommended dosage is 75 mg/day. Depending on tolera-

bility and the need for further clinical effect, the dose may be increased in 75 mg steps every 4 or more days to 150–225 mg/day. When discontinuing Effexor after more than 1 week of therapy, it is generally recommended that the dose be tapered to minimize the risk of discontinuation symptoms. *Clients who have received Effexor for 6 weeks or more should have their dose tapered gradually over a 2-week period.*

Nursing Considerations

Observe the client for signs of hypersensitivity. Note the effectiveness of the drug. Are the symptoms improved? Observe for adverse reactions. Report any adverse reactions to the proper authority. Evaluate the client for history of drug abuse and be aware of the possibility of misuse or abuse. Be aware and ever alert to the possibility of suicide.

Clients' Instruction

Inform the client that Effexor may impair mental and/or physical abilities; therefore, he/she should not operate machinery or drive a motor vehicle. Advise the client to inform the physician if he/she is taking or plans to take any prescription or over-the-counter medication or alcohol. The client should advise the physician if she becomes pregnant or intends to become pregnant or if she is breast-feeding an infant. If the client has high blood pressure, he/she should inform the physician, as Effexor can cause sustained increases in blood pressure. If the client has liver or kidney disease and/or a history of seizures, the physician should be informed before initiation of drug therapy.

Instruct the client to take the medication as ordered. Inform the client to keep the medication out of reach of children.

Inform the client to report any adverse reactions to this medication, especially a rash or hives.

Encourage the client to seek medical attention if symptoms do not improve.

> **Safety Precaution:** Taking Effexor in combination with a monoamine oxidase inhibitor (MAOI) or within 14 days of stopping MAOI therapy can cause serious side effects and/or fatalities. At least 14 days should elapse between discontinuation of an MAOI and initiation of therapy with Effexor. In addition, at least 7 days should be allowed after stopping Effexor before starting an MAOI. Some commonly prescribed MAOIs include Nardil (phenelzine sulfate) and Parnate (tranylcypromine sulfate).

Tricyclic Antidepressants

Tricyclic antidepressants share a chemical configuration that is characterized by a three-ring or tricyclic structure. They are used in the treatment of depression.

Actions

The precise mechanism of action in humans is not known. These agents are believed to block norepinephrine and serotonin uptake shortly after administration. They seem to elevate mood, increase physical activity and mental alertness, and improve appetite and sleep. In 60 to 70 percent of clients with endogenous depression, morbid preoccupation was reduced. Anticholinergic and alpha-adrenergic blocking activities are adverse actions to note.

Uses

Tricyclic antidepressants are used for the relief of symptoms of depression. Endogenous depression is more likely to be alleviated than other depressive states.

Contraindications

Hypersensitivity to tricyclic antidepressants.

Adverse Reactions

The most common adverse reactions of these agents are due to their blocking parasympathetic nerve impulses (anticholinergic) and alpha-adrenergic blocking activities: flushing, diaphoresis, blurred vision, disturbance of accommodation, increased intraocular pressure, constipation, paralytic ileus, urinary retention, and dilatation of urinary tract.

Other adverse reactions that may occur are hypotension, particularly orthostatic hypotension; hypertension; tachycardia; palpitation; confusion; excitement; anxiety; insomnia; numbness, tingling, and paresthesias of the extremities; ataxia; tremors; seizures; skin rash; nausea; vomiting; anorexia; diarrhea; dizziness; fatigue; headache; weight gain or loss; and drowsiness.

> ***Note:*** Cimetidine (Tagamet) may increase the bioavailability of certain tricyclic antidepressants. This drug interaction may produce severe anticholinergic adverse reactions such as dizziness and orthostatic hypotension.

Dosage and Route

The dosage and route is prescribed by the physician and individualized for each client. See Table 22-3 for selected tricyclic antidepressants.

Nursing Considerations

Observe the client for any signs of hypersensitivity. Note the effectiveness of the drug. Are the symptoms improved? Observe for adverse reactions. Report any adverse reactions to the proper authority or to the physician.

During hospitalization, provide for safety measures and monitor vital signs, especially the blood pressure (orthostatic hypotension may occur). Be aware and ever alert to the possibility of suicide.

Clients' Instruction

Inform the client that tricyclic antidepressants may impair mental and/or physical abilities; therefore, one should not operate machinery or drive a motor vehicle. Advise the client not to arise suddenly. Teach the client that alcohol and/or other central nervous system depressants have an additive effect and should not be used while on these medications.

Instruct the client to take the medications as ordered. Inform the client to keep these medications out of the reach of children.

Inform the client to report any adverse reactions to his/her physician. Encourage the client to seek medical attention if symptoms do not improve.

TABLE 22-3 SELECTED TRICYCLIC ANTIDEPRESSANTS

Generic Name	Trade Name	Route	Usual Dosage
amitriptyline HCl	Elavil	Oral	*Adults:* Outpatients: 75 mg/day in divided doses; may be increased to 150 mg/day Hospitalized clients: 100–200 mg daily *Adolescents and Geriatric:* 10 mg tid with 20 mg at bedtime; maximum 100 mg/day
amoxapine	Asendin	Oral	*Adults:* 200–300 mg daily *Geriatric:* 25 mg bid or tid
desipramine HCl	Norpramin	Oral	*Adults:* 100–200 mg daily *Adolescents and Geriatric:* 25–100 mg daily
imipramine HCl	Tofranil	Oral	*Adults:* Outpatients: 75–150 mg daily Hospitalized clients: 100–300 mg daily *Adolescents and Geriatric:* 30–40 mg daily; not to exceed 100 mg/day
nortriptyline hydrochloride	Pamelor	Oral	*Adults:* 25 mg 3–4 times daily; not to exceed 150 mg/day *Geriatric:* 30–50 mg/day in divided doses
trazodone HCl	Desyrel	Oral	*Adults:* Outpatients: Initial dose of 50 mg tid. The dose may be increased by 50 mg/day every 3–4 days. The maximum dose should not exceed 400 mg/day.
trimipramine maleate	Surmontil	Oral	*Adults:* Outpatients: 75–150 mg daily in 2–3 divided doses Hospitalized clients: 100–200 mg daily in 2–3 divided doses *Adolescents and Geriatric:* 50–100 mg/day

Safety Precaution: Tricyclic antidepressants should not be given with monoamine oxidase inhibitors. When replacing a monoamine oxidase inhibitor with one of these agents, a minimum of 14 days should be allowed to elapse after the former is discontinued.

 Note: The possibility of suicide in depressed clients remains until significant remission occurs. Potentially suicidal persons should not have access to a large quantity of these agents.

Monoamine Oxidase Inhibitors (MAOIs)

Monoamine oxidase inhibitors are antidepressants that inhibit the oxidase enzyme that breaks down monoamine transmitters in the body. They may be considered as the drugs of choice in such nonendogenous types of depression as agoraphobia and hysteroid dysphoria. They appear to be less effective than the tricyclic antidepressants in clients with endogenous depression and their use generally requires strict dietary control. See Table 22-4.

Actions

MAOIs inhibit the monoamine oxidase enzyme that catalyzes the inactivation of serotonin, norepinephrine, and dopamine, thereby increasing the brain concentrations of these substances. In theory, this increased concentration of monoamines in the brain stem is the basis for the antidepressant activity of MAOIs. In vivo and in vitro studies demonstrated inhibition of amine oxidase in the brain, heart, and liver.

Uses

MAOIs may be used in agoraphobia, hysteroid dysphoria, and in clients who have not responded to treatment with tricyclic antidepressants.

Contraindications

- In clients with known hypersensitivity to the drug
- In clients with cerebrovascular defects or cardiovascular disorders
- In the presence of pheochromocytoma
- In combination with sympathomimetics
- In combination with meperidine (Demerol)

TABLE 22-4   MONOAMINE OXIDASE INHIBITORS (MAOIs)

Trade Generic Name	Name	Route	Usual Dosage
phenelzine sulfate	Nardil	Oral	*Adults:* Initial dose: 15 mg (one tablet) tid Early-phase treatment: 60 mg/day or up to 90 mg/day Maintenance dose: 15 mg/day or every other day
tranylcypromine sulfate	Parnate	Oral	*Adults:* Starting dose: 30 mg/day in divided doses. If no improvement in 2 weeks, increase by 10 mg/day every 1 to 3 weeks to a maximum of 60 mg/day.

- In combination with cheese or other foods with a high tyramine content
- In clients undergoing elective surgery
- In clients with impaired renal and/or liver function
- In combination with narcotics, alcohol, and hypotensive agents
- Cautious use with anti-parkinsonism drugs

Adverse Reactions

Orthostatic hypotension, drowsiness, dryness of the mouth, blurred vision, dysuria, constipation, restlessness, insomnia, weakness, nausea, diarrhea, abdominal pain, tachycardia, anorexia, edema, palpitation, chills, impotence, headache, dizziness, vertigo, tremors, muscle twitching, and photosensitivity are some of the adverse reactions.

Dosage and Route

The dosage and route is determined by the physician. The dosage is individualized for each client and regulated according to the effectiveness of the medication. The client has to be carefully monitored by the prescribing physician.

Nursing Considerations

Observe the client for any signs of hypersensitivity. Note the effectiveness of the drug. Observe for adverse reactions.

During hospitalization, provide for safety and carefully monitor the client's blood pressure for orthostatic hypotension as well as hypertension.

Safety Precaution: Hypertensive crises may occur with the use of MAOIs and the consumption of large amounts of foods that contain tyramine. These crises may be fatal.

Know the symptoms of marked elevation of blood pressure: occipital headache, which may radiate frontally, palpitation, neck stiffness or soreness, nausea or vomiting, sweating (sometimes with fever and sometimes with cold), and photophobia. Tachycardia or bradycardia, chest pain, and dilated pupils may occur. Notify the physician immediately if these symptoms appear. The medication should be discontinued and measures to lower the blood pressure should be initiated. Be observant for signs of orthostatic hypotension.

Clients' Instruction

Instruct the client to notify the physician immediately if headache, stiff neck, pounding heartbeat, feelings of nausea, or vomiting occur. Instruct the client not to suddenly arise from a lying position. If the client feels dizzy upon arising, instruct him/her to lie back down until the dizziness disappears.

Inform the client not to drink alcoholic or caffeinated beverages or take over-the-counter medications while using MAOIs. Inform the client to be sure to tell the physician about all other medications that he or she may be taking. If the client is seeing more than one physician, each physician should be informed of the client's medication regimen. Advise the client who is taking insulin and/or oral sulfonylureas to monitor blood glucose levels very carefully, as MAOIs may have an additive hypoglycemic effect when taken with these drugs. The client with diabetes should discuss this information with his/her physician.

Be sure that the client understands that large amounts of tyramine can lead to a hypertensive crisis. Provide the client with a list of foods and beverages to *avoid*. You may use the following list:

When taking MAOIs, the following foods and beverages must be *avoided*:	
Cheese	Yeast extracts
Sour cream	Meats prepared with tenderizers
Pickled herring	
Liver	Chianti wine
Canned figs	Sherry
Raisins	Beer
Bananas	Protein foods that are aged
Avocados	
Chocolate	Chicken livers
Soy sauce	Pickles
Fava beans	Yogurt

Note: Effects of MAOIs will continue for as long as 2 weeks after the MAOI is stopped. Foods and beverages containing tyramine must be avoided during this period.

ANTIMANIC AGENT(S)

Lithium is considered the drug of choice for the treatment of the manic episode of bipolar disorder. **Bipolar disorder** is a major affective disorder that is characterized by episodes of mania and depression. It was previously called manic-depressive psychosis. Bipolar disorder is subdivided into three types: manic, depressed, and mixed. In the manic phase, there are excessive emotional displays such as excitement, euphoria, hyperactivity, boisterousness, impaired ability to concentrate, decreased need for sleep, exalted feelings, delusions of grandeur, and overproduction of ideas. In the depressive phase, there is marked apathy, underactivity, and feeling of profound sadness, loneliness, and guilt. In the mixed phase, elements of both mania and depression may be present.

Lithium

Actions

The specific biochemical mechanism of lithium action in mania is unknown. It counteracts mood changes without producing sedation. Studies have shown that lithium alters sodium transport in nerve and muscle cells and effects a shift toward intraneuronal metabolism of catecholamines.

Uses

Specific antimanic drug for prophylaxis and treatment of bipolar disorder (manic-depressive).

Warnings

Generally not given to clients with significant renal or cardiovascular disease, severe debilitation or dehydration, or sodium depletion, since the risk of lithium toxicity is high in such clients. Lithium may cause fetal harm when administered during pregnancy.

Adverse Reactions

Fine hand tremor, polyuria, and mild thirst may occur during initial therapy and may persist throughout the treatment. During the first few days of lithium administration, there may be transient and mild nausea and general discomfort.

Early signs of lithium intoxication are diarrhea, vomiting, drowsiness, muscular weakness, and lack of coordination. These signs may appear at serum lithium levels below 2.0 mEq/L. At higher levels, ataxia, giddiness, tinnitus, blurred vision, and polyuria may occur. Serum lithium levels above 3.0 mEq/L may cause a complex of signs and symptoms involving various organs and systems of the body. Refer to the *Physicians' Desk Reference*, or Delmar's *Nurse's Drug Handbook*™ for further information.

Dosage and Route

The dosage is individualized according to the serum lithium level and the client's clinical response. A threshold level of lithium in body tissues must be reached before it is effective. This may take 3 to 5 days of therapy. Lithium is available as

- Eskalith—300 mg tablets and capsules; 300 mg and 450 mg controlled-release tablets
- Lithobid—300 mg slow-release tablets
- Lithium carbonate—300 mg tablets and capsules
- Lithium Citrate Syrup—8 mEq/5 ml (300 mg of lithium carbonate)

Nursing Considerations

The client should have a complete physical examination before the initiation of lithium therapy.

Close clinical observation and frequent monitoring of serum lithium levels is essential. Serum lithium levels should be determined two to three times weekly during the acute manic phase, then on a monthly basis during maintenance therapy. During the initial stage of therapy, the blood level should be maintained between 1 and 1.5 mEq/L of serum. During maintenance therapy, the blood level should be between 0.6 and 1.2 mEq/L of serum. Observe for adverse reactions. Report to the proper authority or to the physician.

During hospitalization, provide for safety measures and support to the client and his/her family. Establish rapport with the client. Assess the client's mental status: cognitive function, alertness, level of orientation, attention span, memory, language function, and spatial ability.

Clients' Instruction

The client and his/her family should be informed of the early symptoms of lithium intoxication or toxicity and instructed to discontinue the medication and contact the physician immediately.

> *Early Symptoms of Lithium Intoxication:*
> drowsiness, vomiting, muscle weakness, ataxia, dryness of the mouth, lethargy, abdominal pain, dizziness, slurred speech, diarrhea, tremor, and nystagmus

Inform the client that the metallic taste may be temporary and will usually decrease with a lower dose of lithium. Teach the client how to perform good oral hygiene. Advise the client to take the medication as prescribed and not to discontinue the medication unless symptoms of lithium intoxication occur.

To diminish nausea, lithium may be given with meals. Stress the importance of good nutrition and emphasize that the client should maintain a normal intake of sodium and fluids. Lithium may enhance sodium depletion, which could enhance lithium toxicity. Instruct the client to drink 10–12 eight-ounce glasses of water daily to prevent possible toxicity. Advise the client to refrain from drinking caffeinated liquids and alcoholic beverages. Instruct the client not to change the brand of the prescribed medication.

Advise female clients against becoming pregnant during the time they are taking lithium.

Advise the client to inform other health care providers of his/her lithium therapy.

Stress to the client the importance of returning to his/her attending physician, as scheduled, for lithium blood analysis.

ANTIPSYCHOTIC AGENTS

Antipsychotic agents modify psychotic behavior and are sometimes called **neuroleptics**. Many antipsychotic agents are **phenothiazine** (an organic compound used in the manufacture of certain antipsychotic drugs) derivatives. Phenothiazines differ in their ability to produce sedation, extrapyramidal reactions, and anticholinergic effects. Thorazine, the first antipsychotic agent to be introduced in the early 1950s, is a phenothiazine derivative. It is available in a variety of forms and dosages such as tablets (10 mg, 25 mg, 50 mg, 100 mg, 200 mg), sustained-release (SR) capsules (30 mg, 75 mg, 150 mg), syrup (10 mg/5 mL), concentrate (30 mg/mL, 100 mg/mL), suppositories (25 mg, 100 mg), and injection (25 mg/mL).

Some antipsychotic agents are not phenothiazines, but resemble a phenothiazine in action. Others resemble tricyclic antidepressants, while some are miscellaneous compounds. Newer compounds antagonize dopamine and serotonin type 2 in the central nervous system, but they also have antihistaminic, anticholinergic, and alpha-antiadrenergic effects.

Neuroleptics

Actions

The precise mechanism of action is not known. They are believed to control the symptomatology of psychosis by reducing excessive dopamine activity: by blocking postsynaptic dopamine receptors in the cerebral cortex, basal ganglia, limbic system, brain stem, and hypothalamus.

Antipsychotic agents have varying degrees of antihistaminic, anticholinergic, and alpha-antiadrenergic activities. These activities account for a number of the adverse reactions associated with antipsychotic agents.

Uses

Antipsychotic agents are used in the treatment of acute and chronic schizophrenia, organic psychoses, the manic phase of bipolar affective disorder, and psychotic disorders.

Contraindications

Hypersensitivity to the specific antipsychotic agent. Most antipsychotic agents are contraindicated in comatose clients; those receiving large doses of CNS depressants; and in clients with bone marrow depression, blood dyscrasias, or liver damage.

Adverse Reactions

Antipsychotic agents may cause a wide gamut of adverse reactions. Some that may occur are drowsiness, sedation, convulsive seizure, dryness of mouth, constipation, urinary retention, blurred vision, orthostatic hypotension, tachycardia, fainting, dizziness, dystonia, motor restlessness, nasal congestion, toxic psychosis, photosensitivity, jaundice, skin pigmentation, and ocular changes.

Other adverse reactions include extrapyramidal symptoms (EPS)—these symptoms appear to be dose related and are the most frightening to the client. **Dystonia**—difficult or bad muscle tone—may appear as spasm of the neck muscles, torticollis, rigidity of back muscles, carpopedal spasm, trismus, swallowing difficulty, oculogyric crisis, and protrusion of the tongue. **Akathisia** (acathisia)—an inability to sit down. The client has a feeling of restlessness and an urgent need of movement. Pacing, fidgeting, and agitation are classic symptoms of akathisia.

Pseudo-parkinsonism—a neuroleptic-induced reaction. Symptoms may include mask-like expression (facies), drooling, tremors, rigidity, bradykinesia, shuffling gait, postural abnormalities, and hypersalivation. These symptoms may occur within a few weeks to a few months after initiating therapy, and may be controlled by an antiparkinsonism agent.

> **Note:** Levodopa has not been found to be effective in the treatment of pseudo-parkinsonism.

Tardive dyskinesia—a syndrome characterized by rhythmical involuntary movement of the tongue, face, mouth, jaw, trunk and extremities. These symptoms may appear in some clients on long-term therapy. They may also appear after drug therapy has been discontinued. Tardive (lateness) dyskinesias (difficult movement) may occur in clients of any age, but is more common in older women. There is no known effective treatment for this syndrome.

Dosage and Route

The dosage and route of administration is determined by the physician. The dosage is individualized for each client and regulated according to the effectiveness of the medication. See Table 22-5 for selected antipsychotic agents.

Nursing Considerations

The client who takes antipsychotic agents needs special care. It is essential that you understand the client's diagnosis and his/her treatment regimen. Remember that drug therapy is only a part of the treatment plan. The client needs emotional, physical, and social support. It is important that the client's family be included in care planning and implementation.

Observe the client for signs of hypersensitivity and adverse reactions. Notify the proper authorities or physician of any adverse reactions. Note the effectiveness of the medication. Are the symptoms improved? During hospitalization, provide for safety measures, monitor vital signs, and record intake and output when indicated.

Clients' Instruction

Inform the client that antipsychotic agents may impair mental and/or physical abilities; therefore, he/she should not operate machinery or drive a motor vehicle while on these medications. Teach the client that alcohol and/or other central nervous system depressants have an additive effect and should not be used while on these medications.

Instruct the client to take the medications as ordered. If the client is unable to manage his/her own plan of treatment, inform the proper family member or other responsible person of any and all essential information.

Assess the client's mental status: cognitive function, alertness, level of orientation, attention span, memory, language function, spatial ability, the presence of delusions or hallucinations, agitation, and withdrawal. Assess the client's behavioral status: purposefulness of activity, sleeping pattern, eating pattern, appropriate responses, and speech patterns.

Teach the client to report adverse reactions to his/her physician. Inform the client to avoid exposure to ultraviolet rays (sunlight or artificial). Instruct the client not to suddenly arise from a lying position. Inform the client to be sure to tell the physician about all other medications that he/she may be taking. If the client is seeing more than one physician, each physician should be informed of the client's medication regimen.

Encourage the client to eat a balanced diet and to drink sufficient fluids. Keeping the mucous membranes moist will help relieve dryness of the mouth. If desired, the client may suck on ice chips or sugarless hard candy to help moisten the mouth. When the client has constipation, the physician should order an appropriate stool softener and/or laxative.

TABLE 22-5   SELECTED ANTIPSYCHOTIC AGENTS

Generic Name	Trade Name	Route	Usual Dosage
chlorpromazine HCl (see Figure 22-2)	Thorazine	Oral	*Adults:* Excessive anxiety, tension, and agitation: 10 mg tid or qid or 25 mg bid or tid More severe cases: 25 mg tid; daily dosage may be 200–800 mg *Children:* Office clients, outpatients: 0.25 mg/lb of body weight every 4–6 h, prn
clozapine	Clozaril	Oral	Initially 25 mg 1–2 times daily. May be increased by 25–50 mg/day over a period of 2 weeks up to a target dose of 300–450 mg/day
fluphenazine HCl	Permitil	Oral	*Adults:* 0.5–10 mg/day in divided doses every 6–8 hours
haloperidol	Haldol	Oral	*Adults:* Moderate symptomatology: 0.5–2.0 mg bid or tid. Severe symptomatology: 3.0–5.0 mg bid or tid. Geriatric or debilitated: 0.5–2.0 mg bid or tid Chronic or resistant clients: 3.0–5.0 mg bid or tid *Children:* 3–12 years: psychotic disorders: 0.05–0.15 mg/kg/day
loxapine	Loxitane	Oral	Initially 10 mg bid Severely disturbed: up to 50 mg/day Maintenance 20–60 mg/day
mesoridazine	Serentil	Oral	Schizophrenia: Starting dose 50 mg tid, daily dose range 100–400 mg/day
olanzapine	Zyprexa	Oral	Initially 5–10 mg/day. May be increased at weekly intervals by 5 mg/day (not to exceed 15 mg/day)
perphenazine	Trilafon	Oral	Moderately disturbed nonhospitalized psychotic clients: 4–8 mg tid or 1–2 REPETABS bid (initially). Hospitalized psychotic clients: 8–16 mg bid to qid or 1–4 REPETABS bid; avoid dosage in excess of 64 mg daily
prochlorperazine (See Figure 22-3)	Compazine	Oral	*Adults:* Nonpsychotic anxiety: 5 mg 3–4 times daily, psychotic disorders (mild) office clients, outpatients: 5–10 mg 3–4 times daily. Moderate–severe hospitalized or adequately supervised clients: 10 mg 3–4 times daily (initially); 50–75 mg/daily. More severe clients: optimum dosage is 100–150 mg daily
promazine HCl	Sparine	Oral	*Adults:* Psychotic disorders: 10–200 mg at 4–6 hour intervals; dose limit 1000 mg/day *Children:* Over 12 years: 10–25 mg every 4–6 hours
risperidone	Risperdal	Oral	1 mg twice daily, increased by 3rd day to 3 mg twice daily
thioridazine HCl	Mellaril	Oral	*Adults:* 50–100 mg tid (starting dose); maximum to 800 mg a day. Daily dosage range 200–800 mg divided into 2–4 doses *Children:* Ages 2–12 years: 0.5–3.0 mg/kg/day
thiothixene HCl	Navane	Oral	Initially (mild) 2 mg tid Severe 5 mg bid Optimal dose 20–30 mg daily
trifluoperazine HCl	Stelazine	Oral	*Adults:* Nonpsychotic anxiety: 1–2 mg bid Psychotic disorders: 2–5 mg bid *Children:* 6–12 years hospitalized or under close supervision: 1 mg once a day or bid (starting dose)

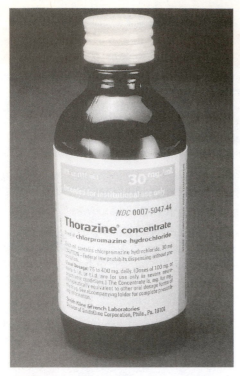

FIGURE 22-2 THORAZINE®
(CHLORPROMAZINE HYDROCHLORIDE) 30 MG/ML
(Courtesy of SmithKline Beecham)

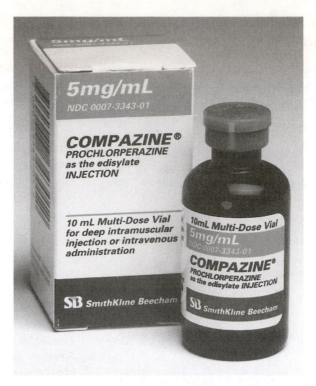

FIGURE 22-3 COMPAZINE® (PROCHLORPERAZINE)
5 MG/ML *(Courtesy of SmithKline Beecham)*

● SPOT CHECK

For each of the psychotropic agents given, list several aspects of client' instruction and nursing considerations.

Psychotropic Agent	Clients' Instruction	Nursing Considerations
Benzodiazepines		
Selective Serotonin Reuptake Inhibitors (SSRIs)		

(continued)

Psychotropic Agent	Clients' Instruction	Nursing Considerations
Tricyclic Antidepressants		
Lithium		

● SELF-ASSESSMENT

Write the answer in the space provided.

Source

p. 257   **1.** List four classifications of drugs that affect psychic function, behavior, or experience. (1) _____, (2) _____, (3) _____, and (4) _____ agents

p. 257   **2.** In the United States, the _____ drugs are among the most widely prescribed medications.

p. 257   **3.** _____ is defined as an involuntary or reflex action of the body to stress, resulting in a feeling of uneasiness, apprehension, worry, or dread.

p. 257   **4.** The most widely prescribed group of drugs for the treatment of the above-mentioned condition are the _____.

p. 258   **5.** On the space provided, choose two of the following agents that do not belong to the group of drugs found in question 4: Xanax, Zoloft, Valium, Asendin, Librium, or Klonopin. The two are _____ and _____.

p. 259   **6.** Symptoms of clinical depression include a deep sense of _____, a noticeable change in _____, a noticeable change in _____ patterns, a loss of _____ in pleasurable activities, fatigue or loss of energy, a feeling of _____, recurrent thoughts of death or suicide, plus other symptoms.

p. 261   **7.** Drugs that specifically block reabsorption of serotonin are known are selective serotonin reuptake inhibitors (SSRIs). The trade names of the most widely known drugs of this group are _____, _____, _____, and Luvox.

p. 264   **8.** _____ may be considered as drugs of choice in such nonendogenous types of depression as agoraphobia and hysteroid dysphoria.

p. 266   **9.** _____ is a major affective disorder characterized by episodes of mania and depression, and the drug of choice for treatment of a client's manic episode is _____.

p. 268   **10.** Extrapyramidal symptoms (EPS) such as dystonia and akathisia appear to be dose related and are most likely to cause fright in a client. The medical term *dystonia* means difficult or bad _____ and the medical term *akathisia* can be defined as _____.

● WEB ACTIVITY

Visit the following Web sites for additional information on psychotropic agents:

http://www.pslgroup.com

http://www.discoveryhealth.com

http://www.medicinenet.com

http://pharmacotherapy.medscape.com

http://www.onhealth.com

http://www.intelihealth.com

http://www.pharminfo.com

http://www.docguide.com

http://www.medscape.com

http://www.mayohealth.org

http://www.rxlist.com

http://www.biopsychiatry.com

http://www.axom.com

http://www.micromedex.com

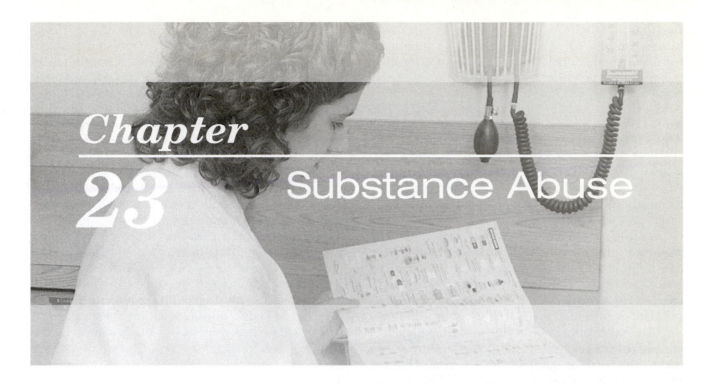

Chapter 23 — Substance Abuse

Objectives

Upon completion of this chapter, you should be able to

- Define the key terms
- Describe the abuse of legal and illegal drugs as well as other substances
- Identify abused substances by street names
- Discuss problems associated with substance abuse
- State the role of the health professional in recognizing substance abuse
- Describe actions one might take when substance abuse is suspected
- List the warning signs of substance abuse in the workplace
- Complete the Spot Check on physiological effects of selected illegal substances
- Complete the Self-Assessment
- Visit indicated Web sites for additional information on substance abuse

Key Terms

abuse	physical dependency
addiction	psychological
anterograde amnesia	dependency
bagging	psychotropic
huffing	tolerance
inhalant	withdrawal

INTRODUCTION

Why do people use drugs? For hundreds of years, humans have sought out substances that relieve pain and/or fight infection as well as those that give pleasure. The modern Western culture in which we live places a reliance on such substances for everything from anxiety relief to a cure for some cancers.

This chapter explores **psychotropic** (mood-altering) drugs and other substances our population has singled out for abuse. In this context, **abuse** can be defined as the misuse of a substance, legal or illegal, sufficient to cause the abuser mental, physical, emotional, or social harm. Abuse, in some instances, can lead to addiction or dependency. **Addiction** or dependency is the compulsive, continued use of a drug. Addiction can involve physical dependence, psychological dependence, or both.

It should be noted that not all drug abuse is related to illegal substances. Between 2 and 3 million Americans are addicted to prescription drugs, and hospital emergencies are as likely to involve legal drugs as they are illegal drugs.

Abused substances take many forms and are introduced into the body in a variety of ways. They can include substances such as marijuana or tobacco, beverages containing alcohol, and pharmacological agents. They may be taken orally, smoked, inhaled, or injected.

Substance abuse can result in the development of drug **tolerance**, a condition wherein the person's body adjusts to the dosage of a particular drug and larger amounts of the drug must be taken in order to achieve the desired effect. Physical dependency is often preceded or accompanied by tolerance. When a person with a physical dependency on a drug is forced to do without it, an illness results. Known as **withdrawal**, this condition may include flu-like symptoms, nausea, shakes, sweats, tremors, and acute craving for the drug.

The abuse of alcohol, nicotine, certain drugs, and other chemical substances is a health and social problem that affects everyone. The cost of substance abuse runs into the billions of dollars, most of which goes to combat crime by drug users, to pay for property and personal injury resulting from accidents involving substance abuse, and for social and psychiatric services to victims of drug abuse. Increased taxation and higher insurance are pocketbook expenses that can be calculated in measurable terms. Not so easily measured is the absenteeism from school or work, the defective products produced by affected workers, and the waste of human potential epitomized by the addict.

How It Begins

A person cannot become addicted to drugs without first starting to use them. Why people try drugs is open to debate, but research has shown that substance abuse occurs among people of all ages and socioeconomic levels. Environmental and social factors such as poverty, family dysfunction, and peer pressure are often cited as reasons for a person's willingness to try drugs as is curiosity about the "feeling" he/she will derive from the experience.

Regardless of the reasons, people who try drugs risk addiction. True, not everyone who drinks becomes an alcoholic and not all substance abusers become drug addicts; however, far too many do. Addictive drugs, including nicotine and alcohol, are dangerous because most people believe that they are immune to addiction. Unfortunately, the body develops a tolerance for most abused substances. Increases in both dosage and frequency of use are needed in order to achieve the same degree of effect that was once possible with smaller or less frequent doses. Abuse with high doses of psychoactive substances leads to dependency. **Physical dependency** occurs when one or more of the body's physiologic functions becomes dependent on the presence of the abused drug. The body experiences withdrawal symptoms if the substance is not taken or ingested. **Psychological dependency** does not involve the body's physiologic functions; rather, it is a psychic craving for the effects produced by the abused substance.

SUBSTANCES BEING ABUSED
Nicotine

According to the National Institute on Drug Abuse (NIDA), nicotine is one of the most heavily used addictive drugs in the United States. Cigarette smoking, since the beginning of the 20th century, has been the method of choice for taking nicotine. Currently, 60 million Americans (including children) are smokers. Like alcohol, tobacco products are legal for adults, yet, according to NIDA, 4.1 million youths between the ages of 12 and 17 unlawfully obtain and use tobacco products.

Nicotine is highly addictive. It is both a stimulant and a sedative to the central nervous system and is absorbed readily from tobacco smoke in the lungs or as a consequence of chewing tobacco. Regular use of tobacco leads to nicotine accumulation in the body, thereby providing a continuous (24-hour) exposure to nicotine's effects on body systems.

It has been demonstrated that stress and anxiety affect nicotine tolerance and dependency. Corticosterone, a hormone released during stress, reduces the effects of nicotine; therefore, with stress more nicotine must be consumed to achieve the same effect. This increases tolerance and leads to dependency. The use of tobacco products, aside from the addictive effects of nicotine, is accompanied by a host of health hazards. In addition to nicotine, cigarette smoke is primarily composed of a dozen or so gases (mainly carbon monoxide) and tar. The tar exposes the user to increased risk for lung cancer, emphysema, and bronchial disorders. The carbon monoxide increases the user's risk of cardiovascular diseases.

Those dependent on nicotine usually find it very difficult to quit because addiction to nicotine results in withdrawal symptoms. When deprived of cigarettes for as little as 24 hours, chronic smokers display increased anger, hostility, aggression, and loss of social cooperation. Approaches commonly employed by those attempting to break the cycle of nicotine dependency include (1) quitting "cold turkey," or abruptly stopping use of tobacco; (2) a gradual cessation program in which the smoker obtains decreasing amounts of nicotine from such sources as a transdermal patch or nicotine chewing gum; and (3) use of medications such as Zyban, which does not replace nicotine but helps to control nicotine craving and the associated urge to smoke.

Club Drugs and Inhalants

Beyond nicotine and alcohol is a plethora of legal and illegal substances sought out by many for their psychotropic effects. On the increase in popularity with young, beginning abusers are two distinct groups of substances: club drugs and inhalants. Club drugs categorize a collection of dangerous substances used by teens and young adults at all-night dances (raves), parties, dance clubs, and bars. According to the National Institute on Drug Abuse (NIDA), uncertainties about the sources, chemicals, and possible contaminants used in the manufacture of many club drugs make it extremely difficult to determine the toxicity and resulting medical consequences of these substances.

Commonly known by abbreviations and street names, the club drugs include MDMA (Ecstacy), GHB, Rohypnol, ketamine, methamphetamine, and LSD. See Table 23-1.

NIDA warns that no club drug is benign. With some of these drugs, users risk long-term neurologic and/or cardiovascular damage, and, because some club drugs are colorless, tasteless, and odorless, they are increasingly being used to intoxicate or sedate others, often preparatory to sexual assault (date rape) or pornographic photography.

Inhalants are breathable chemical vapors that produce psychoactive (mind-altering) effects. Most abused inhalants are legal substances commonly found in the home or workplace. Those most likely to abuse inhalants are young children in middle school experimenting with such substances and teens using nitrous oxide in combination with club drugs while attending raves or all-night dance parties. The popularity of inhalants tends to decrease among users as they grow older and move on to marijuana, LSD, and other illegal substances.

Nearly all inhalants produce effects similar to anesthetics by slowing down the body's functions. In sufficient concentrations, inhalants can cause intoxication lasting from a few minutes to several hours depending on frequency of use. Serious, irreversible effects, including death, can result from the misuse of inhalants. Well documented are instances of brain damage and hearing loss associated with toluene (an ingredient found in paint sprays and some glues) and peripheral neuropathies (limb spasms) associated with the hexane in glues and gasoline or nitrous oxide used in whipping cream or from small metal cylinders. See Table 23-2.

Nationally, estimates on inhalant deaths per year range from 100 to 1,000. Because researchers rely on surveys such as NIDA's *Monitoring the Future Study (MTF),* it is difficult to determine exactly how many young people use inhalants. However, when asked on the 1997 MTF if they had ever used inhalants, 21 percent of 8th-graders, 18.3 percent of 10th-graders, and 16.1 percent of 12th-graders responded yes. In the same survey, almost 12 percent of 8th-graders replied that their use had been within the past year.

Amphetamines

Drugs of the amphetamine group are prescription medications designed for oral use in the treatment of exogenous obesity, narcolepsy, and attention deficit disorder. Amphetamine sulfate, dextroamphetamine sulfate (Dexedrine), methamphetamine sulfate (Desoxyn), methylphenidate HCl (Ritalin), and phenmetrazine HCl (Preludin) have a high potential for abuse and are classed as Schedule II drugs under the Federal Controlled Substances Act. These drugs stimulate the central nervous system and cause increased alertness, elevation of mood, reduction of appetite, and a diminished sense of fatigue.

The misuse and abuse of amphetamines relates to the effects these drugs have upon the central nervous system. They have been taken to avoid sleep while studying or driving, and they have also been taken by athletes in an attempt to improve performance. Primarily, these drugs are abused by those seeking euphoric excitement, or by those who want to counter the effects of depressant drugs. Street names for amphetamines include speed, crystal, bennies, wake-ups, and pep pills.

Euphoria, excitement, anorexia, and insomnia are but a few of the possible effects of amphetamines. Those abusing these drugs may also experience dilated pupils, talkativeness, nervousness, agitation, dizziness, increased blood pressure, palpitations, tachycardia, pallor or flushing, dry mouth, abdominal pain, chills, fever, and fatigue.

TABLE 23-1 CLUB DRUGS

Substances	Street Names	Physiological Effects	Psychological Effects	Route and Appearance
GHB (gamma hydroxybutyrate)	Liquid Ecstacy, Scoop, Somatomax, Georgia Home Boy, Grievous Bodily Harm, G	Sedative, anabolic high dosage can slow heart rate and respiration to dangerous levels	Euphoric, intoxicant, anxiety relief	Oral: liquid, powder, tablet, or capsule
Ketamine (an injectable anesthetic primarily for veterinary use)	Special K, K, vitamin K, Cat Valiums	High dose: delirium, high blood pressure, impaired motor skills, respiratory distress	Weightless feeling, out-of-body or near-death sensation	Liquid or powder that is often snorted or smoked with tobacco or marijuana
MDMA (methylenedioxymethamphetamine)	Ecstacy, XTC, Adam, Clarity, Lover's Speed, X	Stimulant, increased heart rate and blood pressure, involuntary teeth clenching, muscle tension	Sense of alertness, psychedelic effect, hallucinogenic effect, increased stamina, anxiety, paranoia	Oral: tablet or capsule
Methamphetamine	Speed, Ice, Chalk, Meth, Crystal, Crank, Fire, Glass	Decreased appetite, physical activity, excited speech, cardiovascular damage	Short-term rush, flash, euphoria, agitation, aggression	Oral: Powder can be smoked, snorted, or injected.
LSD (lysergic acid diethylamide)	Acid, Boomers, Yellow Sunshine	Weakness, trembling, nausea, numbness, dilated pupils, loss of appetite, sweating	Hallucinogenic effect, hallucinogen persisting perception disorder (flashbacks)	Oral: tablets, capsules, liquid, or licked from absorbent paper
Rohypnol (flunitrazepam)	Rophies, Roofies, Roach, Rope, and the "Date Rape" Drug, the Forget-Me Pill	Sedative-hypnotic, muscle relaxation, decreased blood pressure, dizziness	Anterograde amnesia (lack of recall for events while drugged)	Oral

TABLE 23-2 INHALANTS SUBJECT TO ABUSE

Substances	Physiological Effects	Psychological Effects	Route and Appearance
Medical anesthetic gases: nitrous oxide, chloroform, ether	General anesthetic used by medical professionals, restricts the pumping action of the heart, drops blood pressure, pulse rate increases	Laughing gas, mind-altering effect	Inhaled as vapor, often in large balloons
Volatile hydrocarbons used as solvents in • paint thinner, gasoline • nail polish remover • dry-cleaning fluids • glues, correction fluids, and as aerosol propellants for • spray paint, fabric protectors • whipping cream, cooking oil • hair spray, air freshener or in gases such as • propane, butane, helium	Various effects including respiratory difficulty, heart palpitations, nerve cell damage, loss of sense of smell, irregular heartbeat, double vision, slowed reaction time, loss of consciousness	Various effects including visual hallucinations and severe mood swings, dizziness, anxiety, poor memory, lack of concentration, confusion, intoxication, disorientation in time and space	Sniffing or snorting via the nose, **bagging** (inhaling fumes from a plastic bag) or **huffing** (stuffing an inhalant-soaked rag or sock into the mouth)
Volatile nitrates: amyl nitrate and products sold as room deodorizers that use chemical variants of butyl nitrate	Vasodilation, face flushes, head and neck perspire, reduction in blood pressure, relaxation of involuntary muscles	Rushing sensation, light-headed or dizzy feeling, slowed perception of time	Yellowish/gold liquid in ampules

If amphetamine use is abruptly stopped, the heavy user exhibits withdrawal symptoms. These symptoms usually include fatigue, long but disturbed sleep, irritability, strong hunger, and deep depression that may lead to attempted suicide.

Cocaine

Like amphetamines, cocaine is a central nervous system stimulant. This drug is extracted from the leaves of *Erythroxylon coca*, a plant that can be found in a number of South American countries. Cocaine hydrochloride (HCl), a fine, white crystal-like powder, is the most available form of the drug and is used medically for surface anesthesia of the ear, nose, throat, rectum, and vagina. Cocaine has a high potential for abuse and is classified as a Schedule II drug under the Federal Controlled Substances Act.

As an abused substance, cocaine is usually sniffed or snorted into the nose, although some users inject it or smoke a form of the drug called crack or freebase. Cocaine is readily absorbed through mucous membranes; thus, the reason for snorting it into the nasal passageway. Its effects begin within a few minutes, reach a peak within 15 to 20 minutes, and subside within an hour. These effects include dilated pupils and increases in blood pressure, heart rate, respiratory rate, and body temperature. The drug's high potential for abuse relates to its ability to cause feelings of euphoria, excitement, and a sense of well-being. Other desirable effects are feeling more energetic or alert and a reduction of appetite.

Crack or freebase cocaine is made by chemically converting cocaine HCl to a purified, altered form of the drug more suitable for smoking. This altered form of the drug resembles beige or brownish clumps of sugar which, when smoked, produces an intense feeling of euphoria in less than 10 seconds. This instant "high" lasts only 5 to 25 minutes and is followed, almost immediately, by an equally intense depression. To avoid the depression, there is a strong need to smoke more of the drug. Crack can cause serious psychological dependency in as little as 2 weeks, and, of those addicted to crack, experts predict 9 out of 10 will continue to abuse the drug despite efforts at rehabilitation.

Cocaine hydrochloride, while not as powerful as crack, is a very dangerous dependency-producing drug. The feeling of well-being produced by cocaine can cause some of its users to center their lives around seeking and using this drug. Street names for cocaine include blow, coke, flake, gold dust, nose candy, rock, snow, and white girl. The street name for the combination of cocaine and heroin is speedball.

The adverse effects of cocaine use include perforated nasal septum, chills, fever, runny nose, ventricular fibrillation, cocaine psychosis, and death from respiratory and circulatory failure. See Table 23-3.

Barbiturates

Barbiturates are a group of drugs derived from barbituric acid. Although they may vary in onset of action, potency, and duration of effect, all are central nervous system depressants. Barbiturates are used medically as sedatives, to relieve anxiety, to treat insomnia, and in the control of seizures. Misuse of barbiturate drugs may grow out of poorly supervised prescription use of these agents. Clients may arbitrarily increase the dosage and frequency of use in response to self-perceived needs. Misuse of barbiturates can lead to their abuse because prolonged use results in tolerance and dependency.

Because of their potential for abuse, barbiturates are classified as Schedule II, III, and IV drugs under the Federal Controlled Substances Act. Those classified as Schedule II are amobarbital (Amytal), pentobarbital (Nembutal), and secobarbital (Seconal). Street names for barbiturates are barbs, blues, downers, goof balls, yellow jacket (pentobarbital), red devil (secobarbital), and blue devil (amobarbital). These drugs are generally taken orally in tablet or capsule form, but may be prepared as a solution for intravenous injection.

Relief from anxiety and sedation occurs when dosages of barbiturates are taken as prescribed. Higher doses may produce slurred speech, confusion, poor motor coordination, impaired judgment, and drowsiness. Very high doses can produce coma, respiratory arrest, circulatory collapse, and death.

Abrupt discontinuance of barbiturates can induce withdrawal symptoms that can be fatal. Such symptoms include apprehension, weakness, dizziness, tremors, nausea, vomiting, sweating, disturbed vision, insomnia, hypotension, headache, delirium, and convulsion.

Narcotic Analgesics (Opiates)

Opiates, sometimes referred to as narcotics, are a group of drugs derived from opium, some of which are used medically to relieve pain. Opiates have a high potential for abuse and can cause dependency if abused or when occasional use extends over a long period of time. Opium is a dark brown substance obtained by air-drying the juice of unripe seed pods of Asian poppy plants. A number of other drugs, including morphine, codeine, and heroin, have been

TABLE 23-3 ILLEGAL SUBSTANCES

Substances	Street Names	Physiological Effects	Psychological Effects	Route and Appearance
Cocaine and crack cocaine	Coke, Snow, Blow, Nose Candy, Flake, Crack, Rock, Freebase	Addictive, CNS stimulant, constricted peripheral blood vessels, dilated pupils	Euphoric, hyperstimulation, reduced fatigue, mental clarity	White powder: inhaled or injected White to tan pellets or rocks: smoked
Heroin	Smack, Skag, Junk, H	Addictive, warm flushing of the skin, dry mouth, alternately wakeful and drowsy	Euphoria, heavy feeling in the extremities	Injected, smoked, or inhaled. White to dark brown powder or tar-like substance
Marijuana (*Cannabis sativa*) (ordinary marijuana: 3% THC)	Over 200 slang terms including Pot, Weed, Grass, Dope, Mary Jane, Reefer, Joint, Nail, Herb	Dry mouth, rapid heartbeat, intoxication, red eyes, some loss of balance and a slower reaction time	Intoxicating, euphoric sensation, engrossed with ordinary sights, sounds, or tastes	Green, gray, or brown mix of shredded hemp plant that is smoked or eaten
• Sinsemilla (made from buds and flowering tops of female plants: 7.5–24% THC)				
• Hashish (sticky resin from the female plant: 4–28% THC)	Hash	More pronounced	More pronounced	Brown or black balls or cakes. Eaten or smoked
• Hash oil (tar-like liquid distillate from hashish: 16–43% THC)	Hash oil	More pronounced	More pronounced	Clear to black syrupy liquid that is applied to tobacco and smoked
PCP (phencyclidine)	Angel Dust, Ozone Wack, Rocket Fuel	Dose-related changes in blood pressure, pulse rate, and respiration. Nausea, blurred vision, drooling and dizziness at high dose	Changes in body awareness similar to alcohol intoxication High doses: illusions and hallucinations	Powder that is snorted, eaten, or applied to leafy material and smoked

derived from opium. Other opiates, such as meperidine (Demerol) and hydromorphone hydrochloride (Dilaudid), are synthetic or semisynthetic drugs with morphine-like qualities.

The use of opium is prohibited in the United States. Heroin is a Schedule I drug under the Federal Controlled Substances Act because of its high abuse potential and the lack of any acceptable medical use. Other natural and synthetic opiates are listed as Schedule II drugs that have medical applications.

Heroin, sometimes called junk or smack, accounts for 90 percent of the opiate abuse in the United States in spite of the fact that its sale or possession is illegal. Most street preparations are "cut" with other substances such as sugar or quinine and appear as a white or brownish powder. Because the effects of heroin (or morphine) are significantly diminished when taken orally, intravenous injection is the route of administration preferred by drug abusers. See Table 23-3.

Clients beginning treatment with an opiate, and those misusing these drugs for the first time, may experience nausea, vomiting, itching, and restlessness. This initial unpleasantness precedes a feeling of relaxation, drowsiness, and/or euphoria. With continued use, the unpleasant side effects of these drugs are diminished. Users develop a drug tolerance and larger dosages are required to produce the same effects. Drug dependence is easily established with opiate use. Finding and using the drug often becomes the primary focus in the lives of users. Since heroin use is very expensive, those addicted to this opiate may resort to criminal acts to pay for their habit.

The physical dangers associated with opiate abuse depend on the specific drug used, its source, the dose, and the route of administration. Most of the danger can be attributed to using too much of the drug, use of unsterile hypodermic needles, contamination of the drug itself, or combining the drug with other substances. Infections from contaminated solutions, syringes, and needles can cause tetanus, hepatitis, and acquired immunodeficiency syndrome (AIDS).

When the opiate-dependent person stops taking the drug, withdrawal symptoms become evident within 4 to 6 hours of the last dose. Symptoms include uneasiness, diarrhea, abdominal cramps, chills, sweating, nausea, runny nose, and tearing of the eyes. The intensity of withdrawal symptoms correlates with the dosage taken, the frequency of use, and the length of time that the user has been dependent on the drug. Withdrawal symptoms for most opiates grow stronger approximately 24 to 72 hours after they begin and subside within 7 to 10 days; however, symptoms such as sleeplessness and drug craving can last for months.

Marijuana

Two widely abused substances, marijuana and hashish, are obtained from the hemp plant *Cannabis sativa*. Both drugs owe their popularity to the same psychoactive component, tetrahydrocannabinol, better known as THC. The major differences in these two drugs are their appearance and the amount of THC each contains.

Marijuana is composed of the flowering tops and leaves of the plant. The seeds and stems of the plant may also be included when preparing marijuana for use by drug abusers. It may range in color from grayish green to greenish brown, and vary in texture from fine to coarse. The fine-textured marijuana resembles the spice oregano, whereas the coarse-textured drug looks like tea. The street names for marijuana include Acapulco gold, grass, joint, Mary Jane, pot, reefer, roach, tea, and weed.

Hashish is the dried resin extracted from the flowers, tops, and leaves of the female plant. This gummy extract, when dried, may range in color from light brown to black and in texture from soft to hard. Hashish also differs from marijuana in that an equal amount of hashish can contain five to ten times as much THC, thereby making it a much more potent drug.

Although it is possible to chew or swallow these substances, the most common method of use is by smoking. Marijuana is usually prepared for use as hand-rolled cigarettes (joints), although it may be smoked in special pipes. Hashish is usually smoked in small pipes. Smoking these substances produces the euphoric effect of THC quicker than other methods of administration. The use of marijuana or hashish has been shown to produce moderate tolerance to the effects of THC, thereby requiring increased usage to produce similar effects.

The effects produced by marijuana and hashish are dose related and can be influenced by such factors as the user's level of tolerance for the drug, the method of use, the concurrent use of other drugs such as alcohol, and the user's psychological state of mind. The use of moderate amounts of marijuana or hashish produces feelings of euphoria, relaxation, and drowsiness. The user may become less inhibited, talking and laughing more than usual. Coordination and judgment may be affected in much the same way as they are by alcohol. With larger doses, there is the tendency to misjudge the passage of time, and the user's perceptions of sound, color, and taste may be sharpened or distorted. In very large doses, the effects of cannabis may cause hallucinations. The effects of marijuana and hashish generally last for several hours. About 5 percent of regular users of these drugs will develop some degree of psychological dependence. Physical dependence and withdrawal symptoms are not usually associated with these drugs.

Aside from the euphoric effect that gives these drugs their high potential for abuse, they tend to increase the heart rate, decrease pulmonary function, and increase appetite. To this end, their use may aggravate an existing medical condition such as heart disease or hypertension. Although marijuana has been reported as beneficial in reducing nausea suffered by clients undergoing cancer chemotherapy, it remains classified as a Schedule I drug under the Federal Controlled Substances Act. See Table 23-3.

Phencyclidine (PCP)

Phencyclidine (PCP) was originally developed for use as a surgical anesthetic; however, its unwanted and undesirable side effects caused its experimental use with humans to be discontinued. Today, the only legal use for phencyclidine is with animals through licensed veterinary clinics. Unfortunately, limiting this drug's use to veterinary medicine has not prevented its abuse by those acquainted with its psychoactive properties. PCP is readily available from illegal suppliers because it is easily made. The chemicals needed to manufacture this drug are readily available to illegal labs across the country that are interested in making a profit.

The street names for PCP include angel dust, cosmos, jet, mist, peace pill, rocket fuel, superjoint, tranq, and whack. Since it is cheaply manufactured, PCP is frequently used to "cut" more expensive drugs, thereby increasing the drug dealer's profits. It may be found as a powder, in tablet form, or as a capsule. In that PCP is usually produced illegally, the size, shape, and color of the tablet may vary, making it possible to masquerade it as other popular street drugs.

For the same reasons that researchers discontinued medical use of PCP, many drug abusers have also labeled it as a bad drug. Its effects are often unpredictable, and, since it is produced illegally, one cannot tell how much PCP is in a powder, tablet, or capsule. The most popular method for taking the drug is by sprinkling the powder on a marijuana cigarette and smoking the combination of drugs. Other methods include taking it orally in any of its available forms, or injecting a solution containing the drug.

Users of PCP often have difficulty describing its effects; however, most agree that it gives them a feeling that is different from other drugs. The psychoactive effects are described as hallucinogenic, sometimes pleasant, sometimes not, but usually associated with a world of fantasy. As the effects of the drug wear off, users report feeling depressed, irritated, and somewhat alienated from their surroundings. While under the influence of PCP, users may appear confused, expressionless, or intoxicated. Speech is often confused, vision is distorted, and the user has difficulty thinking and remembering. Some users become violent and aggressive, while others withdraw and resist communicating. High doses of PCP can induce prolonged stupor or even coma for periods of a few days to several weeks. Long-term users of PCP are subject to recurring episodes of anxiety or depression, and regularly experience disturbances in memory, judgment, concentration, and perception, even after they have stopped taking the drug. Accidental death in which the victim fails to perceive danger is more likely to occur while under the influence of PCP than is death by chemical overdose. Users have been known to drown in shallow water, fall from buildings, and die of burns in circumstances that would have been avoided by less disoriented people. See Table 23-3.

Lysergic Acid Diethylamide (LSD)

Lysergic acid diethylamide (LSD), or "acid" as it is sometimes called, is a hallucinogenic agent that has no accepted medical use. As such, LSD is classified as a Schedule I drug under the Federal Controlled Substances Act. The psychoactive effects of the drug are influenced by such factors as the environment in which it is being used, the user's personality, and the user's state of mind at the time the drug was taken. When LSD is taken in pleasant surroundings by a stable, unthreatened personality, the effect on the user can be pleasant and has been described as a "good trip." Alter any of these circumstances and this mood-related drug can provoke unpleasant hallucinations and a "bad trip."

LSD is usually taken orally, often by absorbing the drug in a sugar cube or other substance. Because it is an extremely potent drug, a dose as small as 25 mcg is capable of producing psychoactive effects in some users. Higher doses of LSD have been associated with effects such as alteration of perception wherein the user can "hear" colors, "taste" sounds, and see structural changes as they occur in objects. Those who use LSD may also experience mood changes that range from euphoria to deep depression.

Whether LSD produces lasting physical changes in those who take the drug is a subject that is under examination. There is some evidence that long-term use can cause chromosome damage and lead to subsequent birth defects. Incidences of serious adverse reactions to LSD have rarely been reported when the dosage taken was not excessive. There have been incidences where users suffered prolonged adverse psychological effects from LSD; however, the greatest danger presented by the drug appears to be from accidents and suicide attempts by those under its influence.

RECOGNIZING SUBSTANCE ABUSE

As a member of a health care team, the nurse is likely to encounter clients who are substance abusers. Aside from the usual disease conditions that might cause an individual to seek medical attention, those who abuse drugs are at greater risk of sustaining accidental injury or infection as a result of drug use. Additionally, there are clients who will attempt to simulate a disease condition that could result in a prescription for a dependency-producing drug.

Obvious signs of drug abuse are needle tracks on the arms or other parts of the client's body. They may be observed when taking vital signs or doing other medical procedures. Less obvious indicators of possible drug abuse are jaundice, nasal ulceration, dilated or constricted pupils, slurred speech, confusion, impaired reflex action, neglected appearance, poor hygiene, and early withdrawal symptoms. When substance abuse is suspected, the nurse should reflect a nonjudgmental attitude toward the client and inform the physician at the earliest opportunity. All information obtained from clients, including evidence of drug abuse, is confidential. Those who provide health care are not allowed to disclose such information unless it becomes necessary to do so during a medical emergency.

SUBSTANCE ABUSE IN THE WORKPLACE

According to the National Institute on Drug Abuse (NIDA), 10 to 23 percent of Americans abuse drugs and alcohol at work. Chemical dependency has an overwhelming impact on industry, with the annual cost expressed in absenteeism, waste, theft, lost productivity, and property damage at a cost of $140 billion.

Marijuana and cocaine are the most used illegal drugs, but alcohol and nicotine pose a far wider problem. It is estimated that 6 percent of all workers always have alcohol in their bloodstream. It is believed that one in three Americans use or have recently used drugs at work.

Warning Signs of Substance Abuse in the Workplace

- Performance deteriorates: inconsistent work quality and low productivity; increased mistakes, poor concentration, carelessness
- Poor attendance and absenteeism: absenteeism and tardiness, particularly around weekends; increased physical complaints, vaguely defined illnesses; leaves early for lunch, long breaks, unexplained absences
- Attitude/physical appearance change: loss of pride in work, blames others for mistakes; avoids contact with co-workers and superiors; drastic change in appearance and hygiene; complaints from co-workers about covering up for him/her
- Health/safety hazards: increase in on-the-job accidents, carelessness in handling equipment, disregard for co-workers' safety
- Domestic problems emerge: complaints about family problems, talk of separation or divorce; recurring financial problems

SERVICES AVAILABLE

There are many organizations and help groups for substance abusers. They provide information via pamphlets and Web sites as well as referral assistance. The following list includes addresses, telephone numbers, and Internet Web site addresses for major substance abuse resource groups:

- Al-Anon/Alateen
  Al-Anon Family Group Headquarters, Inc.
  1600 Corporate Landing Parkway
  Virginia Beach, VA 23454
  757-563-1600 (literature)
  888-425-2666 (meeting referral)
  http://www.al-anon.org
- Alcoholics Anonymous
  World Services, Inc.
  475 Riverside Drive
  New York, NY 10115
  212-870-3400 (literature)
  212-647-1680 (meeting referral)
  http://www.alcoholics-anonymous.org

- American Council for Drug Education
    c/o Phoenix House
    164 West 74th Street
    New York, NY 10023
    800-488-DRUG

- Cocaine Anonymous
    World Service Office
    3740 Overland Avenue, Suite C
    Los Angeles, CA 90034
    http://www.ca.org

- Marijuana Anonymous
    World Services
    P.O. Box 2912
    Van Nuys, CA 91404
    800-766-6779

- Mothers Against Drunk Driving
    511 John Carpenter Freeway, Suite 700
    Irving, TX 75062
    800-GET-MADD

- Narcotics Anonymous
    World Services
    P.O. Box 9999
    Van Nuys, CA 91409
    818-773-9999

- National Clearinghouse for Alcohol and Drug Information
    800-729-6686
    http://www.health.org

- National Council on Alcoholism and Drug Dependency
    12 West 21st Street, 7th Floor
    New York, NY 10010
    800-NCA-CALL (will refer to local resources)

- National Institute on Drug Abuse
    800-662-HELP (treatment and referral hotline)
    888-644-6432 (Infofax in English/Spanish)
    http://www.nida.nih.gov
    http://www.drugabuse.gov

● SPOT CHECK

Give the physiological effects of the following illegal substances:

Substances(s)	Physiological Effects
Cocaine	
Heroin	
Marijuana	
Phencyclidine (PCP)	

● SELF-ASSESSMENT

Write the answer in the space provided or circle true or false as instructed.

Source

p. 275 **1.** True or False (circle one) Use of the medication Zyban in a smoking cessation program replaces the nicotine that would otherwise be consumed.

p. 274 **2.** Withdrawal may include flu-like symptoms, nausea, _____, _____, _____, and _____.

p. 276 **3.** Rohypnol has been associated with sexual assaults because it can produce _____, the lack of recall for events while drugged.

p. 275 **4.** The most logical reason why those abusing inhalants are usually young children in middle school is _____.

p. 278 **5.** Give three delivery systems by which a person might take cocaine. The drug may be

(1) _____,

(2) _____, or

(3) _____.

p. 278 **6.** True or False (circle one) All barbiturates are central nervous system depressants.

p. 280 **7.** Other than addiction and overdose, what serious danger is usually present when one becomes an intravenous user of an opiate? _____

p. 281 **8.** Give two reasons why some drug abusers have labeled PCP as a bad drug.

(1) _____

(2) _____

p. 282 **9.** Although some have experienced prolonged psychological effects, the greater dangers posed by LSD appear to be from _____ and _____.

p. 282 **10.** True or False (circle one) Chemical dependency has an overwhelming impact on industry. Marijuana and cocaine are the most used illegal drugs, but alcohol and nicotine pose a far wider problem.

● WEB ACTIVITY

Visit the following Web sites for additional information on substance abuse:

http://www.al-anon.org

http://www.alcoholics-anonymous.org

http://www.ama-assn.org

http://www.ca.org

http://www.health.org

http://www.inhalants.org

http://www.nida.nih.gov

http://www.drugabuse.gov

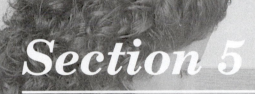

Section 5

EFFECTS OF MEDICATIONS ON BODY SYSTEMS

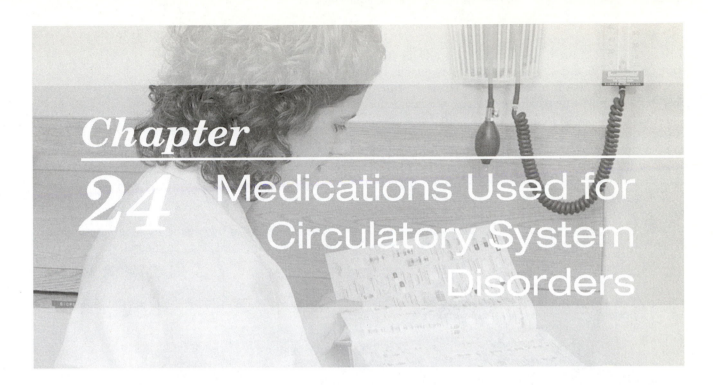

Chapter 24

Medications Used for Circulatory System Disorders

Chapter Outline

- Describe the various drug classifications used for circulatory system disorders
- Identify selected drugs according to each described classification
- State the actions, uses, contraindications, safety precautions, adverse reactions, dosage and route, nursing considerations, clients' instruction, and special considerations for selected drugs
- Complete the Spot Check on selected drugs that are used to treat circulatory system disorders
- Complete the Self-Assessment
- Visit indicated Web sites for additional information on medications used for circulatory system disorders

Objectives

Upon completion of this chapter, you should be able to

- Define the key terms
- List the warnings signs of a heart attack
- State two primary causes of chest pain
- Describe three ways that drugs may affect heart action

Key Terms

angina pectoris
arrhythmia
chronotropic
dromotropic
embolus
hypertension

inotropic
mast cell
pacemaker
plasminogen
vasodilators
vasopressors

INTRODUCTION

In the United States, one out of four adults is at risk for heart disease. Coronary heart disease is the number one cause of death in the United States, outnumbering the deaths from cancer and accidents combined. See Figure 24-1. It is said that every minute an American suffers a heart attack. Of the Americans alive today, 4.8 million have a history of heart attack, angina, or both. This year, 1.5 million Americans will have a heart attack. About 600,000 will die and of this number 350,000 die before they reach medical help. It is said that the average heart attack victim waits 3 hours after symptoms occur to seek help. Many times they try to ignore the symptoms or say "it's just indigestion." It is imperative to seek medical help immediately.

The American Heart Association lists the following as warning signs of heart attack:

- Pressure, fullness, squeezing pain in the center of the chest that lasts 2 minutes or longer
- Pain that spreads to the shoulders, neck, or arms
- Dizziness, fainting, sweating, nausea, or shortness of breath

Chest pain can be caused by a variety of conditions, including angina, myocardial infarction,

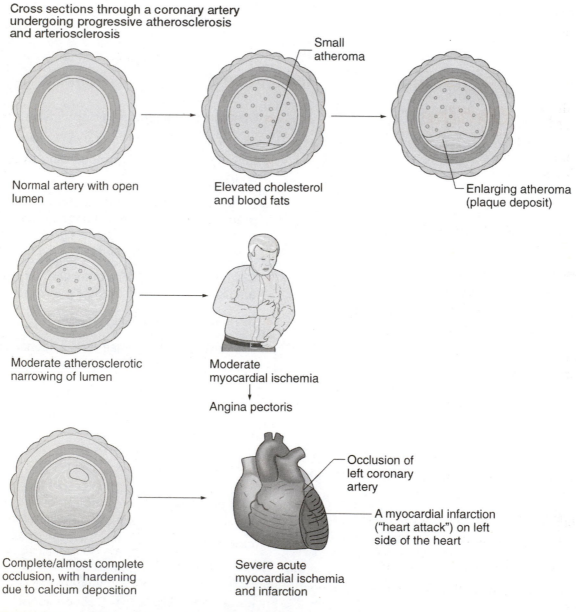

Cross sections through a coronary artery undergoing progressive atherosclerosis and arteriosclerosis

Small atheroma

Normal artery with open lumen

Elevated cholesterol and blood fats

Enlarging atheroma (plaque deposit)

Moderate atherosclerotic narrowing of lumen

Moderate myocardial ischemia

Angina pectoris

Complete/almost complete occlusion, with hardening due to calcium deposition

Severe acute myocardial ischemia and infarction

Occlusion of left coronary artery

A myocardial infarction ("heart attack") on left side of the heart

FIGURE 24-1   THE PROGRESSION OF CORONARY HEART DISEASE

stress, anxiety, and gastrointestinal disorders. It is essential that the physician determine the cause of the pain and treat it appropriately. (See Table 24-1.)

Risk Factors

- Male sex/postmenopausal women
- Family history (heredity)
- Smoking
- Hypertension
- Diabetes mellitus
- Obesity
- Elevated blood cholesterol level
- History of cerebrovascular or occlusive vascular disease
- Physical inactivity
- Stress

WOMEN AND HEART DISEASE

Heart disease is just as likely to develop in postmenopausal women as in men. One in ten American women 45 to 64 years of age has some form of heart disease, and this increases to one in four women over 65. Approximately 9 million American women of all ages suffer from heart disease. Another 2 million women have had a stroke. In the United Sates, heart disease or stroke will claim 500,000 women this year. By comparison, breast cancer kills about 44,000 American women each year.

The common misconception that heart disease is a man's disease may cause many women to be misinformed about heart disease, the risk factors associated with developing heart disease, and lifestyle changes. Recommendations for lifestyle changes include not smoking, eating a diet that includes five or more servings of fruits and vegetables daily and foods low in cholesterol and saturated fats, exercising for at least 30 minutes three times a week, controlling high blood pressure and high blood cholesterol. About one-quarter of American women have blood cholesterol levels high enough to pose a serious risk for heart disease. Blood cholesterol among women tends to rise from the age of 20 onward, but goes up sharply beginning around 40 years of age. It continues to increase until about age 60.

Studies indicate that women who take estrogen after menopause may reduce their risk of developing heart disease. Hormone replacement therapy (HRT) lowers LDL (bad cholesterol), raises HDL (good cholesterol), and helps keep blood vessels relaxed. All of these factors may help prevent heart

TABLE 24-1   TWO PRIMARY CAUSES OF CHEST PAIN

	Angina Pectoris	Myocardial Infarction
Cause(s)	Decreased blood flow through the coronary arteries that causes less oxygen to reach the myocardium	Occlusion of a coronary artery. Area becomes necrotic (infarct). May be caused by an embolus, vasoconstriction of the arteries, or sudden atherosclerotic changes in the vessels.
Predisposing Factors	• atherosclerosis • hypertension • diabetes mellitus • syphilis • rheumatic heart disease	• atherosclerosis • hypertension • diabetes mellitus • obesity • family history • smoking • blood cholesterol level: 　200–239 borderline high 　240 high 　LDL 130–159 borderline/160 high-risk
Symptoms	Sudden, agonizing pain in the substernal region, may radiate to left shoulder and arm, up to jaw; skin cold and clammy; pulse normal; B/P little or no change; anxious, apprehensive	Severe, crushing pain in the substernal region and upper abdomen, radiates to shoulders, arms, jaw; skin cold and clammy; pulse rapid, weak, irregular; nausea and possible vomiting; B/P drops; extremely apprehensive

disease. There are known risks associated with hormone replacement therapy; therefore, it is important for each women to be informed of the benefits and risks and make an educated decision about this type of therapy with the help of her physician.

DRUGS THAT AFFECT THE HEART

Medications that affect heart action may be described as inotropic, chronotropic, and/or dromotropic. **Inotropic** refers to influencing the force of muscular contractility, especially of the myocardium. When a drug exerts a positive inotropic effect, it increases the force of myocardial contraction. When a drug exerts a negative inotropic effect, it decreases the force of myocardial contraction. **Chronotropic** refers to influencing the heartbeat rate. When a drug exerts a positive chronotropic effect, it increases the heart rate. When a drug exerts a negative chronotropic effect, it decreases the heart rate. **Dromotropic** refers to affecting the conductivity of nerve or muscle fibers, especially of the myocardium. When a drug exerts a positive dromotropic effect, it increases the conduction of electrical impulses through the heart muscle. When a drug exerts a negative dromotropic effect, it decreases the conduction of electrical impulses through the heart muscle.

Digitalis

In the treatment of congestive heart failure, therapy usually includes the use of a digitalis drug together with a diuretic, a low-sodium diet, and a reduction of physical activities. This combination of drugs, diet, and change in lifestyle is designed to increase cardiac output while reducing pulmonary congestion and the lower-body edema that is characteristic of this disorder.

Digitalis is obtained by crushing into a powder the dried leaves of the plant *Digitalis purpurea* or purple foxglove. A similar drug, digoxin, is obtained from the leaves of *Digitalis lanatas*. The primary use for these and other digitalis compounds is the treatment of various types of heart failures, and, together, they belong to a chemical classification known as cardiac glycosides. See Table 24-2. These drugs exert a positive inotropic effect on the heart. They strengthen the heart muscle (myocardium), increase the force of systolic contraction, slow the heart, and improve the muscle tone of the myocardium. As a result of these effects on the heart, there is a decrease in venous pressure as the heart takes in larger amounts of venous blood. Improving the effectiveness of the heart's pumping action reduces the size of the heart and increases the flow of blood to the kidneys, thereby causing a diuretic effect and the removal of some excess fluid from the body. Additional fluids are removed through the use of diuretic drugs.

The pharmacologic actions of all digitalis compounds are similar, but these products differ in their potency, onset of action, and the rate at which they are absorbed. Digitalis drugs may be given parenterally, although the oral route is generally preferred.

When first started, an initial or digitalizing dose is often given to bring the serum level of the drug up to the desired level. The effect of the initial dose is then sustained by smaller daily maintenance doses. When a digitalizing dose is not given, the administration of maintenance doses over a period of about 7 days will usually result in sufficient accumulation of the drug to produce the desired serum level. The amount of the initial and maintenance doses may vary, depending upon the size of the client and whether there is normal renal or hepatic function. Frequently, maintenance doses of digitalis drugs must be taken throughout the remainder of a client's lifetime.

Digitalis intoxication can occur when there is excess accumulation of the drug in the body. This can occur when the initial or digitalizing dose is administered too rapidly, or from maintenance doses

TABLE 24-2 DIGITALIS DRUGS (CARDIAC GLYCOSIDES)

Medication	Usual Initial or Digitalizing Dose	Usual Maintenance Dose
digitoxin (Crystodigin) (Digitaline)	Oral, IV: 0.6 mg initially followed by 0.4 mg and then 0.2 mg at 4–6 hour intervals; or 0.2 mg twice daily for 4 days	0.05–0.3 mg daily
digoxin (Lanoxin)	Oral: 0.5–0.75 mg initially, then 0.25–0.5 mg every 6–8 hours until therapeutic levels are obtained IV: 0.4–0.6 mg initially, then 0.25 mg every 4–6 hours until therapeutic levels are reached	0.125–0.5 mg daily

that are larger than necessary. The difference between therapeutic and toxic doses of digitalis is generally not great. Signs of digitalis intoxication have been reported in up to 20 percent of hospitalized clients receiving the drug; therefore, those who administer this medication should observe the client for possible toxic reactions.

Digitalis Preparations

Actions

Digitalis drugs strengthen the heart muscle, increase the force and velocity of myocardial systolic contraction (positive inotropic effect), slow the heart rate (negative chronotropic effect), and decrease conduction velocity through the atrioventricular (AV) node.

Uses

Congestive heart failure, atrial fibrillation, atrial flutter, paroxysmal atrial tachycardia.

Contraindications

Contraindicated in clients with known hypersensitivity to any of its ingredients and in ventricular fibrillation.

Adverse Reactions

Unifocal or multiform ventricular premature contractions, ventricular tachycardia, atrioventricular dissociation, atrial tachycardia, excessive slowing of the pulse (clinical sign of digitalis overdose), complete heart block, anorexia, nausea, vomiting, diarrhea, blurred or yellow vision, headache, weakness, dizziness, apathy, psychosis, gynecomastia, maculopapular rash, drowsiness, confusion, depression.

Dosage and Route

The dosage and route of administration is determined by the physician and individualized for each client. See Table 24-2.

Nursing Considerations

Assess the apical pulse for one minute before administering digitalis drugs. If the pulse is below 60 or the minimum specified, notify the prescribing physician. Monitor intake and output ratio, daily weight, liver function studies, serum electrolytes, creatinine, and drug levels. Be alert for signs of digitalis toxicity and hypokalemia. Evaluate therapeutic response of medication (decreased edema, weight loss, increased urine output, improved heart rate, and rhythm).

Signs and Symptoms of Digitalis Toxicity

The most common early symptoms of digitalis toxicity are anorexia, nausea, vomiting, and arrhythmias. Other signs and symptoms according to body system are:

- *Gastrointestinal:* anorexia, nausea, vomiting, diarrhea, abdominal pain
- *Nervous System:* headache, restlessness, irritability, drowsiness, depression, confusion, disorientation, insomnia, psychosis, convulsions, coma, blurred or yellow vision (yellow halos around lights)
- *Cardiovascular:* bradycardia, tachycardia, atrial tachycardia with varying AV block, ventricular bigeminy, ventricular tachycardia, second-degree AV block, complete AV block
- *Musculoskeletal:* severe weakness

Clients' Instruction

Educate the client

- About possible adverse reactions and the signs and symptoms of digitalis toxicity
- To notify his/her physician without delay if symptoms of digitalis toxicity appear
- About the importance of taking the medication as prescribed
- To not stop taking the drug unless the physician so orders
- To avoid over-the-counter medications unless ordered by the physician
- To include foods high in potassium (unless the client is taking a potassium-sparing diuretic) and low in sodium in his/her diet
- And his/her family about how to take a pulse and how to recognize changes in rate, volume and rhythm, and to withhold the medication if the pulse is below 60 beats per minute
- To weigh him/herself weekly and report a weight gain of 5 pounds or more to the physician
- To wear or carry a Medic Alert ID stating that he/she is on digitalis

Special Considerations

- Potassium-depleting corticosteroids and diuretics may be major contributing factors to digitalis toxicity.

- Rapid intravenous administration of calcium may produce serious arrhythmias in clients receiving digitalis.

- Quinidine, verapamil, and amiodarone cause a rise in serum digoxin concentration, with the implication that digitalis intoxication may result.

- Antacids, kaolin-pectin, sulfasalazine, neomycin, cholestyramine, and certain anticancer drugs may interfere with intestinal digoxin absorption, resulting in expectedly low serum concentration.

- The additive effects of beta-adrenergic blockers or calcium channel blockers and digitalis can result in complete heart block.

- There are numerous precautions and drug interactions associated with digitalis drugs. Please refer to a current edition of the *PDR® Nurse's Drug Handbook™* and/or a *Physicians' Desk Reference* for more information.

Antiarrhythmic Agents

The heartbeat is controlled by neuromuscular tissue within the heart. The sinoatrial (SA) node, located in the upper wall of the right atrium, is considered to be the source of the heartbeat. This specialized network of Purkinje fibers has the property of automaticity and is referred to as the **pacemaker** of the heart.

Normally, impulses from the sinoatrial node cause contraction of both left and right atria. The impulse also stimulates the atrioventricular node below the endocardium of the right atrium, which in turn transmits the impulse to the atrioventricular bundle (Bundle of His) and causes contraction of the left and right ventricles.

Disorders of the SA node that interfere with impulsive formation or disorders of the conduction system (AV node, Bundle of His) result in a variety of cardiac arrhythmias. The term **arrhythmia** means irregularity or loss of rhythm and is used to describe an irregular heartbeat. Some cardiac arrhythmias do not require treatment while others may result in death if not treated by drug therapy or the use of an artificial pacemaker.

Antiarrhythmic drugs are used to control many cardiac arrhythmias. Some of the drugs used to threat this condition are found in Table 24-3.

TABLE 24-3 ANTIARRHYTHMIC DRUGS

Medication	Usual Dosage
bretylium (Bretylol)	Severe ventricular fibrillation: Adult: IV bolus 5 mg/kg, increase to 10 mg/kg repeated every 15 min. Not to exceed 30 mg/kg/day. IV infusion: 1–2 mg/min or 5–10 mg/kg over 10 min every 6 hours (maintenance)
	Ventricular dysrhythmias: Adult: IV infusion 500 mg diluted in 50 ml D5W or NS, infuse over 10–30 min, may repeat in 1 hour, maintain with 1–2 mg/min or 5–10 mg/kg over 10–30 min every 6 hours. IM: 5–10 mg/kg undiluted; repeat in 1–2 hours if needed; may repeat with 3rd dose every 6–8 hours
disopyramide (Norpace)	Oral: 600 mg/day in divided doses (150 mg every 6 hours)
(Norpace CR)	Oral: 600 mg/day in divided doses (300 mg every 12 hours). For clients less than 110 pounds (50 kg) the recommended dosage is 400 mg/day in divided doses (Norpace—100 mg every 6 hours; Norpace CR—200 mg every 12 hours)
flecainide acetate (Tambocor)	Oral: 100 mg every 12 hours with increases of 50 mg bid every 4 days until efficacy is achieved
lidocaine HCl (Xylocaine HCl)	IM: 2 mg/lb (4.3 mg/kg) of 10% solution as needed
procainamide HCl (Pronestyl)	Oral: 50 mg/kg per day in divided doses every 3 hours IM: 0.5–1 g every 4–8 hours
(Procan SR)	Oral (maintenance): 50 mg/kg per day in divided doses every 6 hours starting 2–3 hours after the last dose of standard oral procainamide
propranolol HCl (Inderal)	Oral: 10–30 mg 3–4 times daily before meals and at bedtime IV: 1–3 mg under careful monitoring

(continued)

TABLE 24-3   *(Continued)*

Medication	Usual Dosage
quinidine sulfate (Quinidex Extentabs)	Oral: 200–300 mg 3–4 times daily
tocainide HCl (Tonocard)	Oral: Initial dosage: 400 mg every 8 hours; then 1200–1800 mg/day in a daily regimen of 3 doses
verapamil (Calan)	Oral: 240–480 mg/day in 3–4 divided doses

Clients' Instruction

Educate the client

- About possible adverse reactions and the signs and symptoms of toxicity
- To notify his/her physician without delay if toxic symptoms appear
- About the importance of taking the medication as prescribed
- To not stop taking the drug unless directed by the physician to do so
- To avoid alcohol and over-the-counter medications
- To make body position changes slowly (during early treatment)
- To avoid hazardous activities if dizziness or blurred vision occurs
- And his/her family about how to take a pulse and how to recognize changes in rate, volume, and rhythm and to withhold the medication if the pulse is below 60 beats per minute
- To weigh him/herself weekly and report a weight gain of 5 pounds or more to the physician
- To wear or carry a Medic Alert ID stating what drug he/she is taking

Special Considerations

- There are numerous precautions and drug interactions associated with antiarrhythmic drugs. Please refer to a current edition of the *PDR Nurse's Drug Handbook* and/or a *Physicians' Desk Reference* for information on precautions and drug interactions. See Table 24-4.

TABLE 24-4   CONTRAINDICATIONS AND ADVERSE REACTIONS OF SELECTED ANTIARRHYTHMIC DRUGS

Medication	Contraindications	Adverse Reactions
bretylium (Bretylol)	No contraindications in the treatment of ventricular fibrillation or life-threatening refractory ventricular arrhythmias	Hypotension, postural hypotension, nausea, vomiting, vertigo, syncope, dizziness, bradycardia, substernal pain, initial increase in arrhythmias
flecainide (Tambocor)	Preexisting second- or third-degree AV block, or with rigid right bundle branch block, cardiogenic shock, hypersensitivity	Cardiac arrest, new or worsened arrhythmias, dizziness, dyspnea, headache, nausea, chest pain, asthenia, edema
lidocaine (Xylocaine)	Hypersensitivity, Stokes-Adams syndrome, Wolff-Parkinson-White syndrome, severe degrees of sinoatrial, atrioventricular, or intraventricular block in the absence of an artificial pacemaker	Nervousness, lightheadedness, euphoria, dizziness, drowsiness, vomiting, double vision, respiratory depression, bradycardia, hypotension, cardiovascular collapse
propranolol (Inderal)	Cardiogenic shock, sinus bradycardia and greater than first-degree block, bronchial asthma, congestive heart failure	Bradycardia, CHF, hypotension, intensification of AV block, mental depression, nausea, vomiting, diarrhea, bronchospasm, agranulocytosis

(continued)

TABLE 24-4 *(Continued)*

Medication	Contraindications	Adverse Reactions
quinidine (Quinidex)	Complete AV block, intraventricular conduction defects, hypersensitivity to quinidine, myasthenia gravis	Cinchonism (loss of hearing, ringing in the ear, nausea, dizziness, headache, lightheadedness, disturbed vision), nausea, vomiting, abdominal pain, diarrhea, anorexia, headache, vertigo
tocainide (Tonocard)	Hypersensitivity, second- or third-degree atrioventricular block in the absence of an artificial pacemaker	Tiredness, drowsiness, hypotension, bradycardia, palpitations, chest pain, nausea, vomiting, anorexia, diarrhea, dizziness, vertigo, headache, rash
verapamil (Calan)	Severe left ventricular dysfunction, hypotension (systolic less than 90 mm Hg), cardiogenic shock, sick sinus syndrome and second- or third-degree AV block (except in clients with a functioning artificial ventricular pacemaker), atrial flutter/fibrillation, Wolff-Parkinson-White, Lown-Ganong-Levine syndromes, hypersensitivity	Heart failure, hypotension, elevated liver enzymes, AV block, constipation, dizziness, nausea, edema, headache, pulmonary edema, fatigue

- Antiarrhythmic drugs may cause serious adverse reactions. Emergency equipment, supplies and medications should be readily available for use.
- Treatment of overdose: oxygen, artificial ventilation, dopamine for circulatory depression, diazepam or thiopental for convulsions. Monitor ECG.

VASOPRESSORS AND VASODILATORS

There are many uses for drugs that act to either constrict (narrow) or dilate (widen) the walls of blood vessels. Based simply upon their primary action, these medications can be classified as vasopressors and vasodilators.

Vasopressors are drugs that cause contraction of the muscles associated with capillaries and arteries, thereby narrowing the space through which the blood circulates. This narrowing increases the resistance to blood flow and results in an elevation of blood pressure. Drugs classified as vasopressors are useful in the treatment of clients suffering from shock. See Table 24-5.

Vasopressors
Actions

Dopamine HCl (Intropin; Dopastat) exerts an inotropic effect on the myocardium, resulting in an increased cardiac output. Metaraminol bitartrate (Aramine) has a positive inotropic effect and a peripheral vasoconstriction action. Norepinephrine (Levophed Bitartrate) acts as a peripheral vasoconstrictor (alpha-adrenergic) and as an inotropic stimulator of the heart and dilator of coronary arteries (beta-adrenergic). Phenylephrine HCl (Neo-Synephrine) is a powerful postsynaptic alpha-receptor stimulant with little effect on the beta receptors of the heart.

Uses

Shock, hypotension.

Contraindications

Contraindicated in clients with known hypersensitivity to any of its ingredients. Other contraindications depend upon the drug. For example, Dopamine is contraindicated in ventricular fibrillation, tachydysrhythmias, pheochromocytoma, and during pregnancy, lactation, arterial embolism, and peripheral vascular disease.

Adverse Reactions

Adverse reactions depend upon the drug. For example, dopamine may have the following adverse reactions: headache, palpitations, tachycardia, hypertension, ectopic heart beats, angina, nausea, vomiting, diarrhea, necrosis, tissue sloughing with extravasation, gangrene.

TABLE 24-5   SELECTED VASOPRESSORS

Medication	Usual Dosage	Adverse Reactions
dopamine HCl (Intropin) (Dopastat)	IV: 2–50 mcg/kg/min as needed after dilution with appropriate sterile solution recommended by manufacturer	Ectopic beats, nausea, vomiting, tachycardia, anginal pain, dyspnea, headache, hypotension, and vasoconstriction
metraraminol bitartrate (Aramine)	IM, SC: 2–10 mg IV infusion: 15–100 mg in 500 ml of Sodium Chloride Injection at rate adequate to maintain blood pressure at desired level	Sinus or ventricular tachycardia, or other arrhythmias, especially in clients with myocardial infarction
norepinephrine (Levophed Bitartrate)	IV infusion: 4 ml per 1000 ml of 5% dextrose solution. Give at rate of 8–12 mcg of base per minute.	Occasional bradycardia or headache may indicate overdosage and extreme hypertension
phenylephrine HCl (Neo-Synephrine 1% Injection)	IM, SC: 2–5 mg IV: 0.2 mg	Headache, reflex bradycardia, excitability, restlessness

Dosage and Route

The dosage and route of administration is determined by the physician and individualized for each client. See Table 24-5.

Nursing Considerations

Assess intake and output ratio, and ECG during administration. Monitor blood pressure. Take blood pressure and pulse every 5 minutes after administration. Dosage adjustment according to blood pressure. Administer IV slowly, after reconstituting. Reconstituted solution (refrigerated) may not be stored more than 24 hours. Do not use discolored solution. Check paresthesia and coldness of extremities; peripheral blood flow may decrease. Check injection site for tissue sloughing. Evaluate therapeutic response, increased blood pressure with stabilization.

Clients' Instruction

Educate the client about

- The therapeutic response
- The reason for the medication

Special Considerations for Dopamine HCl

- It should not be used within 2 weeks of MAOIs, since hypertensive crisis may occur.
- Dysrhythmia may occur when used with general anesthetics.
- Beta-blockers may decrease the action of dopamine.

Vasodilators

Vasodilators are medications that cause the relaxation of blood vessels. This action dilates the vessels, thereby increasing their ability to carry blood. This eases resistance to blood flow and lowers blood pressure.

Coronary vasodilators are used primarily for the treatment of **angina pectoris** (chest pain), a condition caused by an insufficient supply of blood to the heart. The treatment of this condition usually involves the nitrate group of drugs. Nitrate tablets are rapidly absorbed through the mucous membrane of the mouth or stomach. See Table 24-6.

Nitrate Preparations

Nitrates include erythrityl tetranitrate, isosorbide dinitrate, nitroglycerin, and pentaerythritol tetranitrate. These drugs are available in various doses and forms. See Table 24-6.

Actions

Increases coronary blood flow by dilating coronary arteries and improving collateral flow to ischemic regions. Produces vasodilation. Reduces myocardial oxygen consumption.

Uses

Angina pectoris, prophylaxis of angina pain, congestive heart failure associated with acute myocardial infarction, control of blood pressure in perioperative hypertension, and in the production of controlled hypotension during surgical procedures.

TABLE 24-6 CORONARY VASODILATORS

Medication	Usual Dosage	Adverse Reactions
amyl nitrate	0.18–0.3 ml by inhalation	Cutaneous vasodilation, marked lowering of systemic pressure, occasional headache, nausea
isosorbide dinitrate (Isordil) (Sorbitrate)	Sublingual: 2.5–5 mg every 3 hours Chewable: 5 mg initially every 2–3 hours Oral: 5–20 mg 4 times daily Oral (sustained-release): 40 mg every 6–12 hours	Headache, hypotension, cutaneous vasodilation with flushing, transient episodes of dizziness
nitroglycerin (Nitro-Bid) (Nitroglyn) (Nitrospan) (Nitrostat) (Transderm Nitro) (Nitrolingual Spray) (Nitrogard)	Topical: Spread in a thin layer over a 2–6 in. area every 3–4 hours when needed. Sublingual: 0.15–0.6 mg under tongue as needed for acute angina Oral (sustained-release): 2.5 mg 3–4 times daily Transdermal: 2.5–20 mg released over a 24-hour period Lingual aerosol: 1–2 metered doses onto or under the tongue Transmucosal: 1 mg placed on the oral mucosa between cheek and gum	Headache, hypotension, cutaneous vasodilation with flushing, and occasional drug rash or exfoliative dermatitis; refer to nitrate preparation for other adverse reactions
pentaerythritol tetranitrate (Peritrate)	Oral (sustained-release): 10–40 mg 4 times daily	Rash, headache, mild gastrointestinal distress, cutaneous vasodilation with flushing, transient episodes of dizziness

Contraindications

Contraindicated in clients with known hypersensitivity to any of its ingredients and in severe anemia, increased intracranial pressure, cerebral hemorrhage.

Adverse Reactions

Headache, tachycardia, nausea, vomiting, apprehension, restlessness, muscle twitching, retrosternal discomfort, palpitations, dizziness, abdominal pain, cutaneous flushing, weakness, drug rash or exfoliative dermatitis.

Dosage and Route

The dosage and route of administration is determined by the physician and individualized for each client. See Table 24-6.

Nursing Considerations

Assess blood pressure, pulse, and respirations during initial therapy. Evaluate pain: time started, activity being performed, duration, severity, and length. Monitor client for adverse reactions. Headache, lightheadedness, and decreased blood pressure are signs that may indicate a need to reduce the dosage. Evaluate therapeutic response.

Clients' Instruction

Educate the client

- About possible adverse reactions
- To avoid hazardous activities if dizziness occurs
- About the importance of taking the medication as prescribed
- To seek medical care immediately if anginal pain is not relieved by 3 tablets in 15 minutes
- To avoid alcohol
- To make position changes slowly to prevent possible fainting
- That Viagra is contraindicated with organic nitrates in any form

Special Considerations

- Most drug interactions with nitrates adversely affect the cardiovascular system. Alcohol may cause severe hypotension; anticholinergics delay sublingual absorption due to dryness of the mouth; antihypertensives and phenothiazines may cause hypotension produced by additive effects of the drugs.

Peripheral vasodilators are used in the treatment of peripheral vascular disease (VD), although many are classified by the Food and Drug Administration as only "possibly effective." They are used for the relief of symptoms of cerebral and peripheral vascular insufficiency. An example is papaverine HCl (Pavabid, Pavagen TD). It is administered orally, 150 mg every 8–12 hours. Some of the adverse reactions are nausea, abdominal distress, anorexia, constipation, headache, drowsiness, and sweating.

ANTIHYPERTENSIVE AGENTS

Hypertension can be defined as a condition wherein the client has a higher arterial blood pressure than that judged to be normal. The primary factor in hypertension is increased resistance to blood flow resulting from the narrowing of peripheral blood vessels. The specific cause for hypertension can be determined for only a small percentage of clients with the condition. When no physical cause can be determined, the client is said to have essential or primary hypertension.

When left untreated, those with elevated blood pressure are at risk for stroke and/or progressive deterioration of cardiac and renal function.

The *Sixth Report of the Joint National Committee on Prevention, Detection, Evaluation, and Treatment of High Blood Pressure* classifies blood pressure for adults age 18 and over as follows:

- Optimal   120/80 mm Hg
- Normal   130/85 mm Hg
- High Normal   130–139/85–89 mm Hg
- Stage 1 Hypertension   140–159/90–99 mm Hg
- Stage 2 Hypertension   160–179/100–109 mm Hg
- Stage 3 Hypertension   180 or greater/110 or greater mm Hg

The decision to initiate drug therapy requires consideration of several factors: the degree of blood pressure elevation, the presence of target organ damage, and the presence of clinical cardiovascular disease or other risk factors, such as smoking, diabetes, and obesity.

The goal of antihypertensive therapy is a blood pressure of 140/90 mm Hg, except in clients with hypertension and diabetes, where the goal is 135/85 mm Hg, and those with renal insufficiency, where the goal is 130/85 mm Hg. Reducing blood pressure with drugs clearly decreases cardiovascular morbidity and mortality.

When the decision has been made to begin antihypertensive therapy and if there are no indications for another type of drug, a diuretic or beta-blocker is generally chosen. If the response to the initial drug choice is inadequate after reaching the full dose, two options for subsequent therapy should be considered.

1. If the client is tolerating the first choice well, add a second drug from another class.
2. If the client is having significant adverse effects or no response, substitute an agent from another class.

Drugs used in the treatment of hypertension may be classified as diuretics, alpha-adrenergic blocking agents, beta-adrenergic blocking agents, calcium channel blockers, direct vasodilators, and angiotensin-converting enzyme (ACE) inhibitors.

Actions

Diuretics act by reducing extracellular fluid volume. *Alpha-adrenergic blockers* interrupt the actions of sympathomimetic agents at alpha-adrenergic receptor sites, relaxing vascular smooth muscle, increasing peripheral vasodilation, and decreasing blood pressure. *Beta-adrenergic blockers* prevent sympathetic nervous system stimulation by inhibiting the action of catecholamines and other sympathomimetic agents at beta-adrenergic receptor sites. *Calcium channel blockers* block the flow of calcium ions into myocardial muscle cells and myocardial pacemaker cells. They produce antianginal effects and act on vascular smooth muscle cells. *Direct vasodilators* act on arteries, veins, or both to reduce blood pressure. They relax smooth muscle, thereby reducing blood pressure. *Angiotensin-converting enzyme (ACE) inhibitors* reduce blood pressure by inhibiting the enzyme that converts angiotensin I to angiotensin II, a potent vasoconstrictor. They also decrease aldosterone release, thereby preventing sodium and water retention. See Table 24-7 for selected antihypertensive agents.

Lifestyle modification is also an important factor in treating hypertension, including reduction in weight and sodium intake, following a regular exercise program, cessation of using tobacco products, and moderation of alcohol intake.

Nursing Considerations

Assess blood pressure for therapeutic response to the prescribed medication. Monitor blood studies (neutrophils, decreased platelets, potassium and sodium levels) and renal studies (protein, BUN, creatinine-increased levels may indicate nephrotic syndrome). Be aware of possible adverse reactions to the prescribed medication.

TABLE 24-7 SELECTED ANTIHYPERTENSIVE AGENTS

Medication	Drug Action	Usual Dosage	Adverse Reactions
amlodipine (Norvasc)	Calcium channel blocker	Oral: 5 mg/day, up to a maximum of 10 mg/day	Nausea, abdominal pain, headache, dizziness, hypotension, palpitations, dry mouth
atenolol (Tenormin)	Beta-1 adrenergic blocking agent	Oral: 50 mg given as one tablet a day	Bradycardia, leg pain, cold extremities, vertigo, postural hypotension, dizziness, fatigue, depression, diarrhea, nausea, dyspnea
captopril (Capoten)	Angiotensin-converting enzyme (ACE) inhibitor	Oral: 12.5–50 mg 3 times daily	Proteinuria, rash, hypotension, loss of taste perception
clonidine HCl (Catapres)	Centrally acting adrenergic agent	Oral: 0.2–0.8 mg daily in 2–3 divided doses	Dry mouth, drowsiness, sedation, anorexia, nausea, constipation, headache
enalapril (Vasotec)	Angiotensin-converting enzyme (ACE) inhibitor	Oral: 5 mg/day, then adjust dosage according to response (range: 10–40 mg/day in 1 or 2 doses)	Nausea, vomiting, diarrhea, headache, dizziness, palpitations, hypotension, cough
eprosartan mesylate (Teveten)	Angiotensin II receptor antagonist	Oral: 600 mg once daily Range: 400–800 mg once or twice daily	Abdominal pain, diarrhea, anorexia, headache, dizziness, hypotension, palpitations
furosemide (Lasix)	Loop diuretic	Oral (Adult): 20–80 mg/day Oral (Child): initial, 2 mg/kg	Anorexia, oral and gastric irritation, nausea, dizziness, anemia, purpura
guanethidine sulfate (Ismelin)	Peripherally acting adrenergic agent	Oral: 10–50 mg/day	Fatigue, nausea, nasal congestion, abdominal distress, weight gain
guanfacine HCl (Tenex)	Alpha-2 adrenergic blocking agent	Oral: 1–2 mg daily, given at bedtime	Sedation, weakness, dizziness, dry mouth, constipation, impotence
hydralazine HCl (Apresoline)	Direct-acting vasodilator	Oral: 10–50 mg 4 times daily	Headache, anorexia, nausea, vomiting, diarrhea, palpitations, tachycardia
lisinopril (Prinivil, Zestril)	Angiotensin-converting enzyme (ACE) inhibitor	Oral: 10 mg once daily, then adjust dosage according to response (range: 20–40 mg/day as a single dose)	Nausea, vomiting, diarrhea, hypotension, palpitations, angina, cough
losartan potassium (Cozaar)	Angiotensin II receptor antagonist	Oral: 50 mg once daily	Diarrhea, dyspepsia, headache, muscle cramps, myalgia, dizziness, cough, insomnia, fatigue, nasal congestion, sinusitis
methyldopa (Aldomet)	Central and peripherally acting adrenergic agent	Oral: 0.5–2.0 g daily divided into 2–4 doses	Drowsiness, dry mouth, nasal congestion, nausea, vomiting, diarrhea

(continued)

TABLE 24-7 *(Continued)*

Medication	Drug Action	Usual Dosage	Adverse Reactions
methyldopa hydrochlorothiazide (Aldoril)	Combination of two antihypertensive agents	Oral: 1 tablet 2 or 3 times/day	Sedation, headache, bradycardia, nausea, rash
metoprolol tartrate (Lopressor)	Beta-adrenergic blocking agent	Oral: 50–100 mg twice daily	Tiredness, dizziness, depression, mental confusion, headache
perindopril (Aceon)	Angiotensin-converting enzyme (ACE) inhibitor	Oral: 4 mg once daily, then adjust dosage according to response (range: 4–8 mg, up to a maximum of 16 mg/day)	Nausea, vomiting, diarrhea, headache, hypotension, palpitations, cough
prazosin HCl (Minipress)	Alpha-1 adrenergic blocking agent	Oral: adjusted according to client's blood pressure Initial dose: 1 mg 2–3 times/day Maintenance dose: slowly increased to a total daily dose of 20 mg given in divided doses	Dizziness, headache, drowsiness, palpitations, nausea
spironolactone (Aldactone)	Potassium-sparing diuretic	Oral: 50–100 mg/day	Gynecomastia, drowsiness, cramping and diarrhea, headache, lethargy
terazosin HCl (Hytrin)	Alpha-1 adrenergic blocking agent	Oral: adjusted according to client's blood pressure Initial dose: 1 mg at bedtime Subsequent dose: slowly increased; range 1–10 mg once a day	Asthenia, back pain, headache, palpitations, postural hypotension, tension, tachycardia, nausea
verapamil HCl (Isoptin SR) (Verelan)	Calcium channel blocker	Oral: 240 mg once daily in the morning	Constipation, dizziness, nausea, hypotension, edema, headache

Clients' Instruction

Educate the client

- To take the medication as prescribed
- That he/she may have to take high blood pressure medicine for the rest of his/her life
- That the medication does not cure hypertension, but helps to control it, and he/she must continue to take the medication even if he/she feels better
- About possible adverse reactions
- To avoid alcohol and over-the-counter drugs (especially cough, cold, and allergy medicines)
- Not to operate hazardous machinery or drive a motor vehicle if dizziness occurs
- About the factors that tend to increase blood pressure: obesity, smoking, consumption of alcohol, stress, lack of exercise, and excessive intake of sodium
- In ways to reduce the factors that may be contributing to hypertension
- Who is taking diuretics that may deplete potassium to eat foods rich in potassium (See Chapter 27 for more information on diuretics.)

DRUGS THAT AFFECT THE BLOOD

A number of medications have been developed that affect the clotting of blood. Simply put, these drugs either assist in the clotting process or work to inhibit the formation of a clot. The formation of a blood clot within a blood vessel is a life-threatening event; therefore, agents that interfere with the clotting process are important. These drugs are the anticoagulants and the thrombolytic agents.

Anticoagulants are used therapeutically after a thrombus or blood clot has formed. They do not alter the size of an existing thrombus; however, they do act to prevent further growth and reduce the possibility of embolization. If a thrombus is detached from the point at which it formed, it becomes an **embolus** moving within the vascular system. An embolus that occludes (blocks) the flow of blood can cause serious damage to an organ, as in the case of a coronary embolism.

Thrombolytic agents will dissolve existing fresh thrombi and emboli. These drugs diffuse into the clot and activate plasminogen that is trapped therein. **Plasminogen** is a protein that is important in the prevention of fibrin clot formation. After a thrombolytic agent has been employed, anticoagulants are used to prevent recurrence of a blood clot.

Heparin

Heparin is a potent anticoagulant. It is produced by **mast cells** (connective tissue cells that contain heparin and histamine) and basophil leukocytes. It inhibits coagulation by forming an antithrombin that prevents conversion of prothrombiin to thrombin and by preventing liberation of thromboplastin from blood platelets. Heparin is poorly absorbed from the gastrointestinal tract; therefore, it must be administered by subcutaneous injection and/or intravenously. Clinically, heparin is used during open heart surgery, during renal hemodialysis, and in the treatment of deep venous thrombosis or pulmonary infarction. Subcutaneous administration of low doses of heparin has been shown to diminish postoperative pulmonary embolism in older adults.

Actions

Prevents conversion of fibrinogen to fibrin.

Uses

Anticoagulant therapy in prophylaxis and treatment of venous thrombosis and its extension. Used for prevention of postoperative deep venous thrombosis and pulmonary embolism, prevention of clotting in arterial and heart surgery, prophylaxis and treatment of peripheral arterial embolism, atrial fibrillation with embolization, disseminated intravascular clotting syndrome, as an anticoagulant in blood transfusions, extracorporeal circulation, and dialysis procedures and in blood samples for laboratory purposes.

Contraindications

Contraindicated in clients with known hypersensitivity to any of its ingredients and in clients with severe thrombocytopenia and uncontrollable active bleeding.

> **Safety Precaution:**
> 1. Use with extreme caution in hemophilia, leukemia with bleeding, peptic ulcer disease, hepatic disease (severe), renal disease (severe), blood dyscrasias, pregnancy, severe hypotension, subacute bacterial endocarditis, and acute nephritis.
> 2. Heparin is not intended for intramuscular use.
> 3. Hemorrhage can occur at almost any site in clients receiving heparin.

Adverse Reactions

Hemorrhage. Local irritation, erythema, mild pain, hematoma, or ulceration may follow deep subcutaneous injection. Hypersensitivity reactions with chills, fever, and urticaria. Other adverse reactions are asthma, rhinitis, lacrimation, headache, nausea, vomiting, and anaphylactoid reactions including shock.

Dosage and Route

The dosage and route of administration (IV or subcutaneous) is determined by the physician and individualized for each client. See Table 24-8.

Nursing Considerations

Parenteral drug products should be inspected visually for particulate matter and discoloration prior to administration. Slight discoloration does not alter potency. *Never administer by intramuscular injection.* Before adding to an infusion solution for continuous intravenous administration, the container should be inverted at least six times to insure adequate mixing and prevent pooling of the heparin in the solution. The dosage of heparin should be adjusted according to the client's coagulation test results; these should be monitored very carefully. *Be aware of signs of bleeding: petechiae, ecchymosis, black tarry stools, bleeding gums, hematuria.*

Clients' Instruction

Educate the client

- About the purpose of the medication
- About adverse reactions

- Not to take aspirin or NSAIDs while on anticoagulant therapy
- To report any symptoms of unusual bleeding or bruising, itching, rash, fever, swelling, or difficulty breathing to his/her physician immediately
- To avoid IM injections and activities leading to injury
- To use a soft toothbrush
- To use an electric razor

Special Considerations

- Heparin sodium is not effective by oral administration and should be given by intermittent intravenous injection, intravenous infusion, or deep subcutaneous injection (do not aspirate).

Oral Anticoagulants

Anticoagulants that are administered orally do not produce an immediate effect. Their action is usually evident within 12 to 24 hours of administration. As with other anticoagulants, the use of these drugs may produce a cumulative effect; therefore, dosages must be individualized and based upon the client's clotting time, using a blood coagulation test. See Table 24-8.

Warfarin Sodium (Coumadin)

Actions

Coumadin acts by inhibiting the synthesis of vitamin K–dependent coagulation factors.

Uses

Indicated for the prophylaxis and/or treatment of venous thrombosis and its extension, pulmonary embolism, atrial fibrillation with embolization, and as an adjunct in the prophylaxis of systemic embolism after myocardial infarction.

Contraindications

Contraindicated in clients with known hypersensitivity to any of its ingredients and in patients where the hazard of hemorrhage might be greater than the potential clinical benefits of anticoagulation such as pregnancy, hemorrhagic tendencies or blood dyscrasias, recent or contemplated surgery, bleeding tendencies associated with active ulceration or overt bleeding, threatened abortion, and in unsupervised senility, alcoholism, and/or psychosis.

TABLE 24-8   ANTICOAGULANTS

Medication	Usual Dosage	Adverse Reactions

enoxaparin (Lovenox)	SC (Adult): prophylaxis before knee/hip surgery:
	  30 mg twice daily starting within 24 hours postop and continued for 7–10 days or until ambulatory (up to 14 days)
	prophylaxis before abdominal surgery:
	  40 mg twice daily starting within 24 hours postop and continued for 7–10 days or until ambulatory (up to 14 days)
	systemic anticoagulation:
	  1 mg/kg every 12 hours
		Hemorrhage, anemia, thrombocytopenia, dizziness, headache, nausea, vomiting, pruritus, rash, urticaria, fever

heparin sodium	(Adult): 5000 U by IV injection, followed by 10,000–2000 U of a concentrated solution Maintenance: 8000–10,000 U every 8 hours or 15,000–20,000 U every 12 hours IV intermittent (Adult): 10,000 units followed by 5000–10,000 units every 4–6 hours IV infusion (Adult): 5000 units by IV injection followed by 20,000–40,000 units daily	Hemorrhage, hematoma, hypersensitivity reaction includes chills, fever, and urticaria
warfarin sodium (Coumadin)	Oral (Adult): 40–60 mg the first day, followed by 2–10 mg daily	Hemorrhage, alopecia, dermatitis, urticaria

Safety Precaution:

1. Hemorrhage can occur at almost any site in clients on anticoagulant therapy.

2. Cautious use during lactation, severe to moderate hepatic or renal insufficiency, trauma that may result in internal bleeding, surgery or trauma resulting in large exposed raw surfaces, and in clients with indwelling catheters, severe to moderate hypertension, known or suspected deficiency in protein C, polycythemia vera, vasculitis, severe diabetes, severe allergic and anaphylactic disorders.

3. A client receiving Coumadin must have frequent lab tests to monitor coagulation factors.

4. There are numerous factors that can affect anticoagulant response. Please refer to a current *Physicians' Desk Reference* and/or a *PDR Nurse's Drug Handbook* for more information.

Adverse Reactions

Hemorrhage. Necrosis of skin and other tissues, alopecia, urticaria, dermatitis, fever, nausea, diarrhea, abdominal cramping, and hypersensitivity reactions.

Dosage and Route

The dosage and route of administration is determined by the physician and individualized for each client. See Table 24-8.

Nursing Considerations

Assess prothrombin time and therapeutic response to medication. Monitor blood pressure, blood studies (hematocrit, platelet count), stools and urine for blood. Be aware of signs of bleeding. Be alert for signs of adverse reactions.

Clients' Instruction

Educate the client

- About the purpose of the medication
- About adverse reactions
- To take the medication as prescribed and to have periodic (monitored) prothrombin time evaluations
- To avoid alcohol, salicylates (aspirin), NSAIDs, large amounts of green vegetables and/or drastic changes in dietary habits, which may affect Coumadin therapy
- That Coumadin may cause a red-orange discoloration of alkaline urine

Special Considerations

- The client should notify the physician if any illness such as diarrhea, infection, or fever develops or if any unusual symptoms develop, such as pain, swelling, prolonged bleeding from cuts, increased menstrual bleeding, nosebleeds, bleeding of gums from brushing of teeth, unusual bleeding or bruising, red or dark brown urine, and/or red or tarry stools.

Antiplatelet Drugs

Antiplatelet drugs help reduce the occurrence of and death from vascular events such as heart attacks and strokes. Aspirin is currently considered to be the reference standard antiplatelet drug and is recommended by the American Heart Association for use in clients with a wide range of cardiovascular disease. Plavix (clopidogrel) is another antiplatelet drug that was approved by the Food and Drug Administration for many of the same indications as aspirin. Plavix may provide valuable therapeutic benefit over aspirin in clients with peripheral arterial disease and in stroke or myocardial infarction clients for whom aspirin treatment is contraindicated or for whom aspirin fails to achieve a therapeutic benefit. The recommended dosage of Plavix is 75 mg tablet once daily.

Aspirin may be recommended by physicians to reduce the risk of a second heart attack, or to reduce the risk of having a heart attack and/or a stroke. Aspirin has been shown to inhibit an essential enzyme that cells use to manufacture prostaglandin production, a hormone-like substance that takes an active role in many cellular activities. By inhibiting prostaglandin production, it also inhibits platelet clumping, the first stage of the blood clotting process.

Aspirin helps keep platelets from sticking together to form clots. With this clotting activity reduced, the blood flows more freely and oxygen is more easily supplied to the heart, brain, and other organs. Clots are less likely to form, thus reducing the possibility of a clot forming and breaking away and lodging in the heart and/or brain.

It is generally recommended that an individual take aspirin (80, 160, or 325 mg) per day to prevent thromboembolic disorders.

Contraindications

Hypersensitivity, gastrointestinal bleeding, bleeding disorders, children under 3 years of age, children with flu-like symptoms, pregnancy, lactation, vitamin K deficiency, peptic ulcer.

Precautions

Anemias, hepatic and/or renal disease, Hodgkin's disease.

Adverse Reactions

Thrombocytopenia, agranulocytosis, leukopenia, neutropenia, hemolytic anemia, increased pro-time, drowsiness, dizziness, confusion, convulsions, headache, flushing, hallucinations, coma, nausea, vomiting, GI bleeding, heartburn, anorexia, rash, urticaria, bruising, ototoxicity, tinnitus, hearing loss, rapid pulse, hyperpnea, hypoglycemia, hypokalemia, hepatotoxicity, renal dysfunction, visual changes.

Nursing Considerations

Assess liver, renal, and blood studies. Monitor prothrombin time and intake and output ratio. Decreased output may indicate renal failure (long-term therapy). Be aware of adverse reactions, especially hepatotoxicity (dark urine, clay-colored stool, jaundice, itching, abdominal pain, fever, diarrhea), allergic reactions (rash, urticaria), renal dysfunction (decreased urine output), ototoxicity (tinnitus, ringing in ears, loss of hearing), visual changes (blurring, halos, corneal, retinal damage), edema in feet, ankles, legs.

Clients' Instruction

Educate the client

- To take the medication as prescribed
- About adverse reactions
- To visit his/her physician on a regular basis
- To have liver, renal, and blood studies performed
- Not to take over-the-counter medications unless prescribed by his/her physician
- To avoid alcohol, caffeine, and nicotine
- To inform dentist or surgeon before surgery or dental work of taking aspirin (may increase the likelihood of bleeding)

Special Considerations

- Client taking anticoagulant drugs should not take aspirin unless prescribed by his/her physician. Frequent lab tests to monitor coagulation factors must be performed on a regular basis and monitored carefully.
- Antacids, steroids, and urinary alkalizers may decrease the effectiveness of the drug.
- Anticoagulants, insulin, and methotrexate may increase the effectiveness of the drug.

Thrombolytic Agents

Approximately 80 percent of all acute myocardial infarctions are caused by a thrombus that occludes a coronary artery. Unless contraindicated, thrombolytic therapy is the treatment of choice for an MI client who reaches the hospital within 6 hours of the onset of chest pain. In some hospitals the time period for administering thrombolytic agents has been extended to 12 and 24 hours.

According to researchers, clients who are 75 years of age and older may respond poorly to treatment with thrombolytics (clot busters) and may be at higher risk of dying if they receive these drugs. The role of these drugs in older adult heart attack clients needs further study. Younger clients clearly benefit from thrombolytics, but one-third of heart attack clients who are older than 75 are unlikely to have any benefit and may be at higher risk of death.

Thrombolytic agents act to dissolve an existing thrombus when administered soon after its occurrence. These agents dissolve the clot, reopen the artery, restore blood flow to the heart, and prevent further damage to the myocardium.

Thrombolytic agents that have been approved for treating acute myocardial infarction are streptokinase (Kabikinase, Streptase), anistreplase (Eminase), alteplase (Activase), urokinase (Abbokinase), which is used to dissolve obstructive thrombi in the peripheral circulation and acute pulmonary emboli, and a single-chain urokinase plasminogen activator that converts to urokinase at the site of the clot. See Table 24-9.

Contraindications

Hypersensitivity, active internal bleeding, recent (within 2 months) cerebrovascular accident, intracranial or intraspinal surgery, intracranial neoplasm, severe uncontrolled hypertension.

Safety Precaution:

1. Bleeding is the most common complication encountered during thrombolytic therapy. Internal bleeding may involve the gastrointestinal tract, genitourinary tract, retroperitoneal or intracranial sites. Superficial or surface bleeding may occur at invaded or disturbed site (venous cutdown, arterial puncture, sites of recent surgical intervention). Intramuscular injections and nonessential handling of the client should be avoided during treatment.
2. Should serious bleeding (not controlled by local pressure) occur, treatment with a thrombolytic agent should be stopped immediately.
3. Each client being considered for therapy must be carefully evaluated and anticipated benefits weighed against potential risks associated with thrombolytic therapy.

TABLE 24-9 THROMBOLYTIC AGENTS

Medication	Usual Dosage	Nursing Considerations
alteplase (Activase)	Bolus dose of 6–10 mg IV over 1–2 minutes, then a lytic dose of 50–54 mg over 60 minutes, followed by a maintenance dose of 40 mg over 2 hours. Total dose: 100 mg IV over 3 hours	Assess vital signs every 30 minutes. Monitor activated partial thromboplastin time every 4 hours for 48 hours. Check cardiac isoenzymes every 3 hours for 12 hours, then every 6 hours for 12 hours. Perform neurological assessment every 30 minutes to detect early signs of intracranial bleeding. Monitor ECG. Be alert for signs of bleeding and/or hypersensitivity.
anistreplase (Eminase)	30 units IV push over 2–5 minutes	Same as above
streptokinase (Kabikinase, Streptase)	1.5 million units IV over 60 minutes by controlled drip	Same as above

Adverse Reactions

Bleeding, allergic reactions, anaphylactic and anaphylactoid reactions, fever.

Dosage and Route

The dosage and route of administration is determined by the physician and individualized for each client. Thrombolytic agents are administered intravenously by a physician, registered nurse, or certified emergency medical technician-paramedic.

Hemostatic Agents

Hemostatic agents may be administered systemically to overcome specific coagulation defects, or applied topically to control surface bleeding. Certain of these drugs are used in the treatment of hemophilia (Proplex) and for hypofibrinogenemia (Vitamin K). Other products, known as locally absorbable hemostatics, are applied topically to control capillary oozing and surface bleeding. Examples of these are gelatin sponge (Gelfoam), oxidized cellulose (Surgicel), microfibrillar collagen (Avitene), and thrombin.

Antianemic Agents: Irons

Oral antianemic agents that are used to treat iron deficiency anemia are ferrous fumarate, ferrous gluconate, and ferrous sulfate. These iron preparations are available in various trade name products such as ferrous fumarate (Femiron, Feostat, Hemocyte, Ircon, Neo-Fer), ferrous gluconate (Fergon), and ferrous sulfate (Feosol, Fer-in-Sol, Slow-Fe).

Actions

Provides the body with iron that is needed for red blood cell development, energy, and oxygen.

Uses

Iron deficiency and iron-deficiency anemia.

Contraindications

Contraindicated in clients with known hypersensitivity and in clients with ulcerative colitis, regional enteritis, hemosiderosis, hemochromatosis, peptic ulcer disease, hemolytic anemia, cirrhosis.

> **Safety Precaution:**
> 1. Oral iron preparations interfere with the absorption of oral tetracycline antibiotics. These products should not be taken within 2 hours of each other.
> 2. Cautious use in pregnancy and/or lactation

Adverse Reactions

Nausea, constipation, epigastric pain, vomiting, diarrhea, tarry stools.

Dosage and Route

The dosage and route of administration is determined by the physician and individualized for each client. See Table 24-10.

Nursing Considerations

Assess hematocrit, hemoglobin, reticulocyte, and bilirubin determinations before initiation of therapy and monthly during treatment. Liquid preparation should be diluted and given through a plastic straw to avoid discoloration of tooth enamel. Store medication in a tight, light-resistant container. Monitor client for signs of toxicity: nausea, vomiting, diarrhea (green then tarry stools), hemateme-

TABLE 24-10   ANTIANEMIC AGENTS: IRON PREPARATIONS

Medication	Usual Dosage
ferrous fumarate	Oral (Adult): 200 mg tid–qid
ferrous gluconate	Oral (Adult): 200–600 mg tid
ferrous sulfate	Oral (Adult): 0.750–1.5 g/day in divided doses, tid
iron dextran (Dex Ferrum)	IV, IM (Adult): Test dose 0.5 ml Less than 50 kg: 100 mg/day More than 50 kg: 250 mg/day
sodium ferric gluconate complex (Ferrlecit)	IV infusion (Adult): Test dose: 2 ml (25 mg) diluted in 50 ml of 0.9% NaCl for injection given over 1 hour Therapeutic dose: 10 ml (125 mg elemental iron) diluted in 100 ml of 0.9% NaCl for injection given over 1 hour

sis, pallor, cyanosis, shock, coma. Assess client's nutritional needs. Evaluate therapeutic response.

Clients' Instruction

Educate the client

- About the purpose of the medication
- About adverse reactions
- To take the medication as prescribed
- To have monthly blood studies evaluated by his/her physician
- To take the medication between meals for best absorption and not to take with milk or antacids
- To take liquid iron preparations through a plastic straw
- That iron may cause dark green or black stools
- About the proper method of storage for the medication
- To include iron-rich foods in his/her diet (Foods rich in iron are liver, beef, veal, lamb, pork, turkey, chicken, oysters, eggs, peanut butter, soybeans, dried apricots, peaches, prunes, dates, figs, raisins, molasses, dried beans, enriched breads and cereals, and dark green leafy vegetables.)

Special Considerations

- Tablets should not be crushed.
- In case of accidental overdose, contact poison control center and seek medical help immediately.
- Do not substitute one iron preparation for another.

Iron Dextran (Dex Ferrum)

Iron dextran (Dex Ferrum) is a parenteral preparation that is available for IM/IV administration. It

is administered only after a test dose of 0.5 ml by preferred route, and if well tolerated, the remaining portion of the dose is administered after a 1 hour wait. The Z-track method of intramuscular injection is used and a 19–20 gauge, 2–3 inch needle is used for the average adult client. For clients who are larger than average, a longer needle is used to insure that the drug is deep in muscle tissue, as the drug may be irritating to subcutaneous tissue and cause discoloration.

Contraindications

Hypersensitivity, all anemias excluding iron deficiency anemia, hepatic disease.

Adverse Reactions

Headache, paresthesia, dizziness, shivering, weakness, convulsions, nausea, vomiting, abdominal pain, rash, pruritus, urticaria, fever, sweating, chills, atrophy/fibrosis at injection site, necrosis, sterile abscess, phlebitis, chest pain, shock, hypotension, tachycardia, dyspnea, leukocytosis.

Nursing Considerations

Assess client for signs of adverse reactions. Monitor cardiac status: chest pain, hypotension, tachycardia. Monitor for hypersensitivity reaction: rash, pruritus, fever, chills, anaphylaxis. Store medication at room temperature in cool environment. Client should remain in the recumbent position for 30 minutes after an injection of Dex Ferrum.

ANTIANEMIC AGENTS USED IN TREATING MEGALOBLASTIC ANEMIAS

Megaloblastic anemias result from decreased erythrocyte formation and the immaturity, fragility, and early destruction of these cells. There is a defective DNA synthesis, usually from vitamin B_{12}.

Folic Acid (Vitamin B₉)

Actions

Increases red blood cell, white blood cell, and platelet formation in megaloblastic anemias.

Uses

Megaloblastic or macrocytic anemia caused by folic acid deficiency; liver disease, alcoholism, hemolysis, intestinal obstruction. Cautious use during pregnancy.

Contraindications

Hypersensitivity, anemias other than megaloblastic/macrocytic anemia, vitamin B_{12} deficiency.

Adverse Reactions

Bronchospasm.

Dosage and Route

Megaloblastic/macrocytic anemia: Oral, IM, SC (Adult and child over 4 years of age): 1 mg every day times 4–5 days.

Nursing Considerations

Assess folate blood levels. Store medication in light-resistant container. Evaluate therapeutic response and nutritional status of client.

Clients' Instruction

Educate the client

- About sources of folic acid (meat, eggs, green leafy vegetables)
- About therapeutic response
- About how to properly store the medication

Cyanocobalamin (Vitamin B₁₂)

Actions

Replaces vitamin B_{12} that the body would normally absorb from the diet.

Uses

Vitamin B_{12} deficiency, pernicious anemia, vitamin B_{12} malabsorption syndrome.

Contraindications

Hypersensitivity, optic nerve atrophy. Cautious use during pregnancy and lactation.

Adverse Reactions

Flushing, optic nerve atrophy, diarrhea, congestive heart failure, peripheral vascular thrombosis, pulmonary edema, itching, rash, hypokalemia.

Dosage and Route

Pernicious anemia (Adult): IM 100–1000 micrograms every day times 2 weeks, then 100–1000 micrograms every month.

Nursing Considerations

Assess gastrointestinal function, blood potassium level, and complete blood count. Be aware of signs of adverse reactions. Evaluate therapeutic response and nutritional status of client.

Clients' Instruction

Educate the client

- About the importance of taking the medication exactly as prescribed by his/her physician
- That treatment is for life when one has pernicious anemia
- About foods rich in vitamin B_{12}

Epoetin Alfa (Epogen)

Epoetin alfa (EPO, Procrit) is a genetically engineered hemopoietin that stimulates the production of red blood cells. It is a recombinant version of erythropoietin and is indicated for treating anemia in clients with chronic renal failure and for the treatment of anemia related to therapy with zidovudine (AZT) in HIV-infected clients, for the treatment of anemia in clients with nonmyeloid malignancies where anemia is due to the effect of concomitantly administered chemotherapy, and for the treatment of anemic clients scheduled to undergo elective, noncardiac, nonvascular surgery who are not donating their own blood.

Contraindications

In clients with uncontrolled hypertension, known hypersensitivity to mammalian cell-derived products and known hypersensitivity to albumin (human).

Safety Precaution:

1. Blood pressure should be properly controlled before initiation of therapy. It must be monitored carefully during therapy.
2. Seizures have occurred in clients with chronic renal failure.
3. Please refer to a current *Physicians' Desk Reference* and/or a *PDR Nurse's Drug Handbook* for additional warnings and precautions.

Adverse Reactions

Hypertension, headache, arthralgia, nausea, edema, fatigue, diarrhea, vomiting, chest pain, skin reactions, asthenia, dizziness, clotted vascular access, seizure, myocardial infarction.

Dosage and Route

Starting dose: 50–100 U/kg three times weekly IV for dialysis clients; IV or SC for nondialysis clients. Reduce dose when (1) target range is reached, or (2) hematocrit increases above 4 points in any 2-week period. Increase dose if hematocrit does not increase by 5–6 points after 8 weeks of therapy, and hematocrit is below target range.

Nursing Considerations

Carefully monitor blood pressure for signs of hypertension. Assess hematocrit for therapeutic range. Do not shake the container as shaking may denature the glycoprotein, rendering it biologically inactive. Inspect parenteral drug product for particulate matter and discoloration. Do not use vial if either or both are apparent. Use aseptic technique. Use only one dose per vial; do not reenter vial. Discard unused portions. Do not administer in conjunction with other drug solutions.

ANTIHYPERLIPIDEMIC AGENTS

Antihyperlipidemic agents are used to lower abnormally high blood levels of fatty substances (lipids) when other treatment regimens fail. Lipids may accumulate in the walls of blood vessels as atherosclerotic plaques and this accumulation can contribute to hypertension, increase the risk of coronary artery disease, and decrease the flow of oxygenated blood to the heart and other body organs. See Table 24-11 and Figure 24-1.

Lipids include sterols (cholesterol and cholesterol esters), free fatty acids (FFA), triglycerides (glycerol esters of FFA), and phospholipids (phosphoric acid esters of lipid substances). Lipids may be exogenous (derived from foods and oils that are high in saturated fat) and endogenous (produced by the liver from the end products of lipid and carbohydrate metabolism).

Saturated fats (usually solid at room temperature) raise low density lipoprotein (LDL) cholesterol, the fatty substance that can accumulate in the walls of blood vessels. Foods high in saturated fats include butter, cheese, chocolate, coconut oil, egg yolk, lard, meats, palm oil, whole milk, shell fish, and sardines. Other types of lipoprotein include very low-density lipoprotein (VLDL) and high-density lipoprotein (HDL). High-density lipoprotein are "H"ighly "D"esirable and are known as the "good type of cholesterol." Elevations in total cholesterol and low-density lipoprotein are associated with the development of coronary heart disease.

Diet, weight and stress management, exercise, and proper treatment of other conditions such as hypertension and diabetes are tried before the physician prescribes an antihyperlipidemic agent. When the blood cholesterol is not lowered by these other means, then one of several medications may be ordered. Lipid-lowering drugs include statins, fibrates, niacin, and bile acid–binding resins. (See Table 24-12.)

- Statins inhibit an enzyme used by the liver to manufacture cholesterol. The statins include atorvastatin (Lipitor), cerivastatin (Baycol), fluvastatin (Lescol), lovastatin (Mevacor), pravastatin (Pravachol), and simvastatin (Zocor). Liver function tests are done prior to starting on a statin drug. Statins can cause liver damage and are contraindicated in clients with active liver disease or unexplained persistently high liver function test. They are not used during pregnancy or lactation.

- Fibrates are fibric acid derivatives used to lower triglyceride levels and increase high-density lipoprotein levels (the good cholesterol). Examples are fenofibrate (Tricor) and gemfibrozil (Lopid). Tricor is contraindicated in clients with hepatic or severe renal dysfunction (including primary biliary cirrhosis), persistent abnormal liver function, preexisting gallbladder disease, and during lactation. Lopid is contraindicated in clients with gallbladder disease, primary bil-

TABLE 24-11 CHOLESTEROL VALUES AND ASSOCIATED RISK LEVEL

Total Cholesterol	LDL	Risk Level
Below 200 mg/dL	Below 130 mg/dL	Desirable level
200–239 mg/dL	130–159 mg/dL	Borderline–High
240 mg/dL	160 mg/dL	High

TABLE 24-12 SELECTED ANTIHYPERLIPIDEMIC AGENTS

Medication	Usual Dosage	Adverse Reactions
atorvastatin calcium (Lipitor)	10 mg once daily	Constipation, flatulence, dyspepsia, abdominal pain
cerivastatin (Baycol)	0.3 mg once daily in evening, orally	Dizziness, headache, insomnia, flatus, myalgia, arthralgia, diarrhea, abdominal cramps, constipation, skin rashes
cholestyramine (Questran)	4 g orally before meals and at bedtime	Headache, dizziness, vertigo, tinnitus, muscle and joint pain, abdominal pain, constipation, nausea, fecal impaction, hemorrhoids, flatulence, vomiting, peptic ulcer, steatorrhea
clofibrate (Atromid-S)	500 mg qid, orally	Nausea, vomiting, dyspepsia, increased liver enzyme studies, stomatitis, flatulence, gastritis, weight gain, hepatomegaly, increased cholelithiasis
colestipol (Colestid)	15–30 g/day in 2–4 divided doses	Constipation, abdominal pain, nausea, fecal impaction, vomiting, hemorrhoids, flatulence, peptic ulcer, steatorrhea
fenofibrate (Tricor)	67 mg/day given with meals, then individualized based on response Maximum daily dose: 200 mg/day	Diarrhea, abdominal pain, constipation, flatulence, dizziness, decreased libido, myalgia, arthralgia, skin rashes
fluvastatin sodium (Lescol)	20 mg once daily at bedtime	Rash, back pain, coughing, dyspepsia, diarrhea, abdominal pain, nausea, constipation, flatulence, dizziness, headache
gemfibrozil (Lopid)	600 mg bid, orally 30 minutes before morning and evening meal	Nausea, flatulence, diarrhea, epigastric pain, abdominal pain
lovastatin (Mevacor) (See Figure 24-2)	20–80 mg daily, orally	Muscle pain and inflammation, increased liver function studies, rhabdomyolysis, acute muscle deterioration, headache, skin rash, pruritus, nausea, diarrhea, constipation, gas
niacin (Nicolar, Nicobid)	300–600 mg daily, orally	Flushing, skin rash, pruritus, GI upset, exacerbation of peptic ulcer, hyperglycemia, hyperuricemia
pravastatin (Pravachol)	10–20 mg once daily at bedtime, orally	Myalgia, muscle cramps, headache, dizziness, vertigo, nausea, vomiting, diarrhea, abdominal pain, palpitations, postural hypotension
simvastatin (Zocor) (See Figure 24-3)	5–10 mg once a day in the evening range 5–40 mg/day single dose in the evening	Muscle cramps, myalgia, tremor, dizziness, headache, vertigo, memory loss, anorexia, vomiting, constipation, diarrhea, alopecia, pruritus, gynecomastia, loss of libido, blurred vision

iary cirrhosis, hepatic or renal dysfunction. It is used with caution during lactation.

● Niacin (vitamin B_3) in large doses decreases lipoprotein and triglyceride synthesis by inhibiting the release of free fatty acids from adipose tissue and decreasing hepatic lipoprotein synthesis. Examples are Nicolar and Nicobid.

Niacin is contraindicated in clients with known hypersensitivity. It is used with caution in clients with liver disease, history of arterial bleeding and/or peptic ulcer disease, gout, glaucoma, and diabetes mellitus. The client may experience a warm flushing in the face and ears within 2 hours after taking niacin. The physi-

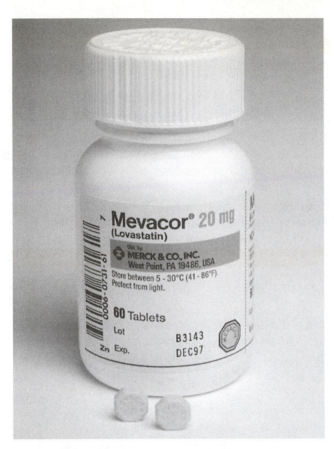

FIGURE 24-2   MEVACOR® (LIOVASTATIN) 20 MG TABLETS
(Courtesy of Merck & Co., Inc.)

cian may advise the client to take one aspirin to help reduce this effect. Alcohol may increase these effects.

- Bile acid–binding resins remove bile acids from the intestine, causing the liver to remove cholesterol from the blood to make more bile acids. Examples are cholestyramine (Questran) and colestipol (Colestid). These drugs are contraindicated in clients with known hypersensitivity and complete biliary obstruction. Some products contain aspartame and should be avoided in clients with phenylketonuria. They are used with caution in clients who have a history of constipation and with extreme caution in children.

Nursing Considerations

Assess lipid and triglyceride blood levels, liver function tests, and renal function tests. Evaluate therapeutic response to medication. Monitor liver function tests at 6 and 12 weeks after starting therapy and with any dosage change, then every 6 months thereafter. If the liver function tests are abnormal (ALT or AST elevated), notify the physician immediately. If the client experiences any unexplained muscle pain, weakness, or tenderness, especially if accompanied by fever or malaise, notify the physician immediately.

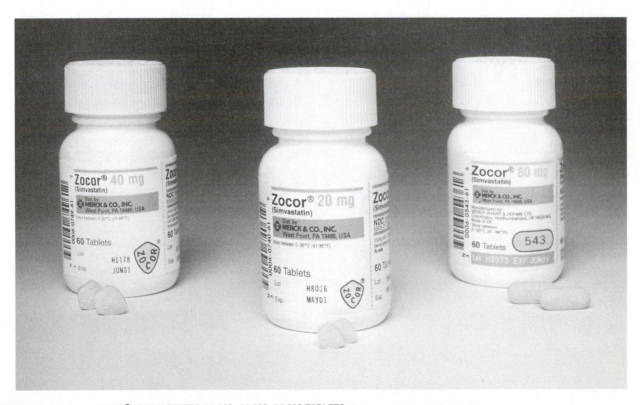

FIGURE 24-3   ZOCOR® (SIMVASTATIN) 20 MG, 40 MG, 80 MG TABLETS *(Courtesy of Merck & Co., Inc.)*

Clients' Instruction

Educate the client

- To take the medication as prescribed
- About adverse reactions
- To report any adverse reactions to his/her physician
- To continue to see his/her physician on a regular basis for cholesterol and liver function tests
- About diet, exercise, lifestyle changes, and stress management

● SPOT CHECK

There are many medications that may be used to treat circulatory system disorders. For each of the selected drugs and/or drug classifications list several aspects of clients' instruction and nursing considerations.

Drug(s)	Clients' Instruction	Nursing Considerations
Digitalis		
Antiarrhythmics		
Vasopressors		
Nitrates		
Antihypertensives		

Drug(s)	Clients' Instruction	Nursing Considerations
Anticoagulants		
Antihyperlipidemics		

● SELF-ASSESSMENT

Write the answer in the space provided or circle true or false as instructed.

Source

p. 289 **1.** Women who take estrogen after menopause may reduce the risk of developing heart disease because this hormone replacement therapy has been shown to

(1) _____ ,

(2) _____ , and

(3) help _____ .

p. 290 **2.** In a few words, distinguish between the following terms descriptive of medications that affect heart action:

- Inotropic agents influence

_____ .

- Chronotropic agents influence

_____ .

- Dromotropic agents affect

_____ .

p. 290 **3.** Signs of digitalis intoxication are not uncommon among hospitalized clients receiving this therapy. Two scenarios for digitalis intoxication are mentioned in the chapter and they are

(1) _____ and

(2) _____ .

p. 294 **4.** True or False (circle one) Vasopressors are drugs that cause contraction of the muscles associated with capillaries and arteries.

p. 295 **5.** A person experiencing angina pectoris might take nitroglycerin. Nitroglycerin is a/an _____ _____ .

p. 297 **6.** One whose arterial blood pressure is higher than normal has _____ , and, when no physical cause can be determined, is said to have _____ .

p. 297 **7.** In a few words, describe the effect associated with the use of a diuretic.

_____

p. 303 **8.** In a few words, describe the effect associated with the use of a thrombolytic agent. _____

p. 302 **9.** The chapter mentions two antiplatelet medications. These are

(1) _____ and

(2) _____ .

p. 307 **10.** In as few words as possible, distinguish between the following antihyperlipidemic agents:

- Statins _____

- Fibrates _____

● WEB ACTIVITY

Visit the following Web sites for additional information on medications used for circulatory system disorders:

http://pharmacology.medscape.com

http://www.discoveryhealth.com

http://www.pslgroup.com

http://www.rxlist.com

http://pharmacotherapy.medscape.com

http://www.docguide.com

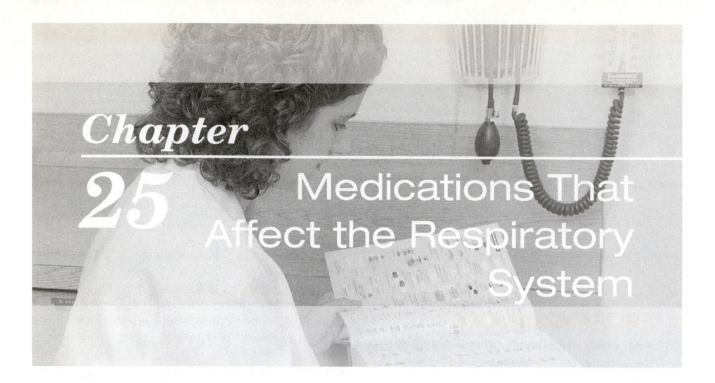

Chapter

25 Medications That Affect the Respiratory System

Chapter Outline

Objectives
Key Terms
Introduction
Antihistamines
Decongestants
Antitussives
Expectorants and Mucolytics
Bronchodilators
Leukotriene Receptor Antagonists (Blockers)
Anticholinergic Agents
Glucocorticoids
Cromolyn Sodium
Tuberculosis
Self-Assessment
Web Activity

- Describe the various drug classifications used for respiratory system disorders
- Identify selected drugs according to each described classification
- Understand the actions, uses, contraindications, safety precautions, adverse reactions, dosage and route, nursing considerations, clients' instruction, and special considerations for selected drugs
- Describe tuberculosis, listing the symptoms, diagnosis, and treatment regimen
- Complete the Spot Check on recommended children's dosages for selected antituberculosis drugs
- Complete the Self-Assessment
- Visit indicated Web sites for additional information on medications used for respiratory system disorders

Objectives

Upon completion of this chapter, you should be able to

- Define the key terms
- Describe the causes of respiratory conditions and/or diseases

Key Terms

allergic rhinitis	mucolytic
allergy	rhinovirus
asthma	SRS-A (slow-reacting
coryza	substance of anaphylaxis,
cough	i.e., leukotrienes)
expectorant	tuberculosis

INTRODUCTION

Respiratory conditions/diseases may be caused by allergies, pathogenic microorganisms such as bacteria and viruses, fungi, environmental and/or hereditary factors. The common cold (**coryza**) is the most frequent infection in all age groups in the United States. It is caused by the **rhinovirus**, one of a species of *picornaviruses*. There are more than 200 rhinoviruses that can infect your nose and throat and cause the common cold. Rhinoviruses affect the average adult two to three times a year and children an average of twelve times a year. There is no cure for the common cold and it generally runs its course with or without treatment. It is estimated that there are 71 million colds a year in the United States.

Some researchers feel that the cold virus is spread by direct contact with an infected person or the things he/she has contaminated. Other researchers say the viruses float through the air, taking root in nasal mucosa of unsuspecting passers-by. Regardless of the method by which the virus is spread, the common symptoms—sniffling, sneezing, hacking cough, and malaise—are experienced by many during a year. Antihistamines, decongestants, antitussives, and analgesics/antipyretics are some of the medications that may be used to treat the symptoms of the common cold. In children, aspirin should not be used as an antipyretic because of the risk of Reye's syndrome.

An over-the-counter (OTC) nasal gel called Zicam may reduce the typical length of the common cold. The gel allows Zicam (zinc ions) to stay within the nasal cavity long enough for it to interact with the virus. The common cold generally lasts an average of 10 to 14 days. In a study of clients who received a high dose of Zicam, cold symptoms resolved in an average of 1.5 days, and in clients receiving a low dose, symptoms resolved in an average of 3.3 days. In the clients who received a placebo, cold symptoms resolved in an average of 9.8 days. Zicam's ability to reduce the duration of the common cold depends on many factors, including how far the infection has progressed and the strength of the individuals' immune system. Zicam comes with an easy-to-use nasal pump and directions for use. It is best if the client consults his/her physician before using this product.

Allergy is an individual hypersensitivity to a substance, usually an antibody-antigen reaction. The most common allergens are pollens, animal dander, house dust, house dust mites, molds, certain drugs, insect stings, and many foods. There are many other substances that act as allergens such as dyes, perfumes, tobacco, feathers, chemicals, metals, and gases. Allergies affect over 25 million Americans.

An allergic condition may manifest itself as **allergic rhinitis** (hay fever), asthma, eczema, conjunctivitis, dermatitis, urticaria/hives, and anaphylaxis. **Asthma** is a chronic disorder of the bronchial airways. It is characterized by narrowed, inflamed, and sensitive bronchial tubes. It is becoming more and more prevalent in children and is the most common chronic medical problem affecting young adults. According to the American Lung Association, the number of deaths attributed to asthma has increased 117 percent since 1979. An estimated 17 million Americans suffer from asthma, including more than 5 million children under the age of 18. Since 1980, asthma in children under the age of 5 has increased by 160 percent. It is the sixth-ranking chronic condition in America and accounts for an estimated 3 million lost workdays for people over 18 years of age. Asthma is the leading cause of school absence due to chronic illness; children with asthma miss 10 million school days each year.

Pathogenic organisms are the cause of many respiratory diseases, such as sinusitis, laryngitis, pharyngitis, pleuritis, bronchitis, pneumonia, tuberculosis, pneumocystis pneumonia, and bronchomycosis. Antimicrobials/antibiotics and antifungals are the drugs of choice for the treatment of respiratory diseases caused by pathogenic microorganisms.

Environmental factors such as smoke, chemicals, metals, and gases may cause certain respiratory diseases such as pneumoconiosis and emphysema (chronic obstructive pulmonary disease). Bronchodilators and mucolytics are the drugs of choice for the treatment of respiratory diseases that may be caused by environmental factors.

Antihistamines, decongestants, antitussives, expectorants, mucolytics, bronchodilators, glucocorticoids, leukotriene receptor antagonists (blockers), cromolyn sodium, and drugs used to treat tuberculosis are described in this chapter.

Safety Precaution: Many of the medications described in this chapter may be given in combination with each other. This is especially true of antihistamines, decongestants, and antitussive agents. When this occurs, one should be aware of the combined effects of the drugs, the possible adverse reactions, contraindications, warnings, and special considerations for each.

ANTIHISTAMINES

Antihistamines are chemical agents that are structurally related to histamine and act to counter its effects by blocking histamine 1 (H_1) receptors. They do not interfere with the production and release of histamine.

Actions

Antihistamines appear to compete with histamine for cell receptor sites on effector cells. Histamine-related allergic reactions and tissue injury are blocked or diminished in intensity.

Uses

The primary use for antihistamine agents is the treatment of allergy symptoms that have resulted from the release of histamine. They are effective in the treatment of perennial and seasonal allergic rhinitis, contact dermatitis, urticaria, pruritus, for amelioration of allergic reactions to substances such as blood, plasma, insect stings, plant poisons, and as an adjunctive therapy during anaphylactic shock. Some antihistamines are used for the prevention and control of motion sickness and others are used in combination with cold remedies to decrease mucus secretion and at bedtime for sedation.

Contraindications

Antihistamines are contraindicated in clients who are known to be hypersensitive to any of its ingredients. They should not be used in newborn or premature infants and during lactation.

> **Safety Precaution:** Antihistamines should be used with considerable caution in clients with narrow-angle glaucoma, stenosing peptic ulcer, liver function problems, pyloroduodenal obstruction, symptomatic prostatic hyperplasia, or bladder-neck obstruction.

Adverse Reactions

The most frequent adverse reactions to antihistamines are sedation, sleepiness, dizziness, disturbed coordination, epigastric distress, and thickening of bronchial secretions. Other adverse reactions are dryness of mouth, nose, and throat, hypotension, headache, palpitations, nervousness, tremor, irritability, vertigo, tinnitus, anorexia, nausea, vomiting, diarrhea, constipation, wheezing, and nasal stuffiness.

Dosage and Route

The dosage and route of administration is determined by the manufacturer, but a physician should be consulted when needed. See Table 25-1 for selected antihistamines.

Nursing Considerations

The nurse should know that many antihistamines have an atropine-like action and therefore should be used with caution in clients with a history of bronchial asthma, increased intraocular pressure, hyperthyroidism, cardiovascular disease, or hypertension.

Clients' Instruction

Educate the client that antihistamines

- May impair mental alertness; therefore, he/she should not operate machinery or drive a motor vehicle, until his/her response to the medication has been determined

- Taken with alcohol or other sedative drugs may enhance drowsiness

- Should not be taken if monoamine oxidase inhibitor(s) or anticoagulants are part of the client's drug regimen

Special Considerations

- The action of oral anticoagulants may be diminished by antihistamines.

- Antihistamines have additive effects with alcohol and other CNS depressants (tranquilizers, sedatives, hypnotics).

- Antihistamines are most likely to cause dizziness, sedation, and hypotension in patients over 60 years of age.

- Antihistamines should only be taken when needed. One may develop tolerance to a certain antihistamine.

- Antihistamines may cause the respiratory tract to dry and mucus to thicken; therefore, one should drink plenty of fluids while taking to thin secretions and keep tissue moist.

DECONGESTANTS

Congestion of the nasal mucosa may occur as a result of infection, allergy, inflammation, or emotional

TABLE 25-1　ANTIHISTAMINES

Medication	Usual Dosage	Adverse Reactions
azatadine maleate (Optimine)	Oral (Adult): 1–2 mg twice daily	Drowsiness, dizziness, epigastric distress, thickening of bronchial secretions
brompheniramine maleate (Dimetane)	Oral (Adult): 16–24 mg/daily or 16–36 mg/daily (time-release form) Oral (Child 6–12): 10–24 mg/day (Child 2–6): 6 mg/day	Drowsiness, dryness of mouth, nose, and throat, thickening of bronchial secretions
cetirizine (Zyrtec)	Oral (Adult): 5–10 mg once daily (Child 6–11): 5 mg once daily	Dizziness, fatigue, pharyngitis, dry mouth
chlorpheniramine maleate (Chlor-Trimeton)	Oral (Adult): 6–16 mg/daily or 8–36 mg/daily (time-release form) IM, IV, SC (Adult): 5–20 mg Oral (Child 6–11): 3–8 mg/day	Drowsiness, excitability in children
clemastine fumarate (Tavist, Tavist-1)	Dosage should be individualized according to the needs and response of the client. Refer to a *Physicians' Desk Reference*.	Drowsiness, urticaria, drug rash, anaphylactic shock, photosensitivity, chills, dryness of the mouth, nose, and throat
diphenhydramine HCl (Benadryl)	Oral (Adult): 25–50 mg 3–4 times daily IV, deep IM (Adult): 10–100 mg 3–4 times daily Oral (Child over 20 lb): 12.5–25 mg 3–4 times daily	Drowsiness, dizziness, epigastric distress, thickening of bronchial secretions
	IV, deep IM (Child): 5 mg/kg/day in 4 divided doses	
fexofenadine (Allegra)	Oral (Adult): 60 mg twice daily Oral (Child 12 and older): 60 mg twice daily	Drowsiness, fatigue, dyspepsia, dysmenorrhea
ketotifen fumarate (Zaditor)	Ophthalmic (Adults and children over 3 years old): 1 drop in the affected eye(s) twice a day, every 8–12 hours	Headache, conjunctival infection, rhinitis, burning or stinging, eye pain, photophobia, rash
loratadine (Claritin)	Oral (Adult): 10 mg once daily Oral (Child 12 and older): 10 mg once daily (Child 2–11): 5 mg once daily	Confusion, drowsiness (rare), paradoxical excitation, blurred vision, dry mouth, GI upset, photosensitivity, rash, weight gain

upset. Decongestants are commonly used for symptomatic relief of nasal congestion.

Actions

Decongestants act by stimulating alpha-adrenergic receptors of vascular smooth muscle. As a result, dilated arterioles in the nasal mucosa are constricted. This reduces blood flow to the affected area, slows the formation of mucus, improves drainage, and opens obstructed nasal passages.

Uses

For the temporary relief of nasal congestion associated with the common cold, hay fever and/or other upper respiratory allergies, and sinusitis.

Contraindications

Decongestants are contraindicated in clients who are allergic to adrenergic agents, narrow-angle glaucoma, and clients who are taking MAOIs or tricyclic antidepressants.

Safety Precaution:

1. If recommended dosage is exceeded, nervousness, dizziness, sleeplessness, rapid pulse, or hypertension may occur.

2. Medication should not be taken more than 7 days. If symptoms do not improve or fever occurs, client should see a physician.

3. Clients with heart disease, hypertension, thyroid disease, glaucoma, diabetes, or prostatic hyperplasia should not take decongestants without the permission of their physician.

4. Clients who are pregnant or breastfeeding should not take decongestants without the permission of their physician.

Adverse Reactions

Rebound nasal congestion, dryness and stinging of the mucosa, sneezing, lightheadedness, headache, anxiety, palpitations, drowsiness, nausea, vomiting, and anorexia.

Dosage and Route

The dosage and route of administration is determined by the manufacturer, but a physician should be consulted when needed. See Table 25-2 for selected decongestants.

Nursing Considerations

Since most decongestants are taken as over-the-counter medications, the implications for client care mainly involve teaching the client about the medication.

Clients' Instruction

Educate the client that

- Long-term use of nasal sprays or solutions increases the risk of sensitization, which often causes a rebound effect or an increase in symptoms
- Decongestants should not be taken if antihypertensive agents, MAOIs, or tricyclic antidepressants are part of the medication regimen

Special Considerations

- Topical decongestants must be administered correctly to avoid systemic absorption.
- Physician should be notified if irregular heartbeat, insomnia, dizziness, or tremors occur.
- Environmental humidification may decrease drying of the mucosa.

TABLE 25-2 DECONGESTANTS

Medication	Usual Dosage	Adverse Reactions
oxymetazoline HCl (Afrin)	Topical (Adults, children over 6 years): 2–3 drops or sprays of 0.5% solution in each nostril twice daily Topical (Children 2–5 years): 2–3 drops of 0.025% solution in each nostril twice daily	Mild adverse effects include dryness and stinging of the mucosa, sneezing, lightheadedness, and headache
phenylephrine HCl (Neo-Synephrine HCl)	Topical (Adults and older children): several drops of a 0.25–1.0% solution in each nostril as needed Topical (Infants): 0.125% solution used as above	Drowsiness, excitability in children, rebound nasal congestion, anxiety
phenylpropanolamine HCl (Propagest)	Oral (Adult): 1 tablet every 4 hours not to exceed 6 tablets in 24 hours Oral (Children, 6–12 years): One-half tablet every 4 hours not to exceed 3 tablets in 24 hours	Nervousness, dizziness, sleeplessness, rapid pulse or high blood pressure can occur at higher doses
pseudoephedrine HCl (Sudafed)	Oral (Adult): 60 mg 3–4 times daily Oral (Child): 4 mg/kg daily in 4 divided doses	Drowsiness, rebound nasal congestion, anxiety, headache, palpitations

ANTITUSSIVES

Cough is a physiologic reflex. It is a protective action that clears the respiratory tract of secretions and foreign substances. Coughing helps to maintain an open airway in individuals with asthma, chronic obstructive pulmonary disease, and cystic fibrosis. In other individuals, coughing may be associated with smoking, viral upper respiratory infections, allergy, and numerous other causes. Often, cough can be alleviated by treating the underlying cause. Although antitussives have no effect on the underlying condition, they ease respiratory discomfort, facilitate sleep, and reduce irritation.

Actions

Nonnarcotic antitussive agents anesthetize the stretch receptors located in the respiratory passages, lungs, and pleura by dampening their activity and thereby reducing the cough reflex at its source. Narcotic antitussive agents depress the cough center that is located in the medulla, thereby raising its threshold for incoming cough impulse.

Uses

For symptomatic relief of cough.

Contraindications

Antitussive agents are contraindicated in individuals who are hypersensitive to any of its ingredients. They should not be used by newborn or premature infants, pregnant women, and during lactation.

Adverse Reactions

Nonnarcotic antitussive agents may produce sedation, headache, mild dizziness, pruritus, nasal congestion, constipation, nausea, and GI upset. Narcotic antitussive agents may produce nausea, vomiting, constipation, lightheadedness, and drowsiness.

Dosage and Route

The dosage and route of administration is determined by the manufacturer, but a physician should be consulted when needed. See Table 25-3 for selected antitussives.

Nursing Considerations

Since most nonnarcotic antitussives are taken as over-the-counter medications, the implications for client care mainly involve teaching the client about the medication. For narcotic antitussives the nurse should monitor the client for signs of improvement, adverse reactions, dependency and/or tolerance.

TABLE 25-3   ANTITUSSIVES

Medication	Usual Dosage	Adverse Reactions
benzonatate (Tessalon)	Oral (Adults, children over 10): 100 mg 3–6 times daily Oral (Children under 10 years): 8 mg/kg/day in 3–6 divided doses	Mild adverse effects include constipation, rash, drowsiness, nasal congestion, headache, and hypersensitivity reactions.
codeine codeine phosphate codeine sulfate	Oral (Adult): 10–20 mg every 4–6 hours (maximum 120 mg/24 hr) Oral (Children 6–12): 5–10 mg every 4–6 hours (maximum 60 mg/day) Oral (Children 2–6): 2.5–5 mg every 4–6 hours (maximum 30 mg/day)	Respiratory and circulatory depression with overdose (particularly with children), nausea, vomiting, constipation, lightheadedness, drowsiness
dextromethorphan hydrobromide	Oral (Adults): 10–20 mg every 4 hours (maximum 120 mg/day) Oral (Children 6–12): 5–10 mg every 4 hours Oral (Children 2–6): 2.5–5 mg every 4 hours	Mild adverse effects include drowsiness, nausea, and dizziness.
diphenhydramine HCl (Benylin)	Oral (Adult): 25 mg every 4 hours (maximum 100 mg/day) Oral (Children 6–12): one-half the adult dose above Oral (Children 2–5): 6.25 mg every 4 hours (maximum 25 mg/day)	Drowsiness, dry mouth, constipation, may interfere with expectoration by making secretions thicker

Clients' Instruction

Educate the client that

- Narcotic antitussive agents may be habit forming and may cause drowsiness
- The medication may impair mental alertness; therefore, he/she should not operate machinery or drive a motor vehicle, until his/her response to the medication has been determined

Special Considerations

- Medication should not be chewed or allowed to dissolve in the mouth as it could anesthetize the throat and lead to choking.
- Liquid medication should not be taken with or followed by water as this could diminish its effect.

EXPECTORANTS AND MUCOLYTICS

Among the drugs used to treat a cough are expectorants and mucolytics. An **expectorant** is an agent that stimulates and decreases the thickness of respiratory tract secretions. **Mucolytics** are drugs that reduce the viscosity of respiratory tract fluids. The actions of these medications are theoretically useful in treating coughs, because such actions should facilitate removal of irritants and phlegm. Despite studies that show some agents to be effective, conclusive evidence of the effectiveness of these medications is yet to be reported.

Expectorants

Actions

Expectorants enhance the output of lower respiratory tract fluids and help make them less viscous. This promotes and facilitates the removal of mucus.

Uses

To help loosen phlegm (mucus) and to thin bronchial secretions to make cough more productive.

Contraindications

Expectorants are contraindicated in clients who are hypersensitive to any of its ingredients and in those with persistent cough.

Adverse Reactions

Drowsiness, nausea, vomiting, and anorexia.

Dosage and Route

The dosage and route of administration is determined by the physician. See Table 25-4 for selected expectorants.

Nursing Considerations

The nurse should monitor the client for signs of improvement and adverse reactions.

TABLE 25-4 EXPECTORANTS AND MUCOLYTICS

Medication	Usual Dosage	Adverse Reactions
Expectorants		
guaifenesin (Robitussin)	Oral (Adult): 100–400 mg every 4 hours (maximum 2400 mg/day) Oral (Children 6–12): 100–200 mg as above (maximum 1200 mg/day) Oral (Children 2–6): 50–100 mg as above (maximum 600 mg/day)	Drowsiness, nausea, vomiting, anorexia
saturated solution of potassium iodide (SSKI)	Oral (Adults): 0.3–0.6 ml diluted in 1 glassful of water, fruit juice, or milk 3–4 times daily	Skin rash, swelling or tenderness of salivary glands
Mucolytics		
acetylcysteine (Mucomyst)	Nebulization face mask, mouth piece, tracheostomy: 3–5 ml of 20% solution, or 6–10 ml of 10% solution 3–4 times/day	Stomatitis, nausea, vomiting, fever, rhinorrhea, drowsiness, clamminess, chest tightness, bronchoconstriction

Clients' Instruction

Educate the client

- On how to cough to facilitate the removal of phlegm and the proper disposal of the coughed-up secretions. (The client should be in the upright position, take several slow, deep breaths, place a tissue over his/her mouth, and then cough. The color, amount, and character of the sputum should be noted. The tissue should be placed in a proper container.)
- To drink plenty of fluids to help keep mucous membranes moist and loosen secretions

Special Considerations

- The client should notify the physician if cough does not improve or if he/she develops a fever, rash, or persistent headache.
- Environmental humidification may decrease drying of the mucosa and help loosen secretions.
- Saturated Solution of Potassium Iodide (SSKI) should be diluted in water or fruit juice before administering.

Mucolytics

Actions

Mucolytics break chemical bonds (disulfide linkage) in mucus, thereby lowering the viscosity.

Uses

As adjuvant therapy for clients who have abnormal viscid or thickened mucus secretions in such conditions as chronic obstructive pulmonary disease(s), cystic fibrosis, and pneumonia.

Contraindications

Contraindicated in clients who are hypersensitive to any of its ingredients.

Safety Precaution:

1. Asthmatics using Mucomyst should be watched carefully. If bronchospasm progresses, immediately discontinue the medication.
2. After proper use, an increased amount of liquefied bronchial secretions may occur. When coughing is inadequate, an open airway must be maintained by mechanical suction.

Adverse Reactions

Most clients tolerate Mucomyst very well. Adverse reactions that may occur are stomatitis, nausea, vomiting, fever, rhinorrhea, drowsiness, clamminess, chest tightness, and bronchospasm.

Dosage and Route

The dosage and route of administration is determined by the physician. See Table 25-4 for Mucomyst.

Nursing Considerations

The nurse should know that this medication should not be mixed with antibiotics, iron, copper, or rubber products.

Clients' Instruction

Educate the client

- About good oral hygienic practices
- That the unpleasant odor experienced with use of Mucomyst will decrease after repeated use, and that discoloration of solution after the bottle is opened does not impair the effectiveness of the medication

Special Considerations

- Medication should be stored in a refrigerator and used within 96 hours of opening.
- Medication should be given $\frac{1}{2}$ to 1 hour before meals for better absorption and to decrease nausea.
- May be used as an antidote for acetaminophen overdose.

BRONCHODILATORS

Bronchodilators are used to improve pulmonary airflow in patients with chronic obstructive pulmonary disease (COPD) and asthma. They may be classified as sympathomimetics (beta-adrenergic agents; Table 25-5), xanthines (phosphodiesterase inhibitors; Table 25-6), leukotriene receptor antagonists (blockers), and anticholinergic agents.

Actions

Sympathomimetics act on beta-2 adrenoreceptors to relax smooth muscle cells of the bronchi. They also produce a vasoconstriction response throughout the body by stimulating alpha receptors. This response reduces edema in the bronchial mucosa. Some sympathomimetics also stimulate beta-1 receptors, and this results in an increased heart rate

TABLE 25-5 SYMPATHOMIMETIC (BETA-ADRENERGIC AGONISTS) BRONCHODILATORS

Medication	Usual Dosage	Adverse Reactions
albuterol (Proventil, Ventolin)	Inhalation (Adult, children 12 and older): 2 inhalations every 4–6 hours Oral: 2 mg or 4 mg 3 or 4 times a day	Palpitations, tachycardia, hypertension, nausea, nervousness
bitolterol mesylate (Tornalate)	Inhalation (Adults, children 12 and older): 2 inhalations every 8 hours to prevent bronchospasm, or 2 inhalations 1–3 minutes apart to treat bronchospasm	Tremors, nervousness, headache, throat irritation, coughing
ephedrine sulfate	Oral, SC, IV (Adults): 25–50 mg every 3–4 hours as needed (Children): 2–6 years: 0.3–0.5 mg/kg every 4–6 hours (Children): 6–12 years: 6.25–12.5 mg every 3–4 hours as needed	tremors, anxiety, insomnia, headache, confusion, anorexia, nausea, dyspnea
epinephrine epinephrine HCl (Adrenalin)	IM, SC (Adult): 0.2–0.5 mg (0.2–0.5 ml of 1:1,000 solution) every 2 hours as necessary IM, SC (Child): 0.01 mg/kg every 4 hours as needed (maximum 0.5 mg/day)	Anxiety, headache, palpitations, tremors, tachycardia
isoproterenol HCl (Isuprel)	Inhalation: 1–2 deep inhalations from nebulizing unit; dose may be repeated up to 5 times daily	Tachycardia, palpitations, headache, nervousness
levalbuterol HCl (Xopenex)	Inhalation (Adults, children 12 and older): Initial: 0.63 mg tid (every 6–8 hours) by nebulization. Those with severe asthma or who do not respond to the 0.63 mg dose may benefit from a dose of 1.25 mg tid.	Dizziness, nervousness, tremor, dyspepsia
metaproterenol sulfate (Alupent)	Inhalation (Adults, children 12 and older): Usual single dose is 2–3 inhalations every 3–4 hours. Total dosage should not exceed 12 inhalations. Oral (Adults): 20 mg 3 or 4 times a day Oral (Children 6–9 years or weight under 60 lb): 10 mg 3–4 times a day	Tachycardia, hypertension, palpitations, nervousness, tremors, nausea and vomiting
salmeterol (Serevent)	Inhalation (Adults, children 12 and older): 50 mcg (2 inhalations) twice daily (12 hours apart). Exercise-induced bronchospasm: 50 mcg (2 inhalations) 30–60 min prior to exercise	Palpitations, tachycardia, elevated blood pressure, tremors, nervousness, headache, throat irritation
terbutaline sulfate (Brethine, Bricanyl)	Oral (Adult): 2.5–5 mg 3 times daily (maximum 15 mg/day) Oral (Adolescent): 2.5 mg 3 times/day (maximum 7.5 mg/day) SC (Adult): 0.25 mg IV infusion: Premature labor: 10 mcg/min initially, then increase rate by 0.005 mg/min every 10 min until contractions cease or a maximum dose of 80 mcg/min is reached. Continue the minimum effective dose for 4–8 hours after contractions cease.	Tremors, nervousness, headache

TABLE 25-6   XANTHINE (PHOSPHODIESTERASE INHIBITOR) BRONCHODILATORS

Medication	Usual Dosage	Adverse Reactions
aminophylline	Oral (Adults): 500 mg, then 250–500 mg every 6–8 hours (Children): 7.5 mg/kg, then 3–6 mg/kg every 6–8 hours Rectal (Adults): 250–500 mg every 6–8 hours IM (Adults): 500 mg as necessary	Anxiety, restlessness, insomnia, headache, palpitations, nausea, vomiting, anorexia, increase in blood pressure
dyphylline (Lufyllin)	Oral (Adults): Up to 15 mg/kg every 6 hours IM (Adult): 250–500 mg (1–2 ml) every 2–6 hours (maximum of 15 mg/kg every 6 hours)	Headache, nausea, palpitations
oxtriphylline (Choledyl)	Oral (Adults): 200 mg 4 times daily (Children): 2–12 years: 3.7 mg/kg 4 times daily	Cardiac arrhythmia, nausea, headache, tachypnea, irritability, diuresis, rash
theophylline (Theo-24)	Oral (Adults): initially 400 mg as single daily dose. Maximum without serum monitoring: 13 mg/kg/day, up to 900 mg/day (Children): 30–35 kg: initially 300 mg once daily	Cardiac arrhythmias, nausea, headaches, diuresis, rash
(Elixophyllin)	Oral (Adults and children): 6 mg/kg initially, followed by 3–4 mg/kg every 4–6 hours	Nausea, vomiting, headache, dizziness, nervousness, epigastric pain

and its force of contraction. Xanthine bronchodilators relax smooth muscle of the bronchial airways and pulmonary blood vessels by blocking phosphodiesterase, which increases cyclic adenosine monophosphate (cAMP). By preventing the breakdown of cAMP, smooth muscles relax and bronchodilation occurs, thus relieving dyspnea. They may also produce cardiac stimulation, coronary vasodilation, stimulation of skeletal muscles, cerebral stimulation, and diuresis.

Uses

Bronchodilators are used in the prevention and relief of bronchospasm in clients with asthma, bronchitis, and emphysema. Investigational: inhibit premature labor.

Contraindications

Bronchodilators are contraindicated in clients who are hypersensitive to any of its ingredients.

Safety Precaution:

1. The potential for paradoxical bronchospasm should be kept in mind, and if it occurs, discontinue the medication immediately.
2. Metered-dose aerosol units are under pressure. Do not puncture and do not use or store near heat or flame.

Adverse Reactions

Palpitations, increase in blood pressure, tremors, nausea, vomiting, dizziness, heartburn, nervousness, urticaria, and headache.

Dosage and Route

The dosage and route of administration is determined by the physician. See Table 25-6 for selected xanthine bronchodilators.

Nursing Considerations

The nurse should be aware that many sympathomimetic bronchodilators may also stimulate beta-1 receptors located in the heart. They may be dangerous to use in clients who have heart disease. Monitor all clients for changes in cardiac function and blood pressure. With xanthine bronchodilators, monitor the client for disruption of cardiac function, insomnia, and hyperexcitability. Be aware of increased potential for convulsive activity. The serum levels of the medication should be checked on a regular basis. Therapeutic range should be 10–20 mcg/ml.

Clients' Instructions

Concerning sympathomimetic bronchodilators, educate the client

● To take the medication as prescribed and not to exceed the dosage

- To notify the physician immediately if symptoms do not improve, if he/she experiences bronchial irritation, dizziness, chest pain, and/or insomnia
- Not to take any other medication unless it is prescribed by the physician
- To drink plenty of fluids, especially water, to help moisten mucous membranes and reduce the thickness of mucus
- That the medication should be protected from light and should be discarded if the color of the solution changes

Regarding xanthine bronchodilators, educate the client that

- Oral xanthine bronchodilators may be taken with food to avoid GI upset, but the medicine should not be crushed or chewed
- Cola drinks, coffee, tea, and chocolate contain xanthine and they should not be consumed while on medication

Special Considerations

- Sympathomimetic bronchodilators should not be used with MAOIs as sympathomimetic activity could be increased and hypertensive crises may occur.
- Clients using antihistamines, tricyclic antidepressants, and thyroid hormone may experience greater sympathomimetic activity with the use of a sympathomimetic bronchodilator.
- Xanthine bronchodilators may enhance CNS stimulation of ephedrine, sympathomimetics, and amphetamines.
- Certain antibiotics (erythromycin, lincomycin, and clindamycin) may increase blood levels of xanthines.
- Xanthines may interact with beta-blocking agents, digitalis, anticoagulants, lithium, and furosemide.

LEUKOTRIENE RECEPTOR ANTAGONISTS (BLOCKERS)

Leukotriene receptor antagonists (blockers) are used for the treatment and management of asthma. These agents block cysteinyl leukotrienes and leukotriene receptor occupation, which have been correlated with the pathophysiology of asthma, including airway edema, smooth muscle contraction, and altered cellular activity associated with the in-

flammatory process contributing to the signs and symptoms of asthma.

Three medications included in this classification are Accolate (zafirlukast), Zyflo (zileuton), and Singulair (montelukast sodium). Accolate and Zyflo are used as long-term control agents in the management of asthma. The dosage of Accolate for adults and children 12 years and older is one 20 mg tablet twice daily. Accolate is also available in a 10 mg nonflavored minitablet specifically designed for children as young as 7 years old. The recommended dosing is one 10 mg minitablet twice daily, even during symptom-free periods. The dosage of Zyflo for adults and children 12 years and older is one 600 mg tablet 4 times daily. Singulair is the first of the leukotriene blockers intended for both adults and children as young as 6 years old, and the first developed for once-daily use. See Figure 25-1.

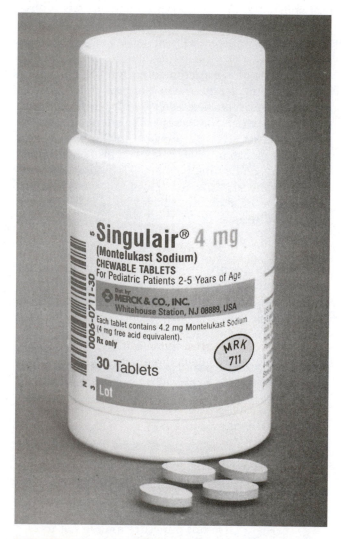

FIGURE 25-1 SINGULAIR® (MONTELUKAST SODIUM) 4 MG TABLETS (*Courtesy of Merck & Co., Inc.*)

Montelukast Sodium (Singulair)

Actions

Singulair is a selective and orally active leukotriene receptor antagonist that inhibits the cysteinyl leukotriene $CysLT_1$ receptor. It is able to block leukotriene action in the lung, resulting in less constriction of the bronchial tissue and less inflammation.

Uses

Indicated for the prophylaxis and chronic treatment of asthma in adults and pediatric clients 6 years of age and older.

Contraindications

Hypersensitivity to any component of this product.

Precautions

Singulair is not indicated for use in the reversal of bronchospasm in acute asthma attacks, including status asthmaticus. Clients should be advised to have appropriate rescue medication available. Singular should not be used as monotherapy for the treatment and management of exercise-induced bronchospasm. Clients who have exacerbations of asthma after exercise should continue to use their usual regimen of inhaled medication.

> **Safety Precaution:** Rare cases in which an inflammatory condition associated with a type of cell called eosinophils has been detected among users of Singulair. Most of the affected clients were taking several asthma medications and Singulair has not been shown to be directly involved with the development of the inflammatory condition.

Adverse Reactions

Asthenia, fatigue, fever, abdominal pain, dyspepsia, gastoenteritis, dizziness, headache, nasal congestion, influenza, rash.

Dosage and Route

The dosage for adults and adolescents 15 years of age and older is one 10 mg tablet daily to be taken in the evening. The dosage for pediatric clients 6 to 14 years of age is one 5 mg chewable tablet daily to be taken in the evening.

Nursing Considerations

The nurse should monitor the client for improvement and adverse reactions. Assist the client and his/her family to identify and eliminate/minimize factors that trigger symptoms.

Clients' Instruction

Educate the client

- To take the medications as prescribed and not to exceed the dosage
- That the drug should be continued during acute attacks as well as during symptom-free periods
- To report if increased use and frequency of inhalers is needed for symptom control
- To continue other prescribed antiasthma medications during this therapy
- To report any unusual side effects, changes in disease, or significant drop in peak flow readings
- To notify physician if pregnancy is suspected or planned
- How to reduce environmental triggers and appropriate steps to minimize or avoid exposure

ANTICHOLINERGIC AGENTS

Inhalational anticholinergic agents inhibit cholinergic receptors in bronchial smooth muscle, resulting in decreased concentrations of cyclic guanosine monophosphate (cGMP). This action produces local bronchodilation. Intranasal local application inhibits secretions from glands lining the nasal mucosa. Atrovent (ipratropium bromide) is an anticholinergic agent prescribed for long-term treatment of bronchial spasms (wheezing) associated with chronic obstructive pulmonary disease (COPD), including chronic bronchitis and emphysema.

The usual starting dose for adults and children 12 years of age and older is 2 inhalations, 4 times a day. Additional inhalations may be taken, but the total should not exceed 12 in 24 hours. For intranasal application (nasal spray 0.03%), the dosage is 2 sprays (42 mcg) per nostril bid–tid for a total daily dose of 168–252 mcg/day. For intranasal application (nasal spray 0.06%), the dosage is 2 sprays (84 mcg) per nostril tid–qid for a total daily dose of 504–672 mcg/day.

Adverse reactions may include blurred vision, cough, dizziness, dry mouth, headache, nausea, nervousness, rash, stomach and intestinal upset, worsening of symptoms.

GLUCOCORTICOIDS

Glucocorticoids are anti-inflammatory agents that are chemically related to the naturally occurring hormone cortisone. There are many uses for glucocorticoids, but inhalational forms are used in the treatment of bronchial asthma, and in seasonal or perennial allergic conditions when other forms of treatment are not effective. Examples of inhalation via metered-dose inhaler steroids are dexamethasone phosphate (Decadron Phosphate Turbinaire), beclomethasone dipropionate (Beclovent, and Vancenase Nasal Inhaler), flunisolide (Aerobid and Nasalide), and triamcinolone acetonide (Azmacort). See Table 25-7 for selected glucocorticoids.

Flonase (fluticasone propionate) and Rhinocort (budesonide) are two examples of anti-inflammatory glucocorticoid nasal medications that are used for the treatment of allergic rhinitis (hay fever). Flonase is a nasal spray, indicated for clients 4 years of age and older, and provides 24-hour relief of nasal allergy symptoms. The usual recommended starting dose is one 50 mcg spray in each nostril once a day, for a total dose of 100 mcg/day. Maximum dose is two sprays (200 mcg) in each nostril once a day. The most common adverse reactions are headache, pharyngitis, and epistaxis. Instructions for use are included with the medication and the client is ad-

vised to follow the directions carefully and use only as directed.

Rhinocort is prescribed as a nasal inhaler. The usual recommended starting dose for adults and children 6 years of age and older is 256 micrograms a day, either as two sprays in each nostril twice a day, morning and evening, or as four sprays in each nostril once a day in the morning. Rhinocort is not recommended for use in children with nasal irritation not due to allergies. The most common adverse reactions are increased coughing, irritation of nasal passages, epistaxis, and sore throat. Because steroids can suppress the immune system, people taking Rhinocort may become more susceptible to infections, and their infections could be more severe. Anyone taking Rhinocort or other corticosteroids who have not had infections such as chickenpox and measles should avoid exposure to them. If the client is taking Rhinocort and is exposed to these illnesses, he/she should notify the physician immediately. Instructions for use are included with the medication and the client is advised to follow the directions carefully and use only as directed.

TABLE 25-7 INHALATIONAL GLUCOCORTICOIDS

Medication	Usual Dosage	Adverse Reactions
beclomethasone (Beclovent)	Inhalation (Adults): 2 inhalations 3–4 times daily or 4 inhalations twice daily. Maximum 20 inhalations daily (Children 6–12): 1–2 inhalations 3–4 times daily or 4 inhalations twice daily. Maximum 10 inhalations daily	Hoarseness, dry mouth, bronchospasm, rash, oral fungal infections
budesonide (Pulmicort)	Inhalation (Adults): 1–2 sprays twice daily (Children 6–12): 1 spray twice daily	Headache, hoarseness, bronchospasm, cough, wheezing, dry mouth, flu-like syndrome
flunisolide (Aerobid)	Inhalation (Adults): 2 inhalations twice daily, morning and evening. Maximum 8 inhalations/day (Children 6–15): 2 inhalations twice daily	Diarrhea, nausea, sore throat, headache, upper respiratory infection, dizziness
fluticasone (Flovent)	Aerosol inhaler (Adults and adolescents): 88–440 mcg twice daily Dry powder inhaler (Adults): 50–250 mg twice daily (Children 4–12): 50–100 mg twice daily	Agitation, depression, fatigue, insomnia, restlessness, nasal stuffiness, sinusitis, nausea
triamcinolone acetonide (Azmacort)	Inhalation (Adults): 2 inhalations 3–4 times daily. Maximum 16 inhalations daily (Children 6–12): 12 inhalations 3–4 times daily. Maximum 12 inhalations daily	Hoarseness, dry mouth and throat, wheezing, cough, oral fungal infections

CROMOLYN SODIUM

Cromolyn sodium inhibits the degranulation of sensitized mast cells that occurs after exposure to specific antigens. It inhibits the release of histamine and **SRS-A** (the slow-reacting substance of anaphylaxis, i.e., leukotrienes). Cromolyn sodium is used for the prophylactic treatment of bronchial asthma and for the prevention and treatment of the symptoms of allergic rhinitis.

TUBERCULOSIS

Tuberculosis is a contagious disease caused by the bacillus *Mycobacterium tuberculosis*. It is spread from person to person by airborne transmission. An infected person releases large and small droplets through talking, coughing, sneezing, laughing, or singing. The large droplets settle, while the small droplets remain suspended in the air and are inhaled by the susceptible person.

Tuberculosis, once called consumption, is not a new disease. At one time it was the number one killer in the United States and it is still a major cause of death worldwide. One of public health's oldest enemies is back, and with a vengeance. An estimated 10 million Americans are infected with the TB bacterium. Compounding the problem are drug-resistant strains of TB that can shrug off as many as seven of the antibiotics traditionally used to treat this disease.

At the present time TB is occurring primarily among AIDS clients, the homeless, drug abusers, prison inmates, and immigrants. Health officials are concerned about the rapid spread of this disease and the risks for the general public. Virtually anyone who comes in contact with an infected person is at risk of contracting TB. Studies show that exposure to an infected person in confined quarters such as in homes and classrooms increases an individual's risk.

Symptoms

Symptoms include a chronic cough, fatigue, low-grade fever, night sweats, weakness, chills, anorexia, weight loss, hemoptysis, and, in the early stages, scanty, whitish, or grayish yellow, frothy sputum.

During the early stages of TB the sputum is expectorated in small quantities, but later when consolidation takes place it becomes more copious, tenacious, and yellowish gray. In the late stages of TB, the sputum becomes mucopurulent, musty, and fetid, containing fibers and tubercle bacilli, and blood-tinged or mixed with blood.

Diagnosis

To determine a diagnosis of tuberculosis, a careful history is taken and a complete physical examination is performed. After evaluation of the client, the physician may order a tuberculin test (if the client has not had a previous positive reaction), chest x-ray, bronchoscopy, or sputum culture for a positive diagnosis.

Treatment

Treatment of TB requires long-term drug therapy (6 to 12 months), often utilizing a regimen that includes a combination of antituberculosis agents. The use of multiple drugs is indicated in all but a few active cases, because any large population of *Mycobacterium tuberculosis* will have naturally occurring mutants that are resistant to each of the drugs administered. Diet and rest are also important aspects of treatment for this disease. See Tables 25-8 and 25-9 for selected antituberculosis agents.

Rifapentine (Priftin) is the first new medication for tuberculosis in 25 years. The drug is important because it makes clients more likely to complete their therapy. Treatment with rifapentine is broken down into two phases: an intensive phase and a continuation phase. In the intensive phase of treatment, rifapentine is administered at 72-hour intervals for 2 months. It must be administered along with at least one other antibiotic accepted for the treatment of tuberculosis. Streptomycin or ethambutol may also be required until the results of susceptibility testing for the specific *M. tuberculosis* isolate are known. Following the intensive phase of treatment, the dose of rifapentine is reduced to one dose per week and should continue to be administered along with an appropriate antibiotic. Susceptibility testing should be conducted at regular intervals during therapy. Clients should be educated as to the importance of compliance during the entire course of therapy, since lack of compliance has been associated with a high incidence of relapse and delayed sputum conversion. Rifapentine may cause serious hepatic damage. It should be administered to clients with liver test function abnormalities only in cases where the advantages of treatment outweigh the disadvantage of delay. Rifapentine may produce a red-orange discoloration of skin, teeth, tongue, urine, sweat, sputum, and tears. This may result in permanent staining of contact lenses. In addition, the effectiveness of oral contraceptives in women may be decreased while taking rifapentine. Women relying on oral contraceptives should consider switching to other forms of birth control. Clients who experience nausea or vomiting after administration of rifapentine should try taking the medication with food.

The effectiveness of treatment can be evaluated by monitoring clients' sputum smear results. It takes about 2 weeks for the drugs to kill enough bacteria so that they cannot infect other people. It takes 6 to 9 months of continuous drug therapy for a cure. Follow-up care is essential. A sputum culture is essential to confirming a diagnosis, determining an infection's susceptibility to drugs, and assessing response to treatment. If the TB bacteria become resistant to two of the drugs that are used to treat tuberculosis, then MDR TB (multidrug-resistant tuberculosis) is suspected and appropriate measures must be instituted promptly to treat and prevent the spread of MDR-TB.

TABLE 25-8 ANTITUBERCULOSIS AGENTS

Medication	Usual Dosage	Adverse Reactions
First-Line Drugs		
ethambutol HCl (Myambutol)	Oral: 15–25 mg/kg/day in a single dose Twice weekly: 50 mg/kg	Optic neuritis, decreased visual acuity and red-green color discrimination, skin rash
isoniazid (INH) (Laniazid) (Nydrazid)	Oral, IM: 300 mg daily in a single dose, or 4–5 mg/kg of body weight per day Twice weekly: 15 mg/kg	Hepatotoxicity, flu-like syndrome, neuropathy, hypersensitivity *Note:* The physician may prescribe pyridoxine to prevent or decrease neuropathy.
isoniazid, rifampin, and pyrazinamide (Rifater)	Oral: Each tablet contains a fixed-dose combination of 50 mg of isoniazid, 120 mg of rifampin, and 300 mg of pyrazinamide. Daily: 99 lb: 4 tabs; 99–120 lb: 5 tabs; above 120 lb: 6 tabs	Same as for isoniazid, rifampin, and pyrazinamide
pyrazinamide (PZA)	Oral: 15–30 mg/kg/day	Hepatotoxicity, hyperuricemia, arthralgia, skin rash, gastrointestinal irritation
rifabutin (Mycobutin)	Oral: 300 mg once daily	Fever, headache, flu-like syndrome, gastrointestinal symptoms, brown-orange discoloration of body fluids *Note:* Interacts with zidovudine and protease inhibitors except indinavir
rifampin (Rifadin, Rimactane)	Oral, IV (Adult): 600 mg/day or 10 mg/kg/day Oral, IV (Child): 10–20 mg/kg/day	Gastrointestinal disturbances, headache, flu-like symptoms, orange-tinged body fluids, fever
rifampin and isoniazid (Rifamate, Rimactane/INH Dual Pack)	Oral: 2 capsules once daily	Gastrointestinal disturbances, headache, flu-like symptoms, hepatotoxicity, neuropathy, hypersensitivity
rifapentine (Priftin)	Oral: Intensive phase: 300 mg at 72-hour intervals for 2 months Continuation phase: 600 mg once a week for 4 months	Hyperuricemia, headache, dizziness, elevation of liver enzymes, neutropenia, pyuria, hematuria, reddish discoloration of body fluids including saliva, rash
streptomycin sulfate	IM: 0.75–1 g daily, then reduced to 1 g 2–3 times weekly	Ototoxicity, nephrotoxicity, hypokalemia
Second-Line Drugs		
ciprofloxacin (Cipro)	Oral, IV: 750–1500 mg daily	Abdominal cramps, nausea, diarrhea, rash, headache, photosensitivity, insomnia

(continued)

TABLE 25-8   *(Continued)*

Medication	Usual Dosage	Adverse Reactions
cycloserine (Seromycin)	Oral: 15–20 mg/kg/day; 250–1000 mg daily in divided doses	Psychosis, personality changes, rash, impaired coordination, depression, increased phenytoin (Dilantin) levels
ethionamide (Trecator-SC)	Oral: 15–20 mg/kg/day; 500–1000 mg daily in divided doses	Gastrointestinal disturbance, arthralgia, hepatotoxicity, hyperthyroidism, metallic taste and distorted sense of smell, severe acne
kanamycin, amikacin, capreomycin	IM, IV: 15–30 mg/kg/day	Renal and auditory toxicity, vestibular toxicity, hypokalemia
levofloxacin (Levaquin)	Oral: 500 mg daily	Nausea, diarrhea, abdominal cramps
ofloxacin (Floxin)	Oral, IV (Adult): 400 mg every 12 hours	Abdominal cramps, nausea, diarrhea

TABLE 25-9   DOSAGE RECOMMENDATIONS FOR THE TREATMENT OF TB IN CHILDREN (12 YEARS OF AGE AND YOUNGER)

Drug	Daily Dose	Twice-Weekly Dose	Thrice-Weekly Dose
Isoniazid	10–20 mg/kg Max. 300 mg	20–40 mg/kg Max. 900 mg	20–40 mg/kg Max. 900 mg
Rifampin	10–20 mg/kg Max. 600 mg	10–20 mg/kg Max. 600 mg	10–20 mg/kg Max. 600 mg
Pyrazinamide	15–30 mg/kg Max. 2 g	50–70 mg/kg	50–70 mg/kg
Ethambutol*	15–25 mg/kg Max. 2.5 g	50 mg/kg	25–30 mg/kg
Streptomycin	20–40 mg/kg Max. 1 g	25–30 mg/kg	25–30 mg/kg

*Ethambutol is generally not recommended for children whose visual acuity cannot be monitored (children under 6 years of age). However, ethambutol should be considered for all children with organisms resistant to other drugs, if susceptibility to ethambutol has been demonstrated or susceptibility is likely.

Some persons are at high risk for drug-resistant TB: persons who have been recently exposed to drug-resistant TB, especially if they are immunocompromised; TB clients who failed to take medications as prescribed; TB clients who were prescribed an ineffective treatment regimen; and clients previously treated for TB.

CDC Guidelines

The Centers for Disease Control and Prevention has published a booklet called *Guidelines for Preventing the Transmission of Tuberculosis in Health-Care Settings.* The following specific actions are used to reduce the risk of tuberculosis transmission:

- Screening client for active TB and TB infection
- Providing rapid diagnostic services
- Prescribing appropriate curative and preventive therapy
- Maintaining physical measures to reduce microbial contamination of the air
- Providing isolation rooms for persons with, or suspected of having, infectious TB
- Screening health care facility personnel for TB infection
- Promptly investing and controlling outbreaks

Transmission-Based Precautions

The Centers for Disease Control and Prevention (CDC) released transmission-based precautions to reduce the risk of airborne, droplet, and contact transmission of pathogens. These precautions are to be used in addition to standard precautions and are intended for clients diagnosed with or suspected of specific highly transmissible diseases, such as tuberculosis. See Tables 25-10 and 25-11.

TABLE 25-10 AIRBORNE PRECAUTIONS, ONE CATEGORY OF TRANSMISSION-BASED PRECAUTIONS

AIRBORNE PRECAUTIONS
(in addition to Standard Precautions)

VISITORS: Report to nurse before entering.

Client Placement

Use **private room** that has
Monitored negative air pressure,
6 to 12 air changes per hour,
Discharge of air outdoors or HEPA filtration if recirculated.
Keep room door closed and client in room.

Respiratory Protection

Wear an **N95 respirator** when entering the room of a client with known or suspected infectious pulmonary **tuberculosis. Susceptible** persons should not enter the room of clients known or suspected to have **measles** (rubeola) or **varicella** (chickenpox) if other immune caregivers are available. If susceptible persons must enter, they should wear an **N95 respirator.** (Respirator or surgical mask not required if immune to measles and varicella.)

Client Transport

Limit transport of client from room to essential purposes only.
Use **surgical mask** on client during transport.

(Courtesy of Brevis Corp.)

TABLE 25-11 DROPLET PRECAUTIONS, ONE CATEGORY OF TRANSMISSION-BASED PRECAUTIONS

DROPLET PRECAUTIONS
(in addition to Standard Precautions)

VISITORS: Report to nurse before entering.

Client Placement
Private room. Cohort or maintain spatial separation of **3 feet** from other clients or visitors if private room is not available.

Mask
Wear mask when working within **3 feet** of client (or upon entering room).

Client Transport
Limit transport of client from room to essential purposes only. Use **surgical mask** on client during transport.

(Courtesy of Brevis Corp.)

● SPOT CHECK

There are several medications that may be used to treat tuberculosis. For each of the selected drugs listed, give the recommended children's dosage.

Drug Daily Dose	Twice-Weekly Dose	Thrice-Weekly Dose
Isoniazid		
Rifampin		
Pyrazinamide		
Ethambutol		
Streptomycin		

● SELF-ASSESSMENT

Write the answer in the space provided or circle true or false as instructed.

Source

p. 313 **1.** A person with an individual hypersensitivity to certain common substances, especially those causing an antibody-antigen reaction, is said to have an _____ .

p. 313 **2.** _____ is the active ingredient in Zicam and interacts with rhinoviruses to reduce the duration of the common cold.

p. 314 **3.** True or False (circle one) Antihistamines are chemical agents that specifically interfere with the production and release of histamine.

p. 314 **4.** True or False (circle one) Persons over 60 years of age are more likely to suffer from antihistamine side effects such as dizziness, sedation, and hypotension than are those under 60.

p. 315 **5.** A client who takes a _____ can anticipate that the medication will cause dilated arterioles in the nasal mucosa to constrict, thereby reducing blood flow to the area, slowing the formation of mucus, improving drainage, and opening obstructed nasal passages.

p. 318 **6.** You purchase Robitussin containing guaifenesin as an _____ . By taking this medication, you can anticipate respiratory secretions to increase in volume and decrease in _____ .

p. 322 **7.** Accolate, Singulair, and Zyflo are three medications used in the treatment of asthma. On the line provided, write the name of the drug whose use is best described. _____ is an asthma-control agent for adults and children 6 and older.

p. 325 **8.** The use of multiple drugs for active cases of TB is indicated due to _____ , a naturally occurring factor associated with a large population of *Mycobacterium tuberculosis*.

p. 326 **9.** The effectiveness of TB treatment can be evaluated by monitoring the client's _____ .

p. 325 **10.** Although TB has long been recognized as a serious disease, _____ is cited in this text as the first new medication for its treatment in over two decades.

● WEB ACTIVITY

Visit the following Web sites for additional information on medications that affect the respiratory system:

http://www.pslgroup.com

http://www.merck.com

http://www.discoveryhealth.com

http://www.medicinenet.com

http://pharmacotherapy.medscape.com

http://www.onhealth.com

http://www.fda.gov/bbs/topics

http://www.cdc.gov

http://www.niaid.nih.gov

Chapter

26 Medications Used for Gastrointestinal System Disorders

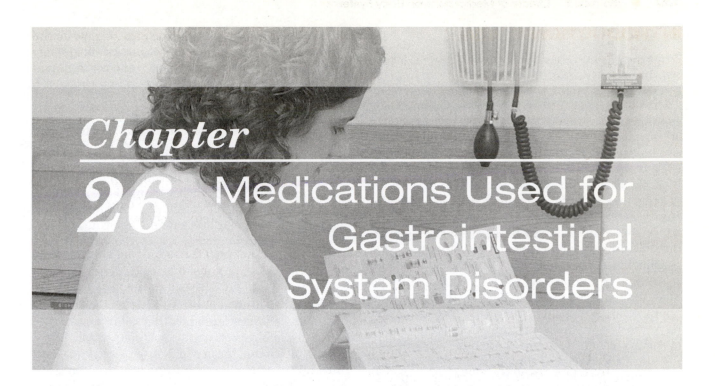

Chapter Outline

Objectives

Key Terms

Introduction

Antiulcer Agents

Ulcers and *Helicobacter pylori* Bacteria

Laxatives

Antidiarrheal Agents

Antiemetics

Emetics

Self-Assessment

Web Activity

- Identify selected drugs according to each described classification

- Understand the actions, uses, contraindications, safety precautions, adverse reactions, dosage and route, nursing considerations, clients' instruction, and special considerations for selected drugs

- State the association of ulcers and *Helicobacter pylori* bacteria

- Complete the Spot Check on selected medications used to treat ulcers

- Complete the Self-Assessment

- Visit indicated Web sites for additional information on medications used for gastrointestinal system disorders

Objectives

Upon completion of this chapter, you should be able to

- Define the key terms

- Describe typical complaints and disorders of the gastrointestinal system

- Describe the various drug classifications used for gastrointestinal system disorders

Key Terms

antacids

antiemetics

Barrett's esophagus

dyspepsia

emetic

erosive esophagitis (EE)

heartburn

Helicobacter pylori (H. pylori)

laxatives

pyrosis

regurgitation

INTRODUCTION

Typical complaints and disorders of the gastrointestinal system include **dyspepsia** (indigestion), **pyrosis** (heartburn), ulcers, nausea, vomiting, diarrhea, constipation, and infection. Many of these complaints may be the result of poor eating habits, stress, overindulgence, alcohol, caffeine, smoking, and nonsteroidal anti-inflammatory drugs (NSAIDs); they can be said to be the result of the client's lifestyle. However, research shows that most ulcers develop as a result of infection with bacteria called *Helicobacter pylori (H. pylori)*. **Heartburn**, a burning sensation in the substernal area, is caused by reflux of acid contents of the stomach into the lower esophagus (gastroesophageal reflux disease, GERD).

About 20 million Americans develop at least one ulcer during their lifetime. Each year ulcers affect about 4 million people, more than 40,000 people have surgery because of persistent symptoms or problems from ulcers, and approximately 6000 people die of ulcer-related complications. According to the American College of Gastroenterology, up to 40 percent of American adults experience heartburn at least once a month and about 7 percent experience heartburn on a daily basis. Twenty-five percent of pregnant women experience daily heartburn and more than 50 percent of them have occasional distress. Recent studies show that heartburn in children is more common than previously recognized, and it may produce recurrent coughing and respiratory problems.

GERD is an all-inclusive term for a range of symptoms that result from the exposure of the esophagus to gastric acid. Heartburn and **regurgitation**, a backward flowing of solids or fluids to the mouth from the stomach, are the most common symptoms, appearing as abdominal pain and burning sensations in the chest. GERD can evolve into **erosive esophagitis (EE)**, a serious condition in which the gastric contents of the stomach pass upward and cause inflammation and tissue damage to the esophagus. If untreated, complications may occur, including hemorrhage, stricture, and **Barrett's esophagus**, inflammation with possible ulceration of the lower part of the esophagus, a condition associated with an increased risk of esophageal cancer.

Medications that are used to treat gastrointestinal system disorders described in this chapter are antiulcer agents, laxatives, antidiarrheal agents, antiemetics, and emetics.

ANTIULCER AGENTS

Antiulcer agents include antacids, histamine H_2-receptor antagonist, mucosal protective medications, and gastric acid pump inhibitors (proton pump inhibitors, PPI). Each of these classifications, along with selected drugs, is described in this chapter.

Antacids

Antacids are drugs that neutralize hydrochloric acid in the stomach. They are used to relieve acid indigestion, gas, heartburn, and in the treatment of peptic ulcers. Ideally, an antacid should neutralize large amounts of acid with a small dose, should have a long-lasting effect, should not interfere with electrolyte balance, and should not cause a secondary increase in gastric acidity. The majority of antacids are classified as nonsystemic agents because they remain largely in the gastrointestinal tract. See Table 26-1. These agents are useful for long-term treatment of ulcers and for occasional relief of gas, indigestion, and other complaints.

Sodium bicarbonate is a systemic antacid. It is readily absorbed, has a rapid onset, and has a short duration of action. For these and other reasons, this antacid is not indicated for use in long-term therapy.

Actions

Antacids act in a variety of ways. They may neutralize gastric acidity, cause hydrogen ion absorption, bind phosphates in the GI tract, buffer the acid, and/or reduce the surface tension of gas bubbles so that the gas may be more easily eliminated.

Uses

Relief of heartburn, acid indigestion, gas, and in the symptomatic relief of hyperacidity associated with peptic ulcer, gastritis, peptic esophagitis, gastric hyperacidity, hiatal hernia, and postoperative gas pain.

Contraindications

Contraindicated in clients with hypersensitivity to any of its ingredients.

Adverse Reactions

Adverse reactions may vary with the type of preparation. See Tables 26-1 and 26-2.

Dosage and Route

The dosage and route of administration is determined by the client and the physician.

Nursing Considerations

The client should not take antacids for more than 2 weeks without the permission of the physician. The client should not exceed the maximum dosage of any antacid or antacid mixture.

TABLE 26-1   NON-SYSTEMIC ANTACIDS

Medication	Usual Dosage	Adverse Reactions
aluminum hydroxide (Amphojel, Basalgel)	Oral: 5–30 ml (1–6 tsp), or 1–2 tablets or capsules, 4–6 times/day, if needed	Constipation, nausea, phosphorus deficiency syndrome
calcium carbonate, precipitated chalk (Tums)	Oral: 0.5–2 g 4–6 times daily, if necessary	Constipation, acid rebound, nausea, flatulence
dihydroxyaluminum sodium carbonate (Rolaids)	Oral: 1–2 tablets 4 or more times per day	Constipation, intestinal concentrations
magaldrate (Riopan)	Oral: 1–2 tablets, or 5–10 ml of suspension 4 times/day	Infrequent diarrhea or constipation
magnesium hydroxide (Milk of Magnesia)	Oral: 5–10 ml, or 1–2 tablets 1 to 3 hours after meals and at bedtime	Diarrhea, nausea, hypermagnesemia
magnesium oxide (Maox)	Oral: 250–1500 mg with water or milk, 4 times/day after meals and at bedtime	Diarrhea, nausea, hypermagnesemia

TABLE 26-2   COMMON ANTACID MIXTURES

Medication	Ingredients	Usual Dosage	Warnings
Gaviscon	aluminum hydroxide, magnesium carbonate (liquid), magnesium trisilicate (tablet)	Oral: 1 or 2 tablespoons, or 2 tablets (chewed), 1 hour after meals and at bedtime	Contraindicated in those with kidney disease, and those taking any form of tetracycline
Gelusil	aluminum hydroxide, magnesium hydroxide, and simethicone	Oral: 2 or more teaspoons or tablets (chewed) after meals and at bedtime	See above
Maalox Plus	aluminum hydroxide, magnesium hydroxide, and simethicone	Oral: 1–4 tablets chewed 4 times a day, 20–60 minutes after meals and at bedtime	See above
Mylanta	aluminum hydroxide, magnesium hydroxide, and simethicone	Oral: 2–4 teaspoons or tablets (chewed), every 2–4 hours between meals and at bedtime	See above

Calcium carbonate and sodium bicarbonate may cause rebound hyperacidity. Clients with renal failure should not use large quantities of antacids containing magnesium. The magnesium cannot be excreted and may produce hypermagnesemia and toxicity.

Clients' Instruction

Educate the client

- That aluminum based and calcium carbonate antacids may cause constipation
- To increase his/her fluid intake to 2000 ml/day while taking an aluminum-based antacid to help relieve constipation, unless contraindicated
- That magnesium-based antacids may cause diarrhea

- To notify the physician if there is any difficulty with constipation and/or diarrhea
- That liquid suspensions must be shaken well before taking
- To store suspensions in a cool place
- That chewable tablets should be chewed thoroughly before swallowing and then followed with 8 ounces of water

Special Considerations

- Antacids should not be used in clients who are taking any form of tetracycline.
- Antacids should be used with caution in geriatric clients, those who have decreased GI motility, bowel obstruction, dehydration, renal disease, sodium-restricted diets, and pregnancy.

- May decrease absorption of cimetidine, iron, benzodiazepines, corticosteroids, anticholinergics, digitalis, and phenytoin (Dilantin)
- Levodopa absorption is increased by antacids.

Antacid Mixtures

Products that combine aluminum and/or calcium compounds with magnesium salts often prove more useful than the single-entity antacids listed in Table 26-1. These agents are commonly used in the treatment of peptic ulcers, acid indigestion, and heartburn. By combining the antacid properties of two single-entity agents, products have been created that provide the antacid action of both, yet tend to counter the adverse effects of each ingredient. For example, a product containing aluminum hydroxide (a cause of constipation) and magnesium hydroxide (a cause of diarrhea) will minimize these effects while offering the sum of the antacid actions of both ingredients. Table 26-2 lists some common antacid mixtures.

Histamine H₂-Receptor Antagonist

Histamine H_2-receptor antagonist inhibits both daytime and nocturnal basal gastric acid secretion and inhibits gastric acid stimulated by food, histamines, caffeine, insulin, and pentagastrin. Four drugs of this type are cimetidine, ranitidine, famotidine, and nizatidine, and they are approved for the treatment of active duodenal ulcer, and for pathological hypersecretory conditions (Zollinger-Ellison Syndrome). See Table 26-3.

Actions

Reduce gastric acid secretion by occupying H_2-receptor sites on parietal cells.

Uses

Active duodenal ulcer, and for pathological hypersecretory conditions (Zollinger-Ellison Syndrome). Short-term treatment of duodenal and gastric ulcers and maintenance therapy.

Contraindications

Contraindicated in clients with known hypersensitivity to any of its ingredients.

Safety Precaution: Should not be used during pregnancy, breast-feeding, and in children under 16 years of age. Cautious use in clients with hepatic disease and/or renal disease.

Adverse Reactions

Histamine H_2-receptor antagonist is generally well tolerated. Adverse reactions vary with the specific drug and the length of use. See Table 26-3. Some adverse reactions that may occur are confusion, headache, depression, dizziness, anxiety, weakness, psychosis, tremors, convulsions, diarrhea, constipation, abdominal cramps, paralytic ileus, jaundice, rash, bradycardia, tachycardia, facial edema, malaise, insomnia, vertigo, gynecomastia, impotence, decreased libido, and/or blood dyscrasia.

TABLE 26-3 HISTAMINE H₂-RECEPTOR ANTAGONIST

Medication	Usual Dosage	Adverse Reactions
cimetidine (Tagamet) (See Figure 26-1)	Active duodenal ulcer: 800 mg at bedtime Maintenance: 400 mg at bedtime Active gastric ulcer: 800 mg at bedtime or 300 mg 4 times a day with meals and at bedtime	Diarrhea, dizziness, somnolence, rash, headache, myalgia, arthralgia, facial edema, bradycardia, constipation, tiredness, confusion, jaundice, gynecomastia, impotence
famotidine (Pepcid)	Acute therapy: 1 (40 mg) tablet at bedtime Maintenance therapy: 1 (20 mg) tablet at bedtime	Headache, dizziness, diarrhea, constipation
nizatidine (Axid)	Active duodenal ulcer: 300 mg at bedtime Alternate dose: 150 mg bid Maintenance therapy: 150 mg at bedtime	Somnolence, sweating, urticaria, confusion, tachycardia, impotence, decreased libido
ranitidine (Zantac)	Active duodenal ulcer: 150 mg bid or 300 mg at bedtime Maintenance therapy: 150 mg at bedtime	Headache, malaise, dizziness, constipation, abdominal pain, diarrhea, insomnia, vertigo, arrhythmias, hepatitis, rash, blood dyscrasia, gynecomastia, impotence

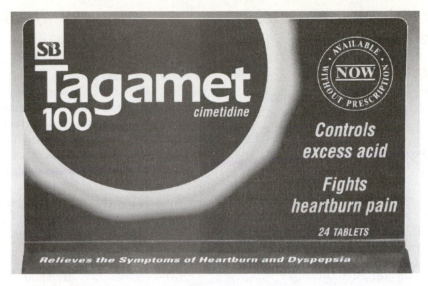

FIGURE 26-1   TAGAMET (CIMETIDINE) RELIEVES THE SYMPTOMS OF HEARTBURN AND DYSPEPSIA *(Courtesy of SmithKline Beecham)*

Dosage and Route

Dosage and route of administration is determined by the physician and individualized for each client. See Table 26-3.

Nursing Considerations

Observe for signs of improvement and/or hypersensitivity. Monitor gastric pH (should be below 5), intake and output ratio, BUN, CBC, liver function tests, creatinine, and prothrombin time.

Clients' Instruction

Concerning cimetidine and ranitidine, educate the client

- That gynecomastia and impotence may occur while using. Explain that both are reversible after discontinuance of the drug(s).

- That the medication may impair mental alertness; therefore, he/she should not operate machinery or drive a motor vehicle, until his/her response to the medication has been determined.

  Regarding famotidine, educate the client

- To report any signs of blood dyscrasia (bleeding, bruising, fatigue, and malaise) to the physician

- That decreased libido may occur while using, but it is reversible after discontinuance of the drug

  For nizatidine, educate the client

- That false-positive tests for urobilinogen with Multistix may occur while taking this medication

- That impotence and decreased libido may occur while using, but they are reversible after discontinuance of the drug

Special Considerations

- Clients with duodenal and/or gastric ulcers should avoid substances that may irritate the mucous membrane of the duodenum or stomach such as caffeine, nicotine, black pepper, alcohol, harsh spices, liquids and foods that are very hot and/or very cold, and over-the-counter medications, especially those that contain aspirin.

- The effect of the medication may be decreased with the use of antacids and ketoconazole (antifungal drug).

- Cimetidine has been reported to reduce the hepatic metabolism of certain drugs, thereby increasing their blood level and delaying their elimination. These drugs include the warfarin-type anticoagulants (Coumadin, Panwarfin), phenytoin (Dilantin), propranolol (Inderal), lidocaine, chlordiazepoxide (Librium), diazepam (Valium), certain tricyclic antidepressants, theophylline, and metronidazole (Flagyl).

- Inhibits the metabolism of calcium channel blocking agents (antianginals and/or antihypertensives) diltiazem, nifedipine, and verapamil

Mucosal Protective Medications

Mucosal-protective medications protect the stomach's mucosal lining from acid, but they do not inhibit the release of acid. Two prescribed protective agents are sucralfate (Carafate) and misoprostol (Cytotec).

Sucralfate (Carafate)

Sucralfate (Carafate) is a cytoprotective agent that is used to prevent further damage by ulcers and to promote the healing process by coating the surface of the damaged mucosa. It exerts its effect through a local rather than systemic action. Following administration, this agent mixes with gastric acid to form a paste-like coating that prevents further damage by ulcerogenic secretions.

Uses

Short-term treatment (up to 8 weeks) of active duodenal ulcer and for maintenance therapy

Contraindications

No known contraindications

Adverse Reactions

Constipation, diarrhea, nausea, vomiting, gastric discomfort, indigestion, flatulence, dry mouth, pruritus, rash, dizziness, sleepiness, vertigo, back pain, headache.

Dosage and Route

Adult dose: 1 g four times a day on an empty stomach. Maintenance therapy: 1 g twice a day. Do not crush to dissolve. Allow to form a slurry (a thin, watery mixture) by adding water.

Interactions

Avoid antacids within 30 minutes of dosing. May reduce absorption of tetracyclines, phenytoin, cimetidine, digoxin, ciprofloxacin, norfloxacin, ranitidine, theophylline. When prescribed, these medications should be given separately and in 2-hour intervals of dosing with sucralfate.

Misoprostol (Cytotec)

Misoprostol (Cytotec) is an antiulcer agent that is used to prevent NSAID (nonsteroidal anti-inflammatory drugs)–induced gastric ulcers. It has not been shown to prevent duodenal ulcers in clients taking NSAIDs. It is contraindicated during pregnancy and childbearing potential because of its abortifacient property. Adverse reactions include diarrhea, abdominal pain, flatulence, headache, and nausea. Dosage for adults is 200 mcg four times a day with food. If not tolerated, 100 mcg can be used. One should avoid magnesium-containing antacids while taking this medication.

Gastric Acid Pump Inhibitors

Gastric acid pump inhibitors (proton pump inhibitors, PPI) are antiulcer agents that suppress gastric acid secretion by specific inhibition of the H+/K+ATPase enzyme at the secretory surface of the gastric parietal cell. Because this enzyme system is regarded as the acid (proton) pump within the gastric mucosa, gastric acid pump inhibitors are so classified, as they block the final step of acid production. This effect is dose related and leads to inhibition of both basal and stimulated acid secretion irrespective of the stimulus. Drugs included in this classification are omeprazole (Prilosec), rabeprazole sodium (Aciphex), lansoprazole (Prevacid), and pantoprazole (Protonix).

Omeprazole (Prilosec)

Uses

Short-term treatment of active duodenal ulcer, erosive esophagitis, poorly responsive symptomatic gastroesophageal reflux disease (GERD), and maintenance of healing or erosive esophagitis. It is indicated for the long-term treatment of pathological hypersecretory conditions (e.g., Zollinger-Ellison, multiple endocrine adenoma, and systemic mastocytosis).

Contraindications

Contraindicated in clients with known hypersensitivity to any component of the formulation.

Adverse Reactions

Headache, diarrhea, abdominal pain, nausea, upper respiratory infection, dizziness, vomiting, rash, constipation, cough, asthenia, back pain.

Dosage and Route

Delayed capsules. Short-term treatment of active duodenal ulcer: Adult oral dose: 20 mg once daily for 4 weeks. Erosive esophagitis or poorly responsive gastroesophageal reflux disease (GERD): Adult oral dose: 20 mg daily for 4 to 8 weeks. Maintenance of healing of erosive esophagitis: Adult oral dose: 20 mg daily. Pathological hypersecretory conditions: Adult oral dose: individualized for each client. The recommended adult oral starting dose is 60 mg once a day. Doses should be adjusted to individual client needs and should continue for as long as clinically indicated. Swallow whole. Do not split, crush, or chew.

Interactions

Decreases metabolism and may increase effects of phenytoin, diazepam, and warfarin. May interfere with absorption of drugs requiring acidic gastric pH, including ketoconazole, esters of ampicillin, and iron salts.

Rabeprazole Sodium (Aciphex)

Uses

Short-term (4–8 weeks) treatment in the healing and symptomatic relief of erosive or ulcerative gastroesophageal reflux disease (GERD) and duodenal ulcers. Maintenance of healing and reduction in relapse of heartburn symptoms in clients with erosive or ulcerative GERD. Long-term treatment of pathological hypersecretory symptoms, including Zollinger-Ellison syndrome.

Contraindications

Contraindicated in clients with known hypersensitivity to any component of the formulation.

Adverse Reactions

Headache, diarrhea, nausea and vomiting, dyspepsia, flatulence, constipation, dry mouth, gastroenteritis, anorexia, insomnia, dizziness, nervousness, vertigo, decreased libido, hypertension, palpitation, dyspnea, asthma, epistaxis, rash, pruritus, cystitis, dysmenorrhea, anemia, agranulocytosis, edema, asthenia, fever, malaise, dry eyes, tinnitus.

Dosage and Route

Tablet, enteric-coated, healing of erosive or ulcerative GERD: Adults: 20 mg once daily for 4–8 weeks. An additional 8 weeks of therapy may be considered for those who have not healed. Maintenance of healing or erosive or ulcerative GERD: Adults: 20 mg once daily. Healing of duodenal ulcers: Adults: 20 mg once daily after the morning meal for up to 4 weeks. Treatment of pathological hypersecretory conditions: Adults, Initial: 60 mg once a day. Adjust dosage to individual client needs (doses up to 100 mg/day bid have been used). Swallow whole. Do not split, crush, or chew.

Lansoprazole (Prevacid)

Uses

In the short-term treatment of symptomatic GERD, erosive esophagitis, maintenance of healed erosive esophagitis, in combination with Biaxin and amoxicillin for *H. pylori* eradication to reduce the risk of duodenal ulcers, active benign gastric ulcers, and hypersecretory conditions including Zollinger-Ellison syndrome.

Contraindications

Contraindicated in clients with known hypersensitivity to any component of the formulation.

Adverse Reactions

Headache, abdominal pain, diarrhea.

Dosage and Route

Delayed-release capsule, 15 mg once daily. Swallow whole. Do not split, crush, or chew.

Pantoprazole Sodium (Protonix)

Uses

Indicated for the short-term treatment in the healing and symptomatic relief of erosive esophatitis (EE) and gastroesophageal reflux disease (GERD). It is also used for treatment of duodenal stomach ulcers and Zollinger-Ellison syndrome.

Contraindications

Contraindicated in clients with known hypersensitivity to any component of the formulation.

Adverse Reactions

Headache, diarrhea, flatulence.

Dosage and Route

Delayed-release tablet, 40 mg once daily. Swallow whole. Do not split, crush, or chew.

ULCERS AND *HELICOBACTER PYLORI* BACTERIA

Helicobacter pylori (H. pylori) is a spiral-shaped bacterium that lives in the stomach and duodenum. It was once believed that the stomach contained no bacteria, but the discovery of *H. pylori* changed this theory. This occurred when Dr. Barry Marshall and Dr. Robin Warren of the Royal Perth Hospital in Western Australia noticed a bacterial infection in the stomach linings of clients with various diseases. Out of 100 clients, 65 percent were tested and found to have the infection, and half of these were found to have ulcers.

In a treatment study among 100 clients whose ulcers would not go away, Dr. Marshall gave half of them Tagamet and the other half received an antibiotic (Flagyl) and an antacid, bismuth. According to the study, the ulcers returned in 95 percent of the clients not treated with an antibiotic. Among those treated with Flagyl and bismuth, the ulcers returned in only 20 percent.

Approximately 90 percent of duodenal ulcers and 70 percent of gastric ulcers are associated with *Helicobacter pylori*. The bacteria settle in the lining of the duodenum or stomach, opening a wound that is then made worse by digestive juices and stomach acids. The wound is said to resemble a flattened volcano or a white-centered, red-rimmed, painful canker sore. By killing the bacteria with antibiotics, it is estimated that 90 percent of the ulcers caused by *H. pylori* can be cured.

The treatment regimen for active duodenal ulcers associated with *H. pylori* may involve a two-drug or a three-drug program. An example of a two-drug program is the use of the antibiotic clarithromycin (Biaxin) and omeprazole (Prilosec). An example of a three-drug program is the use of two antibiotics: metronidazole (Flagyl) and either tetracycline or amoxicillin and Pepto Bismol.

The reported problem associated with this drug regimen is that the client has to complete the full treatment program that involves taking 15 pills a day for a total of at least 2 weeks, and many of the clients quit prematurely. If the treatment is not completed, it is believed that only the weakest of the bacteria are killed, leaving the more resistant ones to cause further damage. The clients have also complained of side effects including changes in taste, a metallic taste in the mouth, nausea, vomiting, diarrhea, and skin rash.

LAXATIVES

Laxatives are used to relieve constipation and to facilitate the passage of feces through the lower gastrointestinal tract. Normally, an active, healthy person who eats a balanced diet does not suffer from constipation. Occasionally, this condition results from travel, emotional stress, and other factors. More often, constipation results from decreased fluid intake, poor diet, lack of physical activity, eating constipating foods, and as a result of certain drugs.

Although relief of constipation is the leading reason for using a laxative, the agents are also used to prepare the bowel prior to surgery and before x-ray or proctoscopic examination of the lower GI tract. Laxatives are used after anthelmintic therapy to speed elimination of parasites, as a means of reducing the strain of defecation in those with cardiovascular weaknesses, and after a barium x-ray study.

Several types of laxatives are in general use. See Table 26-4. These agents have been grouped into

TABLE 26-4   VARIOUS TYPES OF LAXATIVE AGENTS

Medication	Type	Usual Dosage	Onset of Action
polycarbophil (FiberCon)	Bulk-forming	Oral (Adult): 1 g 1–4 times daily or as needed (not to exceed 6 g/24 hr)	Acts within 12–24 hours
psyllium (Metamucil)	Bulk-forming	Oral (Adult): 1–2 tsp/packet/wafer (3–6 g psyllium) in or with a full glass of liquid 2–3 times daily Oral (Children 6 years and older): 1 tsp/packet/wafer (1.5–3 g psyllium) in or with $\frac{1}{2}$–1 glass of liquid 2–3 times daily	Acts within 12–24 hours
mineral oil (Fleet Mineral Oil)	Lubricant	Oral (Adult): 5–45 ml, usually in the evening	Acts within 6–8 hours
glycerin (Fleet Babylax)	Osmotic	Rectal (Adult and children 6 years and older): 2–3 g as a suppository or 5–15 ml as an enema	Acts within 15–30 min
lactulose (Cholac)	Osmotic	Oral (Adult): 15–30 ml/day; maximum dose up to 60 ml/day	Acts within 24–48 hours
polyethylene glycol/electrolyte (GoLYTELY)	Osmotic	Oral (Adult): 30–60 ml single or divided dose or 10–20 ml as concentrate Oral (Children 6–12 years): 15–30 ml as single or divided dose Oral (Children 2–5 years): 5–15 ml as single or divided dose	Acts in 1 hour

(continued)

TABLE 26-4   (*Continued*)

Medication	Type	Usual Dosage	Onset of Action
magnesium hydroxide (Milk of Magnesia)	Saline	Oral (Adult): 30–60 ml single or divided dose or 10–20 ml as concentrate Oral (Children 6–12 years): 15–30 ml as single or divided dose Oral (Children 2–5 years): 5–15 ml as single or divided dose	Acts in 3–6 hours
docusate calcium (Surfak)	Stool softener	Oral (Adult): 240 mg once daily Oral (Children 6–12 years): 50–150 mg once daily	Acts within 24–48 hours (up to 3–5 days)
docusate sodium (Colace)	Stool softener	Oral (Adult and Children 12 years and older): 50–500 mg once daily Oral (Children 6–12 years): 40–120 mg once daily Oral (Children 3–6 years): 20–60 mg once daily Oral (Children under 3 years): 10–40 mg once daily	Acts within 24–48 hours (up to 3–5 days)
bisacodyl (Dulcolax)	Stimulant	Oral (Adult and Children 12 years and older): 5–15 mg (up to 30 mg/day) as a single dose Oral (Children 3 years and older): 5–10 mg (0.3 mg/kg) as a single dose Rectal (Adult and Children 12 years and older): 10 mg single dose Rectal (Children 1–11 years): 5–10 mg single dose Rectal (Children 2 years and older): 5 mg single dose	Acts within 6–12 hours Acts within 15–60 min
senna, sennosides (Ex-Lax Gentle Nature Laxative Pills; Senokot)	Stimulant	Oral (Adult and Children 12 years and older): senna: 0.5–2 g; sennosides: 12–50 mg 1–2 times daily Oral (Children 6–11 years): 50% of the adult dose Oral (Children 1–5 years): 33% of the adult dose Rectal (Adult and Children 12 years and older): 30 mg 1–2 times daily	Acts within 6–12 hours Acts within $\frac{1}{2}$–2 hours

the following classifications: *bulk-forming* agents, which absorb water and expand, and thereby stimulate peristaltic action; *lubricants*, which are various oils that soften the fecal mass and facilitate penetration of the fecal mass by intestinal fluids; *osmotic laxatives*, which help prevent the bowel from absorbing water so that the bulk volume increases; *saline laxatives*, which are salts that draw water into the intestinal lumen osmotically to mix with the stool and stimulate motility; *stool softeners*, which act as detergents, moistening and breaking up the feces; and *stimulant laxatives*, which act by irritating the intestinal mucosa or nerves in the intestinal wall. See Table 26-5.

Special Considerations

- Contraindicated in clients with hypersensitivity to any of the ingredients used in laxative preparations
- Laxatives are contraindicated in clients with abdominal pain, nausea, vomiting, fecal impaction, intestinal obstruction, appendicitis, biliary tract obstructions, and/or acute hepatitis.

TABLE 26-5 CLASSIFICATION OF LAXATIVE AGENTS AND CLIENT INSTRUCTION CONSIDERATIONS

Classification	Example	Client Instruction
Bulk-forming	Metamucil	Do not take dry. Take with 8 ounces of water and follow with 8 ounces of water. If abdominal distention or unusual amount of flatulence occurs, notify your physician. Do not take within 1 hour of antacids, milk, or cimetidine. Report muscle cramps, pain, weakness, dizziness, or excessive thirst to your physician.
Lubricant	Mineral oil	Mineral oil may impair the absorption of fat-soluble vitamins (A, D, E, K). May increase effect of oral anticoagulants. Swallow carefully as access of oil into the pharynx, bronchi, and lung may produce a lipid pneumonia.
Osmotic	Cholac	Caution client that this medication may cause belching, flatulence, or abdominal cramping. Client should notify physician if this becomes bothersome or if diarrhea occurs.
Saline	Milk of Magnesia	Magnesium laxatives should not be taken by clients who have renal insufficiency. Only short-term use is recommended because of possibility of CNS or neuromuscular depression, and/or electrolyte imbalance. Medicine should be followed by 8 ounces of water. Chilling helps taste.
Stimulant	Dulcolax	Tablets should be swallowed. Do not crush or chew. Avoid milk or antacids within 1 hour of taking because the enteric coating may dissolve prematurely.
Stool softener	Colace	May be taken alone or with 8 ounces of water. Store in cool environment, but do not freeze. Swallow tablets whole; do not chew. May be used safely by clients who should avoid straining.

- Side effects may include nausea, vomiting, diarrhea, anorexia, abdominal cramps, and electrolyte imbalance.

- It is stated that approximately $400 million a year is spent on laxatives. Many clients abuse laxatives, so you should evaluate each client for signs of abuse. Laxative abuse causes the colon to become lazy and it stops responding to the defecation reflex, causing true constipation. If the client is abusing laxatives he/she should gradually reduce the dose or use a milder preparation, at the same time slowly increasing fiber and fluid intake until the defecation reflex returns to a normal state.

- Stimulant laxatives discolor alkaline urine red-pink, acid urine yellow-brown, and they may give a reddish color to feces.

- Administration of laxatives should be such that results will not interfere with a client's daily activities.

ANTIDIARRHEAL AGENTS

Diarrhea is characterized by frequent defecation of loose, watery stools. It is not a disease; rather, it is a symptom that has been associated with numerous medical conditions. It may be a sign of incomplete intestinal obstruction. Diarrhea may be caused by infection, intoxication, allergy, malabsorption, inflammation, tumors of the GI tract, food poisoning, and by certain medications.

Diarrhea may be described as acute when it has a sudden and severe onset, or chronic when it is of long-term duration. Acute diarrhea can cause water and salt depletion, resulting in dehydration and electrolyte imbalance.

Since diarrhea is a symptom of an underlying disorder, it is often more important to determine and treat its specific cause than it is to alleviate the diarrhea.

When the specific cause of diarrhea can be diagnosed, therapy may involve the use of an antiprotozoal agent, an antibacterial drug, or an adrenal corticosteroid. Should it become necessary, certain nonspecific antidiarrheal agents may be used to treat severe acute diarrhea when its cause is unknown. Table 26-6 lists some of these agents.

Special Considerations

- When diarrhea is severe or prolonged, the client can become dehydrated and experience electrolyte imbalance. Monitor potassium, sodium, and chloride levels. Increase fluids if not contraindicated. Monitor bowel pattern.

- Clients using antidiarrheal agents should avoid over-the-counter products unless prescribed by their physician.

TABLE 26-6   NONSPECIFIC ANTIDIARRHEAL AGENTS

Medication	Usual Antidiarrheal Dosage	Adverse Reactions
bismuth subsalicylate (Pepto-Bismol)	Oral (Adult): 30 ml or 2 tablets (maximum of 8 doses/day at 30–60 min intervals) (Child 10–14 years): 20 ml as above (Child 6–10 years): 10 ml or 1 tablet (Child 3–6 years): 5 ml or one-half tablet	Temporary darkening of stool and tongue
diphenoxylate HCl with atropine sulfate (Lomotil)	Oral (Adult): 5 mg 3–4 times/day as needed Oral (Child 2–12 years): 0.3–0.4 mg/kg/day of liquid in divided doses Pediatric/Dose 2–3 years 0.75–1.5 mg qid 3–4 years 1–1.5 mg qid 4–5 years 1–2 mg qid 5–6 years 1.25–2.25 mg qid 6–9 years 1.25–2.5 mg qid 9–12 years 1.75–2.5 mg qid	Headache, sedation, dizziness, flushing nausea, dry mouth, blurred vision
kaolin mixture with pectin (Kaopectate)	Oral (Adult): 60–120 ml after each loose stool Oral (Children over 12 years): 45–60 ml after each loose stool 6–12 years 30–60 ml after each loose stool 3–6 years 15–30 ml after each loose stool	Few adverse reactions. In the elderly and debilitated clients, constipation may occur.
loperamide HCl (Imodium)	Oral: 4 mg initially, then 2 mg after each unformed stool; maintenance dose: 4–8 mg/day	Drowsiness, abdominal discomfort or pain, nausea
paregoric (in Parepectolin)	Oral (Adult): 5–10 ml after bowel movement (maximum of 4 doses at 2 hour intervals) Oral (Child): 0.25–0.5 ml/kg 1–4 times/day	Anorexia, nausea, constipation, vomiting, abdominal pain

- Pepto-Bismol tablets should be chewed or allowed to dissolve in the mouth; do not swallow them. While taking this medicine, client should avoid salicylates.

- Lomotil is contraindicated in clients with known hypersensitivity, severe liver disease, pseudomembranous enterocolitis, glaucoma, electrolyte imbalance, and by children under 2 years of age. Precautions in clients with hepatic disease, renal disease, ulcerative colitis, and during pregnancy and lactation. Lomotil is a Schedule V controlled substance. This medication should not be used with MAOIs as hypertensive crisis may occur.

- Imodium is contraindicated in clients with known hypersensitivity, severe ulcerative colitis, and pseudomembranous enterocolitis. Precautions in clients with liver disease, dehydration, bacterial disease, during pregnancy and lactation, and children under 2 years of age.

- Paregoric is contraindicated in clients with known hypersensitivity. Precautions in clients with liver disease, addiction-prone individuals, prostatic hyperplasia, during pregnancy and lactation. Paregoric is a controlled substance, and depending upon the amount of opium, it may be a Schedule II or III drug. The client should not take other CNS depressants while taking this medication.

ANTIEMETICS

Antiemetics are agents that prevent or arrest vomiting. These drugs are the same as those listed in Chapter 30 for the treatment of vertigo, motion sickness, and the nausea associated with the use of antineoplastic agents and radiation. For information on route, dosage, and adverse reactions of the various antiemetic agents, see Table 30-12.

EMETICS

Emetics are used to induce vomiting in people who have taken an overdose of oral drugs or who have ingested certain poisons. An emetic agent should not be given to a client who is unconscious, in shock, or in a semicomatose state. Emetics are also contraindicated in individuals who have ingested strongly caustic substances, such as lye or acid, since their use could result in additional injury to the client's esophagus.

Ipecac syrup is available without a prescription from local pharmacies in amounts up to 30 ml. Some physicians advise parents of young children to keep a small amount of this emetic on hand for use in an emergency. It acts directly on the chemoreceptor trigger zone of the medulla and reflexly on the gas-tric mucosa to cause vomiting. The usual dose for adults is 20 ml followed by 1–2 full glasses of water. For children between 1 and 12 years of age, the usual dose is 15 ml (1 tablespoon) followed by 1–$1\frac{1}{2}$ full glasses of water. The usual dose for infants 9–12 months of age is 2 teaspoonsful followed by $\frac{1}{2}$ to 1 full glass of water. Ipecac syrup will usually cause vomiting within 20 minutes of administration and the dosage can be repeated should vomiting not occur within this time. Activated charcoal may be used after vomiting has subsided to absorb the remaining poison.

● SPOT CHECK

There are several medications that may be used to treat ulcers. For each of the selected drugs listed, give the usual dosage and several adverse reactions.

Drug	Usual Dosage	Adverse Reactions
Tagamet		
Pepcid		
Axid		
Zantac		

(continued)

Drug	Usual Dosage	Adverse Reactions
Carafate		
Cytotec		

● SELF-ASSESSMENT

Write the answer in the space provided or circle true or false as instructed.

Source

p. 332   1. Although we often blame disorders of the gastrointestinal system on lifestyle choices, research has shown that most ulcers are a result of infection with _____ and heartburn is usually caused by _____ (abbreviated GERD).

p. 334   2. Some antacids contain both aluminum hydroxide, which can cause constipation, and magnesium hydroxide, which may cause diarrhea. The advantages of this combination of ingredients are _____.

p. 334   3. On the spaces provided, list the trade names of four histamine H_2-receptor antagonists approved for treatment of active duodenal ulcer. (1) _____ (2) _____ (3) _____ (4) _____

p. 336   4. The trade names of the two mucosal protective medications discussed in this chapter are _____ and _____.

p. 338   5. In a few words, complete the following sentence: The reported problem with multidrug antibiotic treatment for active duodenal ulcers associated with infection is that many clients _____.

p. 338   6. Other than relief of constipation, laxatives are used to prepare _____.

p. 338–339   7. On the lines provided, classify each product by its laxative action.
- Metamucil is a _____ laxative.
- Dulcolax is a _____ laxative.
- Mineral oil is a _____ laxative.
- Cholac is a _____ laxative.
- Milk of Magnesia is a _____ laxative.

p. 340   8. True or False (circle one) The overuse of laxatives can lead to constipation.

p. 340   9. True or False (circle one) Since diarrhea is a symptom of an underlying disorder, diagnosis and treatment for that cause is often more important than alleviation of the diarrhea.

p. 342   10. _____ _____ is an emetic often recommended for at-home emergency use for young children.

● WEB ACTIVITY

Visit the following Web sites for additional information on medications used for gastrointestinal system disorders:

http://pharmacology.medscape.com

http://www.discoveryhealth.com

http://www.pslgroup.com

http://www.rxlist.com

http://pharmacotherapy.medscape.com

http://www.docguide.com

http://www.pharminfo.com

http://www.allsands.com/health

http://www.pylori.com

http://www.diagnosishealth.com

http://www.intelihealth.com

http://www.mediconsult.com

http://www.gastro.org

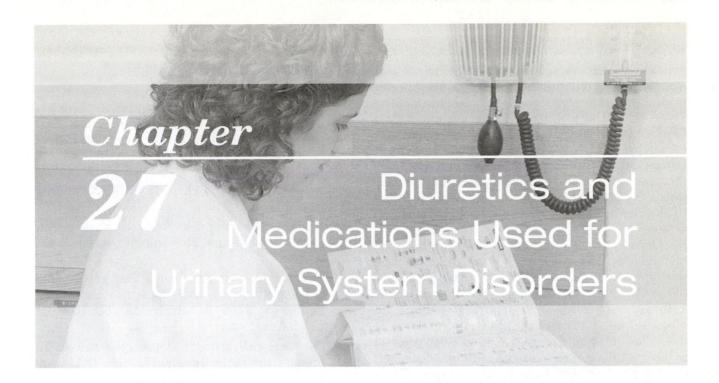

Chapter 27

Diuretics and Medications Used for Urinary System Disorders

Chapter Outline

Objectives

Key Terms

Introduction

Diuretics

Urinary Tract Infections (UTI): Cystitis

Urinary Tract Antibacterials

Urinary Tract Antiseptics

Miscellaneous Agents

Self-Assessment

Web Activity

Objectives

Upon completion of this chapter, you should be able to

- Define the key terms

- List several causes of kidney and urologic diseases

- List the warning signs of kidney and urinary tract disease

- Describe the various drug classifications used for urinary system disorders

- Identify selected drugs according to each described classification

- Understand the actions, uses, contraindications, safety precautions, adverse reactions, dosage and route, nursing considerations, clients' instruction, and special considerations for selected drugs

- Describe cystitis, giving the symptoms, diagnosis, and treatment

- Give the guidelines to help avoid cystitis in the female

- Complete the Spot Check on selected medications used to treat urinary tract infection

- Be familiar with selected agents that discolor urine

- Complete the Self-Assessment

- Visit indicated Web sites for additional information on medications used for urinary system disorders

Key Terms

cystitis	hypertension
diuretics	incontinence
edema	interstitial cystitis (IC)
Escherichia coli (E. coli)	*Klebsiella*
glomerulonephritis	nocturia
hematuria	*Proteus mirabilis*

INTRODUCTION

Diseases and disorders of the urinary system may involve the kidneys, ureters, bladder, and urethra. Approximately 20 million Americans are affected by kidney and urologic diseases. Diabetes mellitus (Type II) is the leading cause of chronic kidney failure, and uncontrolled or poorly controlled high blood pressure is the second leading cause. **Glomerulonephritis**, an inflammatory disease of the glomeruli of the kidney, is the third leading cause. Some of the other conditions that may affect the kidney are kidney stones and polycystic kidney disease.

Urinary tract infections (UTIs), another common disorder of the urinary system, are more common in women than men. They are usually confined to the bladder (**cystitis**), and if they spread to the kidneys, they can lead to nephritis. Urinary **incontinence**, the loss of the ability to retain urine due to lack of sphincter control, is a health problem in older adults. An estimated 3 million older Americans suffer from this condition. Other types of bladder-control problems involve (1) overactive bladder, (2) stress incontinence, and (3) mixed symptoms. These conditions may affect men and women of all ages, and it is estimated that 17 million Americans are affected by bladder problems.

Kidney and urologic diseases continue to be one of the major causes of work loss among men and women. The National Kidney Foundation lists the following warning signs of kidney and urinary tract disease:

- Burning or difficulty during urination
- More frequent urination, particularly at night (**nocturia**)
- Passage of bloody-appearing urine (**hematuria**)
- Puffiness around eyes, swelling of hands and feet, especially in children
- Pain in small of back just below the ribs (not aggravated by movement)
- High blood pressure (**hypertension**)

Medications used to treat urinary system diseases and disorders described in this chapter are diuretics, urinary tract antibacterials, urinary tract antiseptics, and miscellaneous agents.

DIURETICS

Diuretics decrease reabsorption of sodium chloride by the kidneys, thereby increasing the amount of salt and water excreted in the urine. This action reduces the amount of fluid retained in the body and prevents **edema**, a local or generalized collection of fluid in the body tissues. Diuretics are classified according to site and mechanism of action.

- *Thiazide diuretics* appear to act by inhibiting sodium and chloride reabsorption in the early portion of the distal tubule. They may also block chloride reabsorption in the ascending loop of Henle.
- *Loop diuretics* act by inhibiting the reabsorption of sodium and chloride in the ascending loop of Henle.
- *Potassium-sparing diuretics* exert their action in the distal tubule. They inhibit potassium excretion.
- *Osmotic diuretics* are agents that are capable of being filtered by the glomerulus but have a limited capability of being reabsorbed into the bloodstream.
- *Carbonic anhydrase inhibitor diuretics* act to promote the reabsorption of sodium and bicarbonate from the proximal tubule.

Thiazide Diuretics

Thiazide diuretics appear to act by inhibiting sodium and chloride reabsorption in the early portion of the distal tubule. They may also block chloride reabsorption in the ascending loop of Henle.

Uses

Edema, hypertension, diuresis.

Contraindications

Contraindicated in clients who are known to be hypersensitive to any of its ingredients. They should not be used in anuria and/or renal decompensation.

> **Safety Precaution:** Should be used with caution in clients with severe renal disease, impaired hepatic function, or progressive liver disease.

Adverse Reactions

Weakness, hypotension, orthostatic hypotension, pancreatitis, jaundice, diarrhea, vomiting, constipation, nausea, anorexia, aplastic anemia, agranulocytosis, leukopenia, hemolytic anemia, thrombocytopenia, electrolyte imbalance, hyperglycemia, glycosuria, hyperuricemia, muscle spasm, vertigo, dizziness, headache, restlessness, renal failure, blurred vision, xanthopsia, anaphylactic reactions, rash, urticaria, photosensitivity fever.

Dosage and Route

The dosage and route of administration is determined by the physician and individualized for each client. See Table 27-1.

Nursing Considerations

Observe client for evidence of fluid or electrolyte imbalance. Warning signs: dryness of mouth, thirst, weakness, lethargy, drowsiness, restlessness, muscle pains or cramps, muscular fatigue, hypotension, oliguria, tachycardia, nausea and vomiting. Monitor weight, intake and output ratio, blood pressure, respirations, and serum electrolytes.

Clients' Instruction

Educate the client

- To increase fluid intake to 2–3 liters per day unless contraindicated
- To eat potassium-rich foods such as bananas, oranges, prunes, raisins, dried peas and beans, fresh vegetables, nuts, meats, and cereals.
- About warning signs of fluid or electrolyte imbalance
- To contact the physician without delay if warning signs occur
- That the medication should be taken in the morning to avoid nocturia

Special Considerations

- Thiazide diuretics may increase blood sugar in the client with diabetes. Dosage adjustment of oral hypoglycemic agents and insulin may be required.
- Use in pregnancy is not recommended.
- Alcohol, barbiturates, and narcotics may potentiate the occurrence of orthostatic hypotension.
- There may be an additive effect when taken with other antihypertensive agents.
- Electrolyte depletion may be intensified when taken with corticosteroids.
- Clients taking lithium should not take diuretics as they reduce the renal clearance of lithium and add a high risk of lithium toxicity.

Loop Diuretics

Loop diuretics act by inhibiting reabsorption of sodium and chloride in the proximal and distal tubules and in the ascending loop of Henle.

Uses

Edema, hypertension, as adjunctive therapy in acute pulmonary embolism.

Contraindications

Contraindicated in clients who are known to be hypersensitive to any of its ingredients. They should not be used in clients with anuria, electrolyte depletion, hypovolemia, by infants, or during lactation.

> **Safety Precaution:**
>
> 1. Lasix (furosemide) is a potent loop diuretic, and if given in excessive amounts, can lead to profound diuresis with water and electrolyte depletion. Careful medical supervision is required.
> 2. In clients with hepatic cirrhosis and ascites, drug therapy should be initiated in the hospital, after the basic condition is improved.
> 3. Ototoxicity has been reported and is usually associated with rapid injection, severe renal impairment, doses higher than recommended, and when given with other agents that cause ototoxicity.

Adverse Reactions

Anorexia, jaundice, pancreatitis, diarrhea, cramping, constipation, nausea, vomiting, tinnitus, hearing loss, paresthesia, vertigo, dizziness, headache, blurred vision, xanthopsia, aplastic anemia, thrombocytopenia, leukopenia, purpura, photosensitivity, urticaria, rash, pruritus, orthostatic hypotension, hyperglycemia, glycosuria, muscle spasm, weakness, restlessness, thrombophlebitis, fever, necrotizing angiitis.

Dosage and Route

The dosage and route of administration is determined by the physician and individualized for each client. See Table 27-1.

Nursing Considerations

Observe client for evidence of fluid or electrolyte imbalance. Monitor weight, intake and output ratio, blood pressure, respirations, and serum electrolytes.

Clients' Instruction

Educate the client

- To increase fluid intake to 2–3 liters per day unless contraindicated
- To eat potassium-rich foods such as bananas, oranges, prunes, raisins, dried peas and beans, fresh vegetables, nuts, meats, and cereals
- That potassium supplements may be prescribed by the physician

TABLE 27-1 DIURETICS

Medication	Classification	Usual Dosage	Adverse Reactions
acetazolamide (Diamox)	Carbonic anhydrace inhibitor	Oral, IV (Adult): 250–375 mg once daily	Tingling in the extremities, anorexia, polyuria
bumetanide (Bumex)	Loop diuretic	Oral (Adult): 0.5–2 mg/day as a single dose IM, IV (Adult): 0.5–1 mg, may be repeated q 2–3 hr as needed (up to 10 mg/day)	Dizziness, headache, tinnitus, hypotension, dry mouth, nausea, vomiting, dehydration, hypokalemia
furosemide (Lasix)	Loop diuretic	Oral (Adult): 20–80 mg as a single dose Oral (Child): 2 mg/kg as a single dose	Anorexia, vertigo, purpura, anemia, hyperglycemia
torsemide (Demadex)	Loop diuretic	Oral, IV (Adult): Congestive heart failure: 10–20 mg once daily Chronic renal failure: 20 mg once daily Hypertension: 5 mg once daily	Dizziness, headache, ototoxicity, nausea, hypotension, constipation, hypokalemia
mannitol (Osmitrol) (Resectisol)	Osmotic diuretic	IV (Adult): 300–400 mg/kg of a 20–25% solution in 1 dose	Headache, nausea, dizziness, polydipsia, chills, angina pectoris
amiloride (Midamor)	Potassium-sparing diuretic	Oral (Adult): 5–10 mg/day	Dizziness, headache, arrhythmias, constipation, photosensitivity, hyperkalemia
spironolactone (Aldactone)	Potassium-sparing diuretic	Oral (Adult): 50–100 mg daily Oral (Child): 1–2 mg/kg in a single dose or in divided doses	Gynecomastia, cramping and diarrhea, drowsiness, rash, irregular menses
triamterene (Dyrenium)	Potassium-sparing diuretic	Oral (Adult): 100–300 mg daily in divided doses	Diarrhea, nausea, vomiting, weakness, headache, rash, dry mouth
chlorothiazide (Diuril)	Thiazide diuretic	Oral (Adult): 250 mg–1 g as a single dose or in divided doses	Weakness, anorexia, gastric irritation, hyperglycemia, purpura, muscle spasm
chlorthalidone (Hygroton) (Thalitone)	Thiazide diuretic	Oral (Adult): 25–100 mg once daily	Dizziness, hypotension, anorexia, nausea, photosensitivity, hypokalemia, dehydration
hydrochlorothiazide (Esidrix) (HydroDIURIL)	Thiazide diuretic	Oral (Adult): 12.5–100 mg 1–2 times/day Oral (Child): 1–2 mg/kg in 1–2 divided doses	Orthostatic hypotension, muscle spasm, vertigo, pancreatitis, aplastic anemia
indapamide (Lozol)	Thiazide diuretic	Oral (Adult): Hypertension: 1.25–5 mg daily in the morning Edema secondary to congestive heart failure: 2.5 mg daily in the morning	Dizziness, arrhythmias, hypotension, nausea, photosensitivity, hypokalemia
metolazone (Mykrox)	Thiazide-like diuretic	Oral (Adult): 0.5–1 mg/day	Drowsiness, nausea, hypotension, photosensitivity, hypokalemia

- About warning signs of fluid and electrolyte imbalance
- To contact the physician without delay if warning signs occur
- That the medication should be taken in the morning to avoid nocturia

Special Considerations

- Loop diuretics may increase blood sugar in the diabetic client. Dosage adjustment of oral hypoglycemic agents and insulin may be required.
- Some clients may be more sensitive to sunlight while taking loop diuretics.
- Use in pregnancy is not recommended.
- May increase ototoxicity effect of aminoglycosides
- Clients taking lithium should not take loop diuretics as they reduce the renal clearance of lithium and add a higher risk of lithium toxicity.
- There may be an additive effect when taken with other antihypertensive agents.
- Alcohol, barbiturates, and narcotics may potentiate the occurrence of orthostatic hypotension.

Potassium-Sparing Diuretics

Potassium-sparing diuretics exert their action in the distal tubule. They cause increased amounts of sodium and water to be excreted, while potassium is retained.

Uses

Edema, primary hyperaldosteronism, congestive heart failure, cirrhosis of the liver, essential hypertension, hypokalemia.

Contraindications

Contraindicated in clients who are known to be hypersensitive to any of its ingredients. They should not be used in anuria, acute renal disease, hyperkalemia, and during pregnancy or lactation.

> **Safety Precaution:** Potassium supplements and foods rich in potassium should not generally be given with potassium-sparing diuretics. Hyperkalemia could occur. Also, most salt substitutes contain potassium salts; therefore, cautious use should be followed.

Adverse Reactions

Gynecomastia, agranulocytosis, cramping, diarrhea, drowsiness, lethargy, headache, urticaria, rash, pruritus, mental confusion, drug fever, ataxia, impotence, irregular menses or amenorrhea, postmenopausal bleeding, hirsutism, gastritis, vomiting.

Dosage and Route

The dosage and route of administration is determined by the physician and individualized for each client. See Table 27-1.

Nursing Considerations

Observe client for evidence of fluid and electrolyte imbalance. Monitor cardiac function and be alert for signs of hyperkalemia: nausea, diarrhea, muscle weakness, marked ECG changes (elevated T waves, depressed P waves), atrial systole, slow irregular pulse, ventricular fibrillation, cardiac arrest. Treatment of hyperkalemia: IV administration of 20–50 percent glucose and 0.25–0.5 units of regular insulin per gram of glucose. Assess weight, intake and output ratio, vital signs, serum electrolytes, and mental status.

Clients' Instruction

Educate the client

- Not to take potassium supplements or eat foods rich in potassium
- That the medication may cause drowsiness, mental confusion, gynecomastia, and menstrual irregularities
- About the warning signs of fluid and electrolyte imbalance
- To contact the physician without delay if warning signs occur

Special Considerations

- Excessive potassium intake may cause hyperkalemia in clients taking potassium-sparing diuretics.
- When used in combination with other diuretics or antihypertensive agents, potassium-sparing diuretics potentiate their effects. Dosage of such drugs, particularly the ganglionic blocking agents, should be reduced by 50 percent.
- Severe hyperkalemia may occur when ACE inhibitors or indomethacin are administered concurrently with potassium-sparing diuretics.
- Reduces the vascular response to norepinephrine; therefore, cautious use in clients undergoing regional or general anesthesia should be the rule.

● Increases the half-life of digoxin; therefore, clients receiving any form of digitalis should be monitored very carefully while taking any potassium-sparing diuretic.

Osmotic Diuretics

Osmotic diuretics are agents that are capable of being filtered by the glomerulus, but have a limited capability of being reabsorbed into the bloodstream. They act by increasing the osmolality of the plasma, glomerular filtrate, and tubular fluid, thereby increasing the excretion of water, chloride, sodium, and potassium.

Uses

To prevent acute renal failure during trauma or prolonged surgery, to prevent increased cerebral, cerebrospinal, or intraocular pressures during trauma or surgery or disease, and to reduce intraocular pressure in acute glaucoma.

Contraindications

Contraindicated in clients who are known to be hypersensitive to any of its ingredients. They should not be used in anuria, diagnosed acute renal failure, cardiac dysfunction, congestive heart failure, active intracranial hemorrhage, severe dehydration, or severe pulmonary congestion.

Adverse Reactions

Marked diuresis, urinary retention, thirst, dizziness, headache, convulsions, nausea, vomiting, dry mouth, diarrhea, thrombophlebitis, hypotension, hypertension, tachycardia, angina-like chest pains, fever, chills, pulmonary congestion, fluid, electrolyte imbalance, dehydration, loss of hearing, blurred vision, nasal congestion, decreased intraocular pressure.

Dosage and Route

The dosage and route of administration is determined by the physician and individualized for each client. See Table 27-1.

Nursing Considerations

Observe client for evidence of fluid or electrolyte imbalance and signs of circulatory overload. Monitor weight, intake and output ratio, vital signs, and serum electrolytes. Observe IV administration sites for signs of local irritation, extravasation, and/or thrombophlebitis.

Clients' Instruction

Educate the client

● To increase fluid intake to 2–3 liters per day unless contraindicated
● That sucking on ice chips and/or hard candy will help relieve his/her thirst

Special Considerations

● Parenteral mannitol crystallizes at low temperatures. Store at 59° to 89°F, unless otherwise ordered. Do not allow it to freeze. If the medication crystallizes, warm it in a hot-water bath and shake container vigorously, then allow the solution to return to room temperature before administration.
● Do not add whole blood to IV lines used for mannitol.
● Do not mix this medication with any other drug or solution.

Carbonic Anhydrase Inhibitor Diuretics

Carbonic anhydrase inhibitor diuretics act to promote the reabsorption of sodium and bicarbonate from the proximal tubules. They block the action of the enzyme carbonic anhydrase (found in the kidneys, eyes, and other organs), thereby reversing the hydration of carbon dioxide and producing a bicarbonate diuresis that promotes the excretion of water, sodium, and potassium. These effects also decrease the formation of aqueous humor, thus reducing intraocular pressure.

Uses

For adjunctive therapy of chronic simple (open-angle) glaucoma, secondary glaucoma, and preoperatively in acute angle-closure glaucoma where delay of surgery is desired in order to lower intraocular pressure.

Contraindications

Contraindicated in clients who are known to be hypersensitive to any of its ingredients. Should not be used in hepatic insufficiency, renal failure, adrenocortical insufficiency, hyperchloremic acidosis, or in conditions where serum levels of sodium and potassium are depressed, and/or severe pulmonary obstruction.

Adverse Reactions

Anorexia, nausea, vomiting, drowsiness, paresthesia, ataxia, tremor, tinnitus, headache, weakness, nervousness, depression, confusion, dizziness, constipation, hepatic insufficiency, loss of weight, electrolyte imbalance, metabolic acidosis, skin eruptions, pruritus, fever, agranulocytosis, thrombocytopenia, frequency of urination, renal colic, renal calculi, phosphaturia.

Dosage and Route

The dosage and route of administration is determined by the physician and individualized for each client. See Table 27-1.

Nursing Considerations

Observe client for evidence of fluid or electrolyte imbalance. Monitor weight, intake and output ratio, vital signs, and serum electrolytes. Administer medication by mouth or IV if possible, because administration by IM injection is painful. Monitor client for signs of metabolic acidosis.

Clients' Instruction

Educate the client

- To increase fluid intake to 2–3 liters per day unless contraindicated
- To eat potassium-rich foods
- To avoid hazardous activities if drowsiness or dizziness occurs
- About warning signs of fluid or electrolyte imbalance
- To contact the physician without delay if warning signs occur
- That the medication should be taken in the morning to avoid nocturia
- That any eye pain should be reported to the physician without delay

Special Considerations

- If serum potassium is below 3.0, potassium supplements are needed.
- Cautious use in clients receiving high doses of aspirin, and during pregnancy and lactation
- Metabolic acidosis signs and symptoms: headache, fatigue, hypotension, anorexia, nausea, vomiting, dysrhythmia, drowsiness, confusion, seizures, coma, Kussmaul's respirations.

URINARY TRACT INFECTIONS (UTI): CYSTITIS

Cystitis is an inflammation of the urinary bladder. The urinary bladder is a muscular, membranous sac that serves as a reservoir for urine. It is located in the anterior portion of the pelvic cavity and consists of a lower portion, the neck, which is continuous with the urethra, and an upper portion, the apex, which is connected to the umbilicus by the median umbilical ligament. The urethra is the musculomembranous tube extending from the bladder to the outside of the body. The external urinary opening is the urinary meatus. The male urethra is approximately 8 inches long and the female urethra is approximately 1.5 inches long.

Each year, in the United States, approximately 10 million clients seek treatment for urinary tract infections, with cystitis being the most common. Cystitis is most often caused by an ascending infection from the urethra and it is more common in the female, because of the short length of the urethra that promotes the transmission of bacteria from the skin and genitals to the internal bladder. The most common type of bacteria that causes cystitis in the female is *Escherichia coli (E. coli)*, the colon bacillus. This bacillus is constantly present in the alimentary canal and is normally nonpathogenic, but when it enters the urinary tract and is transmitted to the bladder, it can cause infection. Cystitis in men is usually secondary to some other type of infection such as epididymitis, prostatitis, gonorrhea, syphilis, and/or kidney stones. Table 27-2 lists the symptoms of cystitis and the methods used to diagnose the condition.

Treatment

Treatment of cystitis usually consists of taking an antibiotic or antibacterial agent for a specified number of times and days, depending of the type of infection and its severity. The sulfonamides and antibiotics such as penicillins, cephalosporins, tetracyclines, and aminoglycosides are generally the drugs of first choice. Always ask the client if he/she is allergic to any medication before the initiation of drug therapy.

TABLE 27-2   CYSTITIS: SYMPTOMS AND DIAGNOSTIC METHODS

Symptoms	
Urgency	Frequency
Pyuria	Hematuria
Chills and fever	Pain or spasm in the region of the bladder and pelvic area
Burning sensation and pain during urination	
Diagnostic Methods	
History of symptoms	Gram stain
Microscopic urinalysis	Urine culture
Dipstick	

Note: If there is any question about a person's hypersensitivity to an antibiotic and/or sulfa drugs, an appropriate skin test should be performed before the initiation of drug therapy.

The client should be informed about possible adverse reactions to the prescribed medication and be instructed to report any signs to his/her physician. Advise the client to take the medication as prescribed until all of the drug has been taken.

Interstitial Cystitis

Interstitial cystitis (IC) is a painful inflammation of the bladder wall. Approximately 450,000 people suffer from this condition and 90 percent are women. Research showed that the median age of onset was 40, with many women experiencing symptoms as early as their 20s and 30s.

Symptoms can vary from mild to severe and are similar to a urinary tract infection (cystitis). There is usually pelvic pain and pressure, frequent urination, sometimes as often as 50 times a day. Diagnosis is difficult because the standard blood tests, urine tests, and x-rays come up negative. The cause is unknown and IC does not respond to antibiotic therapy. Women with IC often live in chronic pain. They are always tired because they are going to the bathroom often, and their sexual, social, and work life are affected.

Guidelines to Help Avoid Cystitis (Female)

- Drink plenty of fluids (8 glasses or more) a day.
- To avoid contaminating the urinary meatus, females should wipe themselves from front to back.
- Females who have repeated infections (cystitis) should drink a glass of water before engaging in sexual intercourse, and then urinate right after intercourse. This helps flush out any bacteria that could have entered the urethra.
- Have your sexual partner wear a condom.
- Do not use vaginal deodorants, bubble baths, colored toilet paper, and other substances that could cause irritation to the urinary meatus.
- Wear cotton underclothes and keep the genital area dry.

URINARY TRACT ANTIBACTERIALS

Sulfonamides are among the drugs of choice for treating acute, uncomplicated urinary tract infections, especially those caused by *Escherichia coli* and ***Pro-***

teus mirabilis bacterial strains. The sulfonamides may be classified according to the length of time they remain in the body. Using this criterion, these drugs can be separated into three groupings: short-, intermediate-, and long-acting sulfonamides. The short-acting sulfonamides are used in the treatment of urinary infections because they are rapidly absorbed, can be terminated quickly if adverse reactions occur, and produce high levels of the drug in urine.

Sulfonamides

Actions

Sulfonamides exert a bacteriostatic effect against a wide range of gram-positive and gram-negative microorganisms. They prevent the growth of microorganisms by inhibiting the production of dihydrofolic acid in the bacterial cells by competing with para-aminobenzoic acid (PABA).

Uses

Acute, recurrent, or chronic urinary tract infections due to susceptible organisms (*Escherichia coli*, ***Klebsiella-Enterobacter, staphylococcus, Proteus mirabilis***, and *Proteus vulgaris*). Also used in meningococcal meningitis, acute otitis media, trachoma, inclusion conjunctivitis, nocardiosis, and/or chancroid.

Contraindications

Contraindicated in clients who are known to be hypersensitive to any of its ingredients. They should not be used in infants less than 2 months of age, pregnancy and lactation.

Safety Precaution: Should not be used for the treatment of group A beta-hemolytic streptococcal infections.

Adverse Reactions

Agranulocytosis, aplastic anemia, myocarditis, serum sickness, hemolytic anemia, purpura, anaphylaxis, hepatitis, pancreatitis, nausea, vomiting, abdominal pain, diarrhea, anorexia, convulsions, peripheral neuritis, ataxia, vertigo, headache, tinnitus, depression, apathy, arthralgia, myalgia, edema, fever, chills, weakness, fatigue, insomnia, photosensitivity.

Dosage and Route

The dosage and route of administration is determined by the physician and individualized for each client. See Table 27-3.

TABLE 27-3　SELECTED SULFONAMIDES

Medication	Usual Dosage	Adverse Reactions
sulfadiazine (Microsulfon)	Oral (Adult): 2–4 g initially, then 0.5–1 g every 6 hours times 10 days Oral (Child): 74 mg/kg initially, then 150 mg/kg in 4–6 divided doses	Nausea, vomiting, headache, confusion, drug fever, blood dyscrasias
sulfamethoxazole (Gantanol)	Oral (Adult): 1–2 g initially, then 1 g two times a day Oral (Child over 2 months): 50–60 mg/kg initially, then 25–30 mg/kg two times a day (maximum 75 mg/kg/day)	Blood dyscrasias, hemolysis, drug fever, rash, nausea, vomiting, headache
sulfisoxazole (Gantrisin)	Oral (Adult): 2–4 g initially, then 1–2 g every 4–6 hours Oral (Child): 75 mg/kg initially, then 150 mg/kg/day in divided doses every 4 hours (maximum, 6 g daily)	Agranulocytosis, erythema multiform, nausea, emesis, headache, drug fever, chills
MIXTURES trimethoprim and sulfamethoxazole (Bactrim) (Septra)	Oral (Adult): 2 tablets or 4 teaspoons (20 ml) of suspension every 12 hours for 10–14 days Oral (Child): 8 mg/kg of trimethoprim and 40 mg/kg of sulfamethoxazole daily in 2 divided doses every 12 hours for 10 days	Blood dyscrasias, nausea, vomiting, anorexia, rash, urticaria

Nursing Considerations

Before initiation of drug therapy make sure that the client is not allergic to sulfonamides. Monitor the client for any adverse reactions, especially for signs that may indicate serious reactions and/or blood dyscrasia (fever, sore throat, arthralgia, cough, shortness of breath, pallor, purpura, jaundice). Monitor intake and output ratio, kidney function studies, and note the color, character, and pH of the client's urine.

Clients' Instruction

Educate the client

- To drink plenty of fluids
- To take the medication with 8 ounces of water
- To take the medication as ordered and for the full-time period to prevent superimposed infection
- To avoid direct sunlight, as he/she may be more sensitive to burns and photosensitivity while taking sulfonamides
- Not to take over-the-counter medications that contain aspirin and vitamin C unless prescribed by physician

- About signs of serious adverse reactions
- To contact physician without delay if signs of serious adverse reactions occur

Special Considerations

- Sulfonamides may decrease the effectiveness of oral contraceptives. Therefore, the client should use additional methods of birth control.
- Some sulfonamide preparations may produce orange-yellow discoloration of the urine.
- May decrease the absorption of digoxin; therefore, serum digoxin levels should be carefully monitored and dosage adjustment made as necessary.
- Can potentiate the blood sugar lowering activity of sulfonylurea. Blood glucose levels should be monitored and dosage adjustment made as necessary.
- May increase anticoagulant effect of warfarin agents. Coagulation time should be monitored and dosage adjustment made as necessary.
- Can displace methotrexate from plasma protein-binding sites, thereby increasing free methotrexate concentrations

URINARY TRACT ANTISEPTICS

The urinary antiseptics, although used against urinary tract infections, are not usually drugs of first choice in such treatments. The sulfonamides and antibiotics such as penicillins, cephalosporins, tetracyclines, and aminoglycosides are generally the drugs of first choice that are used to treat urinary tract infections.

Urinary antiseptics are most often used in clients who are either intolerant of or unresponsive to one of the first-choice antibiotics. They are also used for the control of chronic urinary infections due to microorganisms that have developed resistance to other drugs.

Actions

Urinary antiseptics may inhibit the growth of microorganisms by bactericidal, bacteriostatic, anti-infective, and/or antibacterial action.

Uses

Treatment of acute and chronic upper and lower urinary tract infections, asymptomatic bacteriuria

caused by susceptible strains of *Escherichia coli, Proteus mirabilis, Morganella morganii, Providencia rettgeri, Proteus vulgaris, Pseudomonas, Enterobacter,* and *Enterococci.*

Contraindications

Contraindicated in clients who are known to be hypersensitive to any of its ingredients. They should not be used in anuria, renal insufficiency, severe dehydration, pregnancy, and lactation. Certain urinary tract antiseptics are contraindicated in children, clients with convulsive disorders, anemia, diabetes, and/or chronic lung disease.

Adverse Reactions

The adverse reactions of urinary antiseptics are listed according to the drug.

Dosage and Route

The dosage and route of administration is determined by the physician and individualized for each client. See Table 27-4.

TABLE 27-4   URINARY ANTISEPTICS

Medication	Usual Dosage	Adverse Reactions
cinoxacin (Cinobac)	Oral (Adult): 1 g daily in 2–4 divided doses for 7–14 days	Nausea, headache, dizziness, rash, pruritus, edema, anorexia, insomnia, photophobia, perineal burning
ciprofloxacin (Cipro)	Oral (Adult): 250–500 mg every 12 hours	CNA stimulation, superinfection, nausea, diarrhea, vomiting, GI discomfort, headache, restlessness, rash, crystalluria
methenamine (Mandelamine) (Hiprex)	Oral (Adult): 1 g 4 times/day after meals and at bedtime Oral (Child 6–12): one-half the adult dose as shown above	Mild gastric irritation, rash, headache, nausea, vomiting
nalidixic acid (NegGram)	Oral (Adult): 4 g/day in 4 divided doses for 2 weeks, reduced to 2 g per day for long-term therapy Oral (Child under 12): 55 mg/kg/day in 4 divided doses	Headache, malaise, weakness, convulsions, photosensitivity, nausea, vomiting
nitrofurantoin (Furadantin) (Macrodantin)	Oral (Adult): 50–100 mg 4 times/day Oral (Child): 5–7 mg/kg/24 hours in 4 divided doses (dose reduced by half if continued past 10 days)	Nausea, vomiting, diarrhea, fever, rash, urticaria
norfloxacin (Noroxin)	Oral (Adult): 400 mg twice a day for 7–10 days. Take 1 hr before or 2 hr after meals with 8 ounces of water.	Crystalluria, dizziness, nausea, headache
trimethoprim (Trimpex)	Oral (Adult): 100–200 mg every 24 hours for 10 days	Rash, pruritus, GI discomfort, blood dyscrasias, drug fever, liver and renal disorders, exfoliative dermatitis

Nursing Considerations

Observe the client for signs of improvement and/or adverse reactions. Monitor intake and output ratio, vital signs, culture and sensitivity tests. Methenamine yields formaldehyde in the presence of an acidic urine, which helps suppress the growth and multiplication of bacteria. This may cause recurrent infection.

Ascorbic acid may be prescribed to help maintain the acidity of urine. Ascorbic acid tablets should not be crushed as they allow the formation of formaldehyde in the stomach, resulting in nausea and belching.

Clients' Instruction

Educate the client

- To increase fluid intake to 2–3 liters per day unless contraindicated
- To report any signs of adverse reactions
- To take his/her medication as prescribed until all of the drug has been taken (It is most important that the client understands this, as many times once the client starts to feel better he/she may discontinue taking the drug, and a relapse can occur.)
- About proper personal hygienic practices

Special Considerations

- A culture and sensitivity test should be performed prior to the initiation of drug therapy to determine the causative type of microorganism.
- A culture and sensitivity test should be performed after the completion of drug therapy to determine the effectiveness of therapy.
- Medication must be taken in equal intervals, day and night, to maintain proper blood levels.

MISCELLANEOUS AGENTS

Miscellaneous agents are used to treat disorders of the lower urinary tract. These agents either stimulate, inhibit, or relax smooth muscle activity and help control involuntary contractions of the bladder muscle. These actions help improve the functions of the urinary bladder, such as storage of urine and its subsequent excretion from the body. See Table 27-5 for selected agents used for urologic disorders. Table 27-6 lists medications and agents that discolor urine.

TABLE 27-5   MISCELLANEOUS AGENTS

Medication	Action	Usual Dosage	Adverse Reactions
bethanechol chloride (Duvoid) (Myotonachol) (Urecholine)	Facilitates bladder emptying	Oral (Adult): 25 mg every 6 hours	Flushing, headache, nausea, vomiting, diarrhea, sweating, salivation
dimethyl sulfoxide (Rimso-50)	Treatment of interstitial cystitis	Intravesical instillation: 50 ml of a 50% solution into the bladder	Garlic-like taste and odor
flavoxate HCl (Urispas)	Reduces dysuria, nocturia, and urinary frequency	Oral (Adult): 100–200 mg 3–4 times/day	Nausea, vomiting, dryness of the mouth, nervousness, blurred vision, vertigo
hyoscyamine sulfate (Cystospaz-M) (Levsin)	Relaxes smooth muscle bladder spasm	Oral (Adult): 1 capsule every 12 hours	Dryness of the mouth, photophobia, constipation
imipramine HCl (Tofranil)	Treatment of nocturnal enuresis in children	Oral (Child): 10 mg nightly for 1 week or as needed	Drowsiness, dryness of the mouth, constipation, nausea, blurred vision
oxybutynin chloride (Ditropan XL)	Relaxes the muscles in the bladder, thereby decreasing the occurrence of wetting accidents	Oral (Adult): One 5 mg tablet once a day	Dry mouth, constipation, sleepiness, headache, diarrhea, nausea, loss of energy, dizziness

(continued)

TABLE 27-5 MISCELLANEOUS AGENTS (*Continued*)

Medication	Action	Usual Dosage	Adverse Reactions
pentosan polysulfate sodium (Elmiron)	Exact mechanism of action is unknown; used for the relief of bladder pain or discomfort associated with interstitial cystitis (CI)	Oral (Adult): 300 mg/day taken as one 100 mg capsule 3 times/day. Should be taken with water and at least 1 hr before meals or 2 hr after meals	Diarrhea, nausea, dizziness, alopecia (reversible upon discontinuation), headache, rash, dyspepsia, abdominal pain, liver function abnormalities
*phenazopyridine HCl (Pyridium)	Analgesic, anesthetic action on the urinary tract mucosa	Oral (Adult): 200 mg 3 times/day after meals. *Stains urine and fabric red-orange.*	Headache, rash, GI discomfort, hemolytic anemia, renal and hepatic toxicity
tolterodine tartrate (Detrol) (See Figure 27-1)	Helps control involuntary contractions of the bladder muscle	Oral (Adult): 2 mg tablet 2 times/day. May be lowered to 1 mg tablet 2 times/day	Dry mouth, headache, constipation, indigestion, dry eyes

*Phenazopyridine may cause the sclera to turn yellow. This may indicate an accumulation of the drug due to decreased renal function.

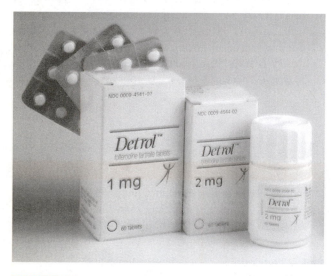

FIGURE 27-1 DETROL™ (TOLTERODINE TARTRATE) 1 MG, 2 MG TABLETS (*Courtesy of Pharmacia Corporation*)

TABLE 27-6 SELECTED AGENTS THAT DISCOLOR URINE

Agent	Color
Aldomet (methyldopa)	Red to black
Aralen (chloroquine)	Rust-yellow to brown
Atabrine (quinacrine HCl)	Yellow
Azulfidine (sulfasalazine)	Orange-yellow
Coumadin sodium (warfarin sodium)	Orange
Desferal (deferoxamine mesylate)	Red
Dilantin (phenytoin)	Pink or red to red-brown
Dopar (levodopa)	Darkening of urine upon standing
Dyrenium (triamterene)	Pale blue fluorescence
Elavil (amitriptyline HCl)	Blue-green
Flagyl (metronidazole)	Darkened urine
Furadantin (nitrofurantoin)	Rust-yellow or brownish
Furoxone (furazolidone)	Brown, orange-brown
Indocin (indomethacin)	Green
Iron (IV)	Blackening
Macrodantin (nitrofurantoin)	Rust-yellow or brownish
Pyridium (phenazopyridine HCl)	Red or orange
Rifadin (rifampin)	Bright red-orange
Robaxin (methocarbamol)	Brown to black to green upon standing
sulfonamides	Rust-yellow or brownish
Vitamin B$_2$ (riboflavin)	Yellow

● SPOT CHECK

There are several medications that may be used to treat urinary tract infections. For each of the selected drugs, give the usual dosage and several adverse reactions.

Drug	Usual Dosage	Adverse Reactions
Gantrisin		
Furadantin		
Hiprex		
Cipro		
Pyridium		

● SELF-ASSESSMENT

Write the answer in the space provided or circle true or false as instructed.

Source

p. 346   **1.** Diuretic medications decrease reabsorption of _____ by the _____, thereby increasing the amount of _____ and water excreted in the urine.

p. 348   **2.** On the lines provided, classify the following products by their diuretic classification:

- Diamox is a _____ diuretic.
- Lasix is a _____ diuretic.
- Osmitrol is a _____ diuretic.
- Midamor is a _____ diuretic.
- Diuril is a _____ diuretic.

p. 349   **3.** True or False (circle one) Potassium supplements and foods such as bananas that are rich in potassium are contraindicated when Aldactone is prescribed.

p. 350   **4.** The use of diuretic agents to reduce intraocular pressure is indicated for persons undergoing treatment for _____.

p. 352   **5.** An appropriate _____ should be performed when there is a question as to a person's hypersensitivity to an antibiotic and/or sulfa drug.

p. 352   **6.** Three reasons are given why short-acting sulfonamides are used in the treatment of urinary infections. In a few words, what are the three reasons given in the chapter?

- Short-acting sulfonamides are _____.
- Short-acting sulfonamides can be _____.
- Short-acting sulfonamides produce _____.

p. 354   **7.** True or False (circle one) Urinary tract antiseptics are usually the drugs of first choice in the treatment of urinary tract infections.

p. 355   **8.** Give a reason why culture and sensitivity tests should be done in the following cases:

- Prior to starting drug therapy to _____
- Upon completion of drug therapy to _____

● WEB ACTIVITY

Visit the following Web sites for additional information on medications used for urinary system disorders:

http://pharmacology.medscape.com

http://www.discoveryhealth.com

http://www.pslgroup.com

http://www.rxlist.com

http://pharmacotherapy.medscape.com

http://www.docguide.com

http://www.pharminfo.com

http://www.allsands.com/Health

http://www.diagnosishealth.com

http://www.intelihealth.com

http://www.mediconsult.com

http://www.kidney.org

http://www.sonic.net

http://www.duj.com

http://www.ichelp.com

http://www.intercyst.org

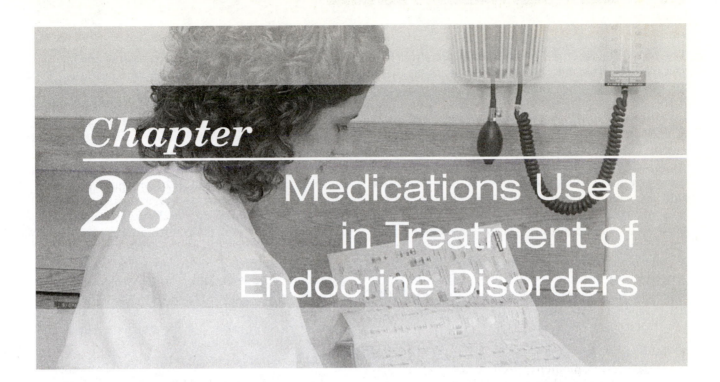

Chapter

28 Medications Used in Treatment of Endocrine Disorders

Chapter Outline

Objectives
Key Terms
Introduction
The Pituitary
The Thyroid
The Parathyroids
The Adrenals
The Islets of Langerhans
Self-Assessment
Web Activity

Objectives

Upon completion of this chapter, you should be able to

- Define the key terms
- Give the location and functions of the endocrine glands described in this chapter
- Describe the various hormones and drugs that are used in endocrine system disorders
- Understand the actions, uses, contraindications, safety precautions, adverse reactions, dosage and route, nursing considerations, clients' instruction, and special considerations for selected drugs

- Describe diabetes mellitus and give the warning signs and symptoms of diabetes, and the signs and symptoms of hypoglycemia and hyperglycemia
- List the types of insulin preparations according to rapid-acting, immediate-acting, and long-acting
- Complete the Spot Check on types of insulin
- List the four classifications of oral hypoglycemic agents and describe how each works
- Identify selected drugs according to each described oral hypoglycemic classification
- Describe hyperglycemic agents
- Complete the Self-Assessment
- Visit indicated Web sites for additional information on medications used for endocrine system disorders

Key Terms

acromegaly	gigantism
cretinism	hormone
diabetes insipidus	hyperglycemia
diabetes mellitus	hypoglycemia
dwarfism	myxedema

INTRODUCTION

The primary glands of the endocrine system are the pituitary, the thyroid, the parathyroids, the islets of Langerhans in the pancreas, the adrenals, the testes, and the ovaries. See Figure 28-1. This chapter covers each of these glands, with the exception of the testes and ovaries, which are discussed as part of the reproductive system in Chapter 31.

The ductless glands of the endocrine system secrete chemical substances known as **hormones** that are carried through the blood. Each of the endocrine glands performs an important part in growth, development, and maintenance of normal body functions. The hormones secreted by these glands act as chemical transmitters that either stimulate or inhibit specific organs of the body. When abnormal production of hormones occurs (too little or too much), the resultant disorders can be life-threatening.

THE PITUITARY

The pituitary is a small gland located at the base of the brain. Sometimes called the *master gland*, the pituitary secretes hormones that are essential for the body's growth and development and the regulation of actions by other endocrine glands. Pituitary hormones are grouped according to the lobe of the gland in which they originate.

An improperly functioning pituitary gland can be caused by a genetic condition or it may be the result of injury, surgery, tumors, or radiation. Disorders of the pituitary relate to the overproduction or underproduction of certain hormones.

● Hyperpituitarism occurs with the overproduction of hormones and can cause **gigantism**, a condition in which there is excessive development of the body or of a body part. If hyperpituitarism occurs after puberty, the feet, hands, and

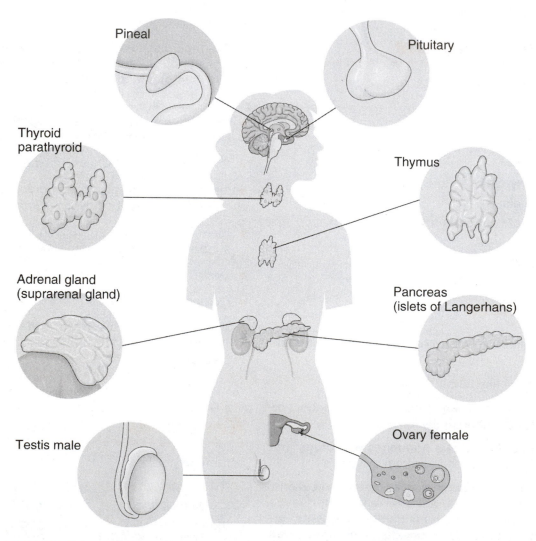

Pineal

Pituitary

Thyroid parathyroid

Thymus

Adrenal gland (suprarenal gland)

Pancreas (islets of Langerhans)

Testis male

Ovary female

FIGURE 28-1 LOCATION OF THE ENDOCRINE GLANDS

face show overgrowth and the resultant condition is known as **acromegaly**. The overproduction of pituitary hormones is often associated with the presence of a tumor. Treatment may involve radiation, chemotherapy, or surgery.

- Hypopituitarism occurs with the underproduction of hormones by the gland. An inadequate supply of pituitary hormones can cause **dwarfism**, a condition of being abnormally small, in the developing child, as well as poor growth and function of the thyroid gland, the sex glands, and the adrenal cortex. Somatropin (Asellacrin) is administered to individuals with this condition following careful screening.

- **Diabetes insipidus** occurs with the underproduction or absence of the hormone vasopressin, also known as antidiuretic hormone (ADH). This condition should not be confused with diabetes mellitus, and is treated by the administration of natural and synthetic substances (Vasopressin, Lypressin) that produce antidiuretic hormone activity.

THE THYROID

The thyroid gland is a large, bilobed gland located in the neck. Two hormones, thyroxine (T_4) and triiodothyronine (T_3), are stored and secreted by the thyroid. When released into the bloodstream, these hormones influence the metabolic rate (the rate at which foods are burned in the tissues). Iodine, which is obtained from the diet, is essential for the production of thyroid hormones.

The amount of hormone produced is also important. If the thyroid produces too much hormone, the resulting condition is known as *hyperthyroidism* and is characterized by a high basal metabolism rate. Should the gland produce too little hormone, a condition known as *hypothyroidism* results and is characterized by a low metabolic rate. The thyroid-stimulating hormone (TSH), thyrotropin, from the anterior lobe of the pituitary gland, regulates the activity of the thyroid and must be present along with an adequate iodine intake for it to function properly. **Cretinism**, a congenital condition that is due to a deficiency in the secretion of thyroid hormones in which there is arrested physical and mental development, and **myxedema**, an acquired condition (in older children and adults) that is due to a deficiency in the secretion of thyroid hormones, in adults are conditions resulting from untreated hypothyroidism. Graves' disease, characterized by bulging eyeballs and other symptoms, is the most common form of hyperthyroidism. Early detection and appropriate replacement therapy with thyroid preparations is necessary in treating hypothyroidism. Antithyroid drugs, radiation, or surgery are used in the treatment of hyperthyroidism.

Thyroid Hormones
Actions

Thyroid hormones increase metabolic rate, cardiac output, oxygen consumption, body temperature, respiratory rate, blood volume, carbohydrate, fat and protein metabolism, and influence growth and development at cellular level.

Uses

Thyroid hormones are used as supplements or replacement therapy in hypothyroidism, myxedema, cretinism, and following a thyroidectomy.

Contraindications

Thyroid hormones are contraindicated in clients with adrenal insufficiency, myocardial infarction, and thyrotoxicosis.

Adverse Reactions

Sweating, alopecia, anxiety, insomnia, tremors, headache, heat intolerance, fever, tachycardia, palpitations, angina, dysrhythmia, hypertension, nausea, diarrhea, increased or decreased appetite.

Dosage and Route

The dosage and route of administration is determined by the physician and individualized for each client. See Table 28-1 for selected drugs used to treat hypothyroidism.

Nursing Considerations

Assess blood pressure and pulse before each dose. If pulse is above 100 beats per minute in adults and in excess of the normal range in children, withhold the medication and notify the physician. Monitor weight gain and/or loss, intake and output ratio, and the child's height and growth rate. Report any signs of hyperthyroidism (loss of weight, palpitations, diaphoresis, tachycardia, and insomnia) to the client's physician. Administer medication at the same time each day, preferably before breakfast, to maintain drug level and help reduce the possibility of insomnia.

Clients' Instruction

Educate the client

- To take the medication as prescribed (best to take before breakfast)

TABLE 28-1   DRUGS USED IN THYROID DISORDERS

Medication	Usual Dosage	Adverse Reactions
Hyperthyroidism		
methimazole (Tapazole)	Oral (Adult): Initial: 15–60 mg in divided doses every 6 hours, then 5–15 mg daily Oral (Child): 0.4 mg/kg/day in 3 doses every 8 hours initially, then 0.2 mg/kg/day	Pruritus, rash, abdominal discomfort, nausea, headache, agranulocytosis
potassium iodide solution (SSKI)	Oral: 0.3 ml 3 times daily	Brassy taste, burning in the mouth, hypersalivation, rash, productive cough, diarrhea
propranolol HCl (Inderal)	Oral: 10–30 mg 3–4 times daily	Bradycardia, bronchospasm, nausea, abdominal cramping, hypotension
propylthiouracil (PTU)	Oral (Adult): 300 mg/day divided into 3 doses at 8-hour intervals; maintenance dosage 100–150 mg/day	Pruritus, nausea, headache, agranulocytosis, abdominal discomfort, rash
strong iodine solution (Lugol's solution)	Oral: 0.3 ml 3 times daily	Brassy taste, diarrhea, rash, hypersalivation, burning in the mouth, cough
Hypothyroidism		
levothyroxine sodium (Levothroid) (Synthroid)	Oral: 50–100 mcg/day, increased by increments of 50–100 mcg/day at 2–3 week intervals until the desired response is maintained	Symptoms of hyperthyroidism may occur with overdose.
liothyronine sodium (Cytomel)	Oral: 25 mcg/day, increased by increments of 12.5–25 mcg/day at 1–2 week intervals until the desired response is maintained	Symptoms of hyperthyroidism may occur with overdose.
liotrix (Thyrolar)	Oral: initially 1 tablet daily, increased by 1 tablet every 2 weeks until the desired desired response is maintained	Symptoms of hyperthyroidism may occur with overdose.
thyroid, USP	Oral: initially 15–30 mg/daily, increased by increments of 15–30 mg/day at 2 week intervals until the desired response is obtained; usual maintenance dose is 60–120 mg in a single dose	Symptoms of hyperthyroidism may occur with overdose.

- To avoid foods and over-the-counter medications that contain iodine
- To report any signs of excitability, irritability, and anxiety to the physician
- That if loss of hair occurs it is generally temporary
- That the child on thyroid hormone therapy will show almost immediate personality and behavior changes

Special Considerations

- When a client's medication regimen includes anticoagulants, the pro-time should be monitored carefully, as the dosage of the anticoagulant may have to be decreased.
- When a client's medication regimen includes insulin, blood glucose level should be monitored carefully, as the dosage of insulin may have to be increased.

- Medication is generally not taken one to several weeks before thyroid function studies.
- To prevent binding of thyroid hormones by cholestyramine, administer at least 4 hours apart.

Antithyroid Hormones

Actions

Inhibits the synthesis of thyroid hormones by decreasing iodine use in manufacture of thyroglobin and iodothyronine. Does not inactivate or inhibit thyroxine or triiodothyronine.

Uses

Antithyroid hormones are used to treat hyperthyroidism, in preparation for thyroidectomy, in thyrotoxic crisis and thyroid storm.

Contraindications

Antithyroid hormones are contraindicated in clients who are hypersensitive to any of the ingredients, and during pregnancy (3rd trimester) and lactation.

Adverse Reactions

Rash, urticaria, pruritus, alopecia, hyperpigmentation, irregular menses, drowsiness, headache, vertigo, fever, paresthesia, neuritis, nausea, diarrhea, vomiting, jaundice, loss of taste, myalgia, arthralgia, nocturnal muscle cramps, agranulocytosis, leukopenia, thrombocytopenia.

Dosage and Route

The dosage and route of administration is determined by the physician and individualized for each client. See Table 28-1 for selected drugs used to treat hyperthyroidism.

Nursing Considerations

Assess blood pressure, pulse, temperature, intake and output ratio, and weight. Observe for signs of improvement and/or hypersensitivity, also edema, bleeding, petechiae, ecchymosis. Evaluate blood work, especially CBC for blood dyscrasia: leukopenia, agranulocytosis, thrombocytopenia. Unless contraindicated encourage client to drink plenty of fluids (3–4 liters/day).

Clients' Instruction

Educate the client

- To follow the prescribed medication regimen
- That the medicine should be stored in a light-resistant container

- To dilute liquid iodine preparation and take through a straw to minimize unpleasant taste
- To report any signs of blood dyscrasia (redness, swelling, sore throat, mouth lesions); signs of overdose (periorbital edema, cold intolerance, mental depression); signs of inadequate dose (tachycardia, diarrhea, fever, irritability) to the physician
- To take his/her pulse daily, measure weight, and be aware of mood changes
- To avoid foods and over-the-counter medications that contain iodine

Special Considerations

- Medication may increase effect of anticoagulants. Pro-time should be monitored carefully.
- Best to administer with meals to decrease gastrointestinal upset and at the same time each day to maintain proper drug level
- Liquid preparations should be diluted and given through a straw to minimize unpleasant taste.
- Medication should be stored in a light-resistant container.

THE PARATHYROIDS

The parathyroid glands are about the size of a pinhead and can be found on either side of the thyroid gland. They secrete *parathormone* in response to lowered serum calcium levels. Parathormone (or PTH) acts in several ways to increase levels of calcium and phosphorus in the body.

A deficiency of parathormone may occur as a consequence of surgery or due to a genetic defect. Symptoms of parathormone deficiency include increased neuromuscular irritability and psychiatric disorders.

THE ADRENALS

Located atop each kidney are the triangular-shaped adrenal glands, each with a tough outer cortex and an inner medulla that secrete hormones. Adrenocorticotropic hormone (ACTH) from the pituitary gland stimulates the adrenals to produce a number of important hormones that regulate fat, salt, and water metabolism; are essential to the development of male secondary sex characteristics; and assist in the regulation of the sympathetic branch of the autonomic nervous system. The adrenal cortex secretes three groups of hormones: the glucocorticoids, the mineralocorticoids, and the androgens. The adrenal medulla synthesizes, stores, and secretes dopamine, epinephrine, and norepinephrine.

Primary adrenocortical insufficiency (Addison's disease) is a progressive condition associated with adrenal atrophy. Symptoms of this disease include hyperpigmentation (copper-colored skin), nausea, vomiting, weight loss, anorexia, weakness, hypotension, and a danger of dehydration. Cortisone and cortisol are the agents most often used in replacement therapy for primary adrenal insufficiency.

THE ISLETS OF LANGERHANS

The word *insulin* comes from the Latin *insula*, which means island. Therefore, it is not surprising that the source of the hormone insulin is the beta cells of the islets of Langerhans. These endocrine glands are masses of cells scattered throughout the pancreas.

Insulin is essential for the proper metabolism of carbohydrates, fats, and proteins. Normally, insulin is released following the rise in blood glucose level that accompanies the ingestion of food. As with other endocrine glands, the oversecretion or undersecretion of hormone results in specific disorders.

When too much insulin is present in the blood, an abnormally low level of blood sugar (glucose) is the result. This condition, known as **hypoglycemia**, is characterized by acute fatigue, marked irritability, and weakness. An overdose of insulin can produce a condition known as insulin shock.

When too little insulin is present in the blood, an abnormally high level of blood sugar is the result. This condition, known as **hyperglycemia**, increases the body's susceptibility to infection and produces symptoms of the disease diabetes mellitus.

Diabetes Mellitus

Diabetes mellitus is a complex metabolic disorder that disrupts the body's ability to produce or use insulin. Insulin is a hormone secreted by the beta cells of the islets of Langerhans. It is essential for the metabolism of carbohydrates, fats, and proteins. Insulin helps convert food into the vital energy source that is needed by the body to help make it function properly. The insulin in the body must be maintained at a certain level, usually between 70 and 110 mg/dL of blood. When the level of insulin is too high, hypoglycemia (low blood sugar) can occur. When the level of insulin is too low, hyperglycemia (high blood sugar) can occur.

Diabetes affects 14 million Americans, with care and treatment costing $20 billion annually. The National Institute of Diabetes and Digestive and Kidney Diseases conducted a 10-year Diabetes Control and Complications Trial on how best to control the complications of insulin-dependent diabetes mellitus (IDDM) and found that those in the intensive-control group who tested their blood sugar four or more times a day and injected insulin three or more times a day, or who used an insulin pump and followed a special diet, showed reductions in complications.

The American Diabetes Association estimates that 7 million Americans have diabetes and do not know it. Are you at risk for diabetes? Do you have any, some, or many of the signs and symptoms of diabetes? (See Table 28-2.) If your answer is yes, you should see a physician and be carefully evaluated and tested for diabetes. For more information on diabetes, you may call 1-800-DIABETES or visit the Web site http://www.diabetes.org.

The National Diabetes Data Group of the National Institutes of Health has categorized the various forms of diabetes mellitus as Type I—insulin-dependent diabetes mellitus (IDDM); Type II—non-insulin-dependent diabetes mellitus (NIDDM); Type III—women who have developed glucose intolerance in association with pregnancy; and Type IV—diabetes associated with pancreatic disease, hormonal changes, the adverse effects of drugs, and other anomalies.

One in ten people who have diabetes are Type I diabetics and must take insulin on a regular basis. Insulin was discovered in 1921 by Sir F. G. Banting. The individual with Type I diabetes is faced with a lifetime commitment of trying to juggle and balance insulin, diet, exercise, other disease processes, stress, and all the other factors that are involved in one's life. Without proper treatment and control,

TABLE 28-2 WARNING SIGNS AND SYMPTOMS OF DIABETES

- Frequent urination (polyuria)
- Excessive thirst (polydipsia)
- Extreme hunger (polyphagia)
- Unexplained weight loss
- Extreme fatigue
- Blurred vision
- Slow-healing wounds
- Tingling or numbing in your feet and/or hands
- Frequent vaginal (female) or skin infections
- Itchy skin
- Irritability
- Drowsiness

diabetes can lead to cardiovascular disease, nephropathy, neuropathy, retinopathy, and death.

Understanding diabetes is the best method for controlling the disease. Through knowledge, self-regulation, discipline, and following the proper medication regimen, diet, exercise program, and weight control, one may be successful in living a full life. Self-monitoring of blood glucose is an important part of managing diabetes. To teach self-monitoring to a client, consider the person's age, cognitive level of understanding, physical ability, and desire to learn the skill. The following are suggestions you may use to teach a client self-monitoring of his/her blood glucose level.

Show and instruct the client how to

- Use the blood glucose monitoring equipment/instrument that the physician has recommended
- Use a prepackaged sterile alcohol swab to cleanse the finger before performing a skin puncture
- Wipe off the first drop of blood with a sterile cotton ball (if recommended)
- Place a drop of blood onto the test strip and how to place the strip onto/into the monitor
- Read the test results
- Record the results and the importance of keeping a daily log, with time(s) and date
- Determine the dosage of insulin based upon the physician's ordered sliding scale
- Properly dispose of used materials

The client should be instructed on when and how many times a day to check his/her blood glucose level. Usually, this is before meals and when one "feels" different than normal. The client should report a high blood glucose level to his/her physician and take insulin as instructed. When the blood glucose level is low, the client should eat some "quick sugar." For example: 1/2 cup of orange juice, milk, or soda; several hard candies; and/or take three glucose tablets.

Refer to Table 28-3 for signs and symptoms of hypoglycemia and hyperglycemia.

Drugs That Affect Blood Glucose Levels

There are many medications that can affect blood glucose levels. The diabetic client needs to know of these medications and the physician should be informed about all drugs that his/her diabetic client takes. Table 28-4 lists some drugs (with examples) that can affect blood glucose levels.

Insulin

Actions

Insulin stimulates carbohydrate metabolism by increasing the movement of glucose and other monosaccharides into cells. It also influences fat and carbohydrate metabolism in the liver and adipose cells. It decreases blood sugar, phosphate, and potassium, and increases blood pyruvate and lactate.

Uses

Insulin is used in insulin-dependent diabetes mellitus (Type I IDDM), non-insulin-dependent diabetes mellitus (Type II NIDDM) when other treat-

TABLE 28-3   SIGNS AND SYMPTOMS: HYPOGLYCEMIA AND HYPERGLYCEMIA

Hypoglycemia	Hyperglycemia
• Tremors (shaking)	• Skin is flushed, hot, and dry
• Fast heartbeat (palpitations)	• Pulse rapid and weak
• Blurred vision	• Drowsiness, loss of consciousness
• Sweating	• Low blood pressure
• Hunger	• Rapid, deep respirations
• Irritability	• Breath has sweet, fruity odor
• Headache	• Thirsty
• Weakness	• Blood sugar above 200 mg/dL
• Confusion	
• Loss of consciousness	
• Convulsions	
• Blood sugar subnormal: 20–50 mg/dL	

TABLE 28-4 DRUGS THAT CAN CAUSE HYPOGLYCEMIA OR HYPERGLYCEMIA

Hypoglycemia	Hyperglycemia
● Alcohol	● Calcium-channel blockers
● Allopurinol (Lopurin, Zyloprim)	● Corticosteroids
● Chloramphenicol (Chloromycetin)	● Diazoxide (Proglycem)
● Clofibrate (Abitrate, Atromid-S)	● Isoniazid (Laniazid, Nydrazid)
● Fenfluramine (Pondimin)	● Levothyroxine (Levoxine, Synthroid)
● Monoamine oxidase inhibitors (MAOIs)	● Oral contraceptives
● Phenylbutazone (Butatab, Butazolidin)	● Phenytoin (Dilantin)
● Salicylates	● Rifampin (Rifadin, Rimactane)
● Sulfonamides	● Thiazide diuretics

ment regimens are not effective, and to treat ketoacidosis.

Contraindications

Insulin is essential for life, and if the client becomes hypersensitive to one type of insulin, another type is prescribed by the physician.

Adverse Reactions

Headache, lethargy, tremors, weakness, fatigue, delirium, sweating, tachycardia, palpitations, blurred vision, hunger, nausea, hypoglycemia, flushing, rash, urticaria, and anaphylaxis.

Dosage and Route

The dosage is individualized for each client and depends upon the client's blood glucose level. The route of administration is parenteral. It cannot be given orally because peptidases in the digestive juices destroy the protein molecule.

Nursing Considerations

To provide essential care to a client with diabetes, the nurse must be familiar with the various types of insulin preparations and their onset of action, peak action, duration of action, and appearance. See Table 28-5.

Clients' Instruction

Client instruction involves a wide scope of activities and the involvement of numerous health professionals. Educate the client

- And his/her family about the person's specific type of diabetes
- About the treatment regimen (medication, diet, exercise, weight control/reduction/management, rest, stress management, and lifestyle modification)
- How to properly test blood sugar and/or urine glucose levels
- How to store and handle insulin
- About the symptoms and treatment for hypoglycemia and hyperglycemia
- When to seek medical attention
- How to properly administer insulin (To teach a client and/or a family member how to administer insulin, you should use the information on subcutaneous injection provided in Chapter 17, Administration of Parenteral Medications.)

To teach other aspects of diabetic care, one should use an appropriate source and seek the assistance of other health professionals. It is not possible to include all the information a nurse needs to know about diabetes and its management in this text, but the following is basic information a nurse should know and be able to teach to the client and his/her family:

- Insulin is given subcutaneously, using a site rotation system.
- While using, most insulin preparations may be stored at room temperature. Other insulin should be stored in a refrigerator, and then warmed to room temperature before use. Always check the expiration date before use. Insulin should be gently rotated in the palms of the hands to mix and should never be shaken.
- The client needs to know that with the initiation of insulin therapy, blurred vision may occur, and that usually vision is stabilized in 1–2 months. The client should not change contact lenses or eye glasses without the advice of the physician.

TABLE 28-5   INSULIN PREPARATIONS

Type of Insulin (Trade Name)	Onset of Action	Peak Action	Duration of Action	Appearance
Rapid-Acting				
insulin injection				
(Regular Insulin)	0.5 hr	2.5–5 hr	6–8 hr	Clear
(Novolin R)	0.5 hr	2.5–5 hr	6–8 hr	Clear
(Humalog)	5–15 min	1–2 hr	4–5 hr	Clear
(Velosulin)	0.5 hr	1–3 hr	6–8 hr	Clear
prompt insulin zinc suspension				
(Semilente Insulin)	1–1.5 hr	5–10 hr	12–16 hr	Cloudy
Intermediate-Acting				
isophane insulin suspension				
(NPH and Lente)	2–4 hr	8–10 hr	18–24 hr	Cloudy
(Humulin L)	1–1.5 hr	4–12 hr	18–24 hr	Cloudy
(Novolin N)	1–1.5 hr	4–12 hr	18–24 hr	Cloudy
(Humulin N)	1–1.5 hr	4–12 hr	18–24 hr	Cloudy
insulin zinc suspension				
(Lente Insulin)	2–2.5 hr	7–15 hr	18–24 hr	Cloudy
(Novolin L)	2–2.5 hr	7–15 hr	18–24 hr	Cloudy
Long-Acting				
(Humulin U)	1–1.5 hr	8–12 hr	18–24 hr	Cloudy
extended insulin zinc suspension				
(Ultralente)	3–5 hr	10–12 hr	36 hr	Cloudy

- The client needs to know that with unusual stress, infection, and/or other health-related conditions, it may be necessary to increase his/her dosage of insulin.
- One should monitor blood glucose levels very carefully and use the correct dose of insulin to maintain proper blood glucose level during times of stress and/or disease.
- The client should always wear or carry a Medic Alert ID. The client should always have the appropriate equipment, medication (Insulin), and candy or lump sugar in his/her possession.
- The client should not use over-the-counter medications without the physician's permission.
- The client should not smoke or drink alcoholic beverages while taking insulin.
- The client needs to know that insulin is a lifetime drug and that its proper use is essential in helping prevent complicating conditions/diseases.

Special Considerations

- The client needs special care and consideration for the prescribed treatment regimen to be an effective lifetime routine.
- Hypoglycemia may be increased with the use of MAOIs, alcohol, beta-blockers, anabolic steroids, guanethidine, salicylate, fenfluramine, tetracycline, clofibrate, and oral hypoglycemics.
- Hyperglycemia may be increased with the use of oral contraceptives, corticosteroids, estrogens, lithium, thiazides, thyroid hormones, triamterene, phenothiazines, and phenytoin.

● SPOT CHECK

For each of the following types of insulin, give the onset of action, peak of action, duration of action, and the normal appearance.

Type of Insulin	Onset	Peak	Duration	Appearance
Regular Insulin				
Semilente Insulin				
NPH and Lente Insulin				
Lente Insulin				
Humulin U				

Oral Hypoglycemic Agents

Oral hypoglycemic agents may be used in conjunction with diet and exercise in the management and treatment of non-insulin-dependent (NIDDM) Type II diabetes. They are classified as sulfonylureas, biguanides, thiazolidinediones, and alpha-glucosidase inhibitors.

- Sulfonylureas (Amaryl, DiaBeta, Diabinese, Dymelor, Glucotrol, Micronase, Orinase, Tolinase) work primarily by stimulating the pancreas to release more insulin.
- Biguanides (Glucophage) work by decreasing the release of glucose by the liver and by making cells more sensitive to insulin.
- Thiazolidinediones (Actos, Avandia) work primarily by making cells more sensitive to insulin.

- Alpha-glucosidase inhibitors (Precose) slow the body's absorption of carbohydrates. This allows the insulin in the body to work better. The medication is taken before each meal.

Sulfonylureas

Agents of the sulfonylurea class of chemical compounds are used to stimulate insulin secretion from pancreatic islet cells in non-insulin-dependent diabetes with some pancreatic function.

Actions

Sulfonylureas stimulate functioning beta cells in the pancreas to release insulin, thereby lowering blood glucose levels. These agents are not effective if the client lacks functioning beta cells.

Uses

Sulfonylureas are used in non-insulin-dependent (NIDDM) Type II stable adult-onset diabetes mellitus.

Contraindications

Sulfonylureas are contraindicated in clients who are hypersensitive to any of its ingredients, juvenile or brittle diabetes, severe renal disease, and severe hepatic disease.

Adverse Reactions

Headache, weakness, paresthesia, nausea, heartburn, vomiting, abdominal pain, diarrhea, hepatotoxicity, cholestatic jaundice, leukopenia, thrombocytopenia, agranulocytosis, aplastic anemia, rash, allergic reaction, pruritus, urticaria, eczema, photosensitivity, erythema, hypoglycemia, and joint pains.

Dosage and Route

The dosage is determined by the physician and individualized for each client. The route of administration is oral. See Table 28-6 for selected oral sulfonylureas.

Nursing Considerations

Monitor the client's blood glucose level and urine test to determine glucose balance. Observe the client for signs of improvement and any adverse reactions.

Clients' Instruction

Educate the client

- And his/her family about the client's specific type of diabetes
- About the treatment regimen (medication, diet, exercise, weight control/reduction/management, rest, stress management, and lifestyle modification)
- About how to properly test blood sugar and/or urine glucose levels
- About the symptoms and treatment for hypoglycemia and hyperglycemia
- About when to seek medical attention
- To take the medication in the morning to prevent hypoglycemic reactions at night
- To be alert for signs of cholestatic jaundice (dark urine, pruritus [severe itching], and yellow sclera). (The physician should be notified immediately if any of these signs occur.)
- To wear a Medic Alert ID
- Not to use over-the-counter medications without the physician's permission
- Not smoke or drink alcoholic beverages while taking oral hypoglycemic agents

TABLE 28-6   SULFONYLUREAS

Medications	Usual Dosage	Adverse Reactions
chlorpropamide (Diabinese)	Oral: 100–500 mg once daily	Hypoglycemia, nausea, vomiting, diarrhea, pruritus
glimepiride (Amaryl)	Oral 1–2 mg once daily, given with breakfast or the first main meal	Hypoglycemia, nausea, vomiting, GI pain, diarrhea, dizziness, headache, pruritus, leukopenia, hemolytic anemia, blurred vision
glipizide (Glucotrol)	Oral: 5 mg initially, then increased by 2.5–5 mg/day until blood glucose level is satisfactory; maximum dose 40 mg daily	Hypoglycemia, nausea and diarrhea, constipation and gastralgia
glyburide (DiaBeta) (Micronase)	Oral: 2.5–5 mg/day initially; maintenance dose ranges from 1.25 to 20 mg/daily	Hypoglycemia, nausea, heartburn, epigastric fullness, allergic skin reactions
tolazamide (Tolinase)	Oral: 100–1000 mg/day in single or divided doses	Hypoglycemia, nausea, heartburn, epigastric fullness
tolbutamide (Orinase)	Oral: 1–2 g/day initially; maintenance dose ranges from 0.25 to 3 g/daily	Hypoglycemia, nausea, heartburn, epigastric fullness, allergic skin reactions

Special Considerations

- The client needs special care and consideration for the prescribed treatment regimen to be an effective lifetime routine.
- The effect of oral hypoglycemic agents may be increased with the use of insulin, MAOIs, and cimetidine.
- The effect of oral hypoglycemic agents may be decreased with the use of calcium channel blockers, corticosteroids, oral contraceptives, estrogens, thiazide diuretics, thyroid preparations, phenothiazines, phenytoin, rifampin, and isoniazid.

Biguanides

Metformin Hydrochloride (Glucophage)

Glucophage is an oral hypoglycemic agent in the chemical group known as biguanides. It can be used alone or in combination with sulfonylurea agents, when glycemia control is inadequate with a sulfonylurea or the client suffers too many adverse reactions.

Actions

Decreases hepatic glucose production, decreases intestinal absorption of glucose, and improves insulin sensitivity (increases peripheral glucose uptake and utilization).

Uses

In the management of non-insulin-dependent diabetes mellitus (NIDDM).

Contraindications

- Renal disease or renal dysfunction
- Should be temporarily withheld in clients undergoing radiologic studies involving parenteral administration of iodinated contrast materials, because use of such products may result in acute alteration of renal function
- Known hypersensitivity to metformin hydrochloride
- Acute or chronic metabolic acidosis, including diabetic ketoacidosis, with or without coma. Diabetic ketoacidosis should be treated with insulin.
- Not recommended for use in pregnancy or for use in children

> **Safety Precaution:** Lactic acidosis is a rare, but serious, metabolic complication that can occur due to metformin accumulation during treatment with Glucophage. When it occurs, it is fatal in approximately 50 percent of cases. Lactic acidosis is characterized by elevated blood lactate levels (>5 mmol/L), decreased blood pH, electrolyte disturbances with an increased anion gap, and an increased lactate/pyruvate ratio. When metformin is implicated as the cause of lactic acidosis, metformin levels >5 microgram/ml are generally found.

Adverse Reactions

Lactic acidosis, diarrhea, nausea, vomiting, abdominal bloating, flatulence, anorexia, unpleasant or metallic taste, rash, dermatitis.

Dosage and Route

Dosage is individualized for each client. The usual starting dose is one 500 mg tablet twice a day with the morning and evening meals. Dosage increases should be made in increments of one tablet every week, given in divided doses, up to a maximum of 2500 mg per day.

Nursing Considerations

Monitor the client's blood glucose level and urine test to determine glucose balance. Observe the client for signs of improvement and any adverse reactions.

Thiazolidinediones (TZDs)

The Food and Drug Administration has approved Avandia (rosiglitazone maleate), Avelox (moxifloxacin hydrochloride), and Actos (pioglitazone hydrochloride) for Type II diabetes. These drugs are a member of a new class of oral diabetes agents called thiazolidinediones (TZDs), which act as insulin sensitizers. In contrast to traditional Type II diabetes medicines, which increase insulin production in the pancreas or decrease glucose output through the liver, these drugs are believed to reduce the amount of insulin needed while improving blood sugar control.

Rosiglitazone Maleate (Avandia)

Avandia is used to treat Type II diabetes by helping the body use the insulin it is already making. It comes in pill form and can be taken either once or twice a day to help control blood sugar levels.

Actions

Avandia helps the body use insulin by making the cells less resistant to insulin so that the sugar can enter the cell.

Uses

It is recommended for Type II diabetes in people over 18 who do not have liver disease or severe heart disease.

Contraindications

Avandia is contraindicated in clients with known hypersensitivity or allergy to any of its components.

Adverse Reactions

Upper respiratory infection, headache, weight gain, edema, anemia.

Dosage and Route

Oral, once a day in the morning or twice a day in the morning and evening.

Clients' Instruction

It is important that the client call the physician immediately if he/she experiences nausea, vomiting, stomach pain, tiredness, lack of appetite, dark urine, or yellowing of the skin. For some women with diabetes, insulin resistance may interfere with their ability to become pregnant. Because Avandia reduces insulin resistance, it may restore their ability to become pregnant. Therefore, the client may need to consider birth-control measures. Although Avandia did not show signs of liver problems in studies, the physician may recommend a liver test before starting it and from time to time while using the drug.

Pioglitazone (Actos)

Actos is the latest member of the thiazolidinedione class of drugs. It is approved for use as sole therapy in diabetics who are unable to control their blood sugar with diet and exercise alone. It is also approved for use in combination with other classes of diabetes-controlling drugs such as sulfonylureas.

Actos (15 mg, 30 mg, or 45 mg) is given orally, once daily. The majority of adverse reactions during clinical trials were mild. The most commonly reported included symptoms of upper respiratory infection, headache, sinusitis, muscle pain, tooth disorder, and sore throat. As observed with other members of this class of drugs, weight gain has been noted. Additionally, mild to moderate edema and anemia were reported in clients taking Actos.

There have been no reported cases of jaundice or liver failure associated with Actos use in the United States. However, it is recommended that clients obtain medical monitoring of liver enzyme levels prior to the start of therapy, every 2 months for the first year of therapy and periodically thereafter. In premenopausal anovulatory clients with insulin resistance, treatment with any thiazolidinedione may result in resumption of ovulation. These clients may be at risk of pregnancy.

Alpha Glucosidase Inhibitors

Acarbose (Precose)

Precose is an oral hypoglycemic agent in the chemical group known as alpha-glucosidase inhibitors. It slows the body's absorption of carbohydrates. This allows the insulin in the body to work better. Precose must be taken with the first bite of food at each meal. It may be used alone or in combination with a sulfonylurea.

Actions

Acarbose blocks the enzymes that digest starches in food. This results in a slower and lower rise of blood sugar throughout the day.

Uses

Acarbose is used in non-insulin-dependent (NIDDM) Type II diabetes.

Contraindications

Acarbose is contraindicated in clients who are hypersensitive to any of its ingredients. Cautious use in clients with inflammatory bowel disease, ulcers of the colon, intestinal obstruction, or chronic intestinal disease.

Adverse Reactions

Alpha-glucosidase inhibitors can cause gastrointestinal symptoms such as cramping, gas, and diarrhea. These symptoms usually pass with time as the body adjusts to the new medication. Other adverse reactions that may occur are rash, hives, or fever.

Dosage and Route

The dosage is determined by the physician and individualized for each client. The route of administration is oral. The usual starting dose is 50 mg three times daily. The maximum dose is 300 mg/day.

Hyperglycemic Agents

Hyperglycemic agents are used to cause an increase in blood glucose of diabetic clients with severe hypoglycemia (insulin shock). In clients with mild hypoglycemia, the administration of an oral carbohydrate (CHO) such as orange juice, candy, or a lump of sugar will generally correct the condition. If comatose, adults may be given 10–30 ml of 50% dextrose solution, IV, and children should receive 0.5–1 ml/kg of 50% dextrose solution, IV.

Glucagon, an insulin antagonist, may be used in the acute management of severe hypoglycemia. It increases blood glucose levels by increasing the breakdown of glycogen to glucose and inhibits glycogen synthesis. It is useful in hypoglycemia only if liver glycogen is available and should be used only with medical supervision. For adults, the dose is 0.5–1 mg, IM, IV, or SC, repeated in 20 minutes when necessary. For children, the dose is 25 mcg/kg up to a maximum dose of 1 mg, IM, IV, or SC, repeated in 20 minutes when necessary. It is contraindicated in individuals with hyperactivity to beef or pork protein and/or glucagon, pheochromocytoma, or a history of insulinoma. Adverse reactions include nausea, vomiting, and an allergic reaction.

Proglycem (diazoxide) is a hyperglycemic agent that may be used in the treatment of hypoglycemia associated with hyperinsulinism or other causes. Oral diazoxide produces a prompt dose-related increase in blood glucose levels by inhibition of pancreatic insulin release. For adults and children, the dose is 1 mg/kg every 8 hours initially; further adjustments are made on the basis of response. Usual maintenance dose is 3–8 mg/kg/day given in divided doses every 8–12 hours. For infants and newborns, the dose is 3.3 mg/kg/day divided into two or three equal doses every 8–12 hours. Proglycem is rapidly absorbed orally and has an onset of action within 1 hour. It has a duration of 8 hours and a half-life between 20 and 36 hours in most individuals. The adverse reactions include taste alterations, anorexia, nausea, vomiting, abdominal pain, constipation, edema, tachycardia, and allergic reaction. It is contraindicated in individuals with hypersensitivity to diazoxide, sulfonamides, and/or thiazides; in clients with coronary or cerebral insufficiency and acute aortic dissection; and in clients who have an inadequate cardiac reserve or compensatory hypertension.

Glucose (Glutose, Insta-Glucose) may be used to correct hypoglycemia in conscious clients. It is well absorbed following oral administration, widely distributed, and rapidly utilized. For adults and children, the oral dose is 10–20 g, and it may be repeated in 10–20 minutes if necessary. Glucose is available as an oral gel and in chewable tablets. It is also available as an intravenous solution for injection. The IV dose for adults is 20–50 ml of 50% solution infused slowly (3 ml/min). The IV dose for infants and neonates is 250–500 mg/kg/dose (as 25% dextrose); repeated doses of 10–12 ml of 25% dextrose may be required.

● SELF-ASSESSMENT

Write the answer in the space provided or circle true or false as instructed.

Source

p. 360   **1.** Endocrine gland secretions are called _____ and act as chemical transmitters that either _____ or _____ specific organs of the body.

p. 360   **2.** Hyperpituitarism occurs with the _____ of hormones and can cause _____ .

p. 361   **3.** True or False (circle one) Thyroid hormones are used as supplements or replacement therapy in cases of adrenal insufficiency and thyrotoxicosis.

p. 363   **4.** On the lines provided, name the three groups of hormones secreted by the adrenal cortex.

   (1) _____

   (2) _____

   (3) _____

p. 364   **5.** In as few words as possible, define the term *hypoglycemia*. _____

p. 364   **6.** In as few words as possible, distinguish between the following types of diabetes:

   ● Type I _____

   ● Type II _____

   ● Type III _____

   ● Type IV _____

p. 367   **7.** Three types of insulin are rapid-acting, intermediate-acting, and long-acting. Identify the following insulins by their type:

   ● Humalog _____

   ● Humulin N_____

   ● Novolin L _____

   ● Novolin R _____

   ● Ultralente _____

p. 368–
371

8. In a few words, distinguish between the actions of the following oral hypoglycemic agents:

- Sulfonylureas act by

_____ .

- Thiazolidinediones act by

_____ .

- Alpha-glucosidase inhibitors act by

_____ .

● WEB ACTIVITY

Visit the following Web sites for additional information on medications used for endocrine system disorders:

http://www.diabetes.org
http://pharmacology.medscape.com
http://www.discoveryhealth.com
http://www.pslgroup.com
http://www.rxlist.com
http://pharmacotherapy.medscape.com
http://www.docguide.com
http://www.pharminfo.com
http://www.allsands.com/Health
http://www.diagnosishealth.com
http://www.intelihealth.com
http://www.mediconsult.com
http://www.onhealth.com/ch1/condctr/diabetes
http://www.mayohealth.org

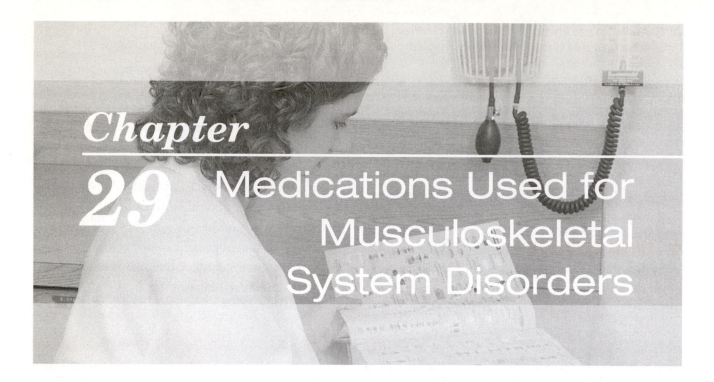

Chapter

29 Medications Used for Musculoskeletal System Disorders

Chapter Outline

Objectives

Upon completion of this chapter, you should be able to

- Define the key terms
- Describe the musculoskeletal system
- Describe the various drug classifications used for musculoskeletal system disorders

- Understand the actions, uses, contraindications, safety precautions, adverse reaction, dosage and route, nursing considerations, client instructions, and special considerations for selected drugs
- Complete the Spot Check on nonsteroidal anti-inflammatory drugs
- Complete the Self-Assessment
- Visit indicated Web sites for additional information on medications used for musculoskeletal system disorders

Key Terms

acetylcholine

acetylcholinesterase

anticholinesterase

autoimmune response

chrysotherapy

cyclooxygenase (COX)

hyperuricemia

inflammation

muscle spasm

neuromuscular junction

INTRODUCTION

The musculoskeletal system is made up of muscles, bones, ligaments, and tendons. The skeleton consists of 206 interconnected bones that give the body its unique shape and provide support for its organs and tissues. There are more than 650 muscles in the body. Those that attach to the skeleton are known as skeletal muscles. The maintenance of normal body posture and the production of movement in response to voluntary control are basic functions of these muscles.

Each skeletal muscle is activated by a motor nerve that has its origin at the spinal cord and terminates in fibers connected to muscle cells. The point at which a motor nerve fiber connects to a muscle cell is known as a **neuromuscular junction**. When an electrical impulse of sufficient strength passes from the spinal cord, over the motor nerve, to this junction, it causes the release of the cholinergic neurotransmitter **acetylcholine** (a cholinergic neurotransmitter that is thought to play an important role in the transmission of nerve impulses at synapses and myoneural junctions). This substance passes across the neuromuscular junction and binds to specialized receptor sites on that part of the muscle opposite the nerve ending. The presence of acetylcholine sends electrical stimulation throughout the muscle, causing it to contract. This action is countered by the presence of **acetylcholinesterase**, an enzyme that inactivates acetylcholine and readies muscle fibers for the next nerve impulse.

Because the musculoskeletal system is made up of living tissues and depends upon neuromuscular activity to function, this chapter will cover medications for the relief of pain and inflammation as well as drugs used to relax or stimulate skeletal muscles. See Chapter 30 for drugs used as analgesics.

ANTI-INFLAMMATORY DRUGS

Inflammation is a normal response to injury, infection, or irritation of living tissue. Redness, tenderness, pain, and swelling of the affected area are characteristics of the inflammatory process. Minor inflammation may occur as the result of a break in the skin or casual contact with a caustic substance. The more severe forms of inflammation are usually associated with rheumatic disorders such as arthritis.

Drugs that relieve the swelling, tenderness, redness, and pain of inflammation are known as anti-inflammatory agents. All but a few of these agents provide only symptomatic relief of pain and inflammation but do not treat its cause.

Steroidal anti-inflammatory agents are chemically related to the naturally occurring hormone cortisone secreted by the adrenal cortex. These agents are most often used in the treatment of local inflammatory disorders. Corticosteroids may be taken orally or injected into a joint or bursa (Table 29-1), or may be applied to the skin for topical treatment of dermatological conditions (Table 29-2). The use of steroidal agents to treat systemic inflammatory disorders is limited by the array of serious side effects caused by these drugs.

TABLE 29-1   CORTICOSTEROIDS FOR ORAL AND PARENTERAL USE

Medication	Oral Dose	Parenteral Dose	Local Injection
betamethasone (Celestone)	0.6–7.2 mg/day	IM, IV: 0.5–9 mg/day	—
cortisone acetate (Cortone)	25–300 mg/day	IM: 20–300 mg/day	—
dexamethasone (Decadron)	0.75–9 mg/day	IM, IV: 0.5–9 mg/day	—
dexamethasone acetate (Decadron-LA)	—	—	0.8–16 mg, rapid onset/long duration
dexamethasone sodium phosphate (Decadron Phosphate)	—	—	0.4–6 mg, rapid onset/short duration
hydrocortisone (Cortef)	20–240 mg/day	IM: 10–150 mg every 12 hours	—
hydrocortisone acetate (Cortef Acetate)	—	Intra-articular: 10–50 mg/dose	25–50 mg, slow onset/long duration
hydrocortisone cypionate (Cortef fluids)	20–240 mg/day	—	—
hydrocortisone sodium (Solu-Cortef)	—	IM, IV: 100–500 mg/day	—

(continued)

TABLE 29-1 *(Continued)*

Medication	Oral Dose	Parenteral Dose	Local Injection
hydrocortisone sodium phosphate (Hydrocortone Phosphate)	—	IM, IV: 15–240 mg/day	—
methylprednisolone (Medrol)	4–48 mg/day	—	—
methylprednisolone acetate (Depo-Medrol) (See Figure 29-1)	—	IM: 40–120 mg every 1–4 weeks	4–80 mg, slow onset/ long duration
methylprednisolone sodium succinate (Solu-Medrol)	—	IM, IV: 10–40 mg, may be repeated every 6 hours	—
prednisolone (Delta-Cortef)	5–60 mg/day	—	—
prednisolone sodium phosphate (Hydeltrasol)	—	IM, IV: 4–60 mg/day	2–30 mg, rapid onset/ short duration
prednisolone tebutate (Hydeltra-TBA)	—	—	8–30 mg, slow onset/ long duration
prednisone (Deltasone)	5–60 mg/day	—	—
triamcinolone (Aristocort)	4–40 mg/day	IM: 40 mg once a week	—
triamcinolone acetonide (Kenalog)	—	—	2.5–15 mg, slow onset/ long duration
triamcinolone diacetate (Amcort)	—	—	5–40 mg, intermediate onset and duration
triamcinolone hexacetonide (Aristospan)	—	—	2–20 mg, slow onset/ long duration

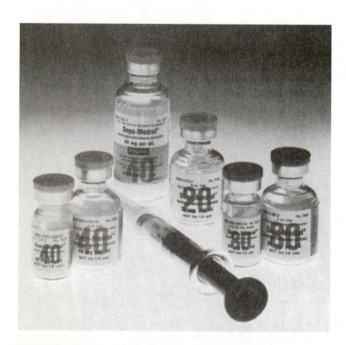

FIGURE 29-1 DEPO-MEDROL® 20 MG, 40 MG, AND 80 MG PER MILLILITER VIALS *(Courtesy of Pharmacia Corporation)*

Corticosteroids (Glucocorticoids)

Actions

Corticosteroids have potent anti-inflammatory effects in disorders of many organ systems. They also cause varied metabolic effects and modify the body's immune responses to assorted stimuli.

Uses

Primary or secondary adrenocortical insufficiency, congenital adrenal hyperplasia, nonsuppurative thyroiditis, hypercalcemia associated with cancer, as adjunctive therapy in psoriatic arthritis, rheumatoid arthritis, ankylosing spondylitis, acute and subacute bursitis, acute nonspecific tenosynovitis, acute gouty arthritis, posttraumatic osteoarthritis, synovitis of osteoarthritis, epicondylitis, and in the treatment of certain collagen, dermatologic, ophthalmic, respiratory, hematologic, gastrointestinal, and neoplastic diseases, during allergic states, edematous states, and cerebral edema.

TABLE 29-2   CORTICOSTEROIDS FOR TOPICAL USE

Medication	Usual Strength
amcinonide (Cyclocort)	0.1% cream
betamethasone (Celestone)	0.2% cream
betamethasone benzoate (Uticort)	0.025% cream, gel, lotion, ointment
betamethasone dipropionate (Diprosone)	0.05–0.1% aerosol, cream, lotion, ointment
betamethasone valerate (Valisone)	0.1–0.15% aerosol, cream, ointment
clobetasol (Temovate)	0.05% cream, ointment
desonide (Tridesilon)	0.05% cream, ointment
desoximetasone (Topicort)	0.25% cream
dexamethasone (Decadrox)	0.01–0.1% aerosol, cream
diflorasone diacetate (Florone)	0.05% cream, ointment

Medication	Usual Strength
fluocinolone acetonide (Fluonid)	0.01–0.2% cream, ointment, solution
fluocinonide (Fluonid)	0.05% cream, 0.005% ointment
flurandrenolide (Cordran)	0.025–0.05% lotion, cream, ointment, tape
halcinonide (Halog)	0.025–0.1% cream, ointment, solution
hydrocortisone (Cort-Dome)	0.125–2.5% aerosol, cream, gel, ointment
hydrocortisone acetate (Cortaid)	0.5–2.5% aerosol, cream, ointment
methylprednisolone acetate (Medrol Acetate)	0.25–1% ointment
triamcinolone acetonide (Aristocort)	0.025–0.5% aerosol, cream, gel, lotion, ointment

Contraindications

Contraindicated in clients with known hypersensitivity to any of its ingredients. They should not be used in clients with systemic fungal infections, idiopathic thrombocytopenia purpura, acute glomerulonephritis, amebiasis, nonasthmatic bronchial disease, and by children under 2 years of age.

Safety Precaution:

1. Corticosteroids may mask some signs of infection and new infections may appear during their use.
2. Prolonged use may produce posterior subcapsular cataracts and glaucoma with possible damage of the optic nerves, and may enhance the establishment of secondary ocular infections due to fungi or viruses.
3. Cautious use during pregnancy, lactation, active tuberculosis, and myocardial infarction
4. Average and large doses of the drug(s) can cause elevation of blood pressure, salt and water retention, and increased excretion of potassium.
5. All corticosteroids increase calcium secretion.

6. Administration of live virus vaccines are contraindicated in clients receiving immunosuppressive doses of corticosteroids.
7. There are many precautions associated with corticosteroids. Please refer to current edition of a *Physicians' Desk Reference* or a *PDR Nurse's Drug Handbook* for information on precautions.

Adverse Reactions

Sodium and fluid retention, congestive heart failure, potassium loss, hypokalemic alkalosis, hypertension, muscle weakness, steroid myopathy, loss of muscle mass, osteoporosis, peptic ulcer, pancreatitis, abdominal distention, poor wound healing, acne, ecchymosis, petechiae, depression, flushing, headache, mood changes, tachycardia, diarrhea, nausea, vertigo, convulsions, menstrual irregularities, development of cushingoid state, hirsutism, glaucoma, weight gain, increased appetite, malaise, hiccups.

Dosage and Route

The dosage and route of administration is determined by the physician and individualized for each client. (See Tables 29-1 and 29-2.)

Nursing Considerations

Observe client for evidence of fluid or electrolyte imbalance and any signs of adverse reactions. Monitor weight, intake and output ratio, vital signs, serum electrolytes, and during long-term therapy monitor blood sugar, urine glucose, and plasma cortisol levels. Protect the client from infection.

Clients' Instruction

Educate the client to

- Take the medication as prescribed
- Be alert for signs of adverse reactions
- Avoid the use of tobacco, alcohol, aspirin, caffeinated beverages, and over-the-counter medications unless he/she has the permission of the physician
- Wear or carry a Medic Alert ID that states he/she is on corticosteroid therapy
- Avoid individuals who have respiratory infections and guard against other types of infection
- Weigh him/herself weekly and report weight gain of 5 pounds or more to the physician
- Include foods high in potassium, low in sodium, and to take in an adequate amount of proteins, vitamins, and calcium in his/her diet

Special Considerations

- Prolonged corticosteroid therapy may result in a cushingoid state. Signs and symptoms include acne, moon face, hirsutism, Buffalo hump, hypertension, protruding abdomen, girdle obesity, amenorrhea, glycosuria, purplish abdominal striae, edema, thinning and atrophy of extremities.
- The effect of corticosteroids may be decreased by barbiturates, rifampin, ephedrine, and/or phenytoin.
- Corticosteroids may decrease the effect of anticoagulants, anticonvulsants, hypoglycemic agents, insulin, isoniazid, and/or neostigmine.
- Corticosteroids may increase digitalis toxicity as a result of increased potassium loss.
- The effect of corticosteroids may be increased by estrogens, salicylates, and/or indomethacin.

Nonsteroidal anti-inflammatory drugs (NSAIDs) are synthetic products that are unrelated to substances produced by the body. See Table 29-3. These agents are widely used in the treatment of inflammation, arthritis, and related disorders. Although the exact mechanism by which these agents act is not fully understood, their anti-inflammatory action is believed to result from inhibition of prostaglandins synthesis.

The most common adverse reactions associated with NSAIDs are nausea, vomiting, abdominal discomfort, diarrhea, constipation, gastric or duodenal ulcer formation, and gastrointestinal bleeding. Hematologic changes can occur and other adverse reactions that may occur are jaundice, toxic hepatitis, visual disturbances, rash, dermatitis, and hypersensitivity reactions. Usually, these adverse reactions are associated with high doses and prolonged drug therapy.

Gastrointestinal disturbances may occur with the use of NSAIDs and can be severe and even fatal, especially in clients with a history of gastric or duodenal ulcers. For the client with diabetes, these agents can affect the blood glucose level; therefore, insulin dosage may require adjustment. For the client taking warfarin, these drugs may potentiate the anticoagulant effect and increase the risk of bleeding. According to research, it is recommended that clients taking warfarin should avoid NSAIDs. If given, these drugs should be introduced slowly and given in lower dosages where feasible. Prothrombin time should be monitored closely, especially during the first 2 weeks. When NSAIDs are stopped, there may be a loss of anticoagulant control.

Safety Precaution: The Food and Drug Administration has indicated new labeling for Tylenol (acetaminophen) and Motrin (ibuprofen) pain relievers. The Motrin label warns of the risk of stomach bleeding for those who drink three or more alcoholic beverages daily and take ibuprofen or other pain relievers. Tylenol's label warns those who drink three or more alcoholic beverages daily that use of acetaminophen may increase their risk of liver damage when taken in larger-than-recommended doses. Both Motrin and Tylenol labels suggest that heavy users of alcohol consult their physicians regarding use of the product.

With Motrin (ibuprofen) there is an additional warning about an allergy alert. Ibuprofen may cause a severe allergic reaction including hives, facial swelling, asthma (wheezing), and/or shock. If an allergic reaction occurs, the client is advised to stop use of the medicine and to seek medical help right away. The client is advised not to use this product if he/she has ever had an allergic reaction to any other pain reliever/fever reducer.

TABLE 29-3   NONSTEROIDAL ANTI-INFLAMMATORY AGENTS

Medication	Usual Anti-inflammatory Dose	Adverse Reactions
acetylsalicylic acid (aspirin)	Oral: 3.6–5.4 g/day in divided doses	GI distress, tinnitus, rapid pulse, pulmonary edema
choline salicylate (Arthropan)	Oral: 1–2 tsp up to 4 times/day	See aspirin
diclofenac (Voltaren)	Oral: 50 mg 2–3 times/day	Dizziness, headache, GI bleeding, heartburn, abdominal pain, diarrhea, acute renal failure, rash, edema
diflunisal (Dolobid)	Oral: 500–1000 mg/day in 2 divided doses	GI distress, dizziness, skin rash, headache, tinnitus
etodolac (Lodine)	Oral: Initially 800–1200 mg/day in divided doses, then 600–1200 mg/day in divided doses. For acute pain: 200–400 mg every 6–8 hours, not to exceed 1200 mg/day	Dyspepsia, GI ulceration, GI bleeding, GI perforation, chills, fever, dizziness, malaise
fenoprofen calcium (Nalfon)	Oral: 300–600 mg 3–4 times/day	GI distress, dizziness, headache, drowsiness, tinnitus
ibuprofen (Motrin, Advil)	Oral: 300–600 mg 3–4 times/day	GI distress, dizziness, headache, drowsiness, tinnitus
indomethacin (Indocin)	Oral, Rectal: 25–50 mg 2–3 times/day. Sustained release: 75 mg once/day	GI distress, dizziness, headache, drowsiness
ketoprofen (Orudis)	Oral: 150–300 mg/day, divided in 3 or 4 doses	Peptic ulcer, GI bleeding, nausea, malaise, diarrhea, anorexia, headache, dizziness, rash, tinnitus
ketorolac (Toradol)	IM: Loading dose: 30–60 mg. Maintenance: 15–30 mg	Drowsiness, nausea, gastrointestinal pain, GI bleeding, GI ulceration
meclofenamate sodium (Meclomen)	Oral: 50–100 mg 3–4 times/day	GI distress
naproxen (Naprosyn)	Oral: 250–500 mg 2 times/day	GI distress, dizziness, headache, drowsiness, tinnitus
naproxen sodium (Aleve)	Oral: 275–550 mg twice daily (up to 1.65 g/day)	GI bleeding, anorexia, constipation, nausea, dizziness, drowsiness, headache, tinnitus, dyspnea, edema, palpitations, tachycardia, cystitis, renal failure, photosensitivity, rash, blood dyscrasias, anaphylaxis
piroxicam (Feldene)	Oral: 20 mg/day as a single or divided dose	GI distress, dizziness, rash, rapid pulse
salsalate (Disalcid)	Oral: 325–1000 mg 2–3 times/day	GI distress, tinnitus, rapid pulse, pulmonary edema
sulindac (Clinoril)	Oral: 150–200 mg 2 times/day	GI distress, dizziness, skin rash
tolmetin sodium (Tolectin)	Oral: 600–1800 mg/day in divided doses	GI distress, lightheadedness, dizziness

● SPOT CHECK

There are many nonsteroidal anti-inflammatory drugs that are used to treat the symptoms of inflammation. For each of the following drugs, give the usual anti-inflammatory dose and several adverse reactions.

Drug(s)	Usual Anti-inflammatory Dose	Adverse Reactions
Acetylsalicylic acid		
Ibuprofen		
Naproxen		
Piroxicam		
Ketorolac		

DISEASE-MODIFYING ANTIRHEUMATIC DRUGS (DMARDs)

Disease-modifying antirheumatic drugs (DMARDs) are also called slow-acting antirheumatic drugs (SAARDs) or second-line drugs. Although nonsteroidal anti-inflammatory drugs reduce pain and inflammation and improve stiffness and mobility in clients with rheumatoid arthritis, they do not slow the progression of joint damage. Disease-modifying antirheumatic drugs may influence the course of the disease progression; therefore, their introduction in early rheumatoid arthritis is recommended to limit irreversible joint damage. Examples of DMARDs are gold preparations (Aurolate, Ridaura, and Solganol), antimalarials (Plaquenil Sulfate), penicillamine (Cuprimine), sulfasalazine (Azulfidine), leflunomide (Arava), and the immunosuppressants methotrexate (Rheumatrex), azathioprine (Imuran), and cyclophosphamide (Cytoxan). See Table 29-4.

TABLE 29-4   DISEASE-MODIFYING ANTIRHEUMATIC DRUGS (DMARDs)

Medication	Usual Anti-inflammatory Dose	Adverse Reactions
auranofin (Ridaura)	Oral: 3 mg twice/day or 6 mg once/day	Loose stools or diarrhea, nausea, rash, pruritus, stomatitis, proteinuria
aurothioglucose (Solganol)	IM: 10 mg the 1st week, 25 mg the 2nd and 3rd weeks, then 50 mg thereafter until a total of 800–1000 mg has been given	Pruritus, "gold dermatitis," ulcerative stomatitis, hypersensitivity reactions, nephrotic syndrome with proteinuria, conjunctivitis
azathioprine (Imuran)	Oral: 1 mg/kg/day for 6–8 weeks, then increase by 0.5 mg/kg/day every 4 weeks until response or up to 2.5 mg/kg/day, then decrease by 0.5 mg/kg/day every 4–8 weeks to minimal effective dose	Retinopathy, anorexia, nausea, vomiting, diarrhea, hepatotoxicity, alopecia, pulmonary edema, rash, anemia, leukopenia, chills, fever
cyclophosphamide (Cytoxan)	Oral: 1–5 mg/kg/day	Pulmonary fibrosis, myocardial fibrosis, hypotension, anorexia, nausea, vomiting, alopecia, hemorrhagic cystitis, hematuria, leukopenia
gold sodium thiomalate (Myochrysine)	IM, (Weekly): 1st injection 10 mg, 2nd injection 25 mg, then 25–50 mg weekly until a cumulative dose of 1000 mg has been given	Hypersensitivity reactions, nephrotic syndrome, stomatitis, dermatitis, colitis
hydroxychloroquine sulfate (Plaquenil Sulfate)	Oral: 200–600 mg daily	GI distress, visual disturbances, retinopathy, vertigo, tinnitus, nerve deafness, dermatologic reactions
leflunomide (Arava)	Oral: Loading dose of one 100 mg tablet/day for 3 days. Daily maintenance dose is 20 mg, and doses higher than this are not recommended.	Nephrotoxicity, diarrhea, alopecia, anorexia, abdominal pain, nausea, gastritis, hypertension, dizziness, rash
methotrexate (Rheumatrex)	Oral: 7.5 mg once weekly, or in 3 divided doses of 2.5 mg/12 hours. Not to exceed 20 mg/week	Nausea, mucositis, GI discomfort, rash, diarrhea, headache, hepato-toxicity, cirrhosis, bone marrow depression with anemia, leukopenia, potentially dangerous lung disease, ulcerative stomatitis
penicillamine (Cuprimine)	Oral: initially 125–250 mg/day. Dosage increases of 125–250 mg/day at 1–3 month intervals, if necessary	Dermatologic reactions, GI distress, thrombocytopenia, cholestatic jaundice, membraneous glomerulopathy
sulfasalazine (Azulfidine)	Oral: 500 mg to 1 g/day (as delayed-release tablet) for 1 week, then increase by 500 mg/day every week up to 2 g/day in 2 divided doses	Ataxia, confusion, dizziness, drowsiness, headache, mental depression, psychosis, restlessness

Gold preparations are used in the long-term treatment of rheumatoid arthritis. These agents have been shown to be effective in reducing the progression of the disease as well as relieving inflammation. The usefulness of gold therapy (**chryso-therapy**) is limited by the toxicity of these drugs. The adverse effects of gold compounds may occur shortly after administration, at any time during the course of therapy, or even after therapy has been discontinued.

The antimalarial drug hydroxychloroquine sulfate has been used as a second-line therapeutic agent for the treatment of rheumatoid arthritis. Treatment with this agent usually requires 6 to 12 months, and is complicated by its potential toxicity and the variability of beneficial effects produced.

Ocular toxicity is the most serious complication, and regular ophthalmologic examinations should accompany therapy with this drug.

Penicillamine, a chelating agent, has been shown to be effective in long-term treatment of rheumatoid arthritis. Its mechanism of action is not fully understood. Because penicillamine causes potentially serious adverse reactions, its use is recommended for those with long-standing progressive disease that has not responded to other agents.

Rheumatrex is a low-dose form of methotrexate approved for adult rheumatoid arthritis. It reduces inflammation, pain, swelling, and stiffness in adult rheumatoid arthritis and is recommended for selected adults with severe, active, classical, or definite rheumatoid arthritis who have had insufficient response to other forms of treatment. The client may see improvement within 3 to 6 weeks.

COX-2 INHIBITORS

Recent advances in the understanding of the underlying causes of inflammation and pain have resulted in the development of a new class of drugs known as COX-2 inhibitors. The first drug of this class to be approved, Celebrex (celecoxib), is used for the treatment of osteoarthritis and rheumatoid arthritis. A second drug, Vioxx (rofecoxib), (see Figure 29-2), is approved for the treatment of both osteoarthritis and acute pain, and a third drug, Mobic (meloxicam), is approved for the treatment of osteoarthritis.

Cyclooxygenase (COX) is an enzyme involved in many aspects of normal cellular function and also in the inflammatory response. Two forms, designated COX-1 and COX-2, have been identified. COX-2 is found in joints and other areas affected by

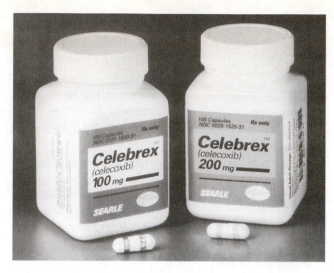

FIGURE 29-3 CELEBREX™ (CELECOXIB) 100 MG, 200 MG CAPSULES *(Courtesy of Pharmacia Corporation)*

inflammation. Inhibition of COX-2 reduces the production of compounds associated with inflammation and pain.

Celecoxib (Celebrex)

Dosage

Osteoarthritis: recommended oral dose is 200 mg/day administered as a single dose or as 100 mg twice/day. Rheumatoid arthritis: recommended oral dose is 100–200 mg twice/day. See Figure 29-3.

Adverse Reactions

Abdominal pain, diarrhea, dyspepsia, flatulence, nausea, back pain, dizziness, headache, insomnia, pharyngitis, rash.

Contraindications

Contraindicated in clients with known hypersensitivity to celecoxib. Celebrex should not be given to clients who have demonstrated allergic-type reactions to sulfonamides. It should not be given to clients who have experienced asthma, urticaria, or allergic-type reactions after taking aspirin or other NSAIDs. Severe, rarely fatal, anaphylactic-like reactions to NSAIDs have been reported in such clients. Celebrex should be used during pregnancy only if the potential benefit justifies the potential risk to the fetus.

Clients' Instruction

Educate the client that

- One need not take the medicine with a meal. A high-fat meal will make the drug act more slowly.

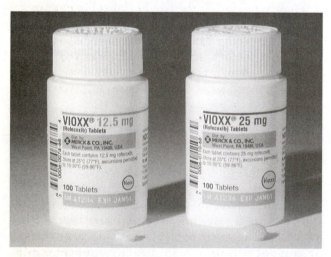

FIGURE 29-2 VIOXX® (ROFECOXIB) 12.5 MG, 25 MG TABLETS *(Courtesy of Merck & Company, Inc.)*

- An antacid will actually make the drug less effective, so do not take with an antacid
- One should take the medicine for at least 5 days to get the full effect
- Celebrex seems to decrease the effect of ACE inhibitors
- Celebrex also interferes with the action of diuretics
- Celebrex might increase lithium blood levels
- Fluconazole increases blood levels of Celebrex
- If the pain is not reduced in a week or two, contact his/her physician

> **Safety Precaution:** Serious gastrointestinal toxicity such as bleeding, ulceration, and perforation of the stomach, small intestine, or large intestine can occur at any time, with or without warning symptoms, in clients treated with nonsteroidal anti-inflammatory drugs. NSAIDs should be prescribed with extreme caution in clients with a prior history of ulcer disease or gastrointestinal bleeding.

ANTITUMOR NECROSIS FACTOR DRUGS

Antitumor necrosis factor drugs have evolved out of the biotechnology industry. Anti-TNF drugs seem to slow, if not halt altogether, the destruction of the joints by disrupting the activity of tumor necrosis factor (TNF), a substance involved in the body's immune response. An **autoimmune response** is a process by which the body's defense system malfunctions and begins to attack itself. It is this process that appears to account for many types of arthritis including rheumatoid arthritis, lupus, myositis, and scleroderma. By blocking TNF, these agents act to preempt the autoimmune response. An example of an anti-TNF agent is etanercept (Enbrel).

Etanercept (Enbrel)

Enbrel (etanercept) binds specifically to tumor necrosis factor (TNF) and blocks its interaction with cell surface TNF receptors. TNF is a naturally occurring cytokine that is involved in normal inflammatory and immune response. Enbrel is indicated for reduction in signs and symptoms of moderately to severely active rheumatoid arthritis in clients who have had an inadequate response to one or more disease-modifying antirheumatic drugs. It can be used in combination with methotrexate in clients who do not respond adequately to methotrexate alone.

Dosage

The recommended dose of Enbrel for adult clients with rheumatoid arthritis is 25 mg given twice weekly as a subcutaneous injection.

Adverse Reactions

Erythema and/or itching, pain, or swelling at the injection site. Upper respiratory infections and sinusitis, headache, dizziness, asthenia, abdominal pain, rash, and dyspepsia.

Contraindications

Enbrel should not be administered to clients with sepsis or with known hypersensitivity to the medication or any of its components.

> **Safety Precaution:** In postmarketing reports, serious infections and sepsis, including fatalities, have been reported with the use of Enbrel. Many of these serious events have occurred in clients with underlying diseases that in addition to their rheumatoid arthritis could predispose them to infections. Clients who develop a new infection while undergoing treatment with Enbrel should be monitored closely. Administration of Enbrel should be discontinued if a client develops a serious infection or sepsis. Treatment with Enbrel should not be initiated in clients with active infections including chronic or localized infections. Physicians should exercise caution when considering the use of Enbrel in clients with a history of recurring infections or with underlying conditions that may predispose clients to infections, such as advanced or poorly controlled diabetes.

AGENTS USED TO TREAT GOUT

Gout is a hereditary metabolic disease that is a form of acute arthritis. It is marked by inflammation of the joints and can affect any joint, but usually begins in the knee or foot. It is believed to be caused by excessive uric acid in the blood (**hyperuricemia**) and deposits of uric acid crystals in and around the joints.

Acute attacks of gout are extremely painful and may persist for several days to several weeks. Acute attacks should be treated as soon as possible. Colchicine, a drug used for gout, may be administered either orally or intravenously. When given orally, an initial dose of 0.5 to 1.2 mg is administered. This dose may be given every 1 to 2 hours until pain is relieved or until nausea, vomiting, and/or diarrhea occur. The total dosage during a 24-hour period should not exceed 4–8 mg. When administered intravenously, an initial dose of 1–2 mg is usually given. This may be followed by doses of 0.5 mg every 6 hours until a satisfactory response is achieved. The total dosage during a 24-hour period should not exceed 4 mg. The major adverse reactions of colchicine are nausea, vomiting, and diarrhea. Other adverse reactions are gastrointestinal bleeding, neuritis, myopathy, alopecia, and bone marrow depression.

Once the acute attack of gout has been controlled, drug therapy to control hyperuricemia can be initiated. The aim of treatment is to reduce the serum urate levels to below 6 mg/dL. Two types of drug therapy may be employed to reduce serum urate levels: uricosuric agents such as probenecid (Benemid) and sulfinpyrazone (Anturane), which increase the urinary excretion of uric acid, and allopurinol (Zyloprim), which prevents the formation of uric acid in the body.

Probenecid and sulfinpyrazone increase uric acid excretion by preventing the reabsorption of uric acid in the renal tubules. Because of this, urate stones may form in the kidneys and the client is advised to drink 10 to 12 eight-ounce glasses of water per day to insure a urine output of more than 1 liter per day. Adverse reactions of probenecid are headache, anorexia, nausea, vomiting, urinary frequency, flushing, and dizziness. Adverse reactions of sulfinpyrazone are nausea and vomiting.

Allopurinol, unlike the uricosuric agents, interferes with the conversion of purines to uric acid by inhibiting the enzyme xanthine oxidase. Two drugs, 6-mercaptopurine (Purinethol) and azathioprine (Imuran), are normally metabolized by the enzyme xanthine oxidase, and their use must be avoided or dosage reduced when allopurinol is prescribed. The major adverse reactions of allopurinol are skin rashes and hepatotoxicity. Other adverse reactions are nausea, vomiting, abdominal pain, and hematologic changes.

SKELETAL MUSCLE RELAXANTS

Skeletal muscle relaxants (Table 29-5) are used to treat painful muscle spasms that may result from musculoskeletal strains, sprains, trauma, or disease. A **muscle spasm** is an involuntary contraction of one or more muscles and is usually accompanied by pain and the limitation of function.

Centrally Acting Muscle Relaxants

Centrally acting muscle relaxants depress the central nervous system and can be administered either orally or by injection. Individuals taking centrally acting muscle relaxants should be aware of the sedative effect of these drugs. Drowsiness, dizziness, and blurred vision may diminish the client's ability to drive a vehicle, operate equipment, or climb stairs. The use of these agents in combination with other CNS depressants (alcohol, narcotic analgesics) may produce an additive effect; therefore, such use must be with caution.

Nursing Considerations

Observe client for signs of improvement and adverse reactions. Monitor CBC, WBC, differential, liver function tests, and EEG in epileptic clients. Administer with meals to decrease GI distress.

Clients' Instruction

Educate the client

- To take the medication as prescribed
- That the drug should be tapered off over 1–2 weeks
- That sudden discontinuance of the medication may cause insomnia, nausea, headache, spasticity, and/or tachycardia
- Not to use alcohol or other CNS depressants while on skeletal muscle relaxants
- To avoid hazardous activities if drowsiness or dizziness occurs
- Not to use over-the-counter medication such as antihistamines, decongestants, and cough preparations unless prescribed by the physician

Special Considerations

- Motor skill impairment, increased sedative effect, and respiratory depression may occur if taken with other CNS depressants (alcohol, narcotics, barbiturates, tricyclic antidepressants, antianxiety agents, and/or anticonvulsants).
- Cyclobenzaprine (Flexeril) may cause hyperpyrexia, excitation, and convulsions if taken with MAOIs.

TABLE 29-5   SKELETAL MUSCLE RELAXANTS

Medication	Type	Usual Dosage	Adverse Reactions
baclofen (Lioresal)	Centrally acting agent	Oral: 5 mg 3 times/day; increased by 5 mg/dose every 3 days until optimum response is obtained (maximum, 80 mg/day)	Hypotension, tinnitus, nasal congestion, blurred vision, nausea, dry mouth, dizziness, drowsiness, weakness
cyclobenzaprine HCl (Flexeril)	Centrally acting agent	Oral: 20–40 mg/day in 2–4 divided doses (maximum, 60 mg/day)	Edema of the face and tongue, pruritus, tachycardia, dry mouth, fatigue, blurred vision
dantrolene sodium (Dantrium)	Peripherally acting agent	Oral (Adult): initial 25 mg/day; increased to 25 mg 2–4 times/day, then by increments to 50–100 mg 4 times/day. Oral (Child): 0.5 mg/kg twice/day; then by increments of 0.5 mg to a maximum of 3 mg/kg 2–4 times/day	Drowsiness, muscle weakness, speech disturbances, tachycardia, diarrhea, nausea, anorexia, abdominal cramps, bloody or dark urine, burning with urination, blurred vision, pruritus, jaundice
diazepam (Valium)	Centrally acting agent	Oral (Adult): 2–10 mg 2–4 times daily. IM, IV (Adult): 2–10 mg as needed. Oral (Child): 1–2.5 mg 3–4 times daily. IM, IV (Child): 1–2 mg as needed	Drowsiness, slurred speech, muscle weakness, vertigo, hypotension, tachycardia, urinary retention, nausea, xerostomia, blurred vision, hiccups, coughing, hepatic dysfunction, jaundice
methocarbamol (Robaxin)	Centrally acting agent	Oral (Adult): 1.5 g 4 times/day, then 1–1.5 g 4 times daily. IM (Adult): 0.5 to 1 g at 8-hour intervals as necessary. IV (Adult): 1–3 g daily	Urticaria, pruritus, nasal congestion, rash, blurred vision, drowsiness, dizziness, headache, nausea

- May decrease the antihypertensive effect of guanethidine (Ismelin) and clonidine (Catapres)
- May increase anticholinergic effects including confusion and hallucinations if taken with cholinergic blocking agents

NEUROMUSCULAR BLOCKING AGENTS

Neuromuscular blocking agents are used to provide muscle relaxation and to reduce the need for deep general anesthesia in clients undergoing surgery. These drugs are also used to facilitate endotracheal intubation, to relieve laryngospasm, and to provide muscle relaxation in clients undergoing electroconvulsive therapy.

Neuromuscular blocking agents are of two types: competitive and depolarizing. The competitive drugs compete with the neurotransmitter acetylcholine for cholinergic receptor sites at the neuromuscular junction. These drugs act by occupying the receptor sites, thereby preventing the stimulation of muscle fibers by acetylcholine and causing paralysis of the affected muscle fibers. The depolarizing drugs are believed to mimic the action of acetylcholine in depolarizing muscle fibers but, because they are not readily destroyed by the enzyme cholinesterase, their prolonged action results

TABLE 29-6 NEUROMUSCULAR BLOCKING AGENTS

Medication	Type	Usual Dosage	Adverse Reactions
atracurium besylate (Tracrium)	Competitive (nondepolarizing)	IV: 0.4–0.5 mg/kg, then 0.08–0.1 mg/kg after 20–45 minutes if needed for maintenance	Increased bronchial secretions, bronchospasm, cyanosis, respiratory depression
gallamine triethiodide (Flaxedil)	Competitive (nondepolarizing)	IV: 1 mg/kg (single dose not to exceed 100 mg), additional dose of 0.5–1 mg/kg after 30 minutes if needed	Tachycardia, hypertension, increased cardiac output
metocurine iodide (Metubine)	Competitive (nondepolarizing)	IV: 1.5–7 mg depending upon the type of anesthetic used, followed by additional 0.5–1 mg if needed	Hypotension, dizziness, increased salivation, respiratory depression
pancuronium bromide (Pavulon)	Competitive (nondepolarizing)	IV: 0.04–0.1 mg/kg followed by an additional 0.01 mg/kg dose at 30–60 minute intervals, if necessary	Increased pulse rate and blood pressure, respiratory depression, salivation
succinylcholine chloride (Anectine)	Depolarizing	IV: 0.6 mg/kg over 10–30 seconds IM: 2.5 mg/kg (maximum, 150 mg)	Arrhythmias, sinus arrest, muscle fasciculations, respiratory depression
tubocurarine chloride (Tubarine)	Competitive (nondepolarizing)	IV: 40–60 units at beginning of surgery, then 20–30 units in 3–5 minutes, if required	Slight dizziness, respiratory depression, increased salivation, bronchospasm
vecuronium (Norcuron)	Competitive (nondepolarizing)	IV (Adults, older children): 0.04–0.1 mg/kg initially, then 0.010–0.015 mg/kg after 20–40 minutes, if needed	Generally well tolerated; rarely: respiratory depression, hyperthermia

in a persistent depolarization block and paralysis of muscle fibers. See Table 29-6.

SKELETAL MUSCLE STIMULANTS

Impaired neuromuscular transmission, thought to result from an autoimmune disorder, produces the condition known as myasthenia gravis. This disease, characterized by progressive weakness of skeletal muscles and their rapid fatiguing, is treated by the use of **anticholinesterase** (a substance that inactivates the action of cholinesterase) muscle stimulants.

Skeletal muscle stimulant drugs (Table 29-7) act by inhibiting the action of acetylcholinesterase, the enzyme that halts the action of acetylcholine at the neuromuscular junction. By slowing the destruction of acetylcholine, these drugs foster accumulation of higher concentrations of this neurotransmitter and increase the number of interactions between acetylcholine and the available receptors on muscle fibers. The increase in the number of transmitter/receptor interactions improves muscle strength but has no curative effect on the cause of the disease.

Nursing Considerations

Observe client for signs of improvement and adverse reactions. Monitor intake and output ratio and vital signs. Atropine sulfate must be available before administration of a skeletal muscle stimulant because of the possibility of a cholinergic crisis (pronounced muscular weakness and respiratory paralysis caused by excessive acetylcholine). May be given with food to decrease GI distress, but better absorption takes place when given on an empty stomach. Discontinue drug if bradycardia, hypotension, bronchospasm, headache, dizziness, convulsions, and/or respiratory depression occurs.

TABLE 29-7   SKELETAL MUSCLE STIMULANTS

Medication	Action	Usual Dosage	Adverse Reactions
edrophonium chloride (Tensilon)	Cholinesterase inhibitor used in diagnosis of myasthenia gravis	IV (Adult): 2–10 mg IM (Adult): 10 mg IV (Child): 1–5 mg IM (Child): 2–5 mg	Uncommon with usual doses; can cause weakness, muscle tension, nausea, diarrhea, respiratory paralysis
neostigmine bromide (Prostigmin Bromide)	Cholinesterase inhibitor	Oral: 15–30 mg 2–4 times/day, increased until maximum benefit is obtained (15–375 mg/day)	Fear, agitation, restlessness, nausea, epigastric discomfort, muscle cramps, fasciculations, pallor
neostigmine methylsulfate (Prostigmin Methylsulfate)	Cholinesterase inhibitor	IM, SC: 0.5 mg with subsequent dose based on individual response	See neostigmine bromide
pyridostigmine bromide (Mestinon)	Cholinesterase inhibitor	Oral: 60–600 mg/day in divided doses IM, IV: 1/30 of oral dose	Acneiform rash, nausea, vomiting, diarrhea, miosis, bronchoconstriction, bradycardia, fasciculation

Clients' Instruction

Educate the client

- To take the medication as prescribed
- To report any signs of cholinergic crisis to the physician without delay
- That skeletal muscle stimulants are used to relieve symptoms and are not a cure for his/her disease

Special Considerations

- These medications should not be given with other cholinergic agents.
- Because of the possibility of cholinergic crisis, emergency equipment and supplies should be available.
- Positive response to the medication includes increased muscle strength, hand grasp, improved gait, and absence of labored breathing.
- The effect of skeletal muscle stimulants may be decreased by aminoglycosides, anesthetics, procainamide (Procan SR), and/or quinidine.
- Skeletal muscle stimulants may decrease the effects of gallamine (Flaxedil), metocurine (Metubine Iodide), pancuronium (Pavulon), tubocurarine (Tubarine), and/or atropine.
- Skeletal muscle stimulants may increase the effects of succinylcholine (Anectine, Quelicin).

● SELF-ASSESSMENT

Write the answer in the space provided.

Source

p. 375 1. Drugs that relieve the swelling, tenderness, redness, and pain of inflammation are known as _____ agents.

p. 375 2. _____ is a naturally occurring hormone that is chemically related to steroidal agents.

p. 379 3. Ibuprofen and acetylsalicylic acid are examples of _____ agents that reduce inflammation.

p. 380 4. Disease-modifying antirheumatic agents may be introduced in persons exhibiting the early stages of rheumatoid arthritis because they _____ and limit _____ .

p. 384 5. The chapter mentions two types of drug therapy that can be used in the treatment of gout. Benemid (probenecid) and _____ increase the urinary excretion of uric acid and Zyloprim (allopurinol) _____ in the body.

p. 382 6. Cyclooxygenase is an _____ that has been linked to the inflammatory response. One form, designated COX-2, is found in _____ and other areas affected by inflammation.

p. 383 **7.** _____ , abbreviated _____ , is involved in the body's immune response and has been linked to the destruction of joints. The chapter offers _____ as an example of a drug used to counter its effects on the joints.

p. 384 **8.** A muscle spasm is an _____ contraction of one or more muscles.

p. 385 **9.** Competitive neuromuscular blocking agents act by _____ , thereby preventing the stimulation of muscle fibers by acetylcholine.

p. 386 **10.** Skeletal muscle stimulant drugs act by inhibiting the action of the enzyme _____ .

● **WEB ACTIVITY**

Visit the following Web sites for additional information on medications used for musculoskeletal system disorders:

http://pharmacotherapy.medscape.com

http://www.arthritis.org

http://www.curearthritis.org

http://www.discoveryhealth.com

http://www.pharminfo.com

http://www.onhealth.com

http://www.healthspotlight.com

http://www.fda.gov

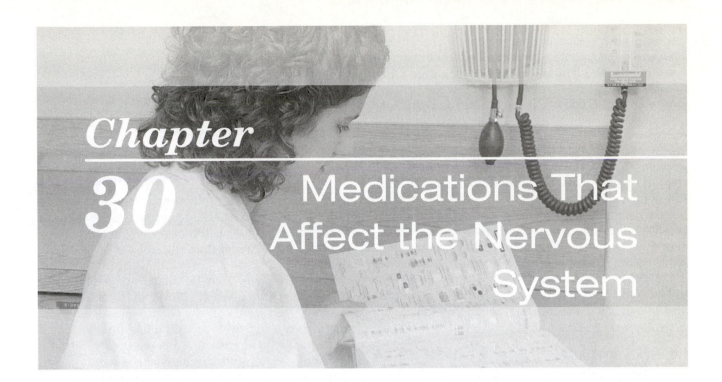

Chapter

30

Medications That Affect the Nervous System

Chapter Outline

- List several alternative methods that may be used for relief of pain
- Explain how to assess a client's pain
- Describe the various drug classifications used for nervous system disorders
- Understand the actions, uses, contraindications, safety precautions, adverse reaction, dosage and route, nursing considerations, clients' instruction, and special considerations for selected drugs
- Complete the Spot Check on selected drugs used to help relieve pain
- Describe Alzheimer's disease, including the symptoms and medications used for this disorder
- Complete the Self-Assessment
- Visit indicated Web sites for additional information on medications used for nervous system disorders

Objectives

Upon completion of this chapter, you should be able to

- Define the key terms
- Describe the nervous system
- Describe acute pain and chronic pain
- State the treatment for acute pain and chronic pain

Key Terms

Alzheimer's disease (AD)
analgesic
anesthetics
antipyretic
epilepsy
hypnotic
insomnia
mydriasis
opiates
opioids
Parkinson's disease
sedative
vertigo

INTRODUCTION

The nervous system is comprised of the brain and spinal cord (the central nervous system or CNS) plus the network of nerves and neural tissues throughout the body (the peripheral nervous system or PNS). See Figure 30-1. The peripheral system connects to the brain and spinal cord by way of 12 pairs of cranial nerves and 31 pairs of spinal nerves. These two systems, functioning as a unit, regulate body functions in relationship to the environment.

Our sense of hearing, taste, equilibrium, touch, smell, and sight all rely on nerves to function properly. Pain receptors alert us to danger from inflammation or hot surfaces. Muscular activity is dependent upon proper stimulation by nerve impulses. Our ability to think, reason, feel emotions, and interact with others is directly related to our neurological processes.

Disorders that interfere with central or peripheral nervous system function are treated with a variety of drugs, some of which are discussed in this chapter. Separate chapters are provided for drugs used primarily with the musculoskeletal system and for mental disorders. (See Chapters 22 and 29.)

PAIN

Pain is a symptom of a physical or emotional condition. The International Association for the Study of Pain defines pain as the sensory and emotional experience associated with actual or potential tissue damage.

A person's pain may be measured by its threshold and its intensity. Pain threshold is the level of stimulus that results in the perception of pain. How one responds to pain is an individual process. Some factors associated with how a person perceives pain are age, gender, and the physical, mental, social, cultural, and emotional makeup of the individual. Pain tolerance is the amount of pain a person can manage without disrupting normal functioning and without requiring pain medication. Intensity is the degree of pain felt by the individual.

In the United States approximately 155 million persons experience an episode of acute pain each year. An estimated 700 million workdays are lost each year because of pain, with a cost of $60 billion. Acute pain may be described as one that comes on suddenly, is severe, and is a warning that something is wrong. Some signs of acute pain are increased heart rate and respiratory rate, increased blood pressure, dilated pupils, sweating (many times profuse), nausea, vomiting, anxiety, and fear. The treatment of acute pain depends upon the cause, but generally it is treated with nonnarcotic analgesics and/or narcotic analgesics.

Chronic pain lasts for a long time. It is a pain that persists beyond the expected time required for the healing of an injury or expected course of recovery. Some signs of chronic pain include disturbances in sleep and eating patterns, irritability, constipation, depression, fatigue, and withdrawal from social activities. Chronic pain is generally managed with analgesics, but the client may wish to try alternative methods for relief.

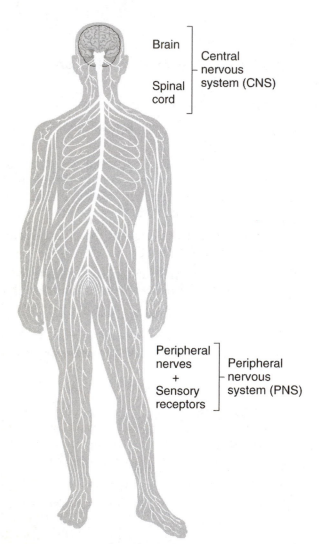

Brain
Spinal cord
⎱ Central nervous system (CNS)

Peripheral nerves
+
Sensory receptors
⎱ Peripheral nervous system (PNS)

FIGURE 30-1 CENTRAL AND PERIPHERAL NERVOUS SYSTEMS

Some Alternative Methods for Relief of Pain

- Behavior modification—relaxation training, biofeedback, and hypnosis
- Surgery—destroying nerves responsible for pain

- Electrostimulation—implanting electrodes at certain sites in the body and then stimulating them to prevent pain messages
- Acupuncture
- Exercise—aerobic exercise increases the secretion of endorphins (natural painkillers)
- Ice—useful for headaches, and in the first 48 hours of an injury (sprains, strains, bumps), because it reduces swelling
- Heat—useful for cramps and muscle aches, and after swelling of an injury has subsided

Chronic intractable pain may be caused by cancer, mental illness, neurologic disorders such as neuralgias, phantom limb pain, nerve entrapment syndromes, spinal cord damage, myofascial syndromes, or thalamic syndrome pain.

New federal guidelines urge doctors to aggressively attack cancer pain, which a study showed severely afflicts one-third of Americans with spreading cancer. The guidelines issued by the Agency for Health Care Policy and Research urge doctors to start clients on mild painkillers, then work up to more potent medicines. The next step is codeine and other weak opiates, followed by morphine and similar powerful drugs. The guidelines say there is no limit on the maximum dose of morphine. Very large doses—several hundred milligrams every 4 hours—may be needed for some clients with extreme pain. Refer to Table 30-1 for a summary of common pain medications.

Assessment of Pain

It is important to obtain an accurate assessment of a client's pain. Because pain is subjective, the client needs to describe in detail the location, intensity, quality, onset, duration, variations, what relieves the pain, and what causes or increases the pain.

- *History of the pain*—questions to ask the client: When did the pain start, how long does the pain last, what increases or decreases the pain, what methods are used to relieve the pain, and how effective are these methods?
- *Physical signs and symptoms*—increased heart rate and respiratory rate, increased blood pressure, dilated pupils, sweating, nausea, vomiting, anxiety, fear
- *Facial expressions*—strained look, clenched teeth, tightly shut lips, tightening of the jaw muscles, furrowed brow, tears
- *Body movements*—protective or guarding movements toward a specific area of the body, limp-

TABLE 30-1 USUAL DOSES AND INTERVALS OF SELECTED DRUGS USED FOR RELIEF OF PAIN

Drug	Dose and Route	Interval
Acetylsalicylic acid	650 mg (oral)	4 hr
Acetaminophen	650 mg (oral)	4 hr
Ibuprofen	400 mg (oral)	4–6 hr
Naproxen	250–500 mg (oral)	12 hr
Codeine	15–60 mg (oral)	4 hr
Hydromorphone	2 mg (oral)	4 hr
Meperidine	50–150 mg (SC, IM, IV)	3–4 hr
Methadone	2.5–10 mg (SC, IM, IV)	6–8 hr
Morphine	10–20 mg (SC, IM)	4 hr

ing, clenched fist, hunched shoulders, doubling over
- *Quality and/or character*—verbal description (aching, burning, prickling, sharp, cutting, throbbing, intense, pressure, mild, moderate, severe, local, deep)

Effectiveness of Treatment

Two methods that are used to monitor treatment effectiveness for pain management are questionnaires and rating scales. The McGill-Melzack Pain Questionnaire measures both sensory and affective dimensions of pain. Rating scales may use numbers, drawings, and/or lines. The number scale may be 0–5 or 0–10 with zero indicating no pain and the upper number signifying the most intense pain. The Wong-Baker face rating scale shows five faces with the numbers 0–5 beneath the picture, with zero indicating no pain and 5 signifying the most intense pain. This is useful for children and for clients who cannot speak English.

Standards for Pain Relief

The American Pain Society has developed Standards for the Relief of Acute Pain and Cancer Pain. Following is a summary of these standards:

1. Acute pain and cancer pain are recognized and effectively treated. Essential to this process is the development of a clinically useful and easy-to-use scale for rating pain and its relief. Clients will be evaluated according to the scales and the results recorded as frequently as needed.

2. Information about analgesics is readily available. This includes data concerning the effectiveness of various agents in controlling pain and the availability of equianalgesic charts wherever drugs are used for pain.

3. Clients are informed on admission of the availability of methods of relieving pain, and that they must communicate the presence and persistence of pain to the health care staff.

4. Explicit policies for use of advanced analgesic technologies are defined. These advances include client-control analgesia, epidural analgesia, and regional analgesia. Specific instructions concerning use of these techniques need to be available for the medical care staff.

5. Adherence to standards is monitored by an interdisciplinary committee. The committee is responsible for overseeing the activities related to implementing and evaluating the effectiveness of these pain standards.

ANALGESICS

Analgesic agents are used to relieve pain caused by disease or other conditions without causing the client to lose consciousness. Morphine, a narcotic derivative of opium, was the forerunner of many natural and synthetic analgesics used today. Because they trace their origin back to opium, the natural and synthetic drugs derived from morphine are known as **opiates**. Other synthetic drugs, not chemically related to morphine, have been developed because they mimic the action of morphine. These drugs, called **opioids**, are also classified as narcotics because they can cause dependency. Table 30-2 lists opiate and opioid narcotic analgesics.

Narcotic Analgesics
Actions

Analgesics inhibit ascending pain pathways in the central nervous system. They increase pain threshold and alter pain perception.

TABLE 30-2   OPIATE AND OPIOID ANALGESICS

Medication	Class/Use	Usual Dosage	Adverse Reactions
codeine phosphate, codeine sulfate	C II analgesic	Oral, SC, IM (Adult): 15–60 mg 4–6 times/day as necessary Oral, SC, IM (Child): 0.5 mg/kg every 4–6 hours as necessary	Dizziness, drowsiness, palpitations, bradycardia, urinary retention, nausea, vomiting, constipation
hydromorphone HCl (Dilaudid)	C II analgesic	Oral, SC, IM, IV (slow): 2 mg every 4–6 hours	Respiratory depression, nausea, hypotension
levorphanol tartrate (Levo-Dromoran)	C II analgesic	Oral, SC: 2–3 mg repeated in 4–6 hours as necessary	As above
meperidine HCl (Demerol)	C II analgesic	Oral, SC, IM, IV (Adult): 50–150 mg every 3–4 hours SC, IM (Child): 1 mg/kg every 4 hours as necessary	Dizziness, weakness, dry mouth, nausea, vomiting, respiratory depression, palpitations, bradycardia
methadone HCl (Dolophine)	C II analgesic	Oral, SC, IM (Adult): 2.5–10 mg every 3–4 hours, if necessary	Drowsiness, nausea, dry mouth, constipation
morphine sulfate	C II analgesic	Oral: 10–20 mg every 4 hours SC, IM: 5–20 mg every 4 hours SC, IM (Child): 0.05–0.2 mg/kg per dose	Deep sleep, respiratory depression, nausea, urinary retention, pruritus, edema, bradycardia, sweating
oxymorphone HCl (Numorphan)	C II analgesic	SC, IM (Adult): 0.5–1.5 mg every 4–6 hours as needed	Nausea, vomiting, euphoria, dizziness
pentazocine HCl (Talwin)	C IV analgesic	Oral: 50 mg every 3–4 hours SC, IM, IV: 30 mg every 3–4 hours	Drowsiness, sweating, dry mouth, nausea, vomiting
propoxyphene HCl, propoxyphene napsylate (Darvon, Darvon-N)	C IV analgesic	Oral (HCl): 65 mg every 4 hours as needed Oral (napsylate): 100 mg every 4 hours as needed	Dizziness, weakness, headache, nausea, vomiting, constipation, abdominal pain

Uses

For the relief of moderate to severe pain, as a preoperative medication, and as support of anesthesia.

Contraindications

Contraindicated in clients with known hypersensitivity to any of its ingredients and those with addiction, also in clients taking MAOIs.

> **Safety Precaution**
>
> 1. Narcotic analgesics can produce drug dependence and have the potential for being abused.
> 2. Must be used with great caution and in reduced dosage in clients who are concurrently taking other narcotic analgesics, general anesthetics, phenothiazines, other tranquilizers, sedative-hypnotics, tricyclic antidepressants, and alcohol. Respiratory depression, hypotension, and profound sedation or coma may result.
> 3. Must be used with extreme caution in clients with head injury, increased intracranial pressure, asthma and other respiratory conditions, acute myocardial infarction, severe heart disease, hepatic disease, and renal disease
> 4. Safe use in pregnancy prior to labor has not been established. Medication will cross the placental barrier and can produce depression of respiration and psychophysiologic functions in the newborn.

Adverse Reactions

Respiratory depression, circulatory depression, lightheadedness, dizziness, sedation, hallucinations, nausea, vomiting, sweating, euphoria, dysphoria, weakness, headache, agitation, tremor, convulsions, dry mouth, constipation, biliary tract spasm, flushing of the face, tachycardia, bradycardia, palpitation, hypotension, syncope, urinary retention, pruritus, urticaria, rash, pain at injection site, visual disturbances.

Dosage and Route

The dosage and route of administration is determined by the physician and individualized for each client. (See Table 30-2.)

Nursing Considerations

Observe client for evidence of respiratory depression (respirations below 12), urinary retention (de-creased output), central nervous system changes (dizziness, drowsiness, hallucinations, euphoria), allergic reactions (rash, urticaria), cardiac dysfunction (tachycardia, bradycardia, palpitation), and constipation. Monitor intake and output ratio, respirations, therapeutic response, need for pain medication, and signs of physical dependence. Protect the client from possible injury. After administration, client should be properly positioned in bed, with siderails up and call bell within easy reach.

Clients' Instruction

Educate the client

- About possible adverse reactions
- To report any symptoms of CNS changes and/or allergic reactions to the physician
- Not to operate machinery or drive a motor vehicle while taking narcotic/analgesics
- To avoid the use of alcohol and other CNS depressants that can enhance the drowsiness caused by analgesics

Special Considerations

- Always assess the client's respiratory rate before administration. Withhold medication and notify the physician if respiratory rate is 12 or below.
- Physical dependency may occur with the long-term use of narcotic analgesics. Withdrawal symptoms include nausea, vomiting, anorexia abdominal cramps, fever, and faintness.
- Federal law requires that all controlled substances be kept separate from other drugs. They are to be stored in a substantially constructed metal box or compartment that is equipped with a double lock. The nurse who is responsible for administering narcotics must keep the narcotics key protected from possible misuse. A separate record book is required for information concerning the administration of controlled substances. This data system must be maintained on a daily basis and kept for a minimum of 2 years (3 years in some states). Narcotics are counted at the end of each shift, and the inventory of controlled drugs must be recorded on an audit sheet. This sheet must be signed for correctness of count by two individuals.
- The client who is receiving a narcotic analgesic via a PCA (patient-controlled analgesia) should be properly instructed in its use and monitored on a regular basis. See Figure 30-2.

Several nonnarcotic analgesic drugs have been developed in an effort to provide alternative agents

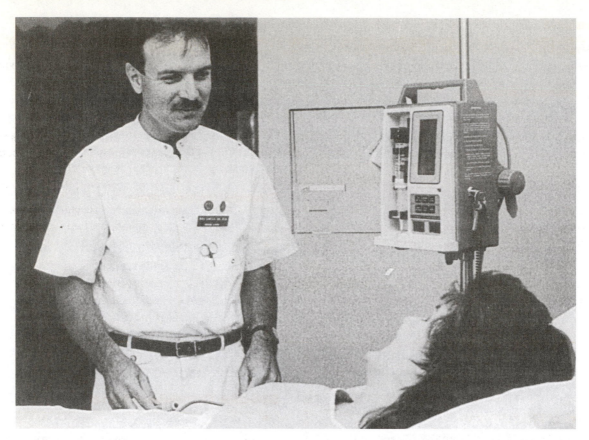

FIGURE 30-2   AN RN INSTRUCTING A CLIENT IN THE USE OF THE PCA (PATIENT-CONTROLLED ANALGESIA) INTRAVENOUS SYSTEM. The system is a portable, computerized pump programmed for the exact amount of medication prescribed by the physician. The system is equipped with a safeguard mechanism that prevents a client from receiving more than the prescribed amount of drug. It also has a locking door on the pump that guards against unauthorized tampering with the dose settings and the prefilled syringe. Note the keys hanging in the lock. These are removed when the unit is set and functioning. To receive the medicine, the client presses a button (held in the nurse's right hand) that is attached to the cord of the pump. When the client presses this button, the syringe dispenses a prescribed dose of drug into the client's IV line. Studies show that less analgesic is required when the client has control over his/her own pain medications.

with less potential for abuse. Like the opiates, these drugs act on the central nervous system. Examples are butorphanol tartrate (Stadol) and nalbuphine HCl (Nubain). They produce adverse reactions similar to those listed in Table 30-2.

Narcotic Antagonist: Naloxone Hydrochloride (Narcan)

Narcan (naloxone hydrochloride) is a narcotic antagonist that prevents or reverses the effects of opioids including respiratory depression, sedation, and hypotension.

Safety Precaution: Should be administered cautiously to persons including newborns of mothers who are known or suspected to be physically dependent on opioids.

Dosage

May be given intravenously, muscularly, and subcutaneously. Narcotic Overdose: initial dose of 0.4 mg to 2 mg IV. Intravenous onset of action is generally apparent within 2 minutes.

TABLE 30-3   ANALGESIC-ANTIPYRETICS

Medication	Actions	Usual Dosage	Adverse Reactions
acetaminophen (Tylenol)	analgesic/antipyretic	Oral (Adult): 325–650 mg at 4 hour intervals Oral (Child): 160–480 mg at 4–6 hour intervals.	Nausea, vomiting, rash, urticaria, anemia, liver damage
aspirin (Bayer)	analgesic/antipyretic, anti-inflammatory antirheumatic	Oral (Adult): 325–650 mg at 4–6 hour intervals Oral (Child): 160–480 mg at 4–6 hour intervals	Gastric irritation, easy bruising, hypersensitivity reactions such as tightness in the chest, bronchospasm, Reyes Syndrome
ibuprofen (Advil) (Motrin) (Nuprin)	anti-inflammatory antirheumatic analgesic/antipyretic	Oral: 200–800 mg 3–4 times per day (maximum, 2400 mg per day)	Headache, dizziness, nausea, vomiting, dyspepsia, leukopenia, flatulence
naproxen (Naprosyn)	anti-inflammatory, analgesic/antipyretic	Oral: 250–500 mg 2 times daily (maximum, 1000 mg/day)	Headache, blurred vision, indigestion, anorexia, agranulocytosis, pruritus

Adverse Reactions

Abrupt reversal of narcotic depression may result in nausea, vomiting, sweating, tachycardia, increased blood pressure, tremulousness, seizures, and cardiac arrest.

ANALGESIC-ANTIPYRETICS

Certain medications act to relieve pain (analgesic effect) and reduce fever (**antipyretic** effect). Although the exact mechanism by which these drugs act is not completely understood, they appear to act peripherally by blocking pain impulse generation. Their antipyretic effect results from direct action on the heat-regulating center in the hypothalamus. In addition to their analgesic-antipyretic properties, all except acetaminophen produce significant anti-inflammatory action. See Table 30-3.

Aspirin or acetaminophen in combination with codeine phosphate or another narcotic analgesic is sometimes prescribed to provide greater relief from pain than is available from aspirin alone. Examples of such combination products include Empirin with Codeine, Percodan, Percodan-Demi, Percocet-5, Tylenol with Codeine, and Phenaphen with Codeine. Tablets and capsules containing these preparations are included in Schedule III of the Controlled Substance Act.

Safety Precaution: The Food and Drug Administration has indicated new labeling for Tylenol (acetaminophen) and Motrin (ibuprofen) pain relievers. The Motrin label warns of the risk of stomach bleeding for those who drink three or more alcoholic beverages daily and take ibuprofen or other pain relievers. Tylenol's label warns those who drink three or more alcoholic beverages daily that use of acetaminophen may increase their risk of liver damage when taken in larger-than-recommended doses. Both Motrin and Tylenol labels suggest that heavy users of alcohol consult their physicians regarding use of the product.

With Motrin (ibuprofen) there is an additional warning about allergy. Ibuprofen may cause a severe allergic reaction including hives, facial swelling, asthma (wheezing), and/or shock. If an allergic reaction occurs, the client is advised to stop use of the medicine and to seek medical help right away. The client is advised not to use this product if he/she has ever had an allergic reaction to any other pain reliever/fever reducer.

● SPOT CHECK

There are many medications that are used to help relieve pain. For each of the following drugs, give the usual dose, route, and the time interval for administration.

Drugs(s)	Dose and Route	Interval
Acetaminophen		
Ibuprofen		
Naproxen		
Codeine		
Meperidine		
Methadone		
Morphine		

SEDATIVES AND HYPNOTICS

Anxiety and insomnia often interfere with job performance and one's ability to interact with others. Sedatives and hypnotics are frequently used in the overall treatment of these disorders. These drugs depress the central nervous system by interfering with the transmission of nerve impulses. Depending upon the dosage, barbiturates, benzodiazepines, and certain other drugs can produce either a sedative or a hypnotic effect. When used as a **sedative**, the dosage is designed to produce a calming effect without causing sleep. Used as a **hypnotic**, the dosage is sufficient to cause sleep. A good hypnotic should have fairly rapid action, produce near normal sleep, and not give the client a delayed effect on the next day.

Barbiturates

The action of barbiturate drugs affects the entire central nervous system. Their use may produce a state ranging from mild sedation to deep sleep and anesthesia, depending upon the drug, the dosage prescribed, and the individual reaction of the client.

Large doses of barbiturates depress the respiratory vasomotor centers in the medulla and can lead to respiratory arrest and death.

Continued use of barbiturates over an extended period of time diminishes their effectiveness. Depending upon the drug, tolerance can develop as soon as a week after first administration, thereby requiring an increase in dosage to sustain the same effect. Psychological and physical dependency can result from the use of these drugs; therefore, they are subject to control under the Federal Controlled Substances Act. The adverse effects commonly associated with barbiturates include residual sedation, vertigo, nausea, and vomiting. Barbiturates used as sedatives and hypnotics are listed in Table 30-4.

Barbiturates differ widely in the duration of their action, which may range from a few seconds (ultra-short-acting) to several days (long-acting). They also differ in onset of action, which can be as little as 30 seconds or as long as 20 to 60 minutes. Short- and intermediate-acting agents are often used in the treatment of insomnia because of their rapid onset and the fact that their use rarely produces a "hangover" effect. Long-acting barbiturates are used as anticonvulsants in clients with epilepsy and as sedatives for a variety of anxiety/tension states.

Actions

As sedatives and hypnotics, barbiturates depress the sensory cortex, decrease motor activity, alter cerebral function, and produce drowsiness, sedation, and hypnosis. They depress activity in brain cells, primarily in the reticular activating system in the brain stem, thus interfering with the transmission of impulses to the cortex.

Uses

Short-term treatment of insomnia, for sedation, as a preoperative medication, and as adjuncts to cancer chemotherapy.

Contraindications

Contraindicated in clients with known hypersensitivity to any of its ingredients. They should not be used in clients with a history of manifest or latent prophyria, respiratory depression, and severe liver impairment.

Safety Precaution

1. Barbiturates may be habit-forming. Tolerance, psychological and physical dependence may occur with continued use.
2. Cautious use in acute and chronic pain
3. Barbiturates can cause fetal damage when administered during pregnancy.
4. Alcohol and other CNS depressants may produce additive CNS depressant effects.
5. There are many precautions associated with the use of barbiturates. Please refer to a current edition of a *Physicians' Desk Reference* or a *PDR Nurse's Drug Handbook* for information on precautions.

Adverse Reactions

Somnolence, agitation, confusion, hyperkinesia, ataxia, CNS depression, nightmares, nervousness, hallucinations, insomnia, anxiety, dizziness, hypoventilation, apnea, bradycardia, hypotension, syncope, nausea, vomiting, constipation, headache, angioedema, rash, exfoliative dermatitis, fever, liver damage, megaloblastic anemia.

Dosage and Route

The dosage and route of administration is determined by the physician and individualized for each client. (See Table 30-4.)

TABLE 30-4   BARBITURATES USED AS SEDATIVES AND HYPNOTICS

Medication	Schedule	Duration	Usual Sedative Dose	Usual Hypnotic Dose
pentobarbital (Nembutal)	C II	Short-acting	Oral: 20–30 mg 2–4 times daily	Oral: 100 mg Rectal: 120–200 mg IM, IV: 100–200 mg
phenobarbital (Luminal)	C IV	Long-acting	Oral: 15–32 mg 2–4 times daily	Oral: 50–100 mg SC, IM, IV: 100–300 mg daily
secobarbital (Seconal)	C II	Short-acting	Oral: 30–50 mg 3 times daily	Oral, IM: 100–200 mg

Nursing Considerations

Observe client for evidence of CNS depression and signs of adverse reactions. Monitor vital signs, blood and hepatic tests, and therapeutic effects. Be alert for signs of drug dependency. Protect the client from possible injury. After administration, the client should be properly positioned in bed, with siderails up and call bell within easy reach. The nurse should be alert for signs of barbiturate toxicity, respiratory dysfunction, and blood dyscrasias such as the following:

- *Barbiturate toxicity:* hypotension, cold and clammy skin, cyanosis of lips, insomnia, nausea, vomiting, hallucinations, delirium, and/or weakness
- *Respiratory dysfunction:* respirations below 12/minute in the adult and pupils dilated
- *Blood dyscrasias:* fever, rash, sore throat, bruising, jaundice, and/or epistaxis

Clients' Instruction

Educate the client

- To take the medication as prescribed
- To be alert for signs of adverse reactions
- To avoid the use of alcohol and other CNS depressants
- Not to smoke, operate machinery, or drive a motor vehicle after taking the medication
- That physical dependency may occur if medication is used for an extended period (45–90 days, depending on dose)
- About alternate methods of relaxation to improve sleep (exercise, reading, warm bath/shower, music, deep breathing, biofeedback, and so forth)

Special Considerations

- Barbiturates are subject to control by the Federal Controlled Substances Act under DEA schedule II. They may be habit-forming and are often abused.
- Emergency supplies and equipment should be readily available for use when administering barbiturates to a client in a hospital setting, long-term-care facility, or other health-related facility.
- Barbiturates may decrease the effect of corticosteroids, oral anticoagulants, griseofulvin, and quinidine.

- The effects of barbiturates may be increased by alcohol, MAOIs, other sedatives, and narcotics.
- Barbiturates should not be mixed with other drugs in solution or syringe.
- Barbiturates should not be used for more than 14 days for insomnia, since they are not effective after that time and tolerance may develop.
- Barbiturates that are used for long-term therapy should not be discontinued quickly as symptoms of withdrawal can be severe and may cause death. Drug must be tapered off over 1–2 weeks.

Other Sedative-Hypnotics

Although benzodiazepines are best known for their use in the relief of anxiety, several drugs in this chemical classification may be used as sedative-hypnotics. These drugs generally reduce incidents of night and early-morning awakening and increase the duration of total sleep time. The onset of action for these drugs is between 15 and 40 minutes and their effect has a duration of 6 to 8 hours. Examples of benzodiazepines used as sedative-hypnotics are flurazepam, lorazepam, oxazepam, temazepam, and triazolam. See Table 30-5.

Other drugs that may be used as sedative-hypnotics are chloral hydrate, one of the oldest hypnotics, zaleplon, and zolpidem. See Table 30-5.

It is recommended that any medication that is used in the treatment of **insomnia** (the inability to obtain the amount of sleep a person needs for optimal functioning and well-being) be used for short-term therapy. Medication should generally be limited to a period of 7 to 10 days.

Sedative-hypnotics have an additive central nervous system (CNS) depressant effect with other CNS depressants including alcohol, antihistamines, antidepressants, opioids, and other sedative-hypnotics.

ANTIPARKINSONIAN DRUGS

Named for British physician James Parkinson, **Parkinson's disease** is a neurologic disorder characterized by the development of a fine, slowly spreading tremor, muscular weakness and rigidity, and the development of disturbances in posture and equilibrium. The cause of the disease is not fully understood, but it is believed to be associated with an imbalance of the neurotransmitters acetylcholine and dopamine in the brain.

Antiparkinsonian drugs are used for palliative

TABLE 30-5   NONBARBITURATE SEDATIVE-HYPNOTIC DRUGS

Medication	Schedule	Usual Sedative Dose	Usual Hypnotic Dose
chloral hydrate (Aquachloral)	C IV	Oral, Rectal (Adult): 250 mg 3 times a day after meals Oral (Child): 8–25 mg/kg/24 hours divided into 2–3 doses	Oral, Rectal (Adult): 500 mg to 1 g before bedtime Oral (Child): 50 mg/kg to a maximum of 1 g
flurazepam HCl (Dalmane)	C IV	No listing	Oral: 15–30 mg at bedtime
lorazepam (Ativan)	C IV	No listing	Oral (Adult): 2–4 mg at bedtime
oxazepam (Serax)	C IV	No listing	Oral (Adult): 15–30 mg at bedtime
temazepam (Restoril)	C IV	No listing	Oral (Adult): 15–30 mg at bedtime Oral (Elderly): 15 mg as an initial dose
triazolam (Halcion)	C IV	No listing	Oral (Adult): 0.25–0.5 mg Oral (Elderly): 0.125–0.25 mg
zaleplon (Sonata)	C IV	No listing	Oral (Adult): 10 mg at bedtime
zolpidem tartrate (Ambien)	C IV	No listing	Oral (Adult): 10 mg at bedtime

relief from such major symptoms as bradykinesia, rigidity, tremor, and disorders of equilibrium and posture. The drug of choice depends upon the severity of the disease at the time of diagnosis and is subject to change with the continuation of the disease. Therapy involves an attempt to replenish dopamine levels and/or inhibit the effects of the neurotransmitter acetylcholine. See Table 30-6.

Actions

These drugs exert an inhibitory effect upon the parasympathetic nervous system. They prolong the action of dopamine by blocking its uptake into presynaptic neurons in the central nervous system.

Uses

Treatment of all forms of parkinsonism.

TABLE 30-6   ANTIPARKINSONIAN DRUGS

Medication	Drug Action	Usual Dosage	Adverse Reactions
amantadine HCl (Symmetrel)	Anticholinergic	Oral: 100 mg twice daily	Dizziness, lightheadedness, irritability, hypotension, edema, anorexia, nausea
benztropine mesylate (Cogentin)	Anticholinergic	Oral: 0.5–6 mg/day if required and tolerated	Sedation, dizziness, tachycardia, nausea, vomiting, urinary retention, dysuria
biperiden HCl (Akineton)	Anticholinergic	Oral: 2 mg 1–4 times daily	Dry mouth, blurred vision, constipation, dizziness
bromocriptine mesylate (Parlodel)	Dopamine receptor agonist	Oral: 1.25 mg 1–2 times daily, increased by 2.5 mg/day in 2–4 week intervals	Orthostatic hypotension, rash, shock, nausea, dizziness, epigastric pain, blurred vision
carbidopa/ levodopa (Sinemet)	Anticholinergic	Oral: 1–6 tablets 3 times daily (tablets contain 10 mg carbidopa and 100 mg levodopa)	No reactions for carbidopa; for levodopa: involuntary movements, nausea, anorexia, urinary retention, dry mouth

(continued)

TABLE 30-6 *(Continued)*

Medication	Drug Action	Usual Dosage	Adverse Reactions
entacapone (Comtan)	COMT inhibitor (catechol-O-methyltransferase)	Oral: 200 mg administered with a levodopa/carbidopa regimen up to a maximum of 8 times/day (1600 mg/day)	Dyskinesia, hyperkinesia, hypokinesia, dizziness, anxiety, somnolence, agitation, hallucinations, nausea, vomiting, diarrhea, abdominal pain, dry mouth, dyspepsia, fatigue, asthenia, back pain, dyspnea, purpura
levodopa (Dopar, Larodopa, L-dopa)	Metabolic precursor of dopamine	Oral: 0.5–8 g daily divided into 2 or more equal doses	Orthostatic hypotension, anorexia, nausea, abdominal distress, increased hand tremor, grinding of the teeth
ropinirole (Requip) (See Figure 30-3)	Dopamine agonist	Oral: 0.25 mg three times a day, then physician increases dose as needed and tolerated. The dose is usually not more than 24 mg/day.	Confusion, dizziness, drowsiness, falling, lightheadedness or fainting, nausea, hallucinations, swelling of legs, twitching, unusual tiredness or weakness, worsening of Parkinson's disease
tolcapone (Tasmar)	COMT inhibitor (catechol-O-methyltransferase)	Oral: 100–200 mg three times/day in addition to current carbidopa/levodopa medications	Abnormal jerky movements, nausea, confusion, dizziness or fainting, especially upon quickly standing or going from a reclining to an upright position, sleep disorders, diarrhea, hallucinations
trihexyphenidyl HCl (Artane)	Anticholinergic	Oral: 1–10 mg daily in 3 or more divided doses	Dry mouth, dizziness, nausea, blurred vision, nervousness

Contraindications

Contraindicated in clients with known hypersensitivity to any of its ingredients. They should not be used in clients with narrow-angle glaucoma, myasthenia gravis, gastrointestinal and/or genitourinary obstructions, and children under 3 years of age.

Safety Precaution

1. Before initiation of drug therapy, client should have a gonioscopic evaluation (inspection of the angle of the anterior chamber of the eye and determination of ocular motility and rotation), and close monitoring of intraocular pressure at regular intervals.
2. Cautious use during pregnancy, lactation, and in the geriatric client
3. Clients with cardiac, liver, or kidney disorders and/or hypertension should be carefully monitored while on an antiparkinsonian drug.

Adverse Reactions

Dryness of the mouth, blurring of vision, dizziness, mild nausea, nervousness, suppurative parotitis, skin rash, dilatation of the colon, paralytic ileus, delusions, hallucinations, paranoia, constipation, drowsiness, urinary hesitancy or retention, tachycardia, dilation of the pupil, increased intraocular tension, weakness, vomiting, headache, angle-closure glaucoma.

Dosage and Route

The dosage and route of administration is determined by the physician and individualized for each client. (See Table 30-6.)

Nursing Considerations

Observe the client for evidence of improvement and signs of adverse reactions. Monitor vital signs, intake and output ratio, gastrointestinal function, and mental status of the client.

Clients' Instruction

Educate the client to

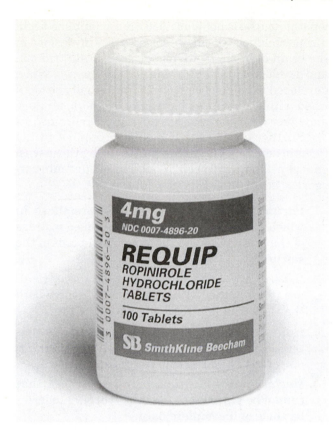

FIGURE 30-3 REQUIP (ROPINIROLE HYDROCHLORIDE) 4 MG TABLETS *(Courtesy of SmithKline Beecham)*

- Take the medication as prescribed
- Be alert for signs of adverse reactions
- Avoid the use of alcohol and over-the-counter medications
- Not operate machinery or drive a motor vehicle after taking the medication

Special Considerations

- Medication should not be discontinued abruptly. It should be tapered off over 1–2 weeks. Sudden withdrawal of medication may precipitate a parkinsonian crisis characterized by anxiety, sweating, and tachycardia, and an exacerbation of tremors, rigidity, and dyskinesia.
- Administer with or after meals to help prevent gastrointestinal upset.
- Anticholinergic effects may be increased by alcohol, narcotics, barbiturates, antihistamines, MAOIs, phenothiazines, and/or amantadine.
- Pyridoxine will reduce the therapeutic effect of levodopa; therefore, only pyridoxine-free multivitamins should be taken when taking levodopa.

Larobec is a vitamin supplement made specifically for clients taking levodopa.

- When taking levodopa, adequate fluid intake and eating bulk-forming foods should be encouraged to minimize the possibility of constipation.
- When taking levodopa, the urine may turn red to black on exposure to air or alkaline substances (toilet bowl cleansers). The client needs to be informed of this so that he/she will not be alarmed.

ALZHEIMER'S DISEASE (AD)

Alzheimer's disease (AD) is a progressive degeneration of brain tissue that usually begins after age 60. It may also rarely affect persons as young as age 30. This disease is marked by a devastating mental decline. Intellectual functions such as memory, comprehension, and speech deteriorate. Attention tends to stray, simple calculations become impossible, and ordinary daily activities grow increasingly difficult, with bewilderment and frustration worsening at night. Dramatic mood swings occur, with outbursts of anger, bouts of fearfulness, and periods of deep apathy. The person with AD, increasingly disoriented, may wander off and become lost. Physical problems, such as odd gait or loss of coordination, gradually develop. Eventually, the client may become totally noncommunicative, physically helpless, and incontinent. The disease is invariably fatal.

In Alzheimer's disease, the paths of communication between brain cells become distorted by deposits of a protein called amyloid. In addition, acetylcholine levels begin to drop, causing more cell-to-cell communication problems. Eventually, the brain cells themselves are affected. They begin to shrivel and die, causing certain areas of the brain to shrink.

Alzheimer's can run its course from insidious onset to death in just a few years, or it may play out over a period of as long as 20 years; the average duration, however, is about 10 years. Among American adults, it is the fourth leading cause of death.

Age and family history are the two most important risk factors for developing this disease. Alzheimer's affects an estimated 4 million older Americans, and, as the baby boomers age, it may eventually affect 14 million by the year 2040. At age 65, approximately 1 percent of persons are stricken, but this increases to more than 30 percent after age 85. In addition to age, there appear to be inherited factors that increase the risk for Alzheimer's disease. Current research links these genetic factors to areas on chromosomes 12 and 19.

Symptoms of the disease include

- Mood changes: depression, paranoia, agitation, anxiety, selfishness, childish behavior
- Disorientation, confusion, inattention, loss of memory for recent events, inability to retain new information
- Increased tendency to misplace things
- Dizziness or impaired equilibrium

Treatment

Alzheimer's disease is incurable. Certain medications seem to slow its general progress to some degree in the early stages, and others can help with mood changes and other specific behavioral problems.

Medications

Medications that may be used to improve global functioning (including activities of daily living, behavior, and cognition) in some clients with Alzheimer's are tacrine (Cognex), donepezil hydrochloride (Aricept), and rivastigmine tartrate (Exelon). These drugs are classified as cholinesterase inhibitors and they work by increasing the brain's levels of acetylcholine, which helps to restore communication between brain cells.

There are several drugs that can be prescribed for specific symptoms associated with this disease. Antipsychotic agents, such as haloperidol (Haldol) and thioridazine (Mellaril), may be prescribed for aggressive behavior and agitation. These agents alter the effect of dopamine in the central nervous system. An antidepressant such as sertraline (Zoloft) may be prescribed for depression and a hypnotic such as zolpidem (Ambien) may be prescribed for sleep.

ANTICONVULSANTS

Epilepsy is the most common of the seizure disorders and affects approximately 1 percent of the population. It is characterized by recurrent abnormal electrical discharges within the brain. An epileptic convulsion may be characterized by sudden, brief episodes of altered consciousness, abnormal motor function, and/or sensory function interference. The disorder may be classified as idiopathic or symptomatic in origin, depending upon whether the cause of the condition is known. The majority of cases are id-

iopathic (cause is not identified) and symptoms begin during childhood or early adolescence. Tiny lesions in the brain at birth, metabolic disease, brain trauma, and developmental defects are possible causes. When developed in adulthood, epilepsy can usually be identified with such causes as trauma, tumors, strokes, and other disease processes affecting the brain.

Further classification has been applied to the types of seizures that are experienced by those with epilepsy. They have been divided into four main categories, some of which have subtypes.

1. *Partial seizures* (focal seizures) are those in which electrical disturbance is localized to areas of the brain near the source or focal point of the seizure.
2. *Generalized seizures* (bilateral, symmetrical) are those without local onset that involve both the right and left hemispheres of the brain.
3. *Unilateral seizures* are those in which the electrical discharge is predominantly confined to one of the two hemispheres of the brain.
4. *Unclassified epileptic seizures* are those that cannot be placed into the other three categories because of incomplete data.

With all types of epilepsy, the objective of drug therapy is to obtain the greatest degree of control over seizures without causing intolerable side effects. Selection of the most appropriate drug for a client with epilepsy depends upon proper diagnosis and classification. The appropriate dosage must be individualized and is related to the size, age, and condition of the client, how the client responds to treatment, and whether the client is taking other medication. See Table 30-7.

Actions

Inhibits spread of seizure activity in the motor cortex.

Uses

Indicated for the control of tonic-clonic and psychomotor (grand mal and temporal lobe) seizures, and prevention and treatment of seizures occurring during or following neurosurgery.

Contraindications

Contraindicated in clients with known hypersensitivity to any of its ingredients. They should not be used in clients with psychiatric disease and during pregnancy/lactation.

TABLE 30-7   ANTICONVULSANTS

Medication	Usual Dosage	Adverse Reactions
carbamazepine (Tegretol)	Oral (Adult): 200 mg twice/day, increased to a maximum of 120 mg/day in 3–4 doses Oral (Child): 100 mg twice/day, increased to a maximum of 1000 mg/day in 3–4 doses	Dizziness, vertigo, drowsiness, edema, arrhythmias, skin rashes, nausea, vomiting, abdominal pain, aplastic anemia, blurred vision
clonazepam (Klonopin)	Oral (Adult): 1.5 mg/day divided into 3 doses, increased by 0.5–1 mg every 3 days until seizures are controlled Oral (Child): 0.01–0.03 mg/kg/day not to exceed 0.05 mg/day in 3 divided doses	Palpitations, bradycardia, hair loss, hirsutism, skin rash, sore gums, drowsiness, ataxia, dysuria
ethosuximide (Zarontin)	Oral: 250 mg twice/day, increased by 250 mg every 4–7 hours until controlled Oral (Child under 6): 250 mg daily	Hiccups, ataxia, dizziness, hyperactivity, anxiety, epigastric distress, nausea, leukopenia
felbamate (Felbatol)	Oral (Adult): 1200 mg/day in 3–4 divided doses, gradually increased to 3600 mg/day Oral (Children): With Lennox-Gastaut syndrome: 15 mg/kg/day; maximum 45 mg/kg/day	Vomiting, constipation, insomnia, headache, fatigue, nausea, dizziness, anorexia, fever
levetiracetam (Keppra)	Oral (Adult): Initial dose 500 mg bid. Can increase dose by 1000 mg/day every 2 weeks up to a maximum daily dose of 3000 mg	Somnolence, dizziness, ataxia, depression, nervousness, vertigo, amnesia, anxiety, hostility, paresthesia, psychotic symptoms, pharyngitis, rhinitis, sinusitis, increased cough, abdominal pain, constipation, diarrhea, dyspepsia, gastoenteritis, gingivitis, nausea, vomiting, headache, anorexia, diplopia, coordination difficulties
phenobarbital sodium (Luminal)	Oral (Adult): 50–100 mg/day IV (Adult): 100–320 mg/day Oral (Child): 16–50 mg 2–3 times daily	Nightmares, insomnia, hangover, dizziness, bradycardia, nausea, coughing, hiccups, liver damage
phenytoin, phenytoin sodium (Dilantin)	Oral (Adult): 100 mg 3 times/day, then gradual increase up to 600 mg/day Parenteral (Adult): 300–400 mg/daily Oral (Child): 4–8 mg/kg/day in 1–3 doses Parenteral (Child): 5 mg/kg in 1–2 doses	Nystagmus, diplopia, blurred or dimmed vision, drowsiness, ataxia, slurred speech, hypotension, nausea, epigastric pain, pruritus, acute renal failure, hyperglycemia, gingival hyperplasia, hirsutism
primidone (Mysoline)	Oral: 250 mg/day, increased by 250 mg weekly (maximum 2 g/day in 2–4 doses) Oral (Child under 8): half of adult dose	Drowsiness, sedation, vertigo, nausea, anorexia, nystagmus, swelling of eyelids, alopecia
valproic acid (Depakene)	Oral: 15 mg/kg/day, increased at 1 week intervals by 5–10 mg/kg/day (maximum recommended dose 60 mg/kg/day)	Breakthrough seizures, sedation, drowsiness, dizziness, ataxia, nausea, hypersalivation, hepatic failure, depression, skin rash

Safety Precaution

1. Abrupt withdrawal of medication in epileptic clients may precipitate status epilepticus.

2. There may be a relationship between anticonvulsants and the development of lymphadenopathy.

3. Acute alcohol intake may increase anticonvulsant drugs serum levels while chronic alcohol use may decrease serum levels.

4. There are many precautions associated with anticonvulsants. Please refer to a current edition of a *Physicians' Desk Reference* or a *PDR Nurse's Drug Handbook* for information on precautions.

Adverse Reactions

Nystagmus, ataxia, slurred speech, mental confusion, dizziness, insomnia, transient nervousness, motor twitching, headache, drug induced dyskinesias similar to those induced by phenothiazines and other neuroleptic agents, nausea, vomiting, constipation, toxic hepatitis, liver damage, fever, measles-like rash, thrombocytopenia, leukopenia, granulocytopenia, agranulocytosis, pancytopenia, lymphadenopathy, coarsening of facial features, enlargement of the lips, liver dysfunction.

Dosage and Route

The dosage and route of administration is determined by the physician and individualized for each client. See Table 30-7.

Nursing Considerations

Observe client for signs of improvement and adverse reactions. Monitor vital signs, weight, blood and liver function studies, intake and output ratio, and drug serum levels.

Clients' Instruction

Educate the client

- To take the medication as prescribed
- To be alert for signs of adverse reactions
- To avoid the use of alcohol and over-the-counter medications

- To not operate machinery or drive a motor vehicle while taking medication
- To wear a Medic Alert ID stating that he/she is an epileptic and on medication
- To see his/her physician on a regular basis
- About support groups and self-help/management programs that can assist in his/her treatment regimen

Teach the client's family how to care for the client during a seizure as per the following:

- Protect from nearby hazards by moving hazard away from the client.
- Do not move or restrain the client.
- Do not put anything in the client's mouth.
- Do not try to hold the client's tongue; it cannot be swallowed.
- Provide for privacy.
- Observe and record the time and length of the seizure: when it started and ended.
- Record if there is loss of bladder or bowel control and/or loss of consciousness.
- Following the seizure, maintain an open airway, turn the client on his/her side, loosen any tight clothing from the neck, reassure the client, and provide for a period of rest.
- Do not give liquid or food until the client is fully conscious and has had an adequate time to recover from the seizure.
- If multiple seizures occur or one seizure lasts longer than 5 minutes, call 911 for help.

Special Considerations

- Some anticonvulsant agents may discolor the urine pink.
- Anticonvulsant medication should not be abruptly discontinued as seizures can occur.
- Drug therapy is individualized for each client and it may involve trying several different drugs and dosages before therapeutic response is reached.
- The effects of anticonvulsants may be decreased by alcohol, antihistamines, antacids, antineoplastics, CNS depressants, rifampin, and/or folic acid.

TABLE 30-8　LOCAL (REGIONAL) ANESTHETIC DRUGS

Medication	Route(s)	Usual Strength of Dosage	Adverse Reactions
bupivacaine HCl (Marcaine HCl)	injection	0.25–0.75% solution	Usually dose related: apnea, hypotension, heart block
dyclonine HCl (Dyclone)	topical	0.5–1% solution	Urticaria, edema, burning, hypotension, blurred vision
lidocaine HCl (Xylocaine HCl)	topical, injection	2.5–5% cream, ointment, jelly 0.5–4% solution	Drowsiness, lightheadedness, euphoria, tinnitus, blurred vision, numbness of lips
procaine HCl (Novocain)	injection	1–10% solution	Nervousness, dizziness, hypotension, postspinal headache
tetracaine HCl (Pontocaine)	topical, injection	0.5–2% ointment, cream 1% solution	Nervousness, blurred vision, drowsiness, nausea, vomiting, chills, hypotension, edema

TABLE 30-9　GENERAL ANESTHETICS

Medication	Brand Name	Route(s)	Remarks
enflurane	Ethrane	Inhalation	Volatile liquid, pleasant odor
etomidate	Amidate	IV injection	Nonbarbiturate hypnotic, rapid onset
fentanyl citrate and droperidol	Innovar	IV injection	Combination drug containing a narcotic analgesic and a major tranquilizer
halothane	Fluothane	Inhalation	Volatile liquid, nonflammable
isoflurane	Forane	Inhalation	Volatile liquid, nonflammable
ketamine	Ketalar	IM, IV injection	Rapid-acting, stimulates muscle tone
methohexital sodium	Brevital	IV injection	Ultra-short-acting barbiturate used for brief operative procedures
methoxyflurane	Penthrane	Inhalation	Volatile liquid, fruity odor
nitrous oxide	—	Inhalation	"Laughing gas," popular anesthetic gas
thiamylal sodium	Surital	IV injection	Rapid-acting barbiturate
thiopental sodium	Pentothal	IV injection, rectal	Ultra-short-acting barbiturate

ANESTHETICS

Anesthetics are drugs that interfere with the conduction of nerve impulses and are used to produce loss of sensation, muscle relaxation, and/or complete loss of consciousness. Local anesthetics block nerve transmission in the area to which they are applied. They produce loss of sensation and motor activity, but do not cause loss of consciousness. See Table 30-8. General anesthetics affect the central nervous system and produce either partial or complete loss of consciousness. They also cause varying degrees of analgesia, skeletal muscle relaxation, and reduction of reflex activity.

General anesthetics should be given only by those who have received adequate training. General anesthetics are of two types: inhalation and injection. Inhalation anesthetics can be further classified as gases or volatile liquids. Table 30-9 is a list of general anesthetic agents.

OPHTHALMIC DRUGS

Medications are used in the eye for the treatment of glaucoma, during diagnostic examination of the eye, and in intraocular surgery. Glaucoma is an eye disease characterized by increased intraocular pressure, which, if not treated, causes atrophy of the optic nerve and blindness. The disease occurs when there is a failure to remove aqueous humor at a rate equal to its production. Drugs used to treat glaucoma either increase the outflow of aqueous humor, decrease its production, or produce both of these actions.

TABLE 30-10 DRUGS USED TO TREAT GLAUCOMA

Medication	Classification	Usual Dosage	Adverse Reactions
acetazolamide (Diamox)	Carbonic anhydrase inhibitor, diuretic	Oral: 250 mg every 6 hours IM, IV: 500 mg repeated in 2–4 hours, if necessary	Paresthesias, drowsiness, tinnitus, nausea, rash, bone marrow depression
demecarium bromide (Humorsol)	Cholinesterase inhibitor, miotic	Topical: 1–2 drops of 0.125% or 0.25% solution 2 times/week up to twice daily	Stinging, burning, ciliary spasm, lacrimation, brow and eye pain, headache
mannitol (Osmitrol)	Osmotic diuretic	IV infusion: 1.5–2 g/kg as a 15–25% solution over 30–60 minutes	Dry mouth, thirst, blurred vision, urinary retention, congestive heart failure
methazolamide (Neptazane)	Carbonic anhydrase inhibitor	Oral: 50–100 mg every 8 hours	Malaise, drowsiness, mild GI disturbances, vertigo
physostigmine sulfate (Eserine Sulfate)	Cholinesterase inhibitor, miotic	Topical: 1 cm strip of 0.25% ointment 1–3 times daily Ophthalmic: 1–2 drops 3 times daily of 0.25–0.5% solution	Headache, eye and brow pain, marked miosis, dimness and blurring of vision, lacrimation

Drugs used to treat glaucoma are listed in Table 30-10.

Mydriatic Drugs

Anticholinergic agents produce dilation of the pupil (**mydriasis**) and interfere with the ability of the eye to focus properly (paralysis of accommodation or cycloplegia). Mydriatic drugs are used primarily as an aid in refraction, during internal examination of the eye, in intraocular surgery, and in the treatment of anterior uveitis and secondary glaucomas.

Sympathomimetic mydriatics produce mydriasis without cycloplegia. Pupil dilation is obtained as the drug causes contraction of the dilator muscle of the iris. These drugs also affect intraocular pressure by decreasing production of aqueous humor while increasing its outflow from the eyes. Mydriatic agents are listed in Table 30-11.

TABLE 30-11 MYDRIATIC AGENTS

Medication	Classification	Usual Dosage	Adverse Reactions
atropine sulfate (Atropisol)	Anticholinergic mydriatic	Topical: 1–2 drops of 0.5–1% solution 1–3 times daily	Blurred vision, photophobia, increased intraocular pressure
dipivefrin (Propine)	Sympathomimetic, adrenergic agonist	Topical: 1 drop of 0.1% solution in eye every 12 hours	Burning, stinging upon application, photophobia
epinephrine HCl (Glaucon)	Sympathomimetic, adrenergic agonist	Topical: 1–2 drops of 0.1% solution in eye	Lacrimation, headache, stinging sensation
naphazoline HCl (Naphcon)	Sympathomimetic, adrenergic agonist	Topical: 1–2 drops of 1% solution every 3–4 hours	Increased intraocular pressure, mydriasis
phenylephrine HCl (Neo-Synephrine)	Sympathomimetic, adrenergic agonist	Topical: 1 drop of 2.5–10% solution 3 times/day	Stinging, browache, sensitivity to light
scopolamine HBr (Hyoscine)	Anticholinergic mydriatic	Topical: 1–2 drops of 0.5–1% solution	Follicular conjunctivitis, local irritation
tropicamide (Mydriacyl)	Anticholinergic mydriatic	Topical: 1–2 drops of 1% solution, repeat in 5 minutes	Photophobia, transient stinging, blurred vision

DRUGS USED IN VERTIGO, MOTION SICKNESS, AND VOMITING

Vertigo describes an illusion of movement. Individuals experiencing vertigo may have the sensation of moving around in space, or know that they are stationary but sense that objects are in motion. Vertigo may be caused by a lesion or other process affecting the brain, the eighth cranial nerve, or the labyrinthine system of the ear. The result is a disturbance of equilibrium wherein the person experiences dizziness, lightheadedness, and possible nausea and vomiting.

Motion sickness is usually associated with travel. Sometimes called seasickness, carsickness, or airsickness, this condition affects large numbers of people and causes nausea and vomiting. About one-third of the population is highly susceptible to motion and another third experiences symptoms when exposed to moderately rough travel conditions. Drugs are used for symptomatic relief rather than for treatment.

Vomiting is a complex reflex that may result from disease, drugs, radiation, toxins, and many other causes that serve to stimulate the vomiting center in the medulla. Since nausea and vomiting are symptoms of underlying causes, every effort should be made to identify and correct the causative condition.

Certain anticholinergic, antihistaminic, and antidopaminergic drugs have been identified as being effective in the treatment of vertigo, motion sickness, and vomiting; however, not all of the drugs in these classifications are effective in these disorders. Those that are effective are listed in Table 30-12.

TABLE 30-12   DRUGS USED IN VERTIGO, MOTION SICKNESS, AND VOMITING

Medication	Uses	Usual Dosage	Adverse Reactions
chlorpromazine (Thorazine)	Nausea, vomiting	Oral: 10–25 mg every 4–6 hours as needed IM: 25–50 mg every 3–4 hours as needed Rectal: One 100 mg suppository every 6–8 hours	Sedation, depressed cough reflex, bizarre dreams, orthostatic hypotension, constipation, blurred vision, nasal congestion, respiratory depression
dimenhydrinate (Dramamine)	Motion sickness, nausea, vomiting, vertigo	Oral: 50–100 mg every 4–6 hours IM, IV: 50 mg	Drowsiness, headache, dizziness, insomnia, hypotension, blurred vision, dry mouth
diphenhydramine HCl (Benadryl)	Motion sickness, vertigo	Oral, IM, IV: 25–50 mg 3–4 times daily at 4–6 hour intervals	Drowsiness, dizziness, headache, fatigue, euphoria, dry mouth, blurred vision, dysuria
meclizine HCl (Antivert)	Nausea, vomiting, motion sickness, vertigo	Oral: 25–100 mg daily in divided doses	Drowsiness, blurred vision, dry mouth, fatigue
promethazine HCl (Phenergan)	Motion sickness, nausea, vomiting	Oral, IM, IV, Rectal suppository: 12.5–25 mg and again at 4–6 hour intervals as needed	Sedation, confusion, dizziness, tremors, anorexia, dry mouth, leukopenia, blurred vision, photosensitivity
scopolamine (Transderm-scop)	Motion sickness, nausea, vomiting	Topical: transdermal delivery of 0.5 mg over 3 days. Apply to dry skin behind one of the ears.	Fatigue, drowsiness, dry mouth, urinary retention, depressed respiration
thiethylperazine maleate (Torecan)	Nausea, vomiting, vertigo	Oral, IM, Rectal suppository: 10 mg 1–3 times/day	Drowsiness, dizziness, dry mouth, and nose, blurred vision, tinnitus, fever
triflupromazine HCl (Vesprin)	Severe nausea and vomiting	Oral: 10–30 mg/day IM: 5–60 mg/day IV: 1–3 mg/day	Xerostomia, constipation, drowsiness, nasal congestion, urinary retention, hypotension

(continued)

TABLE 30-12 *(Continued)*

Medication	Uses	Usual Dosage	Adverse Reactions
trimethobenzamide HCl (Tigan)	Nausea, vomiting	Oral: 250 mg 3–4 times daily Rectal: 200 mg 3–4 times daily IM: 200 mg 3–4 times daily	Allergic skin eruptions, hypotension, blurred vision, headache, drowsiness, diarrhea, acute hepatitis, muscle cramps

● SELF-ASSESSMENT

Write the answer in the space provided or circle true or false as instructed.

Source

p. 391   **1.** Guidelines from the Agency on Health Care Policy and Research urge physicians to treat clients with chronic intractable pain progressively by starting them out on _____, followed by _____, and finally using _____ .

p. 391   **2.** The two methods used to monitor treatment effectiveness for pain management are _____ and _____ .

p. 392   **3.** In a few words, complete the definitions of the following terms:
   • Opiates are _____ .
   • Opioids are _____ .

p. 396   **4.** In a few words, complete the definitions of the following terms:
   • A sedative dosage is designed to _____ .
   • A hypnotic dosage is designed to _____ .

p. 397   **5.** Short- and intermediate-acting barbiturates are used in treating insomnia because of their _____ , and their use rarely cause a _____ effect.

p. 399   **6.** Drug therapy for Parkinson's disease involves an attempt to replace _____ and/or inhibit the effects of the neurotransmitter _____ .

p. 402   **7.** With all types of epilepsy, the objective of drug therapy is to obtain the greatest degree of _____ without causing intolerable _____ .

p. 405   **8.** In a few words, distinguish between the actions of agents classified as
   • General anesthetics _____
   • Local anesthetics _____

p. 405   **9.** True or False (circle one) Drugs used to treat glaucoma either increase the outflow of aqueous humor, decrease its production, or produce both of these actions.

p. 407   **10.** To treat motion sickness with the transdermal application of Scopolamine, one applies the adhesive patch to the dry skin located _____ .

● WEB ACTIVITY

Visit the following Web sites for additional information on medications used for nervous system disorders:

http://pharmacotherapy.medscape.com

http://www.docguide.com

http://www.discoveryhealth.com

http://www.pharminfo.com

http://www.onhealth.com

http://www.healthspotlight.com

http://www.fda.gov

http://www.intelihealth.com

http://www.rxlist.com

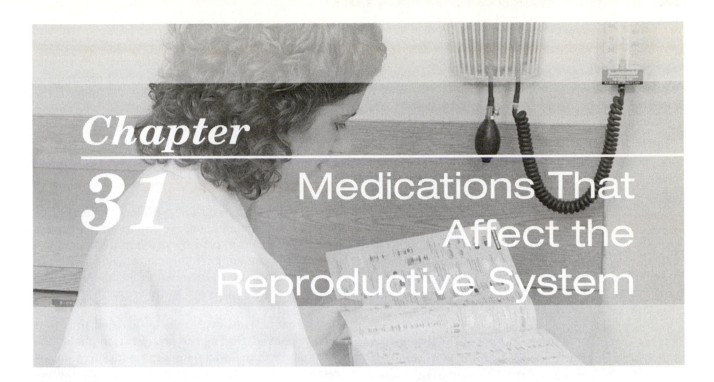

Chapter
31
Medications That Affect the Reproductive System

Chapter Outline

Objectives

Key Terms

Introduction

Female Hormones

Hormone Replacement Therapy

Oral Contraceptives

Male Hormones

Drugs Used During Labor and Delivery

Spot Check

Self-Assessment

Web Activity

Objectives

Upon completion of this chapter, you should be able to

- Define the key terms
- Describe the functions of the ovaries
- Describe the functions of the testes
- Understand the actions, uses, contraindications, safety precautions, adverse reaction, dosage and route, nursing considerations, clients' instruction, and special considerations for estrogen and progesterone preparations

- Describe hormone replacement therapy, giving the benefits and risks
- Describe selected estrogen preparations and/or combination estrogen and progestin that are prescribed for menopausal and postmenopausal women
- Describe how oral contraceptives, when used as directed, prevent the occurrence of pregnancy
- Identify selected oral contraceptives as monophasic, biphasic, triphasic, and progesterone-only preparations
- Understand the actions, uses, contraindications, safety precautions, adverse reaction, dosage and route, nursing considerations, clients' instruction, and special considerations for testosterone preparations
- Describe erectile dysfunction and list several physical causes of this condition
- State the action, uses, contraindications, safety precaution, adverse reactions, dosage and route, and clients' instruction for sildenafil citrate (Viagra)
- Describe the drugs that may be used during labor and delivery
- Complete the Spot Check on hormone replacement therapy pharmaceuticals
- Complete the Self-Assessment
- Visit indicated Web sites for additional information on medications used for reproductive system disorders

Key Terms

cryptorchidism

erectile dysfunction (ED)

hormone replacement therapy (HRT)

hypogonadism

menopause

menstruation

minipill

oxytocic agents

priapism

progestin

INTRODUCTION

The ovaries in the female (Figure 31-1) and the testes in the male (Figure 31-2) are the primary organs of sexual reproduction. With the onset of puberty (ages 9–16 in females, 13–15 in males), the pituitary gland secretes increased amounts of two gonad-stimulating hormones that cause the reproductive organs to mature and begin the production of ova and sperm. Known as follicle-stimulating hormone (FSH) and luteinizing hormone (LH), these secretions continue to exert control over the functions of the reproductive organs after maturation.

The functions of the ovaries are (1) production of ova and (2) secretion of the female sex hormones estrogen and progesterone. The functions of the testes are (1) production of sperm and (2) secretion of the male sex hormone testosterone. The female sex hormones are instrumental in the development of breast tissue, pubic and axillary hair growth, and the preparation of the uterus for pregnancy. In the male, testosterone is essential for the growth and development of male accessory sexual organs, the deepening of the voice, muscular development, the growth of facial, pubic, and axillary hair, and the occurrence of penile erection.

FEMALE HORMONES

One needs to be familiar with the interrelated processes of the menstrual cycle in order to fully appreciate the role played by the female hormones. The onset of the menstrual cycle coincides with puberty, ends during menopause, and in human females occurs monthly on an average of every 28 days.

The menstrual cycle can be divided into four distinct phases. During the proliferation phase, the ovarian (graafian follicle) undergoes maturation, secretes estrogen, and thickening and vascularization of the endometrium occurs. This phase ends when the ovarian follicle ruptures, expelling the ovum into the fallopian tube. Estrogen, due to the source of its secretion, is sometimes referred to as the follicular hormone. The next phase in the cycle is the luteal or secretory phase, which is characterized by continued thickening and vascularization of the endometrium and the secretion of progesterone by the

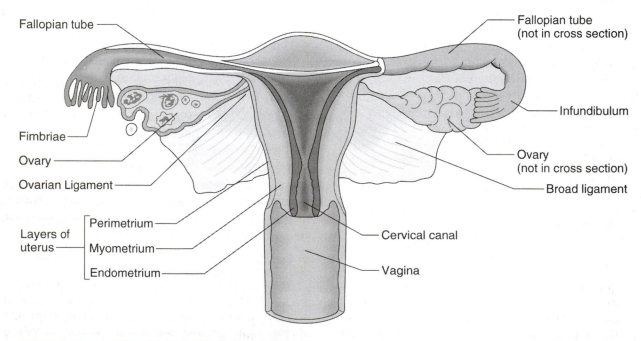

FIGURE 31-1 FEMALE REPRODUCTIVE ORGANS

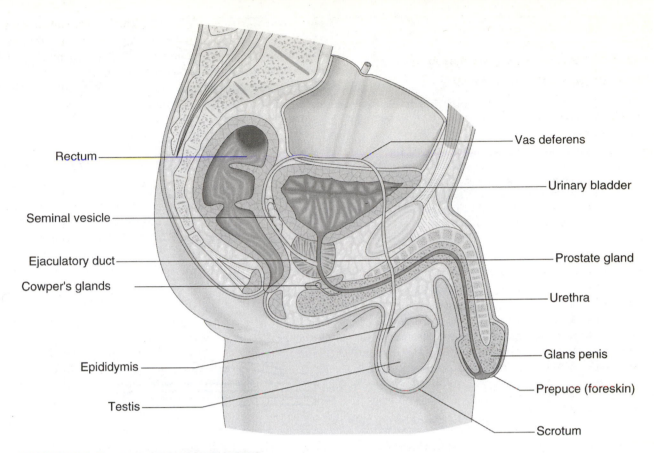

Rectum

Seminal vesicle

Ejaculatory duct

Cowper's glands

Epididymis

Testis

Vas deferens

Urinary bladder

Prostate gland

Urethra

Glans penis

Prepuce (foreskin)

Scrotum

FIGURE 31-2   MALE REPRODUCTIVE ORGANS

corpus luteum, a small yellow body within the ruptured ovarian follicle. Because it is produced by the corpus luteum, progesterone is called the luteal hormone. At this point, the thick, spongy uterine lining is engorged with blood. If conception has not occurred, the cycle enters the premenstrual phase, characterized by constriction of the coiled arteries within the uterine lining, shrinkage of the endometrium, and a decrease in hormonal secretion by the corpus luteum. This phase ends with the start of the menstrual flow. The fourth phase is known as **menstruation**. This is a period of uterine bleeding, containing endometrial cells, blood, and glandular secretions, lasting 4–5 days. After menstruation, the endometrium of the uterus is again thin and the cycle begins anew.

Estrogen

Estrogen preparations are used for a variety of conditions such as in the treatment of amenorrhea, dysfunctional bleeding, hirsutism, and in palliative therapy for breast cancer in men and postmenopausal women and prostatic cancer in men.

They may also be used to relieve the uncomfortable symptoms of menopause. In this instance, estrogen replacement therapy is useful in the prevention of osteoporosis. (See Figure 31-3.)

Actions

Estrogens promote growth, development, and maintenance of the female reproductive system and secondary sex characteristics. They also affect the release of pituitary gonadotropins.

Uses

Menopause, atrophic vaginitis, atrophic urethritis, osteoporosis, hypogonadism, castration, primary ovarian failure, breast cancer, and androgen-dependent carcinoma of the prostate.

Contraindications

Contraindicated in clients with known hypersensitivity to any of its ingredients, known or suspected pregnancy, breast cancer, estrogen-dependent neoplasia, undiagnosed abnormal genital bleeding, thrombophlebitis, thromboembolic disorders.

ESTRADERM®
Estradiol Transdermal System

What is ESTRADERM®?

Estraderm is an estrogen skin patch that relieves menopausal symptoms such as hot flashes, night sweats, and vaginal dryness.

Less than 2 inches in diameter, the wafer-thin patch delivers estradiol, the same estrogen as that produced by a woman's ovaries prior to menopause, through the skin directly to the bloodstream, without first passing through the liver. This avoids changes in hepatic function that may be associated with other forms of estrogen therapy.

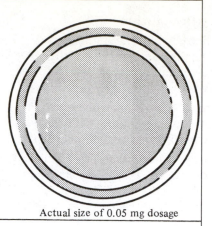

Actual size of 0.05 mg dosage

The ESTRADERM® skin patch is composed of five layers.

1. A sealed backing that holds the drug in the system
2. A reservoir containing estradiol
3. A membrane that controls the release of estradiol
4. A nonallergenic adhesive that keeps the patch on the skin
5. A protective peel strip

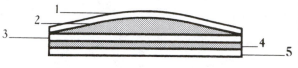

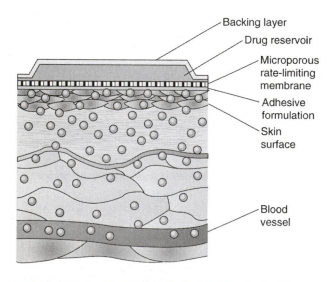

Backing layer
Drug reservoir
Microporous rate-limiting membrane
Adhesive formulation
Skin surface
Blood vessel

Four separate layers are inside the transdermal therapeutic system, a revolutionary way of delivering medicine to the body. Applied like a bandage, the system provides a consistent and controlled amount of medication through the skin, directly into the bloodstream over an extended period of time. The latest application of transdermal technology is Estraderm® (Estradiol Transdermal System), a low-dose estrogen skin patch available by prescription for the relief of such menopausal symptoms as hot flashes, night sweats, and vaginal dryness.

FIGURE 31-3 ESTROGEN CAN BE PROVIDED TRANSDERMALLY. *(Courtesy of CIBA-GEIGY Pharmaceuticals, Summit, New Jersey)*

Safety Precaution

1. Clients who take higher doses of estrogens for a long period of time (5 years or more) may have an increased risk of breast cancer.

2. There is a 2.5-fold increase in the risk of developing gallbladder disease in women receiving postmenopausal estrogens.

3. Large doses of estrogen (5 mg/day) may increase the risk of myocardial infarction in men. This dose is comparable to the dose used to treat cancer of the prostate and breast.

4. If higher doses of estrogen are used, there may be an increase in the risk of developing hypertension.

5. In clients with breast cancer and bone metastases, the administration of estrogen may lead to severe hypercalcemia. If this occurs, the drug should be stopped and appropriate action taken.

Adverse Reactions

Breakthrough bleeding, spotting, breast tenderness and enlargement, nausea, vomiting, abdominal cramps, bloating, cholestatic jaundice, chloasma or melasma, erythema, loss of scalp hair, hirsutism, headache, migraine, dizziness, mental depression, edema, hypertension, intolerance to contact lenses, vaginal candidiasis, changes in weight, hypercalcemia.

Dosage and Route

The dosage and route of administration is determined by the physician and individualized for each client. See Table 31-1.

Nursing Considerations

Observe for signs of improvement and adverse reactions. Weigh daily, and if weight increases by 5 pounds within a week, notify physician. Assess blood pressure every 4 hours and notify physician if a consistent increase is noted in the systolic and/or diastolic readings. Monitor intake and output ratio and liver function studies. Be aware that a client with diabetes may have an increase in urine glucose

TABLE 31-1   ESTROGENS

Medication	Usual Dosage
conjugated estrogens (Premarin)	Oral: 0.3–1.25 mg daily Vaginal: 2–4 g daily
diethylstilbestrol (DES)	Oral: 0.2–0.5 mg daily Vaginal: 0.1–0.5 mg daily for 10–14 days
esterified estrogens (Menest)	Oral: 0.3–1.25 mg daily (cyclic regimen)
estradiol (Estrace)	Oral: 1–2 mg daily
estradiol cypionate in oil (Depo-Estradiol)	IM: 1–5 mg every 3–4 weeks
estradiol hemihydrate (Vagifem)	Vaginal tablet: Treatment of atrophic vaginitis: 1 tablet once daily for 2 weeks; maintenance of 1 tablet twice weekly

estradiol transdermal system
  (Alora, Estraderm)
  (Climara)
  (Fem-Patch)
  (Vivelle)
	
	50–100 mcg/24 hr patch applied twice daily
	50-100 mcg/24 hr patch applied weekly
	25 mg/24 hr patch applied every 7 days
	37.5–100 mcg patch applied twice weekly

estradiol valerate (Clinagen LA, Delestrogen, Dioval, Duragen, Estra-LA, Estro-Span, Gynogen LA, Menaval, Valergen)	Oral: 0.5–2 mg daily or in a cycle IM: 10–20 mg monthly
estropipate (Ogen)	Oral: 0.75–6 mg/day Vaginal: 2–4 g of cream daily

and that the physician should be notified if such occurs. Encourage the client to see the physician on a regular basis.

Clients' Instruction

Educate the client

- To read the package insert (leaflet) that comes with the prescription and to call the physician if there are any questions
- To weigh daily, at the same time of day and with the same amount of clothing on/off
- To notify the physician if there is a weight gain of 5 pounds or more within a week
- To be aware of possible adverse reactions and report any of the following to the physician without delay: abnormal vaginal bleeding, pains in the calves or chest, sudden shortness of breath, severe headache, dizziness, faintness, or changes in vision, breast lumps, jaundice, pain, swelling or tenderness in the abdomen
- To check with the physician before taking calcium supplements
- About breast self-examination
- To see the physician on a regular basis

Special Considerations

- Estrogen replacement therapy is relatively well tolerated by most menopausal women who take the recommended lowest effective dose.
- Estrogens may decrease the action of anticoagulants and oral hypoglycemics.
- Estrogens may increase the action of corticosteroids.
- Anticonvulsants, barbiturates, phenylbutazone, and rifampin may decrease the action of estrogen.
- Possible toxic effect if taken with tricyclic antidepressants

Progesterone

Progesterone is produced by the ovaries and, to a lesser extent, by the adrenal cortex. The primary source of this hormone is the corpus luteum that forms monthly in the ruptured ovarian follicle. Progesterone prepares the uterus for the implantation of the fertilized ovum. It also suppresses ovulation during pregnancy and stimulates the breast to secrete milk following delivery. Natural progesterone, taken orally, is quickly inactivated by the liver; therefore, chemical modification of the progesterone molecule or the use of a synthetic prepa-

ration is necessary to provide a sustained effect. Synthetic preparations are called progestogens/progestins. See Table 31-2.

Progesterone is used to prevent uterine bleeding and is combined with estrogen for treatment of amenorrhea. It is also ordered in cases of infertility, threatened or habitual miscarriage, and for the management of menopausal symptoms.

Actions

Responsible for changes in the uterine endometrium during the second half of the menstrual cycle, development of maternal placenta after implantation, and development of mammary glands.

Uses

Secondary amenorrhea, abnormal uterine bleeding, infertility, threatened or habitual miscarriage.

Contraindications

Contraindicated in clients with known hypersensitivity to any of its ingredients, thrombophlebitis, thromboembolic disorders, cerebral apoplexy, liver disease, breast cancer, reproductive organ cancer(s), undiagnosed vaginal bleeding, missed abortion. Use during pregnancy and lactation is not recommended.

Adverse Reactions

Breast tenderness, galactorrhea, urticaria, pruritus, edema, rash, acne, alopecia, hirsutism, thrombophlebitis, pulmonary embolism, breakthrough

TABLE 31-2 PROGESTOGENS/PROGESTINS

Medications	Available Dosages
medroxyprogesterone acetate	
(Amen)	10 mg
(Cycrin)	2.5 mg, 5 mg, 10 mg
(Provera)	2.5 mg, 5 mg, 10 mg
megestrol acetate	
(Megace)	20 mg, 40 mg, 160 mg
natural progesterone	
(Prometrium)	100 mg
norethindrone acetate	
(Aygestin)	5 mg
(Micronor)	0.35 mg
(Nor-QD)	0.35 mg
(Nortulate)	5 mg
(Nortulin)	5 mg
norgestrel	
(Ovrette)	0.075 mg

bleeding, spotting, amenorrhea, changes in weight, changes in cervical erosion and cervical secretions, cholestatic jaundice, anaphylaxis, mental depression, insomnia, nausea, somnolence.

Dosage and Route

The dosage and route of administration is determined by the physician and individualized for each client. See Table 31-2.

Nursing Considerations

Observe for signs of improvement and adverse reactions. Weigh daily, and if weight increases by 5 pounds within a week, notify physician. Assess blood pressure every 4 hours and notify physician if a consistent increase is noted in the systolic and/or diastolic readings. Monitor intake and output ratio and liver function studies.

Clients' Instruction

Educate the client

- To weigh daily, at the same time of day and with the same amount of clothing on/off
- To notify the physician if there is a weight gain of 5 pounds or more within a week
- To be aware of possible adverse reactions and report any of the following to the physician without delay: abnormal vaginal bleeding, pains in the calves or chest, jaundice, dark urine, clay-colored stools, dyspnea, blurred vision
- About breast self-examination
- To see the physician on a regular basis

Special Considerations

- Progestins may cause fluid retention. Used with caution in clients with epilepsy, migraine, asthma, cardiac disease, and renal dysfunction.
- Clients with mental depression should be carefully observed while using progestins. Discontinue drug if depressive state becomes severe.
- Clients with diabetes should be carefully monitored while taking progestogens. A decrease in glucose tolerance may occur.

HORMONE REPLACEMENT THERAPY

Hormone replacement therapy (HRT) is a medication regimen of providing a woman who has gone through menopause (natural or surgically) with hormones that her body has stopped producing.

At about 50 years of age, women begin experiencing bodily changes that are directly related to hormonal production. The ovaries cease to produce estrogen and progesterone. With decreased production of these female hormones, women enter the phase of life known as **menopause**. Menopause marks the permanent cessation of menstrual activity. It is also referred to as the *climacteric*. Natural menopause will occur in 25 percent of women by age 47, in 50 percent by age 50, in 75 percent by age 52, and in 95 percent by age 55. Menopause may also be surgically produced when a woman has had an oophorectomy.

The symptoms of menopause vary from being hardly noticeable to being severe. They may include irregular periods, hot flashes, vaginal dryness, insomnia, joint pain, headache, emotional instability, irritability, and depression. Breast tissue may lose its firmness, and pubic and axillary hair becomes sparse. Without estrogen, the uterus becomes smaller, the vagina shortens, and vaginal tissues become drier. There may be a loss of bone mass leading to osteoporosis.

Hormone replacement therapy may involve estrogen preparations and/or a combination of estrogen and progestin. Estrogen replacement therapy (ERT) is employed when a woman has had a hysterectomy and does not have a uterus. A combination of estrogen and progestin are employed when a woman has a uterus.

Benefits of Hormone Replacement Therapy

- Relief of uncomfortable menopausal symptoms, such as hot flashes, night sweats, vaginal dryness, irritability, and depression
- Prevention of bone loss and osteoporosis
- May reduce a woman's risk of coronary artery disease and heart disease
- May reduce a woman's risk of developing Alzheimer's disease
- May increase blood levels of high-density lipoproteins (HDL), the good cholesterol

Possible Risks of Hormone Replacement Therapy

The risks depend on the type of treatment prescribed, whether the woman has a uterus, and how long hormones are taken. With short-term therapy of less than 5 years, there are very few risks involved.

- *Endometrial cancer:* If estrogen alone is taken by a woman who has a uterus, there is an increased risk of endometrial cancer. This increased risk can be eliminated by the addition of a progestin to the medication regimen.

- *Breast cancer:* There have been many studies done to evaluate whether hormones cause breast cancer in postmenopausal women. The studies do not agree. Some find no increased risk. Some find a small increased risk after many years (10 to 15 years or more) of regular use. With short-term therapy (less than 5 years), studies show that women are not at increased risk of breast cancer.

Side Effects of Hormone Replacement Therapy

Some of the side effects of estrogen are breast tenderness, edema, nausea, headache, and breakthrough bleeding. Some of the side effects of progestins are fluid retention, acne, anxiety, depression, premenstrual-like symptoms, and irritability.

Hormone Replacement Therapy Pharmaceuticals

There are many pharmaceutical products available for treating the symptoms of menopause and/or providing hormone replacement therapy for postmenopausal women. The following are selected estrogen preparations and/or combination estrogen and progestin prescribed for menopausal and postmenopausal women:

- *Vivelle-Dot (estradiol transdermal system)* is a small ERT patch that comes in four dosage strengths: 0.0375, 0.05, 0.075, and 0.10 mg/day.
- *Cenestin (synthetic conjugated estrogens)* is an oral tablet that is produced from soy and yam plants. It comes in 0.625 mg and 0.9 mg tablets. The commended initial dose is 0.625 mg with titration up to 1.25 mg daily.
- *Prempro (conjugated estrogens/medroxyprogesterone acetate)* is a combination oral tablet that is to be taken once daily. It comes in 0.635 mg/2.5 mg and 0.625 mg/5 mg tablets.
- *Activelle (estradiol/norethindrone acetate)* is a combination oral tablet that is taken once daily. Activelle contains 1 mg estradiol and 0.5 mg norethindrone acetate.
- *CombiPatch (estradiol/norethindrone acetate)* is a single transdermal patch that combines both estrogen and progestin. The patch is changed twice a week.

- *Prometrium (progesterone)* is an oral capsule of micronized progesterone for use with estrogen therapy. It is synthesized from yams and is structurally identical to endogenous (naturally occurring) progesterone found in a woman's body. The suggested dose is 200 mg taken orally once a day, in the evening, for 12 sequential days per 28-day cycle.

ORAL CONTRACEPTIVES

Women who desire to prevent the occurrence of pregnancy may take oral contraceptive pills that are nearly 100 percent effective when used as directed. These pills contain mixtures of estrogen and **progestin** (a large group of drugs that have a progesterone effect on the uterus; synonymous with progesterone) in various levels of strength. The estrogen in the pill inhibits ovulation by suppressing the normal secretion of FSH and LH from the anterior pituitary gland. The progestin inhibits pituitary secretion of LH, causes changes in the cervical mucus that renders it unfavorable to penetration by sperm, and alters the nature of the endometrium.

Most oral contraceptives are taken daily for 20 to 21 days, beginning with the 5th day after menstrual bleeding starts. This cycle is then followed by a week without medication to allow bleeding to occur. An exception to this regimen is a pill that contains only progestin. Called a **minipill**, this product is taken daily and continuously. It acts by interfering with sperm and ovum transport and by adversely affecting the suitability of the endometrium for ovum implant. Progestin-only minipills have been associated with menstrual irregularities (breakthough bleeding) and are slightly less effective than the combination products.

Combination products may contain estrogen and progestin in varying formulations, some having more estrogen, others more progestin. They are available in regular or low-dose strength, again based on the amounts of the two hormones in the product. See Figure 31-4.

Adverse reactions to oral contraceptives are related to their hormone content. Those with high estrogen content tend to cause estrogen-related reactions (nausea, weight gain, edema, swelling of the breast), and those with high progestin content cause progestin-related effects (headache, acne, fatigue). As a rule, those preparations containing the lowest hormone content, but which provide consistently effective contraceptive action, are likely to be preferred because of a lower incidence of adverse reaction.

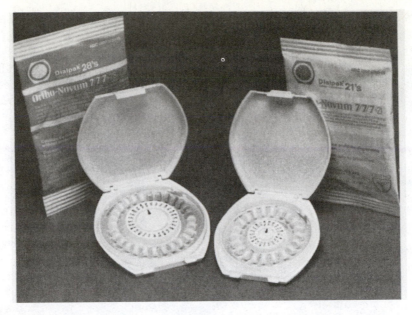

FIGURE 31-4   DIALPAK® ORTHO-NOVUM 7/7/7 *(Courtesy of Ortho Pharmaceutical Corporation)*

Oral contraceptives may be grouped according to the amount of hormone that is available at a given time during the 20–21 day cycle of administration. *Monophasic* preparations provide a fixed concentration of hormones throughout the entire cycle. With *biphasic* preparations, estrogen is available in fixed amounts for the duration of the cycle, but the progestin content is varied. Low levels of progestin are provided during the first half of the cycle and high amounts are included during the last half when endometrial secretions are desired. *Triphasic* preparations vary both the estrogen and progestin dosages within the cycle in an effort to mimic the normal hormonal fluctuation found in women of childbearing age. See Figure 31-5.

An original birth-control pill, Mircette, has a different dosing schedule than other birth-control pills. It comes in a 28-day pill pack containing 26 active white and yellow pills (with hormones) and 2 inactive green pills (without hormones). The regimen begins with 21 days of 20 mcg ethinyl estradiol and 150 mcg desogestrel. The last 7 days in the cycle start with 2 days of placebo pills, followed by 5 days of 10 mcg ethinyl estradiol pills. Also, the total amount of estrogen taken during the month is less than most of the other birth-control pills.

Literature accompanying oral contraceptive preparations usually cautions those who either have or once had any of the following conditions not to take an oral contraceptive:

1. Clots in the legs or lungs
2. Angina pectoris
3. Known or suspected cancer of the breast or sex organs
4. Unusual vaginal bleeding that has not yet been diagnosed
5. Heart attack or stroke
6. Known or suspected pregnancy

Such literature will also include the following statement on cigarette smoking and the use of oral contraceptives:

Safety Precaution: Cigarette smoking increases the risk of serious adverse effects on the heart and blood vessels from oral contraceptive use. This risk increases with age and with heavy smoking (15 or more cigarettes per day) and is quite marked in women over 35 years of age. Women who use oral contraceptives should not smoke.

The choice of an oral contraceptive depends upon a number of factors, including sensitivities to hormones, how the preparation might interact with other drugs being taken, and other considerations. Table 31-3 lists selected oral contraceptive preparations currently in use.

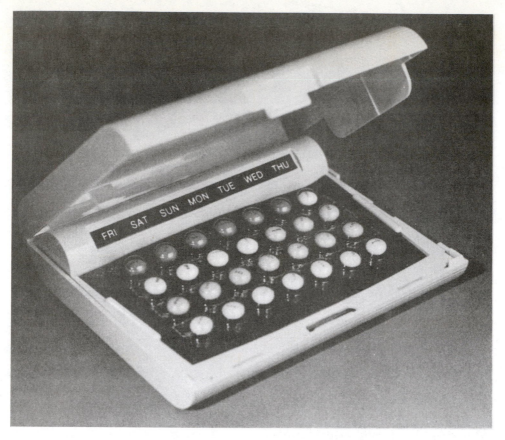

FIGURE 31-5 TRIPHASIL® *(Courtesy of Wyeth Laboratories, Philadelphia, Pennsylvania)*

MALE HORMONES

Adequate secretions of androgenic hormones are necessary to maintain normal male sex characteristics, the male libido, and sexual potency.

Testosterone

Testosterone is the most important androgen and is secreted primarily by the Leydig cells located in the interstitial spaces of the testes. With the advent of puberty (ages 13–15), boys experience a dramatic increase in the amount of testosterone secreted. The increased levels of this hormone stimulate the development of male secondary sex characteristics, initiate the production of sperm, and enhance the functional capacity of the penis and the accessory sex organs in the male. Normal men produce 2.5 to 10 mg of testosterone per day. After the age of 40 there is a gradual decline in the amount of testosterone produced, and by age 80, output is approximately 20 percent of that produced during peak years.

Testosterone is rapidly inactivated by the liver; therefore, longer-lasting testosterone derivatives and synthetic forms of the hormone are available for oral administration, parenteral administration, and as a topical gel and/or transdermal system. These agents are used for replacement therapy in androgen deficiency, for treatment of **hypogonadism** (a condition of defective secretion of the gonads), **cryptorchidism** (failure of the testicles to descend into the scrotum), and for palliative treatment of certain metastatic breast carcinomas in women. See Table 31-4 for selected androgens.

Actions

Testosterone is responsible for growth, development, and maintenance of the male reproductive system and secondary sex characteristics.

Uses

As replacement therapy in primary hypogonadism, hypogonadotropic hypogonadism, to stimulate puberty in carefully selected males, and in impotence. It may be used in women with advanced inoperable metastatic breast cancer who are 1–5 years postmenopausal.

TABLE 31-3   SELECTED ORAL CONTRACEPTIVES

Monophasic Preparations	Biphasic Preparations	Triphasic Preparations	Progesterone Only Preparation
Alesse	Nelova 10/11	Ortho-Novum 7/7/7	Micronor
Brevicon	Ortho-Novum 10/11	Tri-Norinyl	Demulen
Nor-QD		Triphasil	Ovrette
Lo/Ovral			
Modicon			
Nordette			
Norinyl 1+35			
Norlestrin 1/50			
Ovcon-50			

Contraindications

Contraindicated in clients with known hypersensitivity to any of its ingredients, during pregnancy and lactation, in men with cancer of the breast or known or suspected cancer of the prostate, in clients with pituitary insufficiency, history of myocardial infarction, hypercalcemia, prostatic hypertrophy, hepatic dysfunction, nephrosis, and in infants and young children. There are many warnings associated with testosterone preparations. Please refer to a current *Physicians' Desk Reference* or a *PDR Nurse's Drug Handbook* for information on warnings.

> **Safety Precaution:** In geriatric clients, diabetic clients, and those with hypertension, coronary artery disease, renal disease, hypercholesterolemia, gynecomastia, and prepubertal males.

Adverse Reactions

In males: gynecomastia, excessive frequency and duration of penile erection, oligospermia, hirsutism, male-pattern baldness, acne, retention of sodium, chloride, water, potassium, calcium, and inorganic phosphates, nausea, cholestatic jaundice, alterations in liver function tests, hepatocellular neoplasms, peliosis hepatis (liver and spleen may become engorged with blood-filled cysts), suppression of clotting factors II, V, VII, and X, increased or decreased libido, headache, anxiety, depression, generalized paresthesia, increased serum cholesterol, and rarely anaphylactoid reactions. *In females:* amenorrhea, menstrual irregularities, inhibition of gonadotropin secretion, and virilization (deepening of the voice, clitoral enlargement, increased growth of facial and body hair, male-pattern baldness).

Dosage and Route

The dosage and route of administration is determined by the physician and individualized for each client. (See Table 31-4.)

TABLE 31-4   ANDROGENS

Medications	Usual Dosage
testosterone (Andro 100) (AndroGel)	IM: 10–25 mg 2–3 times/week for androgen deficiency Topical gel: Apply once daily to the shoulders, upper arms, and/or abdomen for replacement therapy.
testosterone cypionate in oil (Depo-Testosterone)	IM: 50–400 mg every 2–4 weeks for replacement therapy
testosterone enanthate in oil (Delatestryl)	IM: 50–400 mg every 2–4 weeks for replacement therapy
testosterone propionate in oil (Testex)	IM: 10–25 mg 2–3 times per week for replacement therapy
testosterone transdermal systems (Testoderm® Ⓒ, Androderm® Ⓒ)	Controlled delivery for once-daily application to the scrotum for replacement therapy

Nursing Considerations

Observe for signs of improvement and adverse reactions. Weigh daily, and if weight increases by 5 pounds within a week, notify physician. Assess blood pressure every 4 hours and notify physician if a consistent increase is noted in the systolic and/or diastolic readings. Monitor intake and output ratio, and liver function studies. Monitor electrolytes: sodium, chloride, calcium, potassium, and blood cholesterol level. When used in males to stimulate puberty, assess growth pattern.

Clients' Instruction

Educate the client

- To weigh daily, at the same time of day and with the same amount of clothing on/off
- To notify the physician if 5 pounds or more are gained within a week
- To be aware of possible adverse reactions and report any of the following to the physician. All clients: nausea, vomiting, jaundice, edema. *Males:* frequent or persistent erections of the penis. *Adolescent males:* signs of premature epiphyseal closure. Should have bone development checked every 6 months. *Females:* hoarseness, acne, changes in menstrual periods, growth of hair on face and/or body.
- That buccal tablets should be placed under the tongue or in the space between the cheek and gum; change the site of placement with each dose (rotate between the four locations in the mouth). The tablet should be completely dissolved before the client engages in eating, drinking, or using any tobacco product.
- That oral tablets should be taken with food to minimize possible gastrointestinal distress

Special Considerations

- In clients with diabetes, the effects of testosterone may decrease blood glucose and insulin requirements.
- Testosterone may decrease the anticoagulant requirements of clients receiving oral anticoagulants. These clients require close monitoring when testosterone therapy is begun and then when it is stopped.
- Anabolic steroids (testosterone) may be abused by individuals who seek to increase muscle mass, strength, and overall athletic ability. This form of use is illegal and signs of abuse may include flu-like symptoms, gastrointestinal distress, headaches, muscle aches, dizziness, bruises, needle marks, increased bleeding (nose-bleeds, petechiae, gums, conjunctiva), enlarged spleen, liver, prostate, edema, and in the female increased facial hair, menstrual irregularities, and enlarged clitoris.

Erectile Dysfunction

According to the National Institutes of Health (NIH), erectile dysfunction (impotence) affects as many as 20 million men in the United States. It was once thought to be an unavoidable result of aging, but now erectile dysfunction is understood to be caused by a variety of factors. **Erectile dysfunction (ED)** is the inability to achieve or maintain an erection sufficient for sexual intercourse. It occurs when not enough blood is supplied to the penis, when the smooth muscle in the penis fails to relax, or when the penis does not retain the blood that flows into it. According to studies by the NIH, 5 percent of men have some degree of erectile dysfunction at age 40 and approximately 15 to 25 percent at age 65 or older. Although the likelihood of erectile dysfunction increases with age, it is not an inevitable part of aging. About 80 percent of erectile dysfunction has a physical cause.

Some physical causes of erectile dysfunction are

- *Vascular diseases:* Arteriosclerosis, hypertension, high cholesterol, and other medical conditions can obstruct blood flow.
- *Diabetes:* Can alter nerve function and blood flow to the penis
- *Prescription drugs:* Certain antihypertensive medications, cardiac medications, antihistamines, psychiatric medications, and other prescription drugs can cause erectile dysfunction.
- *Substance abuse:* Excessive use of tobacco, alcohol, and illegal drugs constrict blood vessels and can cause erectile dysfunction.
- *Neurologic diseases:* Multiple sclerosis, Parkinson's disease, and other diseases can interrupt nerve impulses to the penis.
- *Surgery:* Prostate, colon, bladder, and other types of pelvic surgery may damage nerves and blood vessels.
- *Spinal injury:* Interruptions of nerve impulses from the spinal cord to the penis can cause erectile dysfunction.
- *Other:* Hormonal imbalance, kidney failure, dialysis, and reduced testosterone levels can cause erectile dysfunction.

Sildenafil Citrate (Viagra)

Viagra is an oral medication that may be prescribed for erectile dysfunction.

Actions

Viagra increases the body's ability to achieve and maintain an erection during sexual stimulation. It does not protect one from getting sexually transmitted diseases, including HIV.

Uses

Viagra is used to treat erectile dysfunction (impotence) in men.

Contraindications

Viagra was shown to potentiate the hypotensive effects of nitrates, and its administration to clients who are using organic nitrates, either regularly and/or intermittently, in any form is therefore contraindicated. It is also contraindicated in clients with a known hypersensitivity to any component of its ingredients.

> **Safety Precaution:** There is a potential for cardiac risk during sexual activity in clients with preexisting cardiovascular disease. Therefore, treatments for erectile dysfunction, including Viagra, generally should not be used in men for whom sexual activity is inadvisable because of their underlying cardiovascular status. Drug is potentially hazardous in those with acute coronary ischemia but not on nitrates; have congestive heart failure and borderline low blood pressure.

Adverse Reactions

Headache, flushing, dyspepsia, nasal congestion, urinary tract infection, diarrhea, dizziness, rash, abnormal vision (color tinge to vision and increased sensitivity to light or blurred vision), and prolonged erection (**priapism**). Serious cardiovascular events such as myocardial infarction, sudden cardiac death, ventricular arrhythmia, cerebrovascular hemorrhage, transient ischemic attack, and hypertension have been reported postmarketing in association with the use of Viagra. Most, but not all, of these clients had preexisting cardiovascular risk factors.

Dosage and Route

For most clients, the recommended dose is one 50 mg tablet taken orally, as needed, approximately 1 hour before sexual activity. However, Viagra may be taken anywhere from 4 hours to $\frac{1}{2}$ hour before sexual activity. Based on effectiveness and toleration, the dose may be increased to a maximum recommended dose of 100 mg or decreased to 25 mg. The maximum recommended dosing frequency is once per day.

Clients' Instruction

Educate the client

- To have a complete medical history and exam to determine the cause of impotence before taking Viagra

- That men who have medical conditions that may cause a sustained erection such as sickle cell anemia, leukemia, or multiple myeloma or who have an abnormally shaped penis may not be able to take Viagra

- To inform his doctor about all medications that he is taking, as there are several medications that interact with Viagra, such as cimetidine, erythromycin, and ritonavir

- Who experiences symptoms (chest pain, dizziness, nausea) upon initiation of sexual activity to refrain from further activity and contact his physician

- That if an erection persists longer than 4 hours, to seek immediate medical assistance

- That the use of Viagra offers no protection against sexually transmitted diseases

DRUGS USED DURING LABOR AND DELIVERY

Drugs that selectively stimulate contraction of the myometrium are known as **oxytocic agents** because they act on smooth muscle much like the hormone oxytocin, which is secreted by the posterior pituitary gland. They may be used in obstetrics to induce labor at term. They are also used to control postpartum hemorrhage and to induce therapeutic abortion. Three types of oxytocic drugs are in general use; they are synthetic oxytocin, the ergot derivatives, and the prostaglandins. These drugs are also known as uterine stimulants.

When labor begins before term, uterine relaxants may be administered to delay labor until the fetus has gained sufficient maturity as to be likely to survive. Agents used for this purpose are generally administered in cases where spontaneous labor begins after 20 weeks of gestation. The most commonly used uterine relaxants are Ethanol and ritodrine. See Table 31-5.

TABLE 31-5 UTERINE STIMULANTS AND RELAXANTS

Medications	Uses	Usual Dosages	Adverse Reactions
STIMULANTS			
carboprost tromethamine (Prostin/15 M)	Used to induce abortion in weeks 13–20	IM: 250 mcg initially, then repeated at 1.5–3.5 hour intervals as indicated by uterine response	Nausea, diarrhea, vomiting, temperature increase more than, 2°F, flushing, cough, pain, hiccups, chills
dinoprost tromethamine (Prostin F$_2$ Alpha)	Used to terminate pregnancy in weeks 16–20	Intra-amniotic instillation: 40 mg or 8 ml (5 mg/ml)	Headache, dizziness, syncope, bradycardia, renal retention, bronchoconstriction, cough
dinoprostone (Prostin E$_2$)	Used to terminate pregnancy in weeks 12–20	Intravaginal: 1 suppository (20 mg) inserted high into vagina, then another every 3–5 hours until abortion	Same as above
ergonovine maleate (Ergotrate, Maleate)	Used to prevent postpartum and postabortal hemorrhage	IM: 0.2 mg every 2–4 hours up to maximum of 5 doses Oral: 0.2–0.4 mg every 6–12 hours (usually for 48 hours)	Nausea, vomiting, severe hypertensive episodes, bradycardia, allergic phenomena including shock, ergotism
methylergonovine maleate (Methergine)	Used for routine management after delivery of placenta	Oral: 0.2 mg 3–4 times/day in puerperium for 1 week IM: 1 ml every 2–4 hours as necessary after delivery of placenta	Anorexia, dizziness, headache, nervousness, insomnia, blood pressure and pulse changes, tachycardia, visual disturbances, abdominal pain
oxytocin (Pitocin) (Syntocinon)	Used to initiate/ improve uterine contraction at term	IV infusion (drip): 1–2 mU/ minute (0.001–0.002 U/min) with gradual increase by 1–2 mU/minute until normal contraction pattern is established that stimulates normal labor	Fetus: bradycardia, hypoxia, intracranial hemorrhage, neonatal jaundice, death Mother: hypersensitivity leading to uterine hypertonicity, uterine rupture
RELAXANTS			
ethyl alcohol (Ethanol)	Used to suppress premature labor	IV: 1.25 g of absolute alcohol per kg/body weight	Depression of the central nervous system, inebriation
ritodrine HCl (Yutopar)	Used to manage premature labor	IV: 50–100 mcg/minute administered by calibrated constant-rate infusion pump	Altered maternal and fetal heart rates, temporary hypoglycemia, nausea, anxiety

● SPOT CHECK

Give a brief description of each of the following hormone replacement therapy pharmaceuticals.

	Description
Vivelle-Dot	
Cenestin	
Prempro	
CombiPatch	

● SELF-ASSESSMENT

Write the answer in the space provided or circle true or false as instructed.

Source

p. 410 **1.** The pituitary gland secretes two gonad-stimulating hormones known as _____ hormone and _____ hormone.

Fig 31-3 **2.** An estradiol transdermal system delivers estrogen through the skin directly to the bloodstream without first passing through the _____, thereby avoiding changes in _____ sometimes associated with other forms of estrogen therapy.

p. 414 **3.** True or False (circle one) Estrogen replacement therapy is relatively well tolerated by most menopausal women who take the recommended lowest effective dose.

p. 414 **4.** The two terms used to designate preparations of synthetic progesterone are _____ and _____ .

p. 416 **5.** The main ingredients of most oral contraceptive pills are _____ and _____ .

p. 417 **6.** In a few words, describe actions associated with the following oral contraceptives:

● Monophasic preparations

_____

_____

● Biphasic preparations

_____

_____

● Triphasic preparations

_____

_____

p. 415– 416 **7.** The possible risks of hormone replacement therapy include cancer. The text mentions two types of cancer. They are _____ and _____ .

p. 418 **8.** Replacement therapy in androgen deficiency utilizes agents containing the hormone _____ .

p. 421 **9.** The text mentions three uses for oxytocic agents:

(1) They may be used in obstetrics to

_____ .

(2) They may be used to control

_____ .

(3) They may be used to induce

_____ .

p. 420 **10.** True or False (circle one) Erectile dysfunction (impotence) is an unavoidable result of the aging process that responds to drug therapy utilizing Viagra.

● WEB ACTIVITY

Visit the following Web sites for additional information on medications used for reproductive system disorders:

http://pharmacotherapy.medscape.com

http://www.docguide.com

http://www.discoveryhealth.com

http://www.pharminfo.com

http://www.onhealth.com

http://www.healthspotlight.com

http://www.fda.gov

http://www.intelihealth.com

http://www.ortho-mcneil.com/products

http://www.healthnet.com

http://www.pslgroup.com

http://www.organoninc.com

http://www.igha.org

http://www.centerwatch.com/drugs

http://www.midlife-passage.com

http://www.mjbovo.com/Contracept

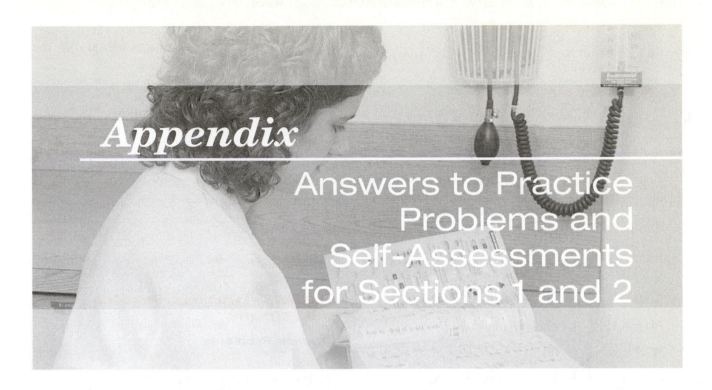

Section 1   Basic Mathematics

Chapter 1   Introduction and Arithmetic Pretest

Arithmetic Pretest

1. a. XV   b. XIX   c. V   d. IV
   e. XX   f. I   g. VIII   h. VII

2. a. 10   b. 6   c. 9   d. 26
   e. 3   f. 24   g. 14   h. 13

3. a. one million, five thousand, two hundred and twenty-one
   b. one hundred twenty-five thousand, nine hundred and thirty-six
   c. forty-eight thousand, two hundred and twenty-four
   d. two thousand one and five-tenths
   e. one million, two hundred thousand

4. a. 2   b. $2\frac{1}{4}$ c. 4
   d. $5\frac{1}{3}$ e. 20   f. $4\frac{7}{15}$

5. a. 500   b. 2,598,000   c. 2,000,000

6. a. 0.216   b. 421.605   c. 1046.069

7. a. $\frac{19}{20}$ b. $\frac{31}{24}$ or $1\frac{7}{24}$ c. $11\frac{11}{8}$ or $12\frac{3}{8}$

8. a. $\frac{1}{6}$ b. $\frac{7}{15}$ c. $2\frac{1}{6}$ d. $3\frac{7}{8}$

9. a. 4   b. 1   c. 6   d. 26

10. a. 1.55   b. 3.50   c. 24.90   d. 89.80

11. a. 267.75   b. 27.505
    c. 589.0401   d. 67.2864

12. a. 2   b. 8   c. 4.071   d. 601

13. a. $\frac{5}{6}$ b. $\frac{3}{4}$ c. 0.75   d. 0.255

14. a. 45.5   b. 35.03
    c. 2.0005   d. 160.003

15. a. 0.7   b. 5.25   c. 2.5   d. 0.25

16. a. 50%   b. 0.7%   c. 75%
    d. 5%   e. 25%   f. 50%

17. a. 3.75   b. 2.50   c. 24
    d. 5.25   e. 50   f. 125

18. a. 4,280   b. 600,000
    c. 6,000,000   d. 40,208
    e. 200,020   f. 503.5 or $503\frac{5}{10}$

Chapter 2   Numerals and Fractions

Practice Problems

1. a. III   b. V   c. VIII
   d. X   e. C   f. VII
   g. L   h. LX   i. 24
   j. 4   k. 16   l. 19
   m. 9   n. 8   o. 20

2. a. $\frac{3}{4}$ b. $\frac{1}{3}$ c. $\frac{1}{4}$
   d. $\frac{1}{2}$ e. $\frac{1}{20}$ f. $\frac{1}{5}$

3. a. $1\frac{1}{3}$ b. $1\frac{1}{3}$ c. $1\frac{1}{2}$
   d. $1\frac{3}{5}$ e. $1\frac{1}{9}$ f. $1\frac{2}{13}$

4. a. $\frac{10}{3}$ b. $\frac{17}{4}$ c. $\frac{17}{3}$
   d. $\frac{67}{10}$ e. $\frac{50}{7}$ f. $\frac{82}{9}$

425

5. Largest   Smallest

a. $\frac{1}{3}$ $\frac{1}{8}$

b. $\frac{1}{4}$ $\frac{1}{150}$

c. $\frac{1}{5}$ $\frac{1}{100}$

d. $\frac{4}{5}$ $\frac{2}{5}$

e. $\frac{10}{40}$ $\frac{2}{40}$

f. $\frac{1}{100}$ $\frac{1}{150}$

g. $\frac{3}{4}$ $\frac{1}{4}$

h. $\frac{1}{2}$ $\frac{1}{5}$

i. $\frac{75}{100}$ $\frac{25}{100}$

j. $\frac{8}{10}$ $\frac{3}{10}$

6. a. $\frac{11}{12}$ b. $\frac{19}{21}$ c. $\frac{24}{16} = 1\frac{1}{2}$

d. $\frac{28}{20} = 1\frac{2}{5}$ e. 99   f. $155\frac{6}{7}$

g. 43   h. $29\frac{5}{6}$ i. $36\frac{29}{30}$

j. $37\frac{1}{3}$ k. $\frac{49}{50}$ l. 1

7. a. $\frac{12}{16} = \frac{3}{4}$ b. $\frac{11}{45}$ c. $\frac{7}{32}$

d. $33\frac{1}{3}$ e. $15\frac{7}{9}$ f. 9

g. $7\frac{7}{10}$ h. $83\frac{4}{8} = 83\frac{1}{2}$ i. $49\frac{38}{25} = 50\frac{13}{25}$

j. $\frac{34}{150}$ k. $\frac{1}{12}$ l. $2\frac{11}{24}$

8. a. $\frac{161}{144}$ b. $\frac{2}{15}$ c. $\frac{28}{32} = \frac{7}{8}$

d. $\frac{410}{12} = 34\frac{1}{6}$ e. $61\frac{1}{9}$ f. $\frac{153}{40} = 3\frac{33}{40}$

g. 21   h. $\frac{126}{5} = 25\frac{1}{5}$ i. 146

j. 12   k. $\frac{1}{2}$ l. $\frac{1}{10}$

m. $\frac{1}{6}$ n. $3\frac{3}{4}$ o. $\frac{95}{48} = 1\frac{47}{48}$

9. a. $\frac{368}{63} = 5\frac{53}{63}$ b. $\frac{6}{5} = 1\frac{1}{5}$ c. $\frac{7}{2} = 3\frac{1}{2}$

d. $\frac{82}{60} = 1\frac{22}{60} = 1\frac{11}{30}$ e. $\frac{275}{2} = 137\frac{1}{2}$

f. $\frac{15}{102} = \frac{5}{34}$ g. 84   h. $\frac{1120}{9} = 124\frac{4}{9}$

i. $\frac{7}{6} = 1\frac{1}{6}$ j. 2   k. 2

l. $\frac{2}{3}$ m. $\frac{3}{5}$ n. $\frac{9}{5} = 1\frac{4}{5}$

o. $\frac{4}{33}$ p. $\frac{27}{32}$

Self-Assessment

1. a. XV   b. XXV   c. L

   d. 4   e. 19   f. 16

2. a. $\frac{11}{2}$ b. $\frac{10}{3}$ c. $\frac{49}{6}$

   d. $\frac{55}{8}$ e. $\frac{14}{3}$ f. $\frac{5}{2}$

3. a. $1\frac{1}{2}$ b. $1\frac{2}{5}$ c. $1\frac{1}{2}$

   d. $7\frac{1}{2}$ e. $1\frac{1}{3}$ f. $1\frac{1}{2}$

4. a. $\frac{1}{2}$ b. $\frac{3}{4}$ c. $\frac{1}{2}$

   d. $\frac{3}{5}$ e. $\frac{1}{4}$ f. $\frac{1}{5}$

5. a. $\frac{7}{8}$ b. $25\frac{1}{3}$ c. $\frac{6}{21}$

   d. 41   e. $\frac{4}{9}$ f. $201\frac{1}{6}$

6. a. $\frac{5}{8}$ b. $15\frac{7}{9}$ c. $\frac{1}{12}$

   d. $22\frac{1}{3}$ e. $\frac{34}{150}$ f. 9

7. a. $\frac{1}{6}$ b. 146   c. 9   d. $16\frac{5}{36}$

8. a. $\frac{2}{3}$ b. $\frac{27}{32}$ c. $\frac{4}{33}$ d. $124\frac{4}{9}$

Chapter 3   Decimal Fractions and Percents

Practice Problems

1. decimal
2. It is used for precise measurement.
3. whole
4. decimals or decimal fractions
5. place value
6. ten
7. one tenth
8. decimal fraction
9. to insure accuracy
10. powers of ten
11. a. one ten-thousandth
   b. two tenths
   c. six one-hundredths
   d. ten one hundred-thousandths
   e. twenty-five thousandths
12. a. twenty-five hundredths
   b. seven-tenths
   c. one hundred and fifty thousandths
   d. four thousand two hundred ten
     thousandths
   e. six hundred-thousandths
13. a. two and five-tenths
     (two point five)
   b. nine and twenty-five hundredths
     (nine point twenty five hundredths)
   c. one hundred twenty-five and forty thousandths
     (one hundred twenty-five point forty
     thousandths)
   d. fifteen and one hundred fifty ten-
     thousandths
     (fifteen point one hundred fifty ten-
     thousandths)
   e. four and five hundred thousandths
     (four point five hundred thousandths)

Practice Problems

1. a. 0.666   b. 0.25   c. 0.75
   d. 0.2   e. 0.875

2. a. $\frac{4}{10}$ b. $\frac{5}{100}$ c. $\frac{10}{1000}$
   d. $\frac{6}{10,000}$ e. $\frac{2}{1,000,000}$

3. a. 1   b. 1   c. 1.35
   d. 0.351   e. 134.26

4. a. 0.06   b. 0.5   c. 40.39
   d. 3.068   e. 0.444   f. 0.13
   g. 0.06   h. 0.21   i. 0.52
   j. 0.44

5. a. 13.175   b. 27.5625   c. 674.98312
   d. 221.9778   e. 0.317504   f. 250,000
   g. 104,000   h. 5200   i. 110
   j. 3

6. a. 7.2   b. 6.02   c. 5.02
   d. 8.02   e. 2.02   f. 0.002
   g. 0.005   h. 0.005   i. 0.004
   j. 3.443

7. a. 100   b. 2000   c. 200
   d. 1000   e. 100,000   f. 8000
   g. 1,000,000   h. 200   i. 5000
   j. 90

8. a. 0.08   b. 0.3   c. 0.1   d. 2
   e. 100   f. 3   g. 70   h. 0.9
   i. 0.03   j. 0.1

9. a. 0.000025   b. 0.00104   c. 0.0052
   d. 0.011   e. 0.03   f. 8.88
   g. 0.0015   h. 0.0000066   i. 0.00007
   j. 0.0001

10. a. 25%   b. $33\frac{1}{3}\%$ c. 40%
    d. $66\frac{2}{3}\%$ e. 12%

11. a. 125%   b. 70%   c. 80%
    d. 495%   e. 12.5%

12. a. $\frac{1}{50}$ and 0.02   b. $\frac{19}{400}$ and 0.0475
    c. $\frac{2}{5}$ and 0.4   d. $\frac{193}{1000}$ and 0.193
    e. $\frac{16}{25}$ and 0.64

13. a. 7.2 and $7\frac{1}{5}$ b. 4.8 and $4\frac{4}{5}$
    c. 3.75 and $3\frac{3}{4}$ d. 52.5 and $52\frac{1}{2}$
    e. 0.2 and $\frac{1}{5}$

Self-Assessment

1. whole
2. decimals or decimal fractions
3. ten
4. $\frac{1}{10}$

5. a. five tenths
   b. ten one-thousandths
   c. five tenths
   d. five hundred-thousandths
   e. two and twenty-hundredths
   f. eight and seventy-five hundredths

6. a. 0.333   b. 0.25

7. a. $\frac{5}{10}$ b. $\frac{5}{100,000}$

8. a. 1   b. 1.74

9. a. 0.52   b. 3.068

10. a. 221.9778   b. 110

11. a. 0.002   b. 0.004   c. 200
    d. 5000   e. 0.1   f. 70

12. a. $33\frac{1}{3}\%$ b. 25%   c. $66\frac{2}{3}\%$

Chapter 4   Ratio and Proportion

Practice Problems

1. a. $1:25$ b. $2:100$ $1:50$
   c. $10:40$ $1:4$ d. $25:75$ $1:3$
   e. $8:64$ $1:8$ f. $1:2$
   g. $1:3$ h. $1:250$
   i. $3:500$ j. $5:2$

2. a. $24 \div 48$ $1 \div 2$ b. $12 \div 6$ $2 \div 1$
   c. $76 \div 304$ $1 \div 4$ d. $5 \div 25$ $1 \div 5$
   e. $2 \div 92$ $1 \div 46$ f. $18 \div 108$ $1 \div 6$
   g. $10 \div 50$ $1 \div 5$ h. $17 \div 51$ $1 \div 3$
   i. $11 \div 22$ $1 \div 2$ j. $55 \div 165$ $1 \div 3$

3. a. $\frac{33}{66}$ $\frac{1}{2}$ b. $\frac{4}{10}$ $\frac{2}{5}$
   c. $\frac{75}{100}$ $\frac{3}{4}$ d. $\frac{22}{88}$ $\frac{1}{4}$
   e. $\frac{43}{86}$ $\frac{1}{2}$ f. $\frac{2}{13}$
   g. $\frac{7}{49}$ $\frac{1}{7}$ h. $\frac{4}{100}$ $\frac{1}{25}$
   i. $\frac{1}{150}$ j. $\frac{12}{36}$ $\frac{1}{3}$

4. a. 0.02   b. 0.08   c. 0.006   d. 0.75
   e. 0.002   f. 0.08   g. 1.25   h. 0.001
   i. 0.005   j. 0.5

5. a. 8   b. 50   c. 2000   d. 24
   e. 8   f. 3   g. 2500   h. 12
   i. 540   j. 20

6. a. 46   b. 28   c. 46   d. 14
   e. 13,990   f. 18   g. 41   h. 85
   i. 15   j. 112

7. a. 4   b. 5   c. 20   d. 0.25
   e. $\frac{5}{9}$ f. 6   g. $\frac{1}{2}$ or 0.5
   h. 3   i. 200   j. $\frac{3}{4}$ or 0.75

8. a. 3 b. 500 c. 5 d. 2
   e. 1000 f. 10 g. $\frac{1}{2}$ or 0.5
   h. 30 i. 1000 j. 5

Self-Assessment

1. a. $1:25, 1 \div 25, 0.04$

   b. $12 \div 6, \frac{12}{6}, 2$

   c. $33 \div 66, \frac{33}{66} (\frac{1}{2}), 0.5$

   d. $1 \div 50, \frac{1}{50}, 0.02$

   e. $25:75, 25 \div 75, 0.333$

2. a. $X = 4$ b. $X = 540$

   c. $X = \frac{6}{10} (\frac{3}{5})$ d. $X = \frac{1}{2}$

   e. $X = \frac{1}{300}$ f. $X = 3$

   g. $X = 20$ h. $X = 10$

   i. $X = 18$ j. $X = \frac{1}{2}$

Chapter 5 Temperature Equivalents

Practice Problems

1. a. 104° b. 95° c. 35° d. 37.2°
2. a. 39° b. 36.5° or 36.6° c. 37.6°
   d. 39.4° e. 40° f. 96.8° g. 99°
   h. 100° i. 101° j. 102.2°

Self-Assessment

1. 97 to 99; 36.1 to 37
2. 212
3. 0
4. a. 37.2 b. 37 c. 38.3
   d. 102.2 e. 96.8 f. 105.8

Section 2 Calculations of Doses and Solutions

Chapter 6 The Metric System

Practice Problems

1. a. meter b. liter c. gram
2. a. kilo b. deci c. micro
   d. hecto e. milli f. deka
   g. centi
3. Decimal fractions
4. 0
5. 39.37
6. a. 0.001 meter b. 0.01 meter
   c. 0.1 meter d. 1 meter
   e. 10 meters f. 100 meters
   g. 1000 meters
7. $2\frac{1}{2}$

8. 1.056
9. 15 or 16
10. one cubic centimeter, one milliliter
11. a. 0.001 L b. 0.01 L c. 0.1 L
    d. 1 L e. 10 L f. 100 L
    g. 1000 L
12. 15 or 0.035
13. a. 0.000001 g b. 0.001 g
    c. 0.01 g d. 0.1 g
    e. 1 g f. 10 g
    g. 100 g h. 1000 g
14. *Volume* a. ml or cc b. L
    Weight a. mcg b. mg
    c. g d. kg
15. a. 1 g b. 0.25 L c. 200 mg
    d. 0.2 ml e. 12 kg
16. a. L b. g c. mg
    d. lb e. mg

Practice Problems

1. a. 0.25 b. 500 c. 2000 d. 0.5
   e. 30 f. 0.0005 g. 0.001 h. 2
   i. 1 j. 4.4
2. a. 0.06 b. 5 c. 0.2 d. 0.001
   e. 6.5 f. 0.0035 g. 4000 h. 0.001
   i. 100 j. 0.00005
3. a. 83.6 b. 95.5 c. 38.6 d. 24.5
4. a. 66 b. 99 c. 143 d. 165
5. 88 lb = 40 kg Dosage = 2000 mg
6. 66 lb = 30 kg Dosage = 200 mg every 8 hours
7. 176 lb = 80 kg Dosage = 80 mg every 8 hours
8. 154 lb = 70 kg Dosage = 700 mg
9. 132 lb = 60 kg Dosage = 300 mg every 8 hours
10. 44 lb = 20 kg Dosage = 1000 mg (in two divided doses of 500 mg each)

Self-Assessment

1. a. meter b. liter c. gram
2. a. kilo b. deci c. micro d. hecto
   e. milli f. deka g. centi
3. $2\frac{1}{2}$
4. 1.056
5. 15 or 16
6. a. liter b. grams c. milligrams
   d. pounds e. milligrams
7. a. 0.001 b. 0.004 c. 5000
   d. 200 e. 0.001 f. 0.0035
8. a. 80 b. 45.45 c. 29.09
9. 55 lb = 25 kg Dosage = 625 mg
10. 110 lb = 50 kg Dosage = 2500 mg (divided into 625 mg every 6 hours)

Chapter 7   Household Measures and Apothecaries' Measurements

Practice Problems

1. a. gtt b. tsp c. T d. oz
  e. tcp f. C g. pt h. qt
  i. gal
2. a. 3 b. 6 c. 1 d. 4
  e. 8 f. 2 g. 5 h. 7
  i. 9
3. a. gtt b. gtt c. T d. oz
  e. oz f. oz g. C h. qt
  i. oz j. pt

Practice Problems

1. a. 150 b. $\frac{5}{8}$ c. 6 d. $7\frac{1}{2}$
  e. $\frac{5}{8}$ f. 160 g. 360 h. 3
  i. $\frac{3}{4}$ j. 80
2. a. 480 b. 45 c. 24 d. $\frac{3}{4}$
  e. $1\frac{1}{2}$ f. $\frac{1}{60}$ g. $\frac{1}{2}$ h. 6
  i. $\frac{3}{8}$ j. $\frac{1}{4}$

Self-Assessment

1. a. gal b. qt c. pt d. C
  e. tcp f. oz g. T h. tsp
  i. gtt
2. a. gtt b. gtt c. oz d. C
  e. T f. T g. oz h. C
  i. pt
3. a. $7\frac{1}{2}$ b. 18 c. 20 d. 9
  e. $\frac{3}{4}$
4. a. gr b. dr c. oz
5. a. $\frac{1}{2}$ b. 45 c. $\frac{1}{60}$ d. 24
  e. $\frac{3}{4}$ f. $\frac{1}{4}$

Chapter 8   Calculating Adult Dosages: Oral Forms

Practice Problems

1. a. $\frac{1}{2}$ tab b. 2 tabs c. 2 tabs
  d. 10 ml e. 2 tabs f. 2 tabs
  g. $\frac{1}{2}$ tab h. 2.5 ml i. $\mathbf{\frac{1}{2}}$ tab
  j. 2 caps
2. a. 2 tabs b. $\frac{1}{2}$ tab c. $\frac{1}{2}$ tab
  d. $1\frac{1}{2}$ tabs e. $\frac{1}{2}$ tab f. 2 tabs
  g. 2 tabs h. 2 tabs i. 1 tab
  j. $\frac{1}{2}$ tab

Self-Assessment Test

1. $\frac{1}{2}$ tab
2. $\frac{1}{2}$ tab
3. 2 tabs
4. $\frac{1}{2}$ tab
5. $1\frac{1}{2}$ tabs
6. 1 tab
7. 2 caps
8. 3 ml
9. 7.5 ml
10. 2.5 ml

Chapter 9   Calculating Adult Dosages: Parenteral Forms

Practice Problems

1. a. 1.5 ml b. 0.2 ml c. 2 ml
  d. 1 ml e. 1 ml
2. a. 1.5 ml b. 1 ml c. 0.7 ml
  d. 0.5 ml e. 1.5 ml f. 0.5 ml
  g. 2.5 ml h. 2 ml i. 0.5 ml
  j. 1 ml
3. a. 0.5 ml b. 0.8 ml c. 1 ml
  d. 32 units

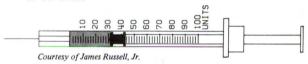

Courtesy of James Russell, Jr.

  e. 64 units

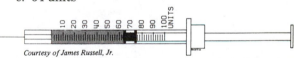

Courtesy of James Russell, Jr.

4. a. 41.6 = 42 gtt/min b. 83.3 = 83 gtt/min
  c. 16.6 = 17 gtt/min d. 17.3 = 17 gtt/min
  e. 18.7 = 19 gtt/min

Self-Assessment

1. 1 ml
2. 2 ml
3. 20 minims
4. 2 ml
5. 12 minims
6. 41.4 = 42 gtt/ml
7. 16.6 = 17 gtt/ml
8. 2 ml
9. 2 ml
10. 0.5 ml
11. 0.75 ml; 9 minims
12. 1 ml

Chapter 10 Calculating Children's Dosages

Practice Problems

1. a. 300 mg q 12 h
   b. 11 mg (22.72 kg) or 11.5 mg (23 kg)
   c. 418 mg or 420 mg
   d. 1145 mg (286 mg/daily)
   e. 141.8 = 142 mg

2. a. 88 mg
   b. 74 mg
   c. 60.29 = 60 mg
   d. 329.4 = 329 units
   e. 147 units

Self-Assessment

1. 20.5 = 21 mg
2. 900 mg
3. 600 mg
4. 88 mg
5. 134.11 mg (134 mg)
6. 82.35 mg (82 mg)
7. 660 mg total amount or 654.54 mg (655 mg) total amount
   220 mg every 8 hours or 218.18 mg (218 mg) every 8 hours
8. 1400 mg total amount or 1418 mg total amount
   350 mg in 4 equal doses or 354.5 mg (355 mg)
9. 78.18 mg (78 mg) every 8 hours
10. 20 mg

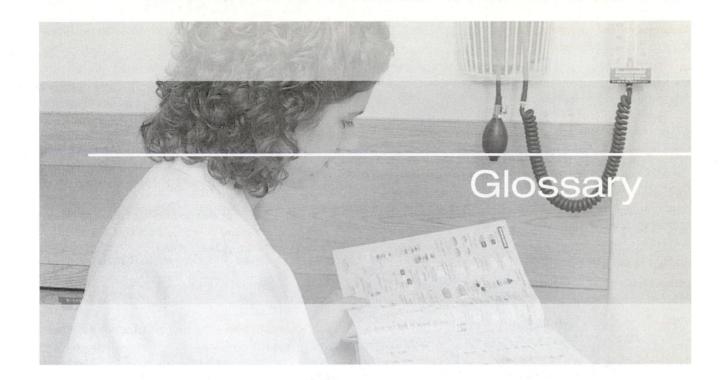

Glossary

Note: Number in parentheses following each term indicates the chapter in which the term is used and described.

A

abuse (23)   The misuse of a substance, legal or illegal, sufficient to cause the abuser mental, physical, emotional, or social harm.

acetylcholine (29)   A cholinergic neurotransmitter that is thought to play an important role in the transmission of nerve impulses at synapses and myoneural junctions.

acetylcholinesterase (29)   An enzyme that inactivates acetylcholine and readies muscle fibers for the next impulse.

acromegaly (28)   A condition in which there is enlargement of the extremities and certain head bones, accompanied by enlargement of the nose and lips.

active immunization (19)   The production of antibodies in response to the administration of a vaccine or toxoid.

addiction (23)   The compulsive, continued use of a drug.

administer (11)   To give.

adverse reaction (12)   An unfavorable or harmful unintended action of a drug.

affective disorder (22)   A condition characterized by a disturbance of mood, accompanied by a manic or depressive syndrome.

akathisia (22)   An inability to sit down. Pacing, fidgeting, and agitation are classic symptoms of akathisia.

allergic rhinitis (25)   Hay fever.

allergy (25)   An individual hypersensitivity to a substance, usually an antibody-antigen reaction.

alopecia (20)   Loss of hair.

Alzheimer's disease (30)   A progressive degeneration of brain tissue that usually begins after age 60.

ampule (9)   A small, sterile, prefilled glass container that holds a hypodermic solution.

analgesic (30)   Agent used to relieve pain caused by disease or other conditions without causing the client to lose consciousness.

anaphylactic shock (18)   A severe allergic reaction, usually to a substance to which the person has become sensitized.

anesthetic (30)   Drug that interferes with the conduction of nerve impulses and is used to produce loss of sensation, muscle relaxation, and/or a complete loss of consciousness.

angina pectoris (24)   Chest pain. A condition caused by an insufficient supply of blood to the heart.

anion (21)   An ion with a negative charge of electricity.

anorexia (20)   Loss of appetite.

antacid (26)   Drug that neutralizes hydrochloric acid in the stomach.

anterograde amnesia (23) Lack of recall for events while drugged.

antibiotic (18) Natural or synthetic substance that inhibits the growth of or destroys microorganisms, especially bacteria.

anticholinesterase (29) A substance that inactivates the action of cholinesterase.

antiemetic (26) Agent that prevents or arrests vomiting.

antioxidant (21) Chemical substance that neutralizes free radicals, the highly reactive and unstable molecules that can cause significant cellular damage.

antipyretic (30) An agent that reduces fever.

antiseptic (18) Substance that prevents or inhibits the growth of microorganisms.

anxiety (22) A feeling of uneasiness, apprehension, worry, or dread.

apothecaries' measurements (7) A system of weights and measures based on 480 grains equal 1 ounce, and 12 ounces equal 1 pound.

application (15) The act of applying (to bring into contact with something).

arrhythmia (24) An irregularity or loss of rhythm; describes an irregular heartbeat.

aspirate (17) To pull back on the plunger in order to ascertain that the needle is not in a blood vessel.

assessment (14) The systematic gathering, organizing, and interpretation of data to determine a client's nursing needs.

asthma (25) A chronic disorder of the bronchial airways. It is characterized by narrowed, inflamed, and sensitive bronchial tubes.

autoimmune response (29) A process by which the body's defense system malfunctions and begins to attack itself.

avitaminosis (21) A deficiency disease that is due to a lack of vitamins in the diet.

B

bactericidal (18) Pertaining to the killing or destruction of bacteria.

bacteriostatic (18) Inhibiting or retarding bacterial growth.

bagging (23) Inhaling fumes from a plastic bag.

barrel (16) The part of the syringe that holds the medication and has graduated markings (calibrations) on its surface for use in measuring medications.

Barrett's esophagus (26) Inflammation with possible ulceration of the lower part of the esophagus.

bevel (16) Flat, slanted surface of a needle.

bipolar disorder (22) A major affective disorder that is characterized by episodes of mania and depression.

body surface isolation (BSI) (14) A system that maintains that personal protective equipment should be worn for contact with all body fluids whether or not blood is visible.

bore (7) The interior or diameter of a tube or needle; a hole.

buccal medicine (15) Medicine placed between the cheek and gum and allowed to dissolve.

C

campylobacteriosis (18) An infectious disease caused by bacteria of the genus *Campylobacter*. It is the most common bacterial cause of diarrheal illness in the United States.

canthus (15) The angle at either end of the slit between the eyelids.

carcinogenic (20) Producing cancer.

cartridge-needle unit (9) A disposable unit containing a premeasured amount of medication. This unit is designed for use in a nondisposable cartridge-holder syringe.

cation (21) An ion with a positive charge of electricity.

Celsius (5) A temperature scale with the freezing point of water at 0° and the boiling point at 100°.

chemotherapy (20) The treatment of disease by using chemical agents, such as cancer drugs that destroy cancer cells.

child (10) Any human between infancy and puberty.

chronotropic (24) Influencing the rate of the heartbeat.

chrysotherapy (29) The use of gold compounds as treatment, especially for rheumatoid arthritis.

common fraction (2) Part of a whole number. It is the result of the process of dividing a number into a numerator separated from the denominator by either a horizontal or diagonal line.

controlled substance (11) A drug that has the potential for addiction and abuse.

controlled substance analogue (11) A substance with a chemical structure substantially similar to the chemical structure of a controlled substance in Schedule I or II.

conversion (6)   The process of changing into another form, state, substance, or product.

coryza (25)   The common cold.

cough (25)   A physiologic reflex. It is a protective action that clears the respiratory tract of secretions and foreign substances.

cretinism (28)   A congenital condition in which there is arrested physical and mental development due to a deficiency in the secretion of thyroid hormones.

cryptorchidism (31)   Failure of the testicles to descend into the scrotum.

cyclooxygenase (29)   An enzyme involved in many aspects of normal cellular function and also in the inflammatory response.

cystitis (27)   Inflammation of the urinary bladder.

cytotoxic (20)   Destructive to cells.

D

decimal (3)   A linear array of numbers based upon ten or any multiple of ten.

decimal fraction (3)   A fraction with an unwritten denominator of 10 or a power of ten. It is expressed by placing a decimal point before the numerator.

dedifferentiation (20)   The process whereby normal cells lose their specialization and become malignant.

denominator (2)   The number below the line in a fraction. It indicates the number of equal parts into which the whole is divided. It is also known as the divisor.

depressant (12)   Drug that decreases cell activity.

diabetes insipidus (28)   A condition caused by inadequate secretion of vasopressin. Classic symptoms are polyuria and polydipsia.

diabetes mellitus (28)   A disorder of carbohydrate metabolism. Classic symptoms are polyuria, polydipsia, and polyphagia. Also glycosuria and hyperglycemia.

diagnosis (14)   Means "through knowledge."

disinfectant (18)   Substance usually of chemical origin, that kills vegetative forms of microorganisms.

dispense (11)   To prepare and give out.

diuretic (27)   Agent that decreases reabsorption of sodium chloride by the kidneys, thereby increasing the amount of salt and water excreted in the urine.

dividend (2)   The number that is divided. It is also known as the numerator.

divisor (2)   The number that is divided into another number or the number by which another can be divided. It is also known as the denominator.

dosage (11)   Amount of medicine that is prescribed for administration.

dromotropic (24)   Affecting the conductivity of nerve or muscle fibers, especially the myocardium.

drug (11)   A medicinal substance that may alter or modify the functions of a living organism.

dwarfism (28)   A condition of being abnormally small.

dyspepsia (26)   Indigestion.

dystonia (22)   Difficult or bad muscle tone. May appear as spasm of the neck muscles, torticollis, rigidity of back muscles, carpopedal spasm, trismus, swallowing difficulty, oculogyric crisis, and protrusion of the tongue.

E

edema (27)   A local or generalized collection of fluid in the body tissues.

electrolyte (21)   Particle that results from disintegration of compounds.

embolus (24)   A detached thrombus (blood clot) moving within the vascular system.

emetic (26)   Agent used to induce vomiting.

endogenous (24)   Originating from within a cell or organism.

enema (15)   The means of delivering a solution or medication into the rectum and colon.

epilepsy (30)   A seizure disorder that is characterized by recurrent abnormal electrical discharges within the brain.

epistaxis (20)   Nosebleed.

erectile dysfunction (ED) (31)   The inability to achieve or maintain an erection sufficient for sexual intercourse.

erosive esophagitis (EE) (26)   A serious condition in which the gastric contents of the stomach pass upward and cause inflammation and tissue damage to the esophagus.

Escherichia coli (E. coli) (18, 27)   A gram-negative bacterium found in normal human bacterial flora; some strains (0157:H7) can cause severe and life-threatening diarrhea.

evaluation (14)   The judgment of anything. An integral part of each step of the nursing process.

exacerbation (20)   The time when the symptoms of a disease process are most severe.

expectorant (25)   An agent that stimulates and decreases the thickness of respiratory tract secretions.

extremes (4)   The outer numbers or the first and fourth terms of the proportion.

F

Fahrenheit (5)   A temperature scale with the freezing point of water at 32° and the boiling point at 212°.

flange (16)   The part located at the end of the barrel of a syringe where the plunger is inserted. It forms a rim around the end of the barrel and has appendages against which one places the index and middle fingers when drawing up solution for injection.

fraction (2)   The result of dividing or breaking a whole number into parts.

fungi (19)   Plant-like organisms that depend upon a host for their existence. These organisms, which include molds and yeast, may be parasitic, or grow in dead and decaying organic matter.

G

gauge (16)   A scale of measurement. The gauge of a needle is determined by the diameter of the lumen.

germicide (18)   Agent that kills or destroys microorganisms.

gigantism (28)   A condition in which there is excessive development of the body or a body part.

glomerulonephritis (27)   An inflammatory disease of the glomeruli of the kidney.

gonioscopic (30)   Inspection of the angle of the anterior chamber of the eye and determination of ocular motility and rotation.

grain (gr) (6)   The smallest unit of weight used in the United States and Great Britain. It is equal to 0.0648 g, which was originally the weight of a grain of wheat.

gram (g) (6)   The metric unit of weight.

Group B Streptococcus (GBS) (18)   A type of bacterium that causes illness in newborn babies, pregnant women, the elderly, and adults with other illnesses such as diabetes or liver disease.

H

heartburn (26)   A burning sensation in the substernal area caused by reflux of acid contents of the stomach into the lower esophagus.

Helicobacter pylori (H. pylori) (26)   A spiral-shaped bacterium that lives in the stomach and duodenum.

helminthiasis (18)   A condition in which there is an intestinal infestation by parasitic worms.

hematuria (27)   Blood in the urine.

hilt (16)   The point at which the shaft attaches to the hub.

homeostasis (21)   The normal fluid state in which positive and negative ions are in balance.

hormone (28)   Chemical substance secreted by the ductless glands of the endocrine system that is carried through the blood.

hormone replacement therapy (HRT) (31)   A medication regimen of providing a woman who has gone through menopause (naturally or surgically) with hormones that her body has stopped producing.

household measure (7)   Approximate measurements.

hub (16)   That part of the needle unit designed to mount onto the syringe.

huffing (23)   Stuffing an inhalant-soaked rag or sock into the mouth.

human immunodeficiency virus (HIV) (19)   A retrovirus that causes acquired immunodeficiency syndrome (AIDS).

hyperglycemia (28)   An abnormally high level of blood sugar. It is generally caused by too little insulin present in the blood.

hypertension (24, 27)   A condition wherein the client has a higher arterial blood pressure than that which is judged to be normal.

hyperuricemia (29)   Excessive uric acid in the blood.

hypervitaminosis (21)   A condition caused by an excessive amount of vitamins, especially from the taking of too many vitamin pills.

hypnotic (30)   An agent that produces sleep.

hypoglycemia (28)   An abnormally low level of blood sugar. It is generally caused by too much insulin present in the blood.

hypogonadism (31)   A condition of defective secretion of the gonads.

hypovitaminosis (21)   A condition due to a lack of vitamins, especially from an inadequate diet. The signs of hypovitaminosis may include fatigue, pain, and aches throughout the body.

hypoxemia (15)   A state when the body does not have an adequate supply of oxygen and irreversible damage to vital organs is possible.

I

immunity (19)   The state of being protected from or resistant to a particular disease due to the development of antibodies.

immunization (19)   The process of inducing or providing immunity artificially by administering an immunobiologic (immunizing agent).

implementation (14)   The process of putting into effect, fulfilling, or carrying through with the plan of action.

incontinence (27)   The loss of the ability to retain urine due to lack of sphincter control.

infancy (10)   The stage of life from the time of birth through the completion of 1 year.

infection (18)   The process or state whereby a pathogenic agent invades the body or a body part, multiplies, and produces injury.

inflammation (29)   A normal response to injury, infection, or irritation of living tissue. Redness, tenderness, pain, and swelling of the affected area are characteristics of the inflammatory process.

inhalant (23)   Breathable chemical vapor that produces psychoactive (mind-altering) effects.

inhalation (15)   The act of drawing breath, vapor, or gas into the lungs.

inhaler (15)   A small handheld apparatus, usually an aerosol unit, that contains a microcrystalline suspension of medication.

inotropic (24)   Influencing of the force of muscular contractility, especially of the myocardium.

inscription (13)   The part of a prescription that states the names and quantities of ingredient to be included in the medication.

insertion (15)   The placement of a suppository into the rectum or vaginal cavity, or a tablet into the mouth, vagina, or rectum.

insomnia (30)   The inability to obtain the amount of sleep a person needs for optimal functioning and well-being.

instillation (15)   The introduction of a drug, usually a liquid form, into a body cavity for temporary retention. Slowly pouring or dropping a liquid into a cavity or onto a surface.

interaction (12)   May occur when one drug potentiates or diminishes the action of another drug.

interstitial cystitis (IC) (27)   A painful inflammation of the bladder wall.

intradermal (9)   Within the epidermal layer of the skin.

intramuscular (9)   Within the muscle.

intravenous (9)   Within a vein.

intravenous solution (9)   Medication intended for intravenous use only; may be supplied in vials, ampules, and ready injectables.

inunction (15)   The application of a drug by rubbing it onto the skin.

ions (21)   Particles that carry electrical charges.

irrigation (15)   A flushing of the mucous lining with a solution for the purpose of removing secretions and soothing the tissues.

K

kiloliter (6)   One thousand liters.

Klebsiella (27)   A genus of bacteria of the family *Enterobacteriacease*. They are frequently associated with respiratory infections and may cause urinary tract infections.

L

laminar airflow (20)   Filtered air flowing along separate planes or layers.

laxative (26)   Drug that is used to relieve constipation and facilitate the passage of feces through the lower gastrointestinal tract.

limbic system (22)   A group of brain structures, including the hippocampus, that is activated by motivated behavior and arousal.

liter (L) (6)   The metric unit of volume.

lowest common denominator (LCD) (2)   The least number into which the denominators of two or more fractions will go evenly.

lozenge (15)   A solid medication that is allowed to dissolve in the mouth. It is used for coughs and sore throats.

lumen (16)   Oval-shaped opening at the beveled tip of a needle.

M

macromineral (21)   Magnesium, sodium, potassium, chlorine, and sulfur.

mast cell (24)   Connective tissue cell that contains heparin and histamine.

means (4)   The inner numbers or the second and third terms of the proportion.

meniscus (14)   The convex or concave upper surface of a column of liquid in a container.

menopause (climacteric) (31)   The period that marks the permanent cessation of menstrual activity.

menstruation (31)   The fourth phase of the menstrual cycle. A period of uterine bleeding, containing endometrial cells, blood, and glandular secretions, lasting 4–5 days.

metastasis (20)   The process whereby malignant cells multiply rapidly and shed into surrounding tissues.

meter (m) (6)   The fundamental unit of length in the metric system.

microgram (mcg, μg) (6)   One-millionth of a gram.

microminerals (21)   Minerals that are required in small amounts. They are also known as trace elements. This group includes iron, copper, iodine, manganese, zinc, fluorine, cobalt, chromium, tin, selenium, vanadium, silicon, nickel, and molybdenum.

microorganism (18)   Any living body not visible to the naked eye. It may be pathogenic or non-pathogenic.

milliliter (ml) (6)   One-thousandth of a liter.

millimeter (mm) (6)   One-thousandth of a meter. It is about the width of the head of a pin.

mineral (21)   Nonorganic substance that is an essential constituent of all body cells.

minim (6)   A small amount of liquid measure. It takes 15 or 16 minims to make one milliliter or one cubic centimeter. A minim is equal to 1/60th of a fluidram or 0.00376 cubic inch.

minipill (31)   An oral contraceptive pill that contains only progestin.

minuend (2)   The number from which another is to be subtracted.

mood (22)   A pervasive and sustained emotion that may play a key role in an individual's perception of the world.

mucolytic (25)   Drug that reduces the viscosity of respiratory tract fluids.

multiple dose (8)   More than one dose per container.

muscle spasm (29)   An involuntary contraction of one or more muscles usually accompanied by pain and the limitation of function.

mutagenic (20)   Causing genetic mutations.

mydriasis (30)   Dilation of the pupil.

myxedema (28)   An acquired condition (in older children and adults) that is due to a deficiency in the secretion of thyroid hormones.

N

neuroleptic (22)   Agent that modifies psychotic behavior.

neuromuscular junction (29)   The point at which a motor nerve fiber connects to a muscle cell.

nitroglycerin (15)   A smooth muscle relaxant with vascular effects manifested predominantly by venous dilatation and pooling.

nocturia (27)   More frequent urination at night.

nomogram (10)   A device graph that shows the relationship among numerical values. One may estimate the body surface area (BSA) of a client according to height and weight by using a nomogram. There are separate nomograms for adults and children.

numerator (2)   The number above the line in a fraction. It is the number of parts into which a number may be divided. It is also known as the dividend.

O

ointment (15)   A semisolid preparation consisting of a drug combined with an oil- or water-soluble base.

oliguria (18)   Decreased amount of urine formation.

opiate (30)   Natural and synthetic drug derived from morphine.

opioid (30)   Synthetic drug not chemically related to morphine that mimics the action of morphine.

oral route (8)   By mouth.

oxygen (15)   A colorless, odorless, tasteless gas that is essential for life.

oxytocic agent (31)   Drug that selectively stimulates contraction of the myometrium.

P

pacemaker (24)   The sinoatrial node (SA), located in the upper wall of the right atrium, is considered to be the source of the heartbeat. This specialized network of Purkinje fibers has the property of automaticity and is referred to as the pacemaker of the heart.

palpate (17)   To feel. Examining by means of touch.

parenteral (9)   Pertaining to the injection of a liquid substance into the body via a route other than the alimentary canal.

Parkinson's disease (30)   A neurologic disorder characterized by the development of a fine, slowly spreading tremor, muscular weakness and rigidity, and the development of disturbances in posture and equilibrium.

passive immunization (19)   The provision of temporary immunity by the administration of pre-formed antitoxins or antibodies.

pathogenic (18)   Disease producing.

percent (3)   Means per hundred; for or out of each hundred. Its symbol, %, is used to indicate that the preceding number is a percentage.

petechiae (20)   Small, purplish, hemorrhagic spots on the skin.

pharmacology (11)   The study of drugs; the science that is concerned with the history, origin, sources, physical and chemical properties, uses, and effects of drugs upon living organisms.

phenothiazine (22)   An organic compound used in the manufacture of certain antipsychotic drugs.

physical dependency (23)   Occurs when one or more of the body's physiologic functions become dependent on the presence of the abused drug.

phytochemical (21)   Any of a hundred natural chemical substances present in plants.

place value (3)   The position of a number to the left or right of a decimal point.

planning (14)   Involves the development of nursing actions designed to enhance the client's responses to treatment or to prevent drug-related problems.

plasminogen (24)   A protein that is found in many body tissues and fluids, important in the prevention of fibrin clot formation.

plunger (16)   The movable cylinder designed for insertion within the barrel.

point (16)   Sharpened end of the needle.

power of ten (3)   The process of multiplying tens together. The number of tens multiplied determines the power.

prescribe (11)   To order or recommend the use of a drug, diet, or other form of therapy.

priapism (31)   Prolonged erection.

progestin (31)   A term used to refer to a large group of drugs that have a progesterone effect on the uterus; synonymous with progesterone.

proof (4)   The stages in resolving the accuracy of your work.

proportion (4)   A way of expressing comparative relationships of a part, share, or portion with regard to size, amount, or number.

proteinuria (18)   Presence of protein (albumin) in the urine.

Proteus (27)   A species of enteric bacilli that may cause urinary tract infections. It is found in the intestines of humans and animals.

pseudo-parkinsonism (22)   A neuroleptic-induced reaction. Symptoms may include mask-like expression (facies), drooling, tremors, rigidity, bradykinesia, shuffling gait, postural abnormalities, and hypersalivation.

psychological dependency (23)   A psychic craving for the effects produced by the abused substance.

psychotropic (23)   Pertaining to mood-altering drugs and other substances.

puberty (10)   The stage of life at which members of both sexes become functionally capable of reproduction. It is a period of rapid physical, mental, and emotional changes that occur from the ages of 13 to 15 in boys and 9 to 16 in girls.

pyrosis (26)   Heartburn.

Q

quotient (4)   The number found when one number is divided by another number.

R

rapport (17)   A feeling of trust and understanding established between the client and those providing health care.

ratio (4)   A way of expressing the relationship of a number, quantity, substance, or degree between two similar components.

RDA (21)   Recommended Daily Allowance. The nutrient level of intake that is considered by the National Research Council (NRC) and Nutrition Board to be adequate for most healthy individuals.

regurgitation (26)   A backward flowing of solids or fluids to the mouth from the stomach.

remission (20)   The time when the symptoms of a disease process are lessened.

rhinovirus (25)   One of a species of *picornaviruses* that causes the common cold in humans.

S

salmonellosis (18)   A common bacterial infection caused by any of more than 2,000 strains of *Salmonella*.

sedative (30)   An agent that produces a calming effect without causing sleep.

shaft (16)   Hollow steel tube through which the medication passes.

side effect (12)   An undesirable action of a drug.

signature (13)   The part of a prescription that gives the directions for the client.

solvent (12)   That in which a substance is dissolved.

SRS-A (25)   The slow-reacting substance of anaphylaxis, i.e., leukotrienes.

stimulant (12)   Drug that increases cell activity.

stomatitis (20)   Inflammation of the mouth.

subcutaneous (9)   Beneath the skin; hypodermic.

sublingual medicine (15)   Medicine that is placed under the tongue.

subscription (13)   The part of a prescription that gives directions to the pharmacist for filling the prescription.

subtrahend (2)   The number that is to be subtracted.

superscription (13)   The part of a prescription that includes the symbol Rx ("take thou").

suppository (15)   A semisolid substance for introduction of medication into the rectum, vagina, or urethra, where it dissolves.

T

tardive dyskinesia (22)   A syndrome characterized by rhythmical involuntary movement of the tongue, face, mouth, jaw, trunk, and extremities.

taut (17)   To pull a surface or draw it tight, such as the skin.

tip (16)   The end of the barrel where the needle is attached.

tolerance (23)   A condition wherein the person's body adjusts to the dosage of a particular drug and a larger amount of the drug must be taken in order to achieve the desired effect.

transdermal system (15)   A small adhesive patch or disk that may be applied to the body near the treatment site.

tuberculosis (25)   A contagious disease caused by the bacillus *Mycobacterium tuberculosis*.

U

unit dose (8)   Premeasured amount of medication that is individually packaged on a per-dose basis.

USRDA (21)   United States Recommended Daily Allowance. The accepted amount of a substance, especially vitamins and minerals, that a person needs each day.

V

vasodilator (24)   Medication that causes the relaxation of blood vessels. This action dilates the vessels, thereby increasing their ability to carry blood. This eases resistance to blood flow and lowers blood pressure.

vasopressor (24)   Drug that causes contraction of the muscles associated with capillaries and arteries, thereby narrowing the space through which the blood circulates. This narrowing increases the resistance to blood flow and results in an elevation of blood pressure.

vertigo (30)   An illusion of movement.

vial (9)   A small, sterile, prefilled glass bottle containing a hypodermic solution.

virus (19)   A parasitic, minute organism that may invade normal cells and cause disease. A virus depends upon the invaded cells for nutrition, metabolism, and reproduction.

viscosity (7)   The state of being thick and sticky.

vitamin (21)   Organic substance that is essential for normal metabolism, growth, and development of the human body.

W

wheal (17)   A slight elevation of the skin that can be produced as a result of an intradermal injection.

withdrawal (23)   When a person with a physical dependency on a drug is forced to do without it, an illness results. This condition may include flu-like symptoms, nausea, shakes, sweats, tremors, and acute craving for the drug.

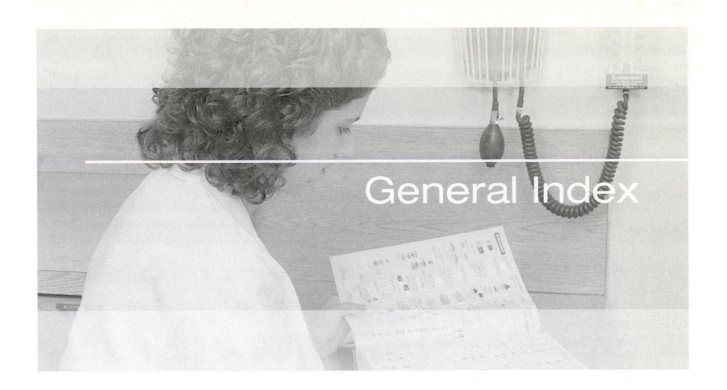

General Index

Note: For specific drugs listed by brand and generic names, refer to the drug index.

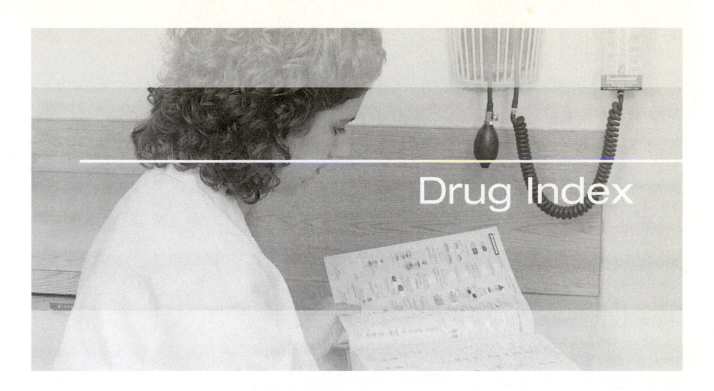

Drug Index

Note: All drugs described in the text are listed here by brand and generic name. For drug classifications and all other topics, refer to the general index.

A

abacavir, **218**
(Ziagen)

Abbokinase, **87, 303**
(urokinase)

Abitrate, **366**
(clofibrate)

acarbose, **87, 368, 371**
(Precose)

Accolate, **87, 322**
(zafirlukast)

Aceon, **299**
(perindopril)

acetaminophen, **85, 86, 378, 395**
(Tylenol)

acetazolamide, **348, 406**
(Diamox)

acetohexamide, **368**
(Dymelor)

acetylcysteine, **87, 318, 319**
(Mucomyst)

acetylsalicylic acid, **85, 86, 302, 379, 391**
(Aspirin)

Achromycin, **197**
(tetracycline hydrochloride)

Aciphex, **86, 337**
(rabeprazole sodium)

Activase, **72, 87, 303, 304**
(alteplase)

Actos, **87, 369, 370, 371**
(pioglitazone hydrochloride)

acyclovir, **86, 214**
(Zovirax)

Adrenalin, **112, 189, 192, 320**
(epinephrine)

adrenaline, **71**

Adriamycin, **239**
(doxorubicin hydrochloride)

Advil, **85, 379, 395**
(ibuprofen)

Aerobid, **324**
(flunisolide)

Afrin, **86, 316**
(oxymetazoline hydrochloride)

Agenerase, **218, 219**
(amprenavir)

Elmiron, **356**
(pentosan polysulfate sodium)

Elspar, **242**
(asparaginase)

Eminase, **87, 303, 304**
(anistreplase)

E-Mycin, **127, 200**
(erythromycin base)

enalapril, **298**
(Vasotec)

Enbrel, **86**
(etanercept)

enflurane, **405**
(Ethrane)

Engerix-B, **87, 224, 229**
(hepatitis B vaccine)

Enovid-E 21, **86**

enoxaparin, **301**
(Lovenox)

entacapone, **400**
(Comtan)

ephedrine sulfate, **320**

epinephrine, **112, 189, 192, 320**
(Adrenalin)

epinephrine hydrochloride, **406**
(Glaucon)

epirubicin hydrochloride, **239, 242**
(Ellence)

Epivir 3TC, **218**
(lamivudine)

epoetin alfa, **306**
(Epogen)
(Procrit)

Epogen, **306**
(epoetin alfa)

eprosartan mesylate, **298**
(Teveten)

Ergamisol, **242**
(levamisole)

ergonovine maleate, **422**
(Ergotrate Maleate)

Ergotrate Maleate, **422**
(ergonovine maleate)

EryPed, **200**
(erythromycin ethylsuccinate)

Ery-Tab, **200**
(erythromycin base)

Erythrocin, **200**
(erythromycin lactobionate)

Erythrocin, **200**
(erythromycin stearate)

erythromycin base, **127, 200**
(E-Mycin)

erythromycin estolate, **200**
(Ilosone)

erythromycin ethylsuccinate, **200**
(EES)

erythromycin gluceptate, **200**
(Ilotycin)

erythromycin lactobionate, **200**
(Erythrocin)

erythromycin stearate, **200**
(Erythrocin)

Eserine Sulfate, **406**
(physostigmine sulfate)

Esidrix, **348**
(hydrochlorothiazide)

Eskalith, **266**
(lithium)

esterified estrogens, **413**
(Menest)

Estrace, **413**
(estradiol)

Estraderm, **83, 412, 413**
(estradiol transdermal system)

estradiol, **413**
(Estrace)

estradiol cypionate in oil, **413**
(Depo-Estradiol)

estradiol hemihydrate, **413**
(Vagifem)

estradiol transdermal system, **413**
(Alora, Climara, Estraderm, Fem-Patch, Vivelle)